Schizophrenia

Second Edition

D0558469

WPA Series
Evidence and Experience in Psychiatry

Other Titles in the *WPA Series* Evidence and Experience in Psychiatry

Volume 1 — Depressive Disorders, Second Edition
Mario Maj and Norman Sartorius

Volume 3 — Dementia, Second Edition
Mario Maj and Norman Sartorius

Volume 4 — Obsessive Compulsive Disorder, Second Edition
Mario Maj, Norman Sartorius, Ahmed Okasha and Joseph Zohar

Volume 5 — Bipolar Disorder
Mario Maj, Hagop S. Akiskal, Juan José López-Ibor and Norman Sartorius

Schizophrenia

Second Edition

Edited by

Mario Maj
University of Naples, Italy

Norman Sartorius
University of Geneva, Switzerland

WPA Series
Evidence and Experience in Psychiatry

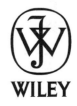

WILEY

Other Wiley Editorial Offices

John Wiley & Sons Inc., 111 River Street, Hoboken, NJ 07030, USA

Jossey-Bass, 989 Market Street, San Francisco, CA 94103-1741, USA

Wiley-VCH Verlag GmbH, Boschstr. 12, D-69469 Weinheim, Germany

John Wiley & Sons Australia Ltd, 33 Park Road, Milton, Queensland 4064, Australia

John Wiley & Sons (Asia) Pte Ltd, 2 Clementi Loop #02-01, Jin Xing Distripark,
Singapore 129809

John Wiley & Sons Canada Ltd, 22 Worcester Road, Etobicoke, Ontario, Canada M9W 1L1

Wiley also publishes its books in a variety of electronic formats. Some content that appears
in print may not be available in electronic books.

British Library Cataloguing in Publication Data

A catalogue record for this book is available from the British Library

ISBN 0-470-84964-9

Typeset in 10/12pt Times by Laserwords Private Limited, Chennai, India
Printed and bound in Great Britain by TJ International, Padstow, Cornwall
This book is printed on acid-free paper responsibly manufactured from sustainable forestry
in which at least two trees are planted for each one used for paper production.

Contents

Review Contributors

Dr Stephen Almond *London School of Economics and Political Science, Department of Social Policy and Administration, Houghton Street, London WC2A 2AE, UK*

Professor Max Birchwood *Northern Birmingham Mental Health NHS Trust, Harry Watton House, 97 Church Lane, Aston, Birmingham B6 5UG, UK*

Professor Robert Cancro *Department of Psychiatry, New York University Medical Center, 22N 550 First Avenue, New York, NY 10016, USA*

Dr Peter Falkai *Department of Psychiatry, University of Bonn, Sigmund Freud Strasse 25, D-53105 Bonn, Germany*

Professor W. Wolfgang Fleischhacker *Department of Psychiatry, Innsbruck University Clinics, Anichstrasse 35, A-6020 Innsbruck, Austria*

Professor Martin Knapp *London School of Economics and Political Science, Department of Social Policy and Administration, Houghton Street, London WC2A 2AE, UK*

Professor Wolfgang Maier *Department of Psychiatry, University of Bonn, Sigmund Freud Strasse 25, D-53105, Bonn, Germany*

Dr Arthur T. Meyerson *Department of Psychiatry, New York University Medical Center, 22N 550 First Avenue, New York, NY 10016, USA*

Dr Mauro Percudani *London School of Economics and Political Science, Department of Social Policy and Administration, Houghton Street, London WC2A 2AE, UK*

Professor Charles B. Pull *Service de Psychiatrie, Centre Hospitalier de Luxembourg, 4 Rue Barblé, Luxembourg*

Dr Judit Simon *London School of Economics and Political Science, Department of Social Policy and Administration, Houghton Street, London WC2A 2AE, UK*

Dr Elizabeth Spencer *Northern Birmingham Mental Health NHS Trust, Harry Watton House, 97 Church Lane, Aston, Birmingham B6 5UG, UK*

Dr Michael Wagner *Department of Psychiatry, University of Bonn, Sigmund Freud Strasse 25, D-53105 Bonn, Germany*

Preface

The gap between research evidence and clinical practice remains substantial in psychiatry. The poor application of findings from research in clinical work is probably due, in part, to the tradition of distance between those engaged in academic pursuits and those working in the service institutions. This separation is not characteristic of psychiatry alone, but is more dangerous in the field of mental health — a field that has been, as a whole, separated from the rest of medicine for a long time. The popularity of psychoanalysis as a self-contained method of thinking about health, illness, social structures, history and other matters may have also contributed to the reluctance to use findings obtained in neuroscience laboratories, and through genetic epidemiology. Other factors might also have been of importance; however, the search for such other reasons must not postpone the effort to bridge the gap and ensure that the vast amount of knowledge is considered and applied in the provision of services to people suffering from mental disorders and in teaching psychiatry to students of medicine and of other health professions.

The diagnosis and treatment of schizophrenia illustrate the gaps existing between currently available knowledge and its application in mental health services. Research in this field has been remarkably active during the last decade: new drugs have been developed which have shown an innovative therapeutic profile; new psychotherapeutic techniques have become available, directly targeted to psychotic symptoms; and new rehabilitative techniques and family interventions have been empirically tested and proposed for clinical use. However, these advances are not adequately reflected in clinical practice. Novel antipsychotics remain underused, and several clinicians feel that clearer guidelines are needed concerning their indications and the choice among them. Cognitive-behavioural psychotherapies, in spite of the empirical evidence of their efficacy, are unknown or ignored in several countries, whereas psychodynamic psychotherapies, whose efficacy is not supported by research findings, remain widely used. Rehabilitation has indeed emerged as a priority in the clinical management of psychotic patients, but the techniques that are used in clinical practice are often different from those that research has validated. Furthermore, several clinicians are dissatisfied with the concept of schizophrenia itself, and feel that the primary psychoses which are seen in clinical practice, especially in outpatient or community settings, are unlikely to represent a single illness.

Yet, all these issues do not emerge from current psychiatric literature. The experience of skilled clinicians is only rarely published in psychiatric journals, while the best of scientific evidence is only infrequently presented in a manner and in a place that would make it immediately accessible to clinicians. Reports on clinical practice in different countries—possibly enriching knowledge by providing a range of experience and a powerful commentary on the applicability of research findings in everyday work—are not easily found in accessible psychiatric literature. In the current era of promotion of evidence-based medicine, these separations between research evidence, experience, and practice are a dangerous anachronism.

The series *Evidence and Experience in Psychiatry* has been initiated as part of the effort of the World Psychiatric Association to bridge gaps within psychiatry and between psychiatry and the rest of medicine. The series aims to be the forum in which major issues for psychiatry and mental health care will be discussed openly by psychiatrists from many countries and different schools of thought. This second volume of the series compares research evidence and clinical experience concerning schizophrenia, with contributions from about one hundred psychiatrists representing twenty-seven different countries.

Mario Maj
Norman Sartorius

1

Diagnosis of Schizophrenia: A Review

Charles B. Pull

Department of Psychiatry, Centre Hospitalier de Luxembourg, Luxembourg

INTRODUCTION

Schizophrenia is a disorder of unknown aetiology. Over the years, a number of different signs and symptoms have been described to define its clinical picture and to separate it from other disorders. Although there have been numerous attempts in recent years to identify clinically useful laboratory tests or biological markers that might confirm the presence of the disorder, the diagnosis continues to rest upon essentially clinical criteria. The present paper reviews the evidence concerning the diagnosis of schizophrenia as described in Chapter V(F) of the *International Classification of Diseases and Related Health Problems* or ICD-10 [1, 2] and the three latest editions of the *Diagnostic and Statistical Manual of Mental Disorders* (DSM-III, DSM-III-R and DSM-IV) [3– 5].

HISTORICAL BACKGROUND

The conceptual history of schizophrenia dates back to the end of the nineteenth century, and to the description of dementia praecox by Emil Kraepelin. Other major influences on the current concept of schizophrenia are those of Bleuler, Schneider, Jaspers and Hughlings Jackson.

In the fifth edition of his textbook [6], Emil Kraepelin established a classification of mental disorders which was based upon the medical model. His goal was to delineate disease entities having a common aetiology, symptomatology, course and outcome. One of these entities he called dementia praecox, because it started early on in life and almost invariably led to psychic impairment. Characteristic symptoms included hallucinations, experiences of influence, disturbances in attention, comprehension and the flow of thought, affective flattening and catatonic symptoms. The aetiology was endogenous,

Schizophrenia, Second Edition. Edited by Mario Maj and Norman Sartorius.

that is, the disorder arose out of inner causes. Dementia praecox was separated from manic-depressive disorder and from paranoia on the basis of
symptom and course criteria. Kraepelin distinguished three forms of the
disorder: hebephrenic, catatonic and paranoid.

Eugen Bleuler [7] acknowledged that "the concept of dementia praecox
comes from Kraepelin and that the grouping and identification of individual
symptoms is almost entirely due to him". Bleuler retained Kraepelin's separation of the disorder from manic-depressive illness and gave the disorder its
present name of schizophrenia. In his view, the course of schizophrenia was
variable, but probably never reached *restitutio ad integrum*. In fact, Bleuler
focused on "fundamental" and "primary" signs and symptoms rather than
on course and outcome. In particular, he emphasized the presence of a
dissociation (*Spaltung*) of mental functions as the essential characteristic
of the disorder. The main aspect of dissociation was a loosening of associations. Other defining features of the disorder were affective blunting
and inappropriate affect, ambivalence, autism and disordered attention. For
Bleuler, schizophrenia was not a unitary disease. The "group of schizophrenias" subsumed multiple disorders that shared a number of clinical features
but differed in aetiology and pathogenesis. In particular, it included a
subgroup designated "simple schizophrenia", in which many of the prominent features of the disorder were absent. Since schizophrenia encompassed
both severe and mild forms, the scope of the concept was much broader than
Kraepelin's.

The writings of Karl Jaspers had a lasting influence on psychiatric nosology,
and in particular on the diagnosis of schizophrenia. In his *Allgemeine
Psychopathologie* [8], Jaspers considered that psychopathological symptoms
were organized in layers or levels, from the more "profound" to the more
"superficial". The most profound level was represented by organic symptoms, then came schizophrenic, affective and neurotic symptoms, and finally
symptoms related to personality disorders. When symptoms from different
levels were present simultaneously, diagnosis was determined by those
symptoms that belonged to the most profound level. One of the major
consequences of this system, which was to become known under the name
"Jaspersche Schichtenregel" (hierarchical rule of levels), was that whenever schizophrenic and affective symptoms were present at the same time,
clinicians opted for a diagnosis of schizophrenia.

For Kurt Schneider, psychiatric diagnosis was based fundamentally on the
clinical picture and not on the course. In his *Klinische Psychopathologie* [9],
Schneider distinguished between psychical abnormalities and diseases.
Diseases were subdivided into psychoses with demonstrable organic aetiology, cyclophrenia and schizophrenia. In his description of psychopathological phenomena, Schneider differentiated between abnormal "experiences"
and abnormal "expressions". Abnormal experiences refer to disturbances in

perceptions, sensations, feelings, impulses and volition. Abnormal expressions concern disturbances in language, writing, mimic and movement. For Schneider, the diagnosis of schizophrenia had to rely essentially on abnormal experiences, with in particular a number of specified experiences that he designated as "first-rank symptoms", and which he considered to be pathognomonic of the disorder.

Hughlings Jackson [10] applied the terms "positive" and "negative" to delineate primary from secondary neurological phenomena. According to Jackson, negative symptoms result directly from damage to brain areas that are responsible for the production of human behaviour, while positive symptoms reflect brain processes that are disinhibited or released by the damaged brain. In 1974, Strauss *et al* [11] proposed to distinguish two symptom profiles in schizophrenia: positive symptoms and negative symptoms. Positive symptoms are defined by the presence of abnormal features such as hallucinations, delusions and disorganized thinking. Negative symptoms are defined by the absence of normal functions, and are characterized by symptoms such as blunted affect, emotional withdrawal and cognitive deficits. In 1980, Crow [12] proposed a typology of schizophrenia based on the positive and negative dichotomy.

CHARACTERISTIC SYMPTOMS OF SCHIZOPHRENIA

The characteristic features of schizophrenia are hallucinations and delusions, disorders of thought and speech, disorders of behaviour, disturbance of emotions and affect, cognitive deficits and avolition.

Hallucinations and delusions are frequently observed at some time during the course of schizophrenia. According to Cutting [13], visual hallucinations occur in 15%, auditory in 50% and tactile in 5% of all subjects, and delusions in more than 90%. Particular diagnostic importance has been attributed to specific delusions and hallucinations.

Kurt Schneider [9] had identified a number of specific delusions and hallucinations that he considered to be pathognomonic of schizophrenia and for which he coined the term "first-rank symptoms". The concept was included in DSM-III, but has been given much less prominence in DSM-III-R and DSM-IV. It has been retained in the ICD-10 definition of schizophrenia. The issue of Schneiderian first-rank symptoms is discussed in detail below.

In DSM-III, DSM-III-R and DSM-IV, bizarre delusions have been attributed major diagnostic importance, in that the presence of any delusion of this kind qualifies for a diagnosis of schizophrenia, even if it is the only symptom. The definition of "bizarre" has, however, been changed in DSM-III-R. In DSM-III, bizarre delusions were defined as false beliefs whose content is patently absurd and which have no possible basis in fact, that is, such delusions would be "impossible". The DSM-III-R definition indicated that such delusions would be "implausible", that is, that they involve a phenomenon that the person's culture would regard as impossible. The concept has remained controversial, in particular because inter-rater reliability in the evaluation of a delusion as bizarre or non-bizarre is poor [14, 15].

The term thought disorder refers to a disorder of the content as well as of the form of a person's thoughts. Delusions are a disorder of the content of a person's thoughts. Disorders in the form of thought may be subdivided in two categories [16]: an intrinsic disturbance of thinking; and a disorder of the form in which thoughts are expressed in language and speech.

The intrinsic disturbance of thinking encompasses concrete thinking, over-inclusion, illogicality and loosening of associations. Disordered language and speech include derailment, tangentiality, neologisms, poverty of speech, poverty in the content of speech, incoherence, pressure of speech, flight of ideas and retarded speech or mutism.

Evaluation of formal thought disorder has been handicapped for many years by the lack of generally accepted definitions of the disturbance. Andreasen [17] provided definitions for 18 varieties of formal thought disorder as well as examples from the speech of patients. The relia-bility of these definitions was found to be quite good for most of the terms defined. Of the 18 definitions, only six had weighted kappa values below 0.6: tangentiality, clanging, echolalia, self-reference, neologisms and word approximations. All other varieties, including derailment, incoherence and poverty of speech, had good to excellent kappa values.

The frequency and specificity of formal thought disorder in schizophrenia vary considerably from one subtype to the other. According to Cutting and Murphy [18], not all patients with schizophrenia had intrinsic thought disorder and those that did tended to have over-inclusive categorization as the most apparent manifestation. According to Andreasen [17], some types of thought disorder, such as neologisms or blocking, occur so infrequently as to be of little diagnostic value. Other types are common in schizophrenia, but do not distinguish patients with schizophrenia from patients with mania (e.g. derailment) or depression (e.g. poverty of speech). As a consequence, formal thought disorder should not be used as a diagnostic criterion for the diagnosis of schizophrenia except in the absence of affective symp-toms.

Disorders of behaviour in schizophrenia include grossly disorganized behaviour and catatonic behaviour. From the beginning, catatonic behaviour has been described among the characteristic features of schizophrenia. Cutting [19] defines catatonia as a set of complex movements, postures and actions whose common denominator is their involuntariness. Catatonic phenomena include: stupor, catalepsy, automatism, mannerisms, stereo-typies, posturing and grimacing, negativism and echopraxia. Catatonic symptoms have been found in 7% [20] and between 5 and 10% [21] of patients with schizophrenia. Catatonic symptoms are not specific to schizophrenia. In particular, they may occur in mania [22].

Anhedonia or loss of feelings, and disorders of affect such as inappropriate affect and blunting or flattening of affect, are among the characteristic disturbances of emotions and affect that are classically associated with the diagnosis of schizophrenia.

Anhedonia or loss of feeling has been proposed as a central [23] or cardinal [24] feature of schizophrenia. Chapman et al [25] designed question-naires of social and physical anhedonia. Physical anhedonia covers pleasures such as admiring the beauty of sunsets, eating, drinking, singing, being massaged. Social anhedonia covers pleasures such as being with friends or being with other people. In a study by Watson et al [26], anhedonia was significantly more frequent in patients with schizophrenia than in patients with alcohol dependency. In a recent study by Blanchard et al [27], patients with schizophrenia reported significantly greater physical and social anhe-donia than controls. In a study by Cook and Simukonda [28], social but not physical anhedonia was significantly higher in patients with schizophrenia than in subjects from a hospital staff control group. Concerning the speci-ficity of anhedonia, Harrow et al [29] found that only chronic, not acute, schizophrenics were significantly anhedonic. According to Schuck et al [30], physical anhedonia was no more prevalent in patients with schizophrenia than in patients with depression.

In a study by Andreasen [31], inappropriate affect occurred in 20% of acutely ill patients with schizophrenia, and flattening of affect in 50% of acute or chronic patients. Inappropriate affect had poor reliability. The symptom appeared significantly more often in patients with schizophrenia than in patients with mania or depression. Affective flattening was found to be common but not omnipresent in patients with schizophrenia, and was also common in depressed patients. Abrams and Taylor [32] documented that affective blunting distinguished between a group of patients with manic symptoms and a group with schizophrenic symptoms.

Cognitive deficits have been listed among the central features of schizo-phrenia since the original descriptions of Kraepelin and Bleuler.

Patients with schizophrenia demonstrate a generalized cognitive deficit, that is, they tend to perform at lower levels than do normal controls across a broad variety of cognitive tests [33]. Braff et al [34] compared patients with schizophrenia with normal controls. Patients with schizophrenia had multiple neuropsychological deficits on tests of complex conceptual reasoning, psycho-motor speed, new learning and incidental memory, and both motor and sensory–perceptual abilities. Saykin et al [35] showed that patients demon-strated generalized impairment relative to controls and a selective deficit in memory and learning compared with other functions. According to Goldberg *et al* [36], patients with schizophrenia perform systematically worse on cognitive measures than patients with affective disorders.

Prominent selective cognitive abnormalities in schizophrenia include deficits in attention, memory and problem solving:

• Attentional dysfunction has been observed in patients with schizophrenia on a number of neuropsychological tests, including tests of immediate attention span, sustained attention, visual search and tracking, selective attention, and executive control of attention [37]. In particular, sustained attention has been investigated in many studies and consistently found to be defective in patients with schizophrenia [38].
• According to Goldberg and Gold [39], patients with schizophrenia demonstrate marked deficits in episodic memory measures; procedural learning that involves motor skills may be relatively intact, and the situation for item-specific implicit memory is unclear.
• Patients with schizophrenia appear to have difficulties in solving problems whose solutions are not readily apparent, or when they must rely upon novel recombinations of existing knowledge [39, 40]. Deficits have been observed in a wide variety of instruments, stimulus materials and response modalities, including the Wisconsin Card Sorting Test [34, 41].

Apathy, abulia, lack of will or avolition are terms that have been applied to characterize a fundamental inability to initiate and persist in goal-directed activities. Avolition is usually included among the characteristic symptoms of schizophrenia. In particular, avolition-apathy is included among the negative symptoms of the disorder [42, 43].

CLUSTERING OF SYMPTOMS

The characteristic symptoms of schizophrenia that have been described above may be classified in many different ways. Prominent among the attempts that have been proposed up to now are Bleuler's classifications in fundamental and accessory symptoms and in primary versus secondary symptoms, as well as Schneider's division in first- and second-rank symptoms. In recent years, the attention of researchers and clinicians alike has focused on the distinction between positive and negative symptoms.

Bleuler identified two sets of symptoms, one descriptive, the other aetiopathogenetic. The two dichotomies are distinct, although they are defined by partially overlapping features. The first set distinguishes between fundamental and accessory symptoms. Fundamental symptoms are present at all times and in all cases. They include disturbances in association and affect, ambivalence and autism (the four A's). All other symptoms encountered in schizophrenia are accessory symptoms, including hallucinations, delusions, catatonia and behavioural problems. Accessory symptoms may be absent at times and even throughout the whole course and they may appear in other types of illness.

The specificity and inter-rater reliability of Bleuler's fundamental symptoms have been questioned in a number of studies [44].

The second set distinguishes between primary and secondary symptoms. Primary symptoms are direct manifestations of the disorder, while secondary symptoms are viewed as psychological reactions of the personality to the disease process. Primary symptoms consist above all in disturbances of associations, while the bulk of the other symptoms described in schizophrenia are secondary symptoms.

For the diagnosis of schizophrenia, Kurt Schneider ascribed a particular importance to 11 abnormal experiences for which he coined the term "first-rank symptoms". Schneider considered that first-rank symptoms were pathognomonic of schizophrenia, provided that they could not be linked in one way or another to an organic cause. Other abnormal experiences that could contribute to the diagnosis were termed "second-rank symptoms". A diagnosis of schizophrenia could also be made when only symptoms of second rank were present. The presence or absence of first- or second-rank symptoms did not carry any theoretical or prognostic significance.

The 11 first-rank symptoms included: thoughts experienced as spoken-aloud or echoed; thought withdrawal, thought insertion and thought broadcasting; voices heard commenting on the patient's thoughts or actions and voices discussing the person in the third person; feelings, impulses and volitional acts experienced as under the control of some external force or agency; somatic passivity and delusional perception. The presence of just one first-rank symptom was considered sufficient for the diagnosis, provided that its presence could be firmly established.

The prevalence of first-rank symptoms has been investigated in a number of studies. The frequency of any first-rank symptom in patients with schizophrenia varied from one study to another, ranging from 28% to 72% [45–47]. According to the results of the International Pilot Study of Schizophrenia [20], the prevalence of first-rank symptoms varied from one participant centre to another, from a low 31% in Moscow to a high 79% in Taipei.

The specificity of first-rank symptoms has been investigated by Abrams and Taylor [48], Carpenter *et al* [49], Taylor and Abrams [50], and Koehler *et al* [51]. According to the results of these studies, first-rank symptoms are not pathognomonic of schizophrenia, but may occur during a depressive or manic episode in a substantial number of patients.

Interest in the positive–negative distinction [52] led to the development of a variety of instruments designed to assess positive and/or negative symptoms. Prominent among these instruments are the Scale for the Assessment of Negative Symptoms (SANS) [53, 54] and the Scale for the Assessment of Positive Symptoms (SAPS) [55]. The SANS includes items that describe different aspects of affective flattening, avolition-apathy, anhedonia-asociality and attentional impairment. The SAPS includes items that describe hallucinations, delusions, bizarre behaviour and formal thought disorder. The first factor analysis on the two scales showed that the correlations between the negative symptoms were quite high, as was the internal consistency of the SANS. The correlations between the positive symptoms were weaker, as was the internal consistency of the SAPS. Subsequent analyses of 15 studies of the SANS and the SAPS led to the conclusion that the symptoms fall into three natural dimensions [43]. While negative symptoms remain more or less the same, positive symptoms subdivide into a first dimension that reflects psychoticism (hallucinations and delusions) and a second dimension that includes disorganized/bizarre behaviour, positive formal thought disorder and disorganized speech, and inappropriate affect.

PRODROMAL SYMPTOMS AND ONSET

It has long been known that schizophrenia does not start with first admission and not even with the first psychotic symptoms. Early manifestations of the disorder have usually been called prodromal signs and symptoms.

During the last decade, the question of when and with what symptoms schizophrenia starts and what type of course it follows until the beginning of the first psychotic episode has led to a considerable number of investigations relative to the signs and symptoms that precede the actual onset of the disorder and the time interval between the first manifestation of the disorder and the first appearance of the full picture.

In 1996, Yung and McGorry [56] published an extensive review on past and current conceptualizations of the prodromal phase of first-episode psychosis, including compilations of definitions, descriptions of symptoms and signs, and patterns and durations. "Prodrome" has been defined as "a heterogeneous group of behaviours temporally related to the onset of psychosis" [57], as the time interval from onset of unusual behavioural symptoms to onset of psychotic symptoms [58], or as the period from first noticeable symptoms to first prominent psychotic symptoms [59]. For Yung and McGorry, "in essence, the prodrome is the period between the most valid estimates of the onset of change in the person and the onset of psychosis". The pre-psychotic period preceding the first onset of a psychosis is sometimes referred to as "initial prodrome" to distinguish this period from the one preceding a relapse in patients with an established diagnosis of psychosis.

To facilitate determination of the duration of the prodromal phase, Häfner [60] distinguishes between five different definitions of onset: first sign of a disturbance, first negative symptom, first positive symptom, first episode, and first admission.

Concerning the sequence of changes that leads to psychosis over time, Yung and McGorry identify two patterns. Pattern 1 consists in non-specific changes, followed by specific pre-psychotic symptoms, then psychosis. Pattern 2 starts with specific changes, followed by neurotic symptoms as a reaction to these, then psychosis. In addition to the previous two patterns, there are variants of patterns of change called "outpost syndromes", that is, clusters of symptoms and behaviours that resemble prodromes but which resolve spontaneously without immediately progressing to psychosis. The symptoms of outpost syndromes have been described by Huber *et al* [61] under the name "basic symptoms".

According to Yung and McGorry, the prodromal features most commonly described in the most methodologically sound first-episode studies include, in descending order of frequency: reduced concentration and attention, reduced drive and motivation, anergia, depressed mood, sleep disturbance, anxiety, social withdrawal, suspiciousness, deterioration in role functioning and irritability.

In Loebel *et al*'s [58] sample, the first psychotic symptoms appeared on average one year, and prodromal signs almost 3 years before first admission. In the Age, Beginning and Course of Schizophrenia (ABC) study [62, 63], the period from the first sign of a mental disturbance and the first hospital-ization averaged 4.2 years for men and 4.9 years for women. The first signs were non-specific indicators such as loss of energy and motivation, difficulty concentrating, anxiety, suspiciousness and social withdrawal. Even the first psychotic symptoms appeared on average 2 years prior to the first hospital-ization. In the Determinants of Outcome of Severe Mental Disorders or DOS study [64], negative manifestations, such as neglect of usual activities, and loss of appetite, sleep or interest in sex were frequently recognized as the first signs of the disorder.

The actual onset rate of the syndrome has been defined by Keith and Matthews [57] as the time interval between the first appearance of charac-teristic schizophrenic symptoms and a full picture of the syndrome. The authors define onset rates as acute (less than 3 months), subacute (less than 6 months), subchronic (less than one year) and chronic (more than one year). Häfner *et al* [65] adopt the following definition: acute (in less than 4 weeks), subchronic (in more than 4 weeks but less than one year), and chronic (in more than one year). According to the results of the ABC study, the chronic onset type was most frequent (68%). The subacute type was observed in 15% and the acute type in 18% of cases.

Although schizophrenia was first described as a disorder beginning in adolescence or early adult life, current investigations confirm that onset can be in childhood as well as in older subjects. According to Häfner [60] and Häfner *et al* [65], schizophrenia is a disorder of (almost) all ages.

In the ABC study, the prodromal phase started before age 30 in 77%, before age 20 in 41%, and before age 10 in 4% of cases. The first psychotic episode began before age 30 in 63%, before age 20 in 17%, and before age 10 in 1% of cases. The same authors report a higher mean age of onset in females, with a difference of 3 to 4 years between males and females. In addition, they describe a second peak of onsets between ages 45 and 50 in females, but not in men. In men, symptom severity decreased with increasing age of onset. In women, symptom severity remained stable except for an increase of negative symptoms with late onset. Within the group of late-onset psychoses, there was no discrimination between schizophrenia and late paraphrenia.

The term "late-onset schizophrenia" was introduced by Manfred Bleuler [66] to identify a form of schizophrenia with onset between the ages of 40 and 60. The concept was hardly used outside of the German-speaking community, and it was commonly admitted that the onset of schizophrenia was restricted to the first half of life. This view has been challenged in recent years. According to a review of the literature by Harris and Jeste [67], onset of schizophrenia in hospitalized patients had been after age 40 in approximately 23% of the patients. Pearlson *et al* [68] found no differences in the prevalence of first-rank symptoms in patients with early-onset or late-onset schizophrenia. Rabins *et al* [69] and Mayer *et al* [70] found no characteristics that clearly separated late-onset from early-onset patients with schizophrenia, but reported that late-onset patients were more frequently female. Finally, Howard *et al* [71], Riecher-Rössler *et al* [72], and Häfner *et al* [65] could not find discriminating empirical criteria in the spectrum of schizophrenia and paranoid disorders of old age sufficient to warrant that the two groups of disorders be separated.

COURSE AND OUTCOME

Although the course and outcome of schizophrenia have been the subject of a great number of studies throughout this century, the issue still remains a topic of considerable debate.

There have been many attempts to classify the courses of schizophrenia, but there is no universally accepted classification in this field. In a recent review, Marengo [73] compares different prototypes that have been proposed over the last 50 years. The author highlights differences in the number of courses described, in the structure of course categories, in the relative emphasis on syndrome character or severity (e.g. severe forms, intermediate forms, etc.) versus syndrome change (e.g. persistent, progressive, etc.), and in documenting specific course features such as illness onset, illness outcome and type of symptoms.

Earlier prototypes listed seven [74], ten [75] and five [76] course categories. Müller's categories [74] described onset, post-onset course and outcome, while Arnold's [75] and Ey's [76] focused on post-onset course and outcome. More recent prototypes identify eight [77, 78] and 12 [61] course categories. Bleuler's and Ciompi's [77, 78] categories are similar and focus on onset, post-onset course and outcome. Huber's [61] classification is more complex, in particular because it is represented in terms of a multilevel typology that includes references to psychotic symptoms, residual symptoms and social impairment.

For future studies on the course of schizophrenia, Marengo [73] recommends that a minimum set of parameters should be documented, including: (a) the rate of syndrome onset; (b) post-onset patterns of psychotic and residual symptoms; (c) post-onset patterns of social, work, and self-care activities; and (d) outcome. For both parameters (b) and (c), Marengo proposes nine patterns.

The course specifiers that are proposed in the current classifications of mental disorders are listed in detail below.

The outcome of schizophrenia has been investigated in many studies throughout the century. The results of these studies remain contradictory.

In 1994, Hegarty *et al* [79] identified a total of 821 studies on the course and outcome of schizophrenia conducted worldwide between 1895 and 1992. Most of these studies did not, however, satisfy at least minimal methodological standards. 320 studies met the inclusion criteria for a meta-analysis. The results showed that only 40.2% of patients were considered improved after follow-ups averaging 5.6 years. Diagnostic criteria have had a consistent and predictable impact on outcome before and during the era of modern biomedical treatment. As was to be expected, outcome was significantly better when patients were diagnosed according to systems with broad criteria (46.5% were improved) rather than narrow criteria (27.3% were improved), in particular because of the introduction, in the latter, of a duration-of-illness criterion.

The results of several reviews of North American and European long-term follow-up studies of schizophrenia [80, 81] have found wide heterogeneity in long-term outcome. Much of the variance in the results from these studies could be linked to sample characteristics, such as broad versus narrow diagnostic criteria and inclusion versus exclusion of dimensions of chronicity in the definition of the disorder.

In 1998, Riecher-Rössler and Rössler [82] discussed the methodological limitations of previous studies and reviewed in detail a number of studies that satisfied certain methodological standards. In a third step, the authors selected and discussed the results of those studies that they considered as methodologically sound, in that they were prospective, standardized and direct investigations of a representative, catchment-area-based sample of first-admitted or first-contact patients diagnosed directly and according to a standardized diagnostic system.

According to Riecher-Rössler and Rössler, there were only three studies that met these criteria: the Buckinghamshire Study [83], the DOS study [64] and the ABC study [62, 63]. Further course (after first admission) was assessed based on treatment parameters, symptomatology, and different levels of psychological impairment and social disability. Duration of follow-up was 2 years [64], 5 years [83], and 10 years [62]. About one third of the patients in the three studies were never rehospitalized during these years. Almost all received medication during this time.

In the Buckinghamshire study, 22% of the patients remained symptom-free over the 5 years following first admission, 35% developed further discrete episodes but were free of symptoms between episodes, and 43% showed persistent florid symptoms. In the DOS study, 50% of the patients had only one episode, 31% two or more episodes followed by remission, and only 16% persistent symptomatology without remission.

In the DOS study, less than one third of the patients suffered more or less severe impairment during the observation period, while more than one third of them showed no impairment in social functioning during at least three-quarters of this period. In the Buckinghamshire study, 45% of the patients showed only minimal, 43% mild to moderate, and 12% severe impairment during the observation period. Finally, in the ABC study, it was shown that impairment often occurred already in the preclinical course of the disorder.

In the conclusion to their review, Riecher-Rössler and Rössler state that the course of schizophrenia may in fact be less unfavourable than implied by other studies in the past. It certainly does not appear systematically to show a progressive deterioration as stated by Kraepelin.

There are, however, other recent studies which show that schizophrenia still is a chronic and frequently disabling disease, and that its outcome is generally worse than that of other functional mental illnesses [80]. In a longitudinal study, Harrow et al [84] compared the course and outcome of schizophrenia versus other psychotic disorders. According to the results of this study, the majority of patients with schizophrenia did not show complete and consistent remission over the long term and experienced significantly poorer functioning than patients with other psychotic disorders at each of three successive follow-ups over 7.5 years. In a study on the natural course of schizophrenic disorders, Wiersma et al [85] present results on the 15-year natural course of the disorder. The study revealed that two-thirds of the subjects had at least one relapse and that after each relapse one of six subjects did not remit from the episode. In addition, one of ten committed suicide.

On the whole, follow-up studies of the course of schizophrenia indicate that there may be very different types of course, ranging from complete cure to severe disabling chronic forms. Some patients experience only one episode of illness, others have several episodes, and still others suffer from chronic symptoms.

DIFFERENTIAL DIAGNOSIS

The signs and symptoms that define schizophrenia may occur in the course of any disease affecting the brain, including a range of mental disorders, substance-induced disorders and general medical conditions.

The redefinition of the boundaries between schizophrenia and mood disorders, either manic or depressive, with psychotic symptoms, has been one of the most important changes in psychiatric nosology during the last two decades. Jaspers' hierarchical rule, according to which priority was to be given to a diagnosis of schizophrenia when both affective and schizophrenic symptoms were present, was abandoned and new rules were adopted to separate the two disorders.

The presence, at the same time, of a manic or depressive episode and mood-incongruent psychotic features, can be conceptualized in three different ways [86– 88]: as forming a particular subtype of a mood disorder, that is, mood incongruent psychotic affective illness (MICPAI); as defining a form of schizoaffective disorder; or as belonging to schizophrenia. In the *DSM-IV Sourcebook*, Kendler [88] has evaluated the three hypotheses regarding the nosologic position of MICPAI. According to this author, the accumulated evidence concerning antecedent validators (family history, demographics) as well as concurrent validators (clinical and biological variables, treatment response and outcome) supports the first hypothesis, that is, MICPAI should be considered a subtype of mood disorder.

The new rules that were adopted to separate schizophrenia from mood disorder also redefined the diagnosis of schizoaffective disorder. The current evidence concerning the status of schizoaffective disorder has been reviewed by Tsuang *et al* [89]. In the "necessarily provisional view" of the authors, schizoaffective disorder is "a genetically heterogeneous condition primarily composed of schizophrenia, unipolar and bipolar disorders and perhaps a residual currently undifferentiated condition".

A considerable number of labels and definitions have been proposed during the last century to designate transient psychotic disorders that are regarded as separate from schizophrenia. Prominent traditional concepts in this field are the *bouffées délirantes* of the French, the reactive or psychogenic psychoses as well as the schizophreniform psychoses of the Scandinavian, and the cycloid psychoses of the German tradition. Although it remains unclear whether transient psychotic disorders are different from schizophrenia, current classification systems have introduced various categories that allow sufficient time for the symptoms to appear, be recognized, and subside, before a diagnosis of schizophrenia can be made [90].

Since the days of Kraepelin, a number of persistent delusional disorders have been regarded as different from schizophrenia. The group includes a variety of conditions in which long-standing delusions constitute the only, or the most conspicuous, clinical characteristic and which do not meet criteria for a diagnosis of schizophrenia. Prominent in this area are the concepts of paranoia and paraphrenia, the *délires chroniques* of the French tradition, as well as a variety of other concepts, either included in the preceding or separated from them, such as delusional jealousy, *folie à deux*, Capgras syndrome, erotomania, Cotard's syndrome, or Kretschmer's *sensitiver Beziehungswahn*. The nosologic position of this group, in particular with regard to schizophrenia, remains uncertain [90].

Schizophrenia spectrum disorders include paranoid, schizoid and schizotypal personality disorder. According to Siever *et al* [91], patients with schizotypal personality disorder demonstrate psychophysiological and cognitive deficits that are similar to, but milder than, those found in schizophrenia. In addition, the symptoms of schizotypal personality disorder seem to be heritable and genetically related to schizophrenia, but there is considerable overlap between schizotypal symptoms and symptoms of personality disorders that are outside the schizophrenia spectrum.

Schizophrenic signs and symptoms may occur in many medical or neurological conditions. Psychotic disorder due to a general medical condition must be excluded when making the diagnosis of schizophrenia.

The causal link between psychoactive substances and an episode of psychosis must also be excluded. The relationship between schizophrenia and substance-induced psychotic disorders may, however, sometimes remain uncertain.

SUBTYPES OF SCHIZOPHRENIA

The classical subtypes of schizophrenia relate back to Kraepelin and Bleuler. They are defined by the predominant symptomatology at the time of evaluation.

The first three classical subtypes of schizophrenia (dementia paranoides, hebephrenia and catatonia) were described as separate illnesses until Kraepelin brought them together under the name dementia praecox. Together with schizophrenia simplex or simple schizophrenia, which was introduced by Bleuler, Kraepelin's paranoid, hebephrenic and catatonic subtypes formed Bleuler's group of schizophrenias. Over the years, additional subtypes, such as latent, undifferentiated, or residual schizophrenia, have been added to the four main types included in Bleuler's original description; some of the subtypes have been renamed, and others have been redefined using slightly different criteria.

In 1974, Tsuang and Winokur [92] suggested that patients with paranoid schizophrenia had fewer psychomotor symptoms and that they were characterized by later onset of illness, less seclusiveness, less distractibility, fewer psychomotor symptoms, a higher incidence of marriage, more children, and less disruption of social and familial relationships. In a review of 32 studies related to intellectual functioning, attention, memory, language, visuo-spatial, and motor functioning, Zalewski *et al* [93] did not find, however, any consistent differences between patients with paranoid and patients with non-paranoid schizophrenia.

In an extensive recent review concerning the classical subtypes of schizophrenia, McGlashan and Fenton [94] have examined the validity of the paranoid, hebephrenic (disorganized), catatonic, simple and undifferentiated subtypes of schizophrenia. The authors review data from familial and genetic studies, subtype stability studies, outcome studies, and neurological and neuropsychological investigations. They conclude that the studies of the last decade lend overall support for the validity of the paranoid, and, albeit with less force, for the validity of the disorganized and undifferentiated subtypes. According to the same review, catatonia is not specific to schizophrenia, but can still characterize a subtype of this disorder. Finally, there is evidence to support the validity of simple schizophrenia.

In 1989, Black and Boffeli [95] provided a historical overview of simple schizophrenia, reviewed its modern successors, and provided recommendations and diagnostic criteria for its inclusion in DSM-IV. The category has been included in DSM-IV, although with different criteria and only in an appendix listing diagnostic categories which need further study.

New approaches to the subtyping of schizophrenia include the type I–type II or positive–negative dichotomy and the proposition of a dimensional model.

Crow [12] proposed a typology for schizophrenia which is based on the positive–negative symptom dichotomy. According to this author, the two types may reflect two aetiologically and prognostically distinct pathological processes. The main symptoms of the positive syndrome (or type I) are hallucinations and delusions. This type may be associated with biochemical imbalance involving dopaminergic overactivity. The main symptoms of the negative syndrome (or type II) are affective flattening and poverty of speech. This type may be associated with structural or anatomical abnormality reflected in ventricular enlargement and cortical atrophy.

In an appendix on criteria sets provided for further study, the DSM-IV [5] introduces a dimensional alternative to the classical subtypes of schizophrenia that have been described above. This alternative is based upon a three-factor dimensional model. The three factors included in the model are a psychotic, a disorganized and a negative one. The psychotic factor includes delusions and hallucinations; the disorganized factor includes disorganized speech, disorganized behaviour, and inappropriate affect; and the negative factor comprises affective flattening, alogia and avolition. According to the authors of DSM-IV, there are studies which suggest that the severity of symptoms within each of the three factors tends to vary together, both cross-sectionally and over time, whereas this is less true for symptoms across factors.

EXPLICIT DIAGNOSTIC CRITERIA FOR SCHIZOPHRENIA

In the early 1970s, a group of researchers at the Washington University School of Medicine in St Louis, led by Robins and Guze [96], introduced a method that attempted to enhance the reliability as well as the validity of psychiatric diagnosis [97]. For a limited number of diagnostic categories, the authors proposed research definitions that were based on clinical description, laboratory studies, exclusion of other diagnoses, follow-up studies and family studies. In addition, each category was defined by inclusion as well as exclusion criteria that were explicit, descriptive and either monothetic or polythetic. In the following years, the method was to be adopted not only for the definition of specific diseases, but for the definition of each category in psychiatric classifications.

The St Louis or Feighner definition of schizophrenia [97] rests upon three criteria: the presence of a chronic illness with at least 6 months of symptoms, in the absence of a period of depressive or manic symptoms sufficient to qualify for affective disorder; the presence of delusions or hallucinations or verbal production that makes communication difficult because of the lack of a logical or understandable organization; and at least three of the following manifestations: being single, poor premorbid social adjustment or work history, family history of schizophrenia, absence of alcoholism or drug abuse within one year of onset of psychosis, and onset of illness prior to age 40.

The St Louis criteria had a major influence on the development of other diagnostic criteria that have been elaborated over the years, in particular because all subsequent criteria sets have been moulded on the format of the initial St Louis criteria.

The Research Diagnostic Criteria (RDC) [98] were developed as part of a collaborative project on the psychobiology of depression that was sponsored by the National Institute of Mental Health (NIMH). The RDC provide explicit criteria for depressive disorders, schizophrenia and several other disorders.

The RDC for schizophrenia consist of a polythetic symptom criterion, a duration criterion and an exclusion criterion. The symptom criterion lists eight symptoms or groups of symptoms. The first seven symptom groups are

Schneiderian first-rank symptoms and other delusions or hallucinations, the last one gives diagnostic value to formal thought disorder if accompanied by either blunted or inappropriate affect, delusions or hallucinations of any type, or grossly disorganized behaviour. The duration criterion requires that signs of the illness have lasted at least 2 weeks from the onset of a noticeable change in the subject's usual condition, and the exclusion criterion describes the differential diagnosis with affective disorders: at no time during the active period of illness being considered did the subject meet the full criteria for either probable or definite manic or depressive syndrome to such a degree that it was a prominent part of the illness.

The RDC have been used extensively by researchers since they were first introduced and up to the present day. They may be applied on the basis of a comprehensive clinical examination or, preferably, a semi-structured interview, the Schedule for Affective Disorders and Schizophrenia (SADS) [99].

Over the years, a number of other explicit diagnostic criteria for schizophrenia have been developed by individual authors. Astrachan *et al* [100] have developed a schizophrenia index that attempts to define the concept of schizophrenia as proposed in DSM-II. Carpenter *et al* [101] have derived a flexible system for the diagnosis of schizophrenia, that was based on data from the International Pilot Study of Schizophrenia. Taylor and Abrams [102] have elaborated criteria that attempt to correct several aspects of the Feighner criteria. Pull *et al* [103] have produced diagnostic criteria that describe the concept of schizophrenia held by French psychiatrists until recently (Kellam [104]. Berner *et al* [105] have developed the Vienna Research Criteria, based on the attributes of a fundamendal syndrome that the authors qualify as endogenomorphic–schizophrenic.

In the third edition of the *Diagnostic and Statistical Manual of Mental Disorders* (DSM-III) [3] the method introduced by the St Louis group was first applied to define each of the disorders of a classification. The method was refined in the DSM-III-R [4] and DSM-IV [5] and was adopted in the research version of the ICD-10 [2].

THE DIAGNOSIS OF SCHIZOPHRENIA IN CURRENT CLASSIFICATIONS

The two major current classifications in psychiatry are Chapter V(F) of the *International Classification of Diseases and Related Health Problems* or ICD-10 [1, 2] and the fourth edition of the *Diagnostic and Statistical Manual of Mental Disorders* or DSM-IV [5]. Although major efforts have been made in the preparation of the two systems to ensure as much compatibility as possible, some differences have remained, also in the diagnosis of schizophrenia.

ICD-10

In the ICD-10, the diagnosis of schizophrenia depends upon the presence of characteristic symptoms, a minimum duration of those symptoms, and a differentiation from affective, other psychotic, organic or substance-induced disorders. The ICD-10 diagnostic criteria for research of schizophrenia are shown in Table 1.1.

TABLE 1.1   ICD-10 research diagnostic criteria for schizophrenia

---

G1. Either at least one of the syndromes, symptoms, and signs listed under (1) below, or at least two of the symptoms and signs listed under (2) should be present for most of the time during an episode of psychotic illness lasting for at least 1 month (or at some time during most of the days).

(1) At least one of the following must be present:

(a) thought echo, thought insertion or withdrawal, or thought broadcasting;

(b) delusions of control, influence, or passivity, clearly referred to body or limb movements or specific thoughts, actions, or sensations; delusional perception;

(c) hallucinatory voices giving a running commentary on the patient's behaviour, or discussing the patient among themselves, or other types of hallucinatory voices coming from some part of the body;

(d) persistent delusions of other kinds that are culturally inappropriate and completely impossible (e.g. being able to control the weather, or being in communication with aliens from another world).

(2) Or at least two of the following:

(a) persistent hallucinations in any modality, when occurring every day for at least 1 month, when accompanied by delusions (which may be fleeting or half-formed) without clear affective content, or when accompanied by persistent over-valued ideas;

(b) neologisms, breaks, or interpolations in the train of thought, resulting in incoherence or irrelevant speech;

(c) catatonic behaviour, such as excitement, posturing or waxy flexibility, negativism, mutism, and stupor;

(d) "negative" symptoms, such as marked apathy, paucity of speech, and blunting or incongruity of emotional responses (it must be clear that these are not due to depression or to neuroleptic medication).

G2. Most commonly used exclusion clauses

(1) If the patient also meets criteria for manic episode (F30.−) or depressive episode (F32.−), the criteria listed under G1 (1) and G1 (2) above must have been met before the disturbance of mood developed;

(2) The disorder is not attributable to organic brain disease (in the sense of F00–F09), or to alcohol- or drug-related intoxication (F1x.0), dependence (F1x.2), or withdrawal (F1x.3 and F1x.4).

The ICD-10 recognizes that no strictly pathognomonic symptoms can be identified. Characteristic symptoms are divided into eight groups that have special importance for the diagnosis and often occur together. The first four groups are comprised of typical delusions and hallucinations; the last four groups are comprised of less typical delusions and hallucinations, as well as neologisms, breaks or interpolations in the train of thought, catatonic behaviour, and negative symptoms such as marked apathy, paucity of speech, and blunting or incongruity of emotional responses.

The delusions and hallucinations described in the first three groups are all Schneiderian first-rank symptoms, while the delusions listed in the fourth group are defined as culturally inappropriate and completely impossible (they probably correspond to the definition of bizarre delusions in other classifications).

The requirement for a diagnosis of schizophrenia is that a minimum of one symptom belonging to any one of the first four groups, or symptoms from at least two of the last four groups, should have been clearly present for most of the time during a period of one month or more.

While adopting a one-month duration of typical psychotic symptoms, the ICD-10 rejects the assumption that schizophrenia must be of comparatively long duration. According to the authors of the ICD-10, a substantial proportion of patients who have clear and typical schizophrenic symptoms lasting for more than one month but less than 6 months, have been shown to make good, if not complete, recoveries from the disorder. According to the authors of the ICD-10, in the present state of ignorance, there appear to be no advantages in restricting the diagnosis of schizophrenia by specifying a longer overall duration of the disorder and it seems best to avoid any assumptions about necessary chronicity.

The authors of the ICD-10 recognize that before the appearance of typical schizophrenic symptoms, there may be a period of weeks or months characterized by the appearance of a prodrome of non-specific symptoms. If a prodrome typical of and specific to schizophrenia could be identified, described reliably, and shown to be uncommon in patients with other psychiatric disorders and in subjects with no disorder at all, it would be justifiable to include such a prodrome among the optional criteria for schizophrenia. It was considered that insufficient information was available on this issue at present to justify the inclusion of a prodromal state as a contributor to the diagnosis in ICD-10.

As a general rule, interference with the performance of social roles has not been used as a diagnostic criterion in ICD-10. This decision has been retained for the diagnosis of schizophrenia, with the exception of simple schizophrenia, in which marked decline in social, scholastic or occupational performance is part of the concept.

According to ICD-10, the course of schizophrenia is variable. The course may be specified after at least one year has elapsed since onset of the disorder. The following patterns are listed: continuous; episodic with progressive deficit; episodic with stable deficit; episodic remittent; incomplete remission; complete remission; other.

Concerning differential diagnosis, the ICD-10 provides clear guidelines on how to differentiate schizophrenia from affective and schizoaffective disorders, other transient or persistent psychotic disorders, as well as any organic or substance-induced mental disorder. The diagnosis of schizophrenia should not be made in the presence of extensive depressive or manic symptoms unless it is clear that schizophrenic symptoms antedated the affective disturbance. If both schizophrenic and affective symptoms develop together and are evenly balanced, the diagnosis of schizoaffective disorder should be made, even if the schizophrenic symptoms by themselves would have justified the diagnosis of schizophrenia.

The separation of acute and transient psychotic disorders and schizophrenia rests upon the presence and duration of symptoms of the schizophrenic type. If such symptoms are present and persist for more than one month, the diagnosis should be changed to schizophrenia.

In persistent delusional disorders, delusions must be present for at least 3 months and the general criteria for schizophrenia are not fulfilled.

Finally, schizophrenia should not be diagnosed in the presence of overt brain disease or during states of drug intoxication or withdrawal.

The ICD-10 describes seven subtypes of schizophrenia: paranoid, hebephrenic, catatonic, post-schizophrenic depression, undifferentiated, residual and simple.

DSM-IV

In DSM-IV, the diagnosis of schizophrenia depends upon the presence of characteristic symptoms, a minimum duration of those symptoms, a minimum duration of the disorder, the presence of social/occupational dysfunction, and a differentiation from mood, schizoaffective, other psychotic disorders, general medical conditions, substance-induced disorders and pervasive developmental disorder. The DSM-IV diagnostic criteria of schizophrenia are shown in Table 1.2.

According to DSM-IV, there are no strictly pathognomonic symptoms of schizophrenia. Characteristic symptoms are conceptualized as falling into two broad categories: positive and negative. There are four groups of positive symptoms — delusions, hallucinations, disorganized speech, and grossly disorganized or catatonic behaviour — and one group of negative symptoms, which includes affective flattening, alogia and avolition.

TABLE 1.2. DSM-IV diagnostic criteria for schizophrenia

A. *Characteristic Symptoms*
Two (or more) of the following, each present for a significant portion of time during a 1-month period (or less if successfully treated);

(1) delusions
(2) hallucinations
(3) disorganized speech (e.g. frequent derailment or incoherence)
(4) grossly disorganized or catatonic behavior
(5) negative symptoms, that is, affective flattening, alogia, or avolition.

Note: Only one Criterion A symptom is required if delusions are bizarre or hallucinations consist of a voice keeping up a running commentary on the person's behavior or thoughts, or two or more voices conversing with each other.

B. *Social/occupational dysfunction*
For a significant portion of the time since the onset of the disturbance, one or more major areas of functioning such as work, interpersonal relations, or self-care are markedly below the level achieved prior to the onset (or when the onset is in childhood or adolescence, failure to achieve expected level of interpersonal academic, or occupational achievement).

C. *Duration*
Continuous signs of the disturbance persist for at least 6 months. This 6-month period must include at least 1 month of symptoms (or less if successfully treated) that meet Criterion A (i.e. active phase symptoms) and may include periods of prodromal or residual symptoms. During these prodromal or residual periods, the signs of the disturbance may be manifested by only negative symptoms or two or more symptoms listed in Criterion A present in an attenuated form (e.g. odd beliefs, unusual perceptual experiences).

D. *Schizoaffective and Mood Disorder exclusion*
Schizoaffective Disorder and Mood Disorder With Psychotic Features have been ruled out because either (1) no Major Depressive, Manic or Mixed Episodes have occurred concurrently with the active-phase symptoms, or (2) if mood episodes have occurred during active-phase symptoms, their total duration has been brief relative to the duration of the active and residual periods.

E. *Substance/general medical condition exclusion*
The disturbance is not due to the direct physiological effects of a substance (e.g. a drug of abuse, a medication) or a general medical condition.

F. *Relationship to a Pervasive Developmental Disorder*
If there is a history of Autistic Disorder or another Pervasive Developmental Disorder, the additional diagnosis of Schizophrenia is made only if prominent delusions or hallucinations are also present for at least a month (or less if successfully treated).

The DSM-IV diagnostic criteria for schizophrenia require the presence of symptoms from at least two of the groups listed above. Symptoms from only one group are required if delusions are bizarre or hallucinations consist of a voice keeping up a running commentary on the person's behaviour or thoughts, or two or more voices conversing with each other. Each of the symptoms must be present for a significant portion of time during a one-month period (or less if successfully treated).

According to DSM-IV, schizophrenia is accompanied by marked social or occupational dysfunction for a significant portion of the time since the onset of the disturbance. The dysfunction must be present in at least one major area such as work, interpersonal relations or self-care.

DSM-IV requires that continuous signs of the disturbance persist for at least 6 months. This 6-month period may include periods when only negative or less severe symptoms are present. Such periods are referred to as prodromal or residual, depending on whether they precede or follow the one-month period of characteristic symptoms described above.

Classification of course can be applied only after at least one year has elapsed since the initial onset of active-phase symptoms. According to DSM-IV, the course of schizophrenia is variable. The manual lists the following course specifiers: episodic with inter-episode residual symptoms; episodic with no inter-episode residual symptoms; continuous; single episode in partial remission; single episode in full remission; other or unspecified pattern.

Concerning differential diagnosis, DSM-IV emphasizes the distinction between schizophrenia and mood disorders. If psychotic symptoms occur exclusively during periods of mood disturbance, the diagnosis is mood disorder with psychotic features. If mood episodes have occurred during active-phase symptoms, and if their total duration has been brief relative to the duration of active and residual periods, the diagnosis is schizophrenia.

If a mood episode is concurrent with the active-phase symptoms of schizophrenia, and if mood symptoms have been present for a substantial portion of the total duration of the disturbance, and if delusions or hallucinations have been present for at least 2 weeks in the absence of prominent mood symptoms, the diagnosis is schizoaffective disorder.

The differentiation between schizophrenia, brief psychotic disorder and schizophreniform disorder rests upon a criterion of duration: less than one month for brief psychotic disorder; more than one month but less than 6 months for schizophreniform disorder; at least 6 months for schizophrenia.

The differential diagnosis between schizophrenia and delusional disorder rests on the nature of the delusions (in delusional disorder they are non-bizarre) and the absence of other characteristic symptoms of schizophrenia such as hallucinations, disorganized speech and behaviour, or prominent negative symptoms.

Schizophrenia and pervasive developmental disorder are distinguished by a number of criteria, including in particular the presence of prominent delusions and hallucinations in the former but not in the latter.

Finally, the diagnosis is not made if the disturbance is due to the direct physiological effects of a substance or a general medical condition.

DSM-IV describes five subtypes of schizophrenia: paranoid, disorganized, catatonic, undifferentiated and residual. Post-psychotic depressive disorder of schizophrenia and simple deteriorative disorder or simple schizophrenia are described in Appendix B, among conditions requiring further study.

In both the ICD-10 and the DSM-IV there is a distinction between positive and negative characteristic symptoms of schizophrenia. According to the definition provided in DSM-IV, "the positive symptoms appear to reflect an excess or distortion of normal functions, whereas the negative symptoms appear to reflect a diminution or loss in normal functions".

In both ICD-10 and DSM-IV, positive symptoms include hallucinations and delusions, disorganized thought and speech, as well as disorganized and catatonic behaviour. In both systems, negative symptoms include affective flattening or blunting of emotional responses, alogia or paucity of speech, and apathy or avolition.

The reliability and validity of psychiatric diagnoses that are based on explicit diagnostic criteria have been investigated in a number of studies during recent decades. According to Kendell [106], psychiatric diagnoses are now as reliable as the clinical judgements made in other branches of medicine. High reliability does not, however, by itself predict high validity. In fact, reliability can be high while validity remains trivial. In a critique of the DSM-IV operational diagnostic criteria for schizophrenia, Maj [107] discusses several important issues. According to Maj, the symptomatological criterion does not characterize schizophrenia as a syndrome, the five groups of symptoms it mentions are all given the same weight, there is no clear indication concerning the threshold above which the clinical manifestations listed in the criterion should be regarded as symptoms, and the concept of bizarre delusions has been kept despite the empirical evidence of the poor reliability in the evaluation of a delusion as bizarre or non-bizarre. Most of these critiques can also be addressed to the ICD-10 criteria for schizophrenia. In addition to the preceding critiques, Maj also critically analyses the chronological criterion (6 months) used in DSM-IV, the definition of the functional criterion, and the aetiologic component implied in the exclusion criteria.

ASSESSMENT INSTRUMENTS FOR THE DIAGNOSIS OF SCHIZOPHRENIA

Traditional psychological tests continue to be routinely applied in psychiatric settings to assess patients with a potential diagnosis of schizophrenia. The most widely used include questionnaires such as the Minnesota Multiphasic Personality Inventory and projective tests such as the Rorschach test and the Thematic Apperception Test (TAT). The value of traditional tests in diagnosing schizophrenia in the absence of clinical findings has been questioned [108].

A considerable number of instruments have been constructed for the assessment of patients with schizophrenia or other psychotic disorders.

The ninth version of the Present State Examination [109] was used in the International Pilot Study of Schizophrenia or IPSS [20]. The PSE includes a considerable number of items for the assessment of psychotic signs and symptoms and provides detailed definitions for each item.

For close to 50 years the most popular and universally used psychiatric rating scale in the field of schizophrenia has been the Brief Psychiatric Rating Scale or BPRS [110], which continues to be used widely, although often under an expanded, or otherwise modified form.

A number of standardized, semi-structured as well as fully structured instruments have been developed to facilitate the collection of data on the basis of which it will be decided whether a patient meets the requirements specified in the criteria for a specified disorder. Over the years, the various instruments have been revised, and adapted to fit the criteria and algorithms of the latest versions of ICD-10 and DSM-IV.

Prominent among structured instruments are the Diagnostic Interview Schedule or DIS [111, 112] and the Composite International Diagnostic Interview or CIDI [113, 114]. Both the DIS and the CIDI are fully structured diagnostic interviews, which can be used by lay interviewers after proper training. They are intended for use in epidemiological studies in general populations. There are computer programs for the CIDI and the DIS that enable users to enter, clean, and score the interview. Both the DIS and the CIDI have a section which contains relevant questions to assess the presence or absence of each single criterion required for a diagnosis of schizophrenia in ICD-10 and DSM-IV. The inter-rater reliability of the instruments is quite high, also for those questions that are listed in the schizophrenia section. The concordance of CIDI and DIS positive or negative diagnoses made independently by clinicians is, however, far less perfect.

Prominent among semi-structured interviews are the SADS [99], the Structured Clinical Interview for DSM (III, III-R, IV) or SCID [115, 116], the Schedules for Clinical Assessment in Neuropsychiatry or SCAN [117, 118] and the International Personality Disorder Examination or IPDE [119, 120]. All of these instruments have been field tested and were found to be reliable and applicable in different cultures.

The SADS was developed to facilitate the application of the Research Diagnostic Criteria or RDC. It exists in three different forms: SADS regular for the assessment of the present episode; SADS-L for the assessment of lifetime diagnoses; and SADS-C for the assessment of change.

The SCID is an instrument that was developed for the assessment of pathology and collection of data required for making diagnoses according to DSM criteria. It was first published for use with DSM-III, then revised for DSM-III-R, and finally for DSM-IV.

The SCAN is a set of instruments aimed at assessing, measuring and classifying the psychopathology and behaviour associated with the major psychiatric disorders of adult life, including schizophrenia and other psychotic disorders. It contains, in particular, the tenth version of the Present State Examination (PSE-10) and is accompanied by a comprehensive glossary. The SCAN yields diagnoses according to both ICD-10 and DSM-IV.

The IPDE assesses phenomenology relevant to the diagnosis of personality disorder according to ICD-10 and DSM-IV. It includes, in particular, items for the assessment of paranoid, schizoid and schizotypal personality disorder.

Various scales have been developed for rating specific individual aspects of schizophrenic symptomatology. For example, Andreasen [31] developed a scale for evaluating the presence of flattening of affect and inappropriate affect, and Chapman *et al* [25] have proposed an instrument for evaluating social as well as physical anhedonia.

Different scales have been proposed for the assessment of positive and negative symptoms in schizophrenia. The most prominent are the SANS [53, 54], the SAPS [55] and the Positive and Negative Syndrome Scale or PANSS [121, 122].

The SANS is a 25-item scale for the assessment of negative symptoms. The items may also be scored (from 0 to 5) on a summary sheet on which they are presented under five headings: affective flattening, alogia, avolition-apathy, anhedonia-asociality, and attentional impairment.

The SAPS is a 34-item scale for the assessment of positive symptoms. The items may also be scored (from 0 to 5) on a summary sheet on which they are presented under four headings: hallucinations, delusions, bizarre behaviour and positive formal thought disorder.

The PANSS is a 30-item instrument for assessing the prevalence of positive and negative syndromes in schizophrenia. It provides specific interview guidelines and assessment criteria, and includes two additional scales that consider positive and negative syndromes relative to one another and relative to general severity of psychopathology. Each item and each level of symptom severity are defined. The ratings provide summary scores on a seven-item positive score, seven-item negative scale, 16-item general psychopathology scale, and a composite (positive minus negative) index.

BIOLOGICAL INDICATORS

During the last two decades, a considerable number of biological indices have been investigated with the aim to find measurable indicators of, and confirmatory tests for, the disorder. According to Szymanski *et al* [123], the most promising biological indicators are pursuit eye movement dysfunctions, abnormalities in electrodermal activity, abnormalities in event-related brain voltage potentials, deficits in attention and information processing, and abnormal findings from brain imaging procedures.

According to a review by Clementz and Sweeney [124], between two-thirds and three-quarters of patients with schizophrenia show an impairment in smooth pursuit eye movements. The impairment is significantly higher in patients with schizophrenia than in normal controls and in other psychotic or non-psychotic control subjects [125, 126]. In addition, abnormal pursuit eye movements have been found in one third to more than one half of first-degree relatives of persons with schizophrenia, in contrast to only a small proportion of relatives of persons with other psychiatric disorders. Abnormal pursuit eye movements are, however, not entirely specific for schizophrenia. In particular, they may be observed in bipolar disorder [127]. According to Matthysse *et al* [128] and Holzman *et al* [129], eye movement impairment may be one possible manifestation of a genetically determined latent trait, with schizophrenic symptoms being one of several possible phenotypic expressions of that trait. On the whole, eye movement dysfunction is "a robust candidate in the search for a trait marker but not a confirmatory test for schizophrenia" [123].

Measures of evoked potentials have been widely found to be abnormal in patients with schizophrenia. St Clair *et al* [130] have reported smaller P300 amplitudes as well as delays in latency in patients with schizophrenia versus control subjects. According to Pfefferbaum *et al* [131], reduced auditory- and visual-evoked P300 amplitudes may be correlated with negative symptoms, while increased auditory P300s have been associated with positive symptoms [132]. Abnormalities in P300 are, however, not specific for schizophrenia, since they have also been found in patients with other psychiatric disorders, in particular in patients with schizotypal or borderline personality disorders [133, 134] and in patients with dementia [135].

Other investigations on event-related brain voltage potentials (ERPs) have found abnormalities in N100 and contingent negative variation as well as defects in sensory gating. The results of these studies are, however, conflicting and non-specific [123].

Studies on electrodermal activity have shown that 40–50% of patients with schizophrenia are non-responsive with the phasic skin conductance orienting response (SCOR) test versus 5–10% of non-psychiatric control subjects [136]. This type of response is, however, not specific for schizophrenia, since it has also been found in other psychiatric disorders, in particular in mood disorders [136]. Attempts to link non-response to positive or negative symptoms have yielded mixed results [137–140]. Recent studies on the SCOR test in patients with schizophrenia have identified two subgroups: a large subgroup of low to moderately aroused phasic SCOR non-responders; and a smaller subgroup of SCOR responders in which electrodermal tonic arousal is abnormally high [141, 142]. According to Dawson *et al* [143], phasic SCOR non-responding may qualify as a vulnerability indicator for schizophrenia, whereas tonic electrodermal arousal qualifies as a state-sensitive indicator.

Impairment in sustained focused attention as measured by continuous performance tests (CPT) may be a strong neuropsychological risk indicator for schizophrenia. According to Erlenmeyer-Kimling and Cornblatt [144], 40–50% of patients with schizophrenia show impaired performance. According to the same authors and to Nuechterlein *et al* [145], more complex CPT versions show significant differences between high-risk children and control subjects. In a recent review of more than forty studies that used various versions of the CPT, Cornblatt and Keilp [146] concluded that impaired attention is detectable in patients with schizophrenia, regardless of clinical state; that the disturbance is detectable before onset of the disorder; and that it is apparently heritable. The authors concede that attentional disturbances are also found in patients with other disorders such as mood disorders and children with attention deficit disorder, but report that there are particular patterns of impairment that appear to be specific to schizophrenia. They conclude that abnormal attention as shown with different versions of the CPT is highly promising as an indicator of a biological susceptibility to schizophrenia.

Structural and functional neuroimaging studies are providing new insights into schizophrenia [147]. Computerized tomography (CT) and magnetic resonance imaging (MRI) studies have shown an enlargement of lateral cerebral ventricles in some but not all patients with schizophrenia. In a meta-analysis of CT and MRI studies, Raz and Raz [148] found convincing evidence that mean ventricular volume in patients is larger than in normal controls, but that the magnitude of the effect is relatively small. There is also evidence that the smaller cerebral tissue volumes found in patients with schizophrenia are due to deficits in the volume of grey matter, with temporal and frontal regions showing greater deficits than parietal and occipital areas [147, 149, 150]. The question of whether the brain abnormalities in patients with schizophrenia are static or progressive, or whether they are static in some patients and progressive in others is still being debated [151].

Functional imaging techniques, such as positron emission tomography (PET) or single photon emission computer tomography (SPECT) have recently been reviewed by Liddle [152]. According to the reviewer, functional imaging studies have provided strong evidence for widespread disturbance of brain function, especially in the association cortex of frontal and temporal lobes.

Studies on the neurochemistry of schizophrenia, in particular on potential neurotransmitter-related enzymatic activity markers, have not yielded any consistent results up to now [123, 153].

In 1987, Garver [154] identified the following criteria for a trait marker to detect biological risk for psychosis: (a) it should distribute differently in patients with psychosis than in control populations; (b) it should have a greater prevalence in family members of identified patients with psychosis than in the general population and be associated with psychotic spectrum disorder in family members; (c) it should correlate with subsequent development of psychotic spectrum disorder in high-risk children and occur preceding the development of clinical manifestations of psychotic spectrum disorder; (d) it should be reliable and stable over time.

Although some biological indicators, including in particular those listed above, show promise for meeting Garver's criteria, none of them meets them completely. According to Szymanski *et al* [123], there are no biological indicators at present that can be employed in establishing a diagnosis of schizophrenia. According to these authors, longitudinal studies in high-risk populations utilizing multiple biological measures may, however, eventually define psychiatric syndromes with greater precision than clinical criteria or single biological markers.

SUMMARY

This chapter has reviewed the evidence regarding the diagnosis of schizophrenia. There are several areas where evidence is consolidated, others where evidence is uncertain, and quite a few that are completely open to research.

Consistent Evidence

It is now well established that schizophrenia is a heterogeneous group of syndromes which differ in symptomatology, course and outcome. Although some of the symptoms are more characteristic of the disorder than others, there are no specific or pathognomonic symptoms of schizophrenia. Characteristic symptoms may be subdivided into positive and negative symptoms. Prominent among positive symptoms are hallucinations, delusions and major disturbances in the form of thought. Prominent among negative symptoms are affective flattening, avolition and alogia.

Standardized and structured instruments are available for the assessment of characteristic signs and symptoms and for making a diagnosis of schizophrenia.

There is convincing evidence that schizophrenia is a disorder of all ages. Although onset of the disorder is usually in adolescence or early adulthood, schizophrenia may start in childhood and in late life. It has also been clearly established that there usually have been non-psychotic symptoms, often for several years, before the appearance of characteristic psychotic symptoms. Prominent pre-psychotic manifestations include symptoms related to impairment of cognitive functioning, in particular impairment of attention.

Outcome studies have consistently shown that the course of schizophrenia is poor in at least 50% of cases, but that a substantial proportion of patients make good, if not complete, recoveries from the disorder.

Incomplete Evidence

The current definitions of schizophrenia, as described in the explicit diagnostic criteria provided in ICD-10 and DSM-IV, are, at best, validated in part only. Owing to the polythetic nature of the symptom criteria, both the ICD-10 and the DSM-IV criteria define a group of disorders which is possibly extremely heterogeneous.

Although there is some evidence to support the distinction between the paranoid subtype and the non-paranoid subtypes, there is little evidence to support the differentiation of the individual classical subtypes of schizophrenia. Alternatives to the classical subtyping of schizophrenia, such as the three-factor dimensional descriptors that are proposed in DSM-IV to describe current and lifetime symptomatology, have not been fully investigated up to now.

While there is substantial evidence supporting the importance of a differentiation between positive and negative symptoms, there is considerably less evidence supporting the type I–type II or positive–negative dichotomy of schizophrenia. In particular, further studies are needed to determine whether the development of prominent negative symptoms justifies a diagnosis of schizophrenia (simple schizophrenia) in a patient who has never shown any positive symptoms.

Inclusion of prodromal or residual signs and symptoms in the definition of the disorder remains controversial, since no prodromal or residual manifestations have as yet been identified that are typical and specific of schizophrenia.

Attempts to differentiate schizophrenia more clearly from non-schizophrenic psychotic disorders, either acute or chronic, have not been conclusive. There also remain unsolved questions with regard to the distinction between schizophrenia and mood disorders, whenever schizophrenic and mood symptoms are present, either simultaneously or consecutively, in the same patient.

There is, up to now, only limited information on schizotypal disorder, and additional studies are needed to clarify the relationship between schizophrenia, schizotypal disorder and the other schizophrenia spectrum personality disorders.

Areas Still Open to Research

Very promising results have been obtained on biological indicators, such as abnormalities in eye movement, electrodermal activity, event-related brain potentials, disturbances in attention and information processing, and brain imaging. However, the importance of these abnormalities for diagnostic purposes remains, at best, controversial. The validity of the same abnormalities as trait markers for schizophrenia also needs to be confirmed by further studies.

ACKNOWLEDGEMENTS

The author wishes to thank Pascale Straus, Caroline Pull and Jacques Nickels for their help with the manuscript.

REFERENCES

1. World Health Organization (1992) *The ICD-10 Classification of Mental and Behavioural Disorders. Clinical Descriptions and Diagnostic Guidelines.* World Heath Organization, Geneva.
2. World Health Organization (1993) *The ICD-10 Classification of Mental and Behavioural Disorders. Diagnostic Criteria for Research.* World Health Organization, Geneva.
3. American Psychiatric Association (1980) *Diagnostic and Statistical Manual of Mental Disorders*, 3rd edn. American Psychiatric Association, Washington, DC.
4. American Psychiatric Association (1987) *Diagnostic and Statistical Manual of Mental Disorders*, 3rd edn, revised. American Psychiatric Association, Washington, DC.
5. American Psychiatric Association (1994) *Diagnostic and Statistical Manual of Mental Disorders*, 4th edn. American Psychiatric Association, Washington, DC.
6. Kraepelin E. (1896) *Psychiatrie. Ein Lehrbuch für Studierende und Ärzte.* 5. Auflage. A. Abel, Leipzig.
7. Bleuler E. (1911) Dementia Praecox oder die Gruppe der Schizophrenien. In *Handbuch der Geisteskrankheiten* (Ed. G. Aschaffenburg). Deuticke, Leipzig.
8. Jaspers K. (1911) *Allgemeine Psychopathologie.* 1. Auflage. Springer, Berlin.
9. Schneider K. (1950) *Klinische Psychopathologie.* G. Thieme, Stuttgart.
10. Jackson J.H. (1869) Certain points in the study and classification of diseases of the nervous system. Reprinted in J. Taylor (1932) *Selected Writings of John Hughlings Jackson*, vol. 2. Hodder & Stoughton, London.
11. Strauss J.S., Carpenter W.T., Bartko J.J. (1974) The diagnosis and understanding of schizophrenia: II. Speculations on the processes that underlie schizophrenic symptoms and signs. *Schizophr. Bull.*, **11**: 61–76.
12. Crow T.J. (1980) Molecular pathology of schizophrenia: More than one disease process? *Br. Med. J.*, **280**: 66–68.
13. Cutting J. (1990) *The Right Cerebral Hemisphere and Psychiatric Disorders.* Oxford University Press, Oxford.
14. Kendler K.S., Glaser W.M., Morgenstern H. (1983) Dimensions of delusional experience. *Am. J. Psychiatry*, **140**: 466–469.
15. Flaum M., Arndt S., Andreasen N.C. (1991) The reliability of "bizarre" delusions. *Compr. Psychiatry*, **32**: 59–65.

16. Andreasen N.C. (1982) Should the term "thought disorder" be revised? *Compr. Psychiatry*, **23**: 291–299.
17. Andreasen N.C. (1979) Thought, language and communication disorders. *Arch. Gen. Psychiatry*, **36**: 1315–1330.
18. Cutting J., Murphy D. (1988) Schizophrenic thought disorder. *Br. J. Psychiatry*, **152**: 310–319.
19. Cutting J. (1995) Descriptive psychopathology. In *Schizophrenia* (Eds S.R. Hirsch, D.R. Weinberger), pp. 15–27. Blackwell Science, Oxford.
20. World Health Organization (1973) *Report of the International Pilot Study of Schizophrenia*, vol. 1. World Health Organization, Geneva.
21. Guggenheim F.G., Babigian H.M. (1974) Catatonic schizophrenia: epidemiology and clinical course. *J. Nerv. Ment. Dis.*, **158**: 291–305.
22. Abrams R., Taylor M.A. (1976) Catatonia: a prospective clinical study. *Arch. Gen. Psychiatry*, **33**: 579–581.
23. Rado S. (1956) *Psychoanalysis of Behaviour: Collected Papers*. Grune & Stratton, New York.
24. Meehl P.E. (1962) Schizotaxia, schizotypy, schizophrenia. *Am. Psychol.*, **83**: 651–657.
25. Chapman L.J., Chapman J.P., Raulin M.I. (1980) Scales for physical and social anhedonia. *J. Abnorm. Psychol.*, **85**: 374–382.
26. Watson C.G., Jacobs L., Kucala T. (1979) A note on the pathology of anhedonia. *J. Clin. Psychol.*, **35**: 740–743.
27. Blanchard J.B., Nueser K.T., Bellack A.S. (1998) Anhedonia, positive and negative affect, and social functioning in schizophrenia. *Schizophr. Bull.*, **24**: 413–424.
28. Cook M., Simukonda F. (1981) Anhedonia and schizophrenia. *Br. J. Psychiatry*, **139**: 523–525.
29. Harrow M., Grinker R.R., Holzman P.S., Kayton L. (1977) Anhedonia and schizophrenia. *Am. J. Psychiatry*, **134**: 794–797.
30. Schuck J., Leventhal D., Rothstein H., Irizarry V. (1984) Physical anhedonia and schizophrenia. *J. Abnorm. Psychol.*, **93**: 342–344.
31. Andreasen N.C. (1979) Affective flattening and the criteria for schizophrenia. *Am. J. Psychiatry*, **136**: 944–947.
32. Abrams R., Taylor M.A. (1978) A rating scale for emotional blunting. *Am. J. Psychiatry*, **135**: 226–229.
33. Binder J., Albus M., Hubmann W., Scherer J., Sobizack N., Franz U., Mohr F., Hecht S. (1997) Neuropsychological impairment and psychopathology in first-episode schizophrenic patients related to the early course of illness. *Eur. Arch. Psychiatry Clin. Neurosci.*, **248**: 70–77.
34. Braff D.L., Heaton R., Kuck J., Cullum M., Moranville J., Grant I., Zisook S. (1991) The generalized pattern of neuropsychological deficits in outpatients with chronic schizophrenia with heterogeneous Wisconsin Card Sorting test results. *Arch. Gen. Psychiatry*, **48**: 891–898.
35. Saykin A.J., Gur R.C., Gur G.E., Mozley D., Mozley L.H., Resnick S.M., Kester B., Stafiniak P. (1991) Neuropsychological function in schizophrenia: Selective impairment in memory and learning. *Arch. Gen. Psychiatry*, **48**: 618–624.
36. Goldberg T.E., Gold J.M., Greenberg R., Griffin S., Schulz C., Pickar D., Kleinman J.E., Weinberger D.R. (1993) Contrasts between patients with affective disorder and patients with schizophrenia on a neuropsychological screening battery. *Am. J. Psychiatry*, **150**: 1355–1362.
37. Kremen W.S., Seidman L.J., Pepple J.R., Lyons M.J., Tsuang M.T., Faraone J.V. (1994) Neuropsychological risk indicators for schizophrenia: A review of family studies. *Schizophr. Bull.*, **20**: 103–118.

38. Cornblatt B.A., Keilp J.G. (1994) Impaired attention, genetics, and the patho-physiology of schizophrenia. *Schizophr. Bull.*, **20**: 31–46.
39. Goldberg T.E., Gold J.M. (1995) Neurocognitive deficits in schizophrenia. In *Schizophrenia* (Eds S.R. Hirsch, D.R. Weinberger), pp. 146–162. Blackwell Science, Oxford.
40. Gold J.M., Herman B.P., Wyler A., Randolph C., Goldberg T.E., Weinberger D.R. (1994) Schizophrenia and temporal lobe epilepsy: a neuropsychological study. *Arch. Gen. Psychiatry*, **51**: 265–272.
41. Goldberg T.E., Greenberg R., Griffin S., Gold J.M., Kleinman J.E., Pickar D., Schulz C., Weinberger D.R. (1993) Impact of clozapine on cognitive impairment and clinical symptoms in patients with schizophrenia. *Br. J. Psychiatry*, **162**: 43–48.
42. Andreasen N.C. (1985) Positive vs. negative schizophrenia. A critical evalua-tion. *Schizophr. Bull.*, **11**: 380–389.
43. Andreasen N.C., Roy M.-A., Flaum M. (1995) Positive and negative symp-toms. In *Schizophrenia* (Eds S.R. Hirsch, D.R. Weinberger), pp. 28–45. Blackwell Science, Oxford.
44. Wing J.W., Nixon J. (1975) Discriminating symptoms in schizophrenia. A report from the International Pilot Study of Schizophrenia. *Arch. Gen. Psychiatry*, **32**: 853–859.
45. Mellor C.S. (1970) First rank symptoms in schizophrenia. *Br. J. Psychiatry*, **117**: 15–23.
46. Carpenter W.T., Strauss J.S. (1974) Cross-cultural evaluation of Schneider's first-rank symptoms of schizophrenia: a report from the International Pilot Study of Schizophrenia. *Am. J. Psychiatry*, **131**: 682–687.
47. Taylor M.A. (1972) Schneiderian first rank symptoms and clinical prognostic features for schizophrenia. *Arch. Gen. Psychiatry*, **26**: 64–67.
48. Abrams R., Taylor M. (1973) First-rank symptoms, severity of illness, and treatment response in schizophrenia. *Compr. Psychiatry*, **14**: 353–355.
49. Carpenter W.T., Strauss J.S., Muleh S. (1973) Are there pathognomonic symp-toms in schizophrenia? *Arch. Gen. Psychiatry*, **131**: 682–687.
50. Taylor M.A., Abrams R. (1975) Acute mania: clinical and genetic study of res-ponders and non-responders to treatments. *Arch. Gen. Psychiatry*, **32**: 863–865.
51. Koehler K., Guth W., Grimm G. (1977) First-rank symptoms of schizophrenia in Schneider-oriented German centers. *Arch. Gen. Psychiatry*, **34**: 810–813.
52. Andreasen N.C., Olsen S.A. (1982) Negative vs. positive schizophrenia: defini-tion and validation. *Arch. Gen. Psychiatry*, **39**, 789–794.
53. Andreasen N.C. (1982) Negative symptoms in schizophrenia: definition and reliability. *Arch. Gen. Psychiatry*, **39**: 784–788.
54. Andreasen N.C. (1983) *The Scale for the Assessment of Negative Symptoms (SANS)*. University of Iowa, Iowa.
55. Andreasen N.C. (1984) *The Scale for the Assessment of Positive Symptoms (SAPS)*. University of Iowa, Iowa.
56. Yung A.R., McGorry P.D. (1996) The prodromal phase of first-episode psycho-sis: past and current conceptualizations. *Schizophr. Bull.*, **22**: 353–370.
57. Keith S.J., Matthews S.M. (1991) The diagnosis of schizophrenia: a review of onset and duration issues. *Schizophr. Bull.*, **17**: 51–67.
58. Loebel A.D., Lieberman J.A., Alvir J.M.J., Mayerhoff D.I., Geisler S.H., Szy-manski S.R. (1992) Duration of psychosis and outcome in first-episode schizo-phrenia. *Am. J. Psychiatry*, **149**: 1183–1188.
59. Beiser M., Erickson D., Fleming J.A.E., Iacono W.G. (1993) Establishing the onset of psychotic illness. *Am. J. Psychiatry*, **150**: 1349–1354.

60. Häfner H. (1996) The epidemiology of onset and early course of schizophrenia. In *New Research in Psychiatry* (Eds H. Häfner, E.M. Wolpert), pp. 33–61. Hogrefe & Huber, Göttingen.
61. Huber G., Gross G., Schüttler R., Linz M. (1980) Longitudinal studies of schizophrenic patients. *Schizophr. Bull.*, **4**: 592–605.
62. Häfner H., Riecher-Rössler A., Maurer K. (1991) Geschlechtsunterschiede bei schizophrenen Erkrankungen. *Fortschr. Neurol. Psychiatrie*, **59**: 343–360.
63. Häfner H., Maurer K., Löffler W., Riecher-Rössler A. (1993) The influence of age and sex on the onset and course of early schizophrenia. *Br. J. Psychiatry*, **162**: 80–86.
64. Jablensky A., Sartorius N., Ernberg G., Anker M., Korten A., Cooper J.E., Day R., Bertelsen A. (1992) Schizophrenia: manifestations, incidence and course in different cultures. A World Health Organization ten-country study. *Psychol. Med.* (Suppl. 20).
65. Häfner H., Hambrecht M., Löffler W., Munk-Jorgensen P., Riecher-Rössler A. (1998) Is schizophrenia a disorder of all ages? A comparison of first episodes and early course across the life-cycle. *Psychol. Med.*, **28**: 351–365.
66. Bleuler M. (1943) Die spätschizophrenen Krankheitsbilder. *Fortschr. Neurol. Psychiatrie*, **15**: 259–290.
67. Harris M.J., Jeste D.V. (1998) Late-onset schizophrenia: an overview. *Schizophr. Bull.*, **14**: 39–55.
68. Pearlson G.D., Kreger L., Rabins P.V., Chase G.A., Cohen B., Wirth J.B., Schlepfer T.B., Tune L.E. (1989) A chart review study of late-onset and early-onset schizophrenia. *Am. J. Psychiatry*, **146**: 1568–1574.
69. Rabins P., Pauker S., Thomas J. (1984) Can schizophrenia begin after age 44? *Compr. Psychiatry*, **25**: 290–294.
70. Mayer C., Kelterborn G., Naber D. (1993) Age of onset in schizophrenia: relations to psychopathology and gender. *Br. J. Psychiatry*, **162**: 665–671.
71. Howard R., Castle D.J., Wessely S., Murray R.M. (1993) A comparative study of 470 cases of early-onset and late-onset schizophrenia. *Br. J. Psychiatry*, **163**: 352–357.
72. Riecher-Rössler A., Rössler W., Först H., Meise U. (1995) Late-onset schizophrenia and late paraphrenia. *Schizophr. Bull.*, **21**: 345–354.
73. Marengo J. (1994) Classifying the courses of schizophrenia. *Schizophr. Bull.*, **20**: 519–536.
74. Müller C. (1951) Katamnestische Erhebungen über den spontanen Verlauf der Schizophrenie. *Monatsschr. Psychiatrie Neurol.*, **122**: 257–276.
75. Arnold O.H. (1955) *Schizophrener Prozess und schizophrene Symptomegesetze.* Maudrich, Vienna.
76. Ey H. (1959) Unity and diversity of schizophrenia: clinical and logical analysis of the concept of schizophrenia. *Am. J. Psychiatry*, **115**: 706–714.
77. Bleuler M. (1978) *The Schizophrenic Disorders: Long-term Patient and Family Studies.* Yale University Press, New Haven.
78. Ciompi L. (1980) The natural history of schizophrenia in the long term. *Br. J. Psychiatry*, **138**: 413–420.
79. Hegarty J.D., Baldessarini R.J., Tohen M., Waterhaux C., Oepen G. (1994) One hundred years of schizophrenia: a meta-analysis of the outcome literature. *Am. J. Psychiatry*, **151**: 1409–1416.
80. McGlashan T.H. (1988) A selective review of recent North American long-term follow-up studies of schizophrenia. *Schizophr. Bull.*, **14**: 515–542.

81. Harding C.M. (1988) Course types in schizophrenia: an analysis of European and American studies. *Schizophr. Bull.*, **14**: 633–643.
82. Riecher-Rössler A., Rössler W. (1998) The course of schizophrenic psychoses: what do we really know? A selective review from an epidemiological perspective. *Eur. Arch. Psychiatry Clin. Neurosci.*, **248**: 189–202.
83. Shepherd M., Watt D., Falloon I., Smeeton N. (1989) The natural history of schizophrenia: a five-year follow-up study of outcome and prediction in a representative sample of schizophrenics. *Psychol. Med.*, **15** (Suppl.): 1–46.
84. Harrow M., Sands J.R., Silverstein M.L., Goldberg J.F. (1997) Course and outcome for schizophrenia versus other psychotic patients: a longitudinal study. *Schizophr. Bull.*, **23**: 287–303.
85. Wiersma D., Nienhuis F.J., Slooff C.J., Giel R. (1998) Natural course of schizophrenic disorders: a 15-year followup of a Dutch incidence cohort. *Schizophr. Bull.*, **24**: 75–85.
86. Pull C.B. (1981) Dépression et schizophrénie. *Encéphale*, **7**: 343–346.
87. Pull C.B. (1993) Troubles affectifs et psychoses. *Halopsy*, **11**: 2–5.
88. Kendler H.K. (1994) The nosologic validity of mood-incongruent psychotic affective illness. In *DSM-IV Sourcebook*, vol. 1. (Eds T.A. Widiger, A.J. Frances, H.A. Pincus, M.B. First, R. Ross, W. Davis), pp. 461–475. American Psychiatric Association, Washington, DC.
89. Tsuang M.T., Levitt J.J., Simpson J.C. (1995) Schizoaffective disorder. In *Schizophrenia* (Eds S.R. Hirsch, D.R. Weinberger), pp. 46–57. Blackwell Science, Oxford.
90. Pull C.B. (1995) Atypical psychotic disorders. In *Schizophrenia* (Eds S.R. Hirsch, D.R. Weinberger), pp. 15–27. Blackwell Science, Oxford.
91. Siever L.J., Bergman A.J., Keefe R.S. (1995) The schizophrenia spectrum personality disorders. In *Schizophrenia* (Eds S.R. Hirsch, D.R. Weinberger), pp. 87–105. Blackwell Science, Oxford.
92. Tsuang M.T., Winokur G. (1974) Criteria for subtyping schizophrenia: clinical differentiation of hebephrenic and paranoid schizophrenia. *Arch. Gen. Psychiatry*, **81**: 43–47.
93. Zalewski C., Johnson-Selfridge M.T., Ohriner S., Zarrella K., Seltzer J.C. (1998) A review of neuropsychological differences between paranoid and nonparanoid schizophrenia patients. *Schizophr. Bull.*, **24**: 127–145.
94. McGlashan T.H., Fenton W.S. (1994) Classical subtypes for schizophrenia. In *DSM-IV Sourcebook*, vol. 1 (Eds T.A. Widiger, A.J. Frances. H.A. Pincus, M.B. First, R. Ross, W. Davis), pp. 419–440. American Psychiatric Association, Washington, DC.
95. Black D., Boffeli T. (1989) Simple schizophrenia: past, present, future. *Am. J. Psychiatry*, **146**: 1267–1273.
96. Robins E., Guze S. (1970) Establishment of diagnostic validity in psychiatric illness: its application to schizophrenia. *Am. J. Psychiatry*, **7**: 983–987.
97. Feighner J.P., Robins E., Guze S., Woodruff R.A., Winokur G., Munoz R. (1972) Diagnostic criteria for use in psychiatric research. *Arch. Gen. Psychiatry*, **26**: 57–63.
98. Spitzer R.L., Endicott J., Robins E. (1978) *Research Diagnostic Criteria (RDC) for a Selected Group of Functional Disorders*, 3rd edn. New York State Psychiatric Institute, New York.
99. Endicott J., Spitzer R.L. (1978) A diagnostic interview: the Schedule for Affective Disorders and Schizophrenia. *Arch. Gen. Psychiatry*, **35**: 837–844.
100. Astrachan B.M., Harrow M., Adler D., Brauer L., Schwartz A., Schwartz C. (1972) A checklist for the diagnosis of schizophrenia. *Br. J. Psychiatry*, **121**: 529–539.

101. Carpenter W.T., Strauss J.S., Bartko J.J. (1973) Flexible system for the diagnosis of schizophrenia: Report from the WHO International Pilot Study of Schizophrenia. *Science*, **182**: 1275–1278.
102. Taylor M.A., Abrams R. (1978) The prevalence of schizophrenia: a reassessment using modern diagnostic criteria. *Am J. Psychiatry*, **16**: 467–478.
103. Pull M.C., Pull C.B., Pichot P. (1987) Des critères empiriques pour les psychoses. III. Algorithmes et arbres de décision. *Encéphale*, **13**: 59–66.
104. Kellam A.M.P. (1989) French empirical criteria for the diagnosis of non-affective non-organic psychoses. *Br. J. Psychiatry*, **155**: 153–159.
105. Berner P., Gabriel E., Katschnig H., Kieffer W., Koehler K., Lenz G., Simhandl C. (1983) *Diagnostic Criteria for Schizophrenia and Affective Psychoses*. American Psychiatric Press, Washington, DC.
106. Kendell R.E. (1993) Diagnosis and classification. In *Companion to Psychiatric Studies*, 5th edn (Eds R.E. Kendell, A.K. Zealley), pp. 277–294. Churchill Livingstone, Edinburgh.
107. Maj M. (1998) Critique of the DSM-IV operational diagnostic criteria for schizophrenia (Editorial). *Br. J. Psychiatry*, **172**: 458–460.
108. Lipton A.A., Cancro R. (1995) Schizophrenia: clinical features. In *Comprehensive Textbook of Psychiatry* (Eds H.I. Kaplan, B.J. Sadock), pp. 968–987. Williams & Wilkins, Baltimore.
109. Wing J.K., Cooper J.E., Sartorius N. (1974) *The Description and Classification of Psychiatric Symptoms. An Instruction Manual for the PSE and Catego System*. Cambridge University Press, Cambridge.
110. Overall J.E., Gorham D.R. (1962) The Brief Psychiatric Rating Scale. *Psychol. Rep.*, **10**: 799–812.
111. Robins L.N., Helzer J.E., Croughan J., Ratcliff C.S. (1981) National Institute of Mental Health Diagnostic Interview Schedule. Its history, characteristics, and validity. *Arch. Gen. Psychiatry*, **38**: 381–389.
112. Robins L., Cottler L., Bucholz K., Compton W. (1995) *Diagnostic Interview Schedule for DSM-IV (DIS-IV)*. Washington University in St Louis, St Louis.
113. Robins L.N., Wing J.E., Wittchen H.U., Heiger J.E., Babor T.F., Burke J., Farmer A., Jablensky A., Pickens R., Regier D.A. (1988) The Composite International Diagnostic Interview: an epidemiological instrument suitable for use in conjunction with different systems and in different cultures. *Arch. Gen. Psychiatry*, **45**: 1069–1077.
114. World Health Organization (1997) *The Composite International Diagnostic Interview (CIDI) Version 2.1*. World Health Organization, Geneva.
115. Spitzer R.L., Williams J.B.W., Gibbon M., First M.B. (1992) The Structured Clinical Interview for DSM-III-R (SCID). I: History, rationale and description. *Arch. Gen. Psychiatry*, **49**: 624–629.
116. Williams J.B.W., Gibbon M., First M.B., Spitzer R.L. (1992) The Structured Clinical Interview for DSM-III-R (SCID). II: Multisite test–retest reliability. *Arch. Gen. Psychiatry*, **49**: 630–636.
117. Wing J.E., Babor T., Brugha T., Burke J., Cooper J.E., Giel R., Jablensky A., Regier D., Sartorius N. (1990) SCAN: Schedules for Clinical Assessment in Neuropsychiatry. *Arch. Gen. Psychiatry*, **47**: 589–593.
118. World Health Organization (1997) *Schedules for Clinical Assessment in Neuropsychiatry (SCAN) Version 2.1*. World Health Organization, Geneva.
119. Loranger A.W., Sartorius N., Andreoli A., Berger P., Buchheim P., Channabasavanna S.M., Coid B., Dahl A., Diekstra R.F., Ferguson B. *et al* (1994) The International Personality Disorder Examination (IPDE): The WHO/ADAMHA

International Pilot Study of Personality Disorders. *Arch. Gen. Psychiatry*, **5**: 215–224.

120. Loranger A.W., Janca A., Sartorius N. (1997) *Assessment and Diagnosis of Personality Disorders. The ICD-10 International Personality Disorder Examination (IPDE).* Cambridge University Press, Cambridge.

121. Kay S.R. (1987) The Positive and Negative Syndrome Scale (PANSS) for Schizophrenia. *Schizophr. Bull.*, **13**: 261–276.

122. Kay S.R. (1991) *Positive and Negative Syndromes in Schizophrenia. Assessment and Research.* Brunner/Mazel, New York.

123. Szymanski S., Kane J., Lieberman J. (1994) Trait markers in schizophrenia. Are they diagnostic? In *DSM-IV Sourcebook*, vol. 1 (Eds T.A. Widiger, A.J. Frances, H.A. Pincus, M.B. First, R. Ross, W. Davis), pp. 477–490. American Psychiatric Association, Washington, DC.

124. Clementz B.A., Sweeney J.A. (1990) Is eye movement dysfunction a biological marker for schizophrenia? A methodological review. *Psychol. Bull.*, **108**: 77–92.

125. Holzman P.S. Solomon C., Levin S., Waterhaux C.S. (1984) Pursuit eye movement dysfunction in schizophrenia: family evidence for specificity. *Arch. Gen. Psychiatry*, **41**: 136–139.

126. Holzman P.S. (1987) Recent studies of psychophysiology in schizophrenia. *Schizophr. Bull.*, **13**: 49–75.

127. Lipton R.B., Levin S., Holzman P.S. (1980) Horizontal and vertical smooth pursuit eye movements, the oculocephalic reflex, and the functional psychoses. *Psychiatry Res.*, **3**: 193–203.

128. Matthysse S., Holzman P.S., Lange K. (1986) The genetic transmission of schizophrenia: application of Mendelian latent structure analysis to eye tracking dysfunctions in schizophrenia and affective disorder. *J. Psychiatr. Res.*, **20**: 57–67.

129. Holzman P.S., Kringlen E., Matthysse S., Flanagan S.D., Lipton R.B., Cramer G., Levin S., Lange K., Levy D.L. (1988) A single dominant gene can account for eye tracking dysfunction and schizophrenia in offspring of discordant twins. *Arch. Gen. Psychiatry*, **45**: 641–647.

130. St Clair D., Blackwood D., Muir E. (1989) P300 abnormality in schizophrenic subtypes. *J. Psychiatr. Res.*, **23**: 49–55.

131. Pfefferbaum A., Fird J.M., White P.M., Roth W.T. (1989) P3 in schizophrenia is affected by stimulus modality, response requirements, medication status and negative symptoms. *Arch. Gen. Psychiatry*, **46**: 1035–1044.

132. Shenton M.E., Faux S.F., McCarley R.W, Ballinger R., Coleman M., Torello M., Duffy F.H. (1989) Correlations between abnormal auditory P300 topography and positive symptoms in schizophrenia: a preliminary report. *Biol. Psychiatry*, **25**: 710–716.

133. Blackwood D.H.R., St Clair D.M., Kutcher S.P. (1986) P300 event related potential abnormalities in borderline personality disorder. *Biol. Psychiatry*, **21**: 557–560.

134. Kutcher S.P., Blackwood D.H.R., St Clair D.M., Gaskell D.F., Muir W.J. (1987) P3 abnormality in borderline personality disorder and schizophrenia. *Arch. Gen. Psychiatry*, **44**: 645–650.

135. Goodin D.S., Squires K.S., Starr A. (1978) Long latency event related components of the auditory evoked potential in dementia. *Brain*, **101**: 635–648.

136. Holzman P.S. (1987) Recent studies of psychophysiology in schizophrenia. *Schizophr. Bull.*, **13**: 49–75.

137. Straube E. (1979) On the meaning of electrodermal nonresponding in schizophrenia. *J. Nerv. Ment. Dis.*, **167**: 601–611.

138. Bernstein A., Taylor K., Starkey P., Juni S., Lubowsky J., Paley H. (1981) Bilateral skin conductance, finger pulse volume, and EEG orienting response to tone of differing intensities in chronic schizophrenics and controls. *J. Nerv. Ment. Dis.*, **169**: 513–528.
139. Alm I., Lindström L.H., Ost L.G., Ohman A. (1984) Electrodermal nonresponding in schizophrenia: relationships to attentional, clinical, biochemical, computed tomographic, and genetic factors. *Int. J. Psychophysiol.*, **1**: 195–208.
140. Green M.F., Nuechterlein K.H., Satz P. (1989) The relationship of symptomatology and medication to electrodermal activity in schizophrenia. *Psychophysiology*, **26**: 148–157.
141. Öhman A. (1981) Electrodermal activity and vulnerability to schizophrenia: A review. *Biol. Psychol.*, **12**: 87–145.
142. Dawson M.E., Nuechterlein K.H. (1984) Psychophysiological dysfunctions in the developmental course of schizophrenic disorders. *Schizophr. Bull.*, **10**: 204–232.
143. Dawson M.E., Nuechterlein K.H., Schell A.M. (1992) Electrodermal anomalies in recent-onset schizophrenia: relationships to symptoms and prognosis. *Schizophr. Bull.*, **18**: 295–311.
144. Erlenmeyer-Kimling L., Cornblatt B. (1987) High-risk research in schizophrenia: a summary of what has been learned. *J. Psychiatr. Res.*, **21**: 401–411.
145. Nuechterlein K.H., Edell W.S., Norris M., Dawson M.E. (1986) Attention vulnerability indicators, thought disorder, and negative symptoms. *Schizophr. Bull.*, **12**: 408–428.
146. Cornblatt B.A., Keilp J.G. (1994) Impaired attention, genetics, and the pathophysiology of schizophrenia. *Schizophr. Bull.*, **20**: 31–46.
147. Zipursky R.B., Kapur S. (1998) New insights into schizophrenia from neuroimaging. *Curr. Opin. Psychiatry*, **1**: 33–37.
148. Raz S., Raz N. (1990) Structural brain abnormalities in the major psychoses: a quantitative review of the evidence from computerized imaging. *Psychol. Bull.*, **108**: 93–108.
149. Lim K.O., Sullivan E.V., Zipursky R.B., Pfefferbaum A. (1996) Cortical gray matter volume deficits in schizophrenia: a replication. *Schizophr. Res.*, **20**: 157–164.
150. Zipursky R.B., Seeman M.V., Bury A., Langevin R., Wortzman G., Katz R. (1997) Deficits in gray matter volume are present in schizophrenia but not bipolar disorder. *Schizophr. Res.*, **26**: 85–92.
151. Woods B., Yurgelun-Todd D., Goldstein J.M., Seidman L.J., Tsuang M.T. (1996) MRI brain abnormalities in chronic schizophrenia: one process or more? *Biol. Psychiatry*, **40**: 585–596.
152. Liddle P.F. (1995) Brain imaging. In *Schizophrenia* (Eds S.R. Hirsch, D.R. Weinberger), pp. 425–439. Blackwell Science, Oxford.
153. Owen F., Simpson M.D.C. (1995) The neurochemistry of schizophrenia. In *Schizophrenia* (Eds S.R. Hirsch, D.R. Weinberger), pp. 358–378. Blackwell Science, Oxford.
154. Garver D.L. (1987) Methodological issues facing the interpretation of high-risk studies: biological heterogeneity. *Schizophr. Bull.*, **13**: 525–529.

Commentaries

1.1
The Diagnosis of Schizophrenia: Practice and Concept
John S. Strauss[1]

The outstanding review by Prof. Pull provides an extremely scholarly and useful perspective on current diagnostic practices in schizophrenia and on their history. It is impressive to look back even a few decades in psychiatry to see what a tremendous advance these practices have made in promoting diagnostic reliability. And reliability is not merely the basis for measurement and scientific study, as important as these are. In a more subtle but even more crucial way, reliability is basic for communication generally. For example, at a meeting among international schizophrenia experts (I was just a trainee) held in the 1960s, the leader, Martin Katz, asked to show a film of a patient with a severe mental disorder to see if the participants would all diagnose the patient the same way. Everyone seemed to feel that was totally unnecessary and protested, so it was only with extreme persistence that Martin was allowed to proceed. He asked each of us to write down our diagnosis on a piece of paper. After the film, Martin asked for a show of hands for our diagnoses as he read off several diagnostic categories. We were amazed and appalled at how much disagreement there was. We had assumed that when we were using the term "schizophrenia" we were all talking about the same thing.

Since that time, developments in operational diagnostic criteria and their use in diagnostic practice throughout the world have greatly increased our ability to communicate. But diagnostic practice is only one leg of the two-legged beast (or beasts) we are trying to understand and treat. The other leg is "concept". What is the nature of the thing or things we are trying to diagnose? Prof. Pull touches on several possibilities in the discussions on validity. But the notion of validity often implies a sense that the nature of the underlying "thing" is known at least roughly.

It was the magic of Kraepelin that he put together under the rubric "dementia praecox" "things" that by appearance looked almost entirely different. Many of his most influential contemporaries actually used a kind of

[1] 50 Burton Street, New Haven, CT 06515, USA

operational diagnostic practice, grouping together into "syndromes" symptoms that they believed to occur together. Kraepelin emphasized the concept of psychiatric "diseases" focusing on the underlying process that he believed united the diverse syndromes, in the case of dementia praecox, the clue to process he believed was deteriorating course.

As Prof. Pull notes, it is now clear that the course and outcome of schizophrenia, the descendant of Kraepelin's notion of dementia praecox, are extremely diverse. The problem is where does that leave us? We have made crucial advances in developing the practice of operational and reliable diagnosis. But what is the thing we are diagnosing? Is it a "thing" at all? Or is it a related group of "things" as Bleuler supposed? Or is it many different "things"? And the further question, of course, is if there is a "thing" (or things), then what is its (their) nature? In a sense, having gone through a cycle since the time of Kraepelin, and having a great deal more information than was available to him, we are back at some of the very issues he faced.

In the difficult bootstrapping task, trying to diagnose a thing reliably when we are not entirely sure what that thing is, we have much company. In fact, the search for the thing or things has been ongoing with many major shifts since Kraepelin's time, major shifts that are suggested in Prof. Pull's review. And, as is almost always the case in the history of science, shifts in concepts, in methods, and in practices of labelling, occur at the same time, whether these changes are noticed overtly or not. Bleuler lived on the grounds where his patients lived and was influenced by Freud, and for these and other reasons saw things somewhat differently from Kraepelin. Bleuler enlarged the concept considerably, changed its name, and focused more on what he believed to be underlying psychological mechanisms. Although Bleuler may have improved the concept of dementia praecox in some ways, he made it at the same time far more vague. Jaspers and his interest in levels shifted the focus of observation again and changed the rules for weighting the importance of observations made. Schneider returned somewhat more to the pre-Kraepelinian attempt to identify diagnostically crucial symptom groups.

Where are we now in this evolving spiral of diagnostic practice and concept? Somewhat mixed as have been all our predecessors, but with our contemporary emphasis on diagnostic symptoms, we are more allied, I think, to the pre-Kraepelinian and the Schneiderian approaches than to many others. Many might disagree, but then it is often difficult to locate one's own position in historical patterns of change.

Where should we be? In my opinion ours is not such a bad location, basic communication being as crucial as it is. If only we could be a bit more humble than we sometimes are, and if only we could see ourselves more clearly and promote more diversity of orientation, given the serious shortcomings in present knowledge. Especially given current trends in medical practice towards briefer contact with patients and the fact that many psychiatric researchers do not see patients at all, I think it particularly crucial that we re-emphasize the importance, depth and complexity of patient experiences and subjectivity as a basis for data, and for the understanding and improved diagnosis of the processes underlying the "thing" for which we search.

1.2
Should Schizophrenia as a Disease Entity Concept Survive into the Third Millennium?
Timothy J. Crow[1]

Charles Pull has put together a masterly overview of the recent litera-ture on nosology and outcome of the disease entity that we have been persuaded by E. Kraepelin and E. Bleuler to identify as "dementia praecox" or "schizophrenia". Arguably, the entity is still as well established as the lynch-pin of psychiatric thought and practice at the turn of the millennium as it was at the end of the nineteenth century. Other conditions, a fortiori the affective psychoses, are defined by reference to schizophrenia — these are diagnoses to be considered when schizophrenia has been excluded. Without the concept of schizophrenia it is difficult to see how discussions of psychi-atric diagnosis and practice could take place. The structure of textbooks and examinations depend upon it. Take away this cornerstone and it seems that the framework of psychiatry as a discipline is at risk of crumbling away.

And yet the edifice is built on sand. It sways and shudders in the wind. And with every creak of the timbers there is a rush in the profession to shore it up, for fear of what might happen without it. The prospect of psychiatry without the concept of schizophrenia is awful to contemplate.

But the fundamental flaw is easy to see, was apparent to Kraepelin, and was formally demonstrated in the literature some 17 years ago. It is simply that the concept has no boundaries. In 1920 Kraepelin [1] wrote of, "the difficulties which prevent us from distinguishing reliably between manic-depressive insanity and dementia praecox. No experienced psychiatrist will deny there is an alarmingly large number of cases in which it seems impossible, in spite of the most careful observation, to make a firm diagnosis . . . it is becoming increasingly clear that we cannot distinguish satisfactorily between these two illnesses and this brings home the suspicion that our formulation of the problem may be incorrect." The failure of the concept was formally demonstrated by Endicott *et al* [2] when they applied seven different sets of operational criteria to a consecutive series of 46 patients admitted to the Psychiatric Institute in New York who met any of the criteria for a diagnosis

---

[1]*University Department of Psychiatry, Warneford Hospital, Oxford OX3 7JX, UK*

of schizophrenia. By the most liberal criteria 44 patients were diagnosed as suffering from schizophrenia; by the most restrictive only six. Yet all of these criteria can be traced back through Bleuler to Kraepelin. Something is fundamentally wrong with the concept. What it is is clear from Endicott et al's seminal contribution and from the direction of recent research on psychosis. Endicott et al [2] showed that the differences between different sets of criteria are to a large extent related to whether or not patients with an affective component to their illness are included. By the more liberal criteria some who by modal Research Diagnostic Criteria (RDC) will be diagnosed as manic-depressive will be given a diagnosis of schizophrenia. Nothing in the recent literature, nosological, pathophysiological or genetic, appears to challenge the concept of a continuum of psychosis [3–5].

But there is the further problem of specifying what it is a continuum of. This is implicit in the now extensive literature on dimensions of psychopathology, and, indeed, was implicit in the two-syndrome concept, in so far as this was taken to describe separate dimensions of pathophysiology. If we really had discrete disease entities why would we also have dimensions? What could these be other than a single dimension of severity? Alongside this issue must be placed the body of evidence that symptoms apparently characteristic of psychoses are common in the general population [6]. Where is the line to be drawn?

I incline [7] to the view that Kretschmer [8] put his finger on the nub of the problem when he framed his challenge to the original Kraepelinian concept: "we can never do justice to the endogenous psychoses so long as we regard them as isolated unities of disease, having taken them out of their natural heredity environment, and forced them into the limits of a clinical system. Viewed in a large biological framework, however, the endogenous psychoses are nothing other than marked accentuations of normal types of temperament."

This is the challenge that no one has taken up. What is "the natural heredity environment" and "its large biological framework"? These questions impinge upon the origins of man, and the nature of human diversity. In their solution the epidemiological characteristics of psychosis are crucial. With the use of Schneider's nuclear symptoms in the World Health Organization (WHO) Ten Country study, Jablensky et al [9] concluded that: "schizophrenic illnesses are ubiquitous, appear with similar incidence in different cultures and have features that are more remarkable by their similarity across cultures than by their difference."

Thus the predisposition to psychosis is intrinsic to human populations. The biological disadvantage, that is, associated with such genetic predisposition must be balanced by an advantage; the relevant variation is inseparable from being human. It must, I have argued, be related to the speciation characteristic, the capacity for language. Schizophrenia, according to this view, is "the price that *Homo sapiens* pays for language" [10]. Nuclear symptoms themselves can be conceived as anomalies of the transition from thought to speech [11, 12]. They represent "language at the end of its tether". My response to Kretschmer's challenge therefore is that the "natural heredity environment" is the genetic change (the "speciation event") associated with the transition between a precursor hominid and *Homo sapiens*, and that this variation may be associated with unusual characteristics — specifically, I suspect the variation is "epigenetic" (associated with gene expression) rather than with variation in the DNA sequence [13]. The "larger biological framework" is the capacity for language and the associated revolution in brain function (hemispheric differentiation) that allowed the transition to take place.

The focus on "schizophrenia" as a disease entity, as widely promoted by psychiatric textbooks, and the drive to develop increasingly refined sets of diagnostic criteria, does no justice to the nature of psychosis. These phenomena are intrinsic to human populations and tell us about the genetic origin of the characteristic that defines the species, the capacity for language. The nuclear symptoms of schizophrenia can be regarded as a window on the transition from thought to speech [12]. By the same logic the whole range of psychotic manifestations, including the affective psychoses, tells us about the variation that relates to the core characteristic of the human brain — hemispheric differentiation [11]. By attempting to understand these phenomena, we can hope to unravel what is distinctive about the function of the brain in *Homo sapiens* and why it is so diverse.

REFERENCES

1. Kraepelin E. (1920) Die Erscheinungsformen des Irreseins. *Zeit. Gesam. Neurol. Psychiatrie*, **62**: 1–29.
2. Endicott J., Nee J., Fleiss J., Cohen J., Williams J.B.W., Simon R. (1982) Diagnostic criteria for schizophrenia: reliabilities and agreement between systems. *Arch. Gen. Psychiatry*, **39**: 884–889.
3. Crow T.J. (1990) Nature of the genetic contribution to psychotic illness — a continuum viewpoint. *Acta. Psychiatr. Scand.*, **81**: 401–408.
4. Crow T.J. (1994) Con: The demise of the Kraepelinian binary system as a prelude to genetic advance. In *Genetic Approaches to Mental Disorders*, pp. 163–192 (Eds E.S. Gershon, C.R. Cloninger). American Psychiatric Press, Washington, DC.
5. Crow T.J. (1995) A continuum of psychosis, one human gene and not much else — the case for homogeneity. *Schizophr. Res.*, **17**: 135–145.
6. Verdoux H., van Os J., Maurice-Tison S., Gay B., Salamon R., Bourgeois M. (1998) Is early adulthood a critical developmental stage for psychosis proneness? A survey of delusional ideation in normal subjects. *Schizophr. Res.*, **29**: 247–254.
7. Crow T.J. (1998) From Kraepelin to Kretschmer leavened by K. Schneider: the transition from categories of psychosis to dimensions of variation intrinsic to *Homo sapiens*. *Arch. Gen. Psychiatry*, **55**: 502–504.
8. Kretschmer E. (1925) *Physique and Character*. Kegan Paul, Trench, Trubner, London.

9. Jablensky A., Sartorius N., Ernberg G., Anker M., Korten A., Cooper J.E., Day R., Bertelsen A. (1992) Schizophrenia: manifestations, incidence and course in different cultures. A World Health Organization Ten Country Study. *Psychol. Med.*, **20** (Suppl.), 1–97.
10. Crow T.J. (1997) Is schizophrenia the price that *Homo sapiens* pays for language? *Schizophr Res.*, **28**: 127–141.
11. Crow T.J. (1998) Sexual selection, timing and the descent of man: a theory of the genetic origins of language. *Curr. Psychol. Cogn.*, **17**: 1079–1114.
12. Crow T.J. (1998) Nuclear schizophrenic symptoms as a window on the relationship between thought and speech. *Br. J. Psychiatry*, **173**: 103–109.
13. Crow T.J. (1998) Why cerebral asymmetry is the key to the origin of *Homo sapiens*: how to find the gene or eliminate the theory. *Curr. Psychol. Cogn.*, **17**: 1237–1278.

1.3
On Defining Schizophrenia
Josef Parnas[1]

Operational criteria were developed as a provisional and pragmatic tool, but are increasingly reified and gradually elevated to a status of unquestionable truth. A brief critical survey of the diagnostic criteria of schizophrenia (ICD-10, DSM-IV) is therefore due. It may be helpful to realize that these criteria represent *a convention* of unknown validity as compared to potential rival definitions. The first-rank symptoms (FRS) are assigned a strong prominence, due to their presumed simplicity and reliability, and their attractiveness as model medical symptoms. However, the reliability of FRS, though reasonable *within* one research group, is much weaker *between* the groups [1]. Schneider was quite laconic in the sole description available in the English translation. Consequently, what psychiatrists consider as representing a FRS varies in important respects [2]. This variation is, moreover, not only due to linguistic limitations. Today we know that FRS do not arise suddenly fully-fledged but are antedated by subtle, anomalous subjective experiences [3]. FRS are termini of progressive spatialization and externalization of these anomalous experiences, usually completed by a delusional elaboration. Reliability problems arise when investigators define a FRS using different cut-off points on these FRS continua [1, 2]. But even the patient himself, at the incipient illness stages, may vacillate in the felt concreteness of his inner change, and hence hesitate as to whether his verbalized explications are only metaphors or should be taken literally.

The pathognomonic status of delusions with "impossible" (bizarre) content was justified by an appeal to Jaspers' notion of "incomprehensibility" of

[1] *University Department of Psychiatry, Hvidovre Hospital, 2650 Hvidovre, Denmark*

delusions in schizophrenia. However, this notion was embedded in a more overarching context of accessibility to empathic understanding. Impossibility of content is neither definitive nor exhaustive of "incomprehensibility". In fact, the diagnostic ineptitude of the sheer delusional content, commonly recognized in the German-speaking psychiatry already by 1930, stimulated interest in *the form of experience* in the arising delusion (e.g. delusional perception), in order to seize the experiential aspects suggestive of schizophrenia [4]. Recently, it has been proposed [5] that typicality of schizophrenic delusions lies partly in the fact that their content transpires a profoundly altered *form of experiencing*: blurred Self-world articulation, solipsistic access to the mind's own constituting activity and a mutation of the ontological axioms of experiencing. In conclusion, attributing to bizarre delusions a sufficient diagnostic efficacy is phenomenologically unfounded and historically inexact.

The second criterion of the ICD-10 (and its DSM-IV equivalents) is formulated on a severity level that fails to diagnose cases clinically considered as incipient disorganized and paranoid schizophrenia, with definite formal thought disorder and peculiarities of rapport, but below the stipulated severity level. In brief, the criteria work best with chronic patients, but definitely less so with first admission cases or cases identified in the population.

Defining schizophrenia equals specification of its validity criteria. No robust extraclinical marker is available and attempts to subtype have been dramatically unsuccessful. Factor analyses do not help because they rarely tell news. They aggregate intercorrelated items, entered in the first place, as *reiterations* of the clinically important aspects. Thus, the three-component structure was mathematically demonstrated already in 1948 [6].

It is logically impossible to assess the diagnostic import of a symptom, by looking at its distributions, if the symptom itself is a part of the very category definition. It does not make sense to claim that, say, thought insertion is more frequent in schizophrenia than in bipolar illness, if one believes, in the first place, that this symptom is highly diagnostic of schizophrenia. That is why many such studies are viciously circular or, at best, uninformative. *An access is needed to the definition, which is independent of single symptoms.* Given the lack of markers and singly typical course patterns, we can only turn to the original definition of what schizophrenia was considered to be. We need to distinguish *criteria*, defining the *essence* of schizophrenia, from *symptoms*, which may, but need not, be present. It was considered to be of essence of schizophrenia to *persist*, but persistence was conceived of as a *persistence of trait phenomena* (e.g. autistic tendencies) and thus not exhaustively reducible to chronicity of psychosis or debilitating course. This essence was perceived as a change at the very core of mental life and variously designated [7]. We can propose, more specifically, that the essence of schizophrenia, marking the extension of its spectrum concept, entails an alteration of the basic, pre-personal configuration of the Self and its intentional relation to the world. Modifications of the medical model are needed in order to investigate this hypothesis more closely. First, we must abandon the view that schizophrenia and its carrier can be separated in the way as one separates an infection from its victim, that is, that the subjectivity (Self) of the subject and his illness can be treated as independent regions. The second modification follows from the first: studying subjectivity calls for a suitable methodology, specifically developed to address first person data, namely phenomenology in its continental sense [5].

REFERENCES

1. Koehler K. (1979) First rank symptoms of schizophrenia: questions concerning clinical boundaries. *Br. J. Psychiatry*, **134**: 236–248.
2. Crichton P. (1996) First-rank symptoms or rank-and-file-symptoms. *Br. J. Psychiatry*, **169**: 537–550.
3. Klosterkötter J. (1988) *Basissymptome und Endphänomene der Schizophrenie. Eine Empirische Untersuchung der Psychopathologischen Übergangsreihen Zwischen Defizitären und Produktiven Schizophreniesymptomen*. Springer, Berlin.
4. Kunz R. (1931) Die Grenze der psychopathologische Wahninterpretationen. *Zeit. Gesam. Neurol. Psychiatrie*, **135**: 671–715.
5. Bovet P., Parnas J. (1993) Schizophrenic delusions: a phenomenological approach. *Schizophr. Bull.*, **19**: 579–597.
6. Wittman P., Sheldon W. (1948) A proposed classification of psychotic behavior reactions. *Am. J. Psychiatry*, **105**: 124–128.
7. Parnas J., Bovet P. (1991) Autism in schizophrenia revisited. *Compr. Psychiatry*, **32**: 1–15.

1.4
Diagnosis and Pathophysiology of Schizophrenia

Peter F. Liddle[1]

A century of research and clinical practice have confirmed many of the features of schizophrenia delineated by Kraepelin and Bleuler, but fundamental attributes such as the time course and prognosis remain uncertain. A number of developments in research methodology, such as the use of standardized diagnostic criteria, attention to the problems of sampling bias, and the development of multivariate statistical techniques, have enhanced the rigour of clinical research. However, until there is a diagnostic method that is not only reliable but also valid, it will remain difficult to draw definitive conclusions.

[1] *Department of Psychiatry, University of British Columbia, 2255 Wesbrook Mall, Vancouver, V6T 2A1, Canada*

This is illustrated by the Buckinghamshire 5-year follow-up study [1], which employed the Present State Examination (PSE) criteria for diagnosis in a carefully ascertained sample. Among its findings was the observation that 16% of cases have a single episode of illness, with no residual deficits. However, despite the meticulous design of the study, the validity of this conclusion depends utterly on the validity of the PSE criteria employed to ascertain the cases. These criteria assign substantial weight to Schneiderian first-rank symptoms. At the time the study was performed, these were widely regarded as the best criteria available, but they have subsequently been superseded by ICD-10 and DSM-IV. A similar study employing the DSM-IV criteria, which demand a persistent illness lasting at least 6 months before the diagnosis of schizophrenia is made, would probably find a smaller proportion of cases having very good outcome. How are we to determine whether or not the DSM-IV criteria are more valid than the PSE criteria?

It is unlikely this dilemma will be resolved until markers for the essential pathological process or processes of schizophrenia are identified. There are potentially two types of marker that might be applicable in clinical practice: genetic markers and measurements of brain function. At this stage, the prospect of a genetic marker that reliably predicts the occurrence of the disease is not strong. With regard to measurements of brain function, a multitude of different abnormalities have been reported in schizophrenia, but in most instances the range of values observed in schizophrenia overlaps the range in healthy subjects. Nonetheless, there are signs of convergence on answers to several questions about the nature of the pathophysiology of schizophrenia.

First, which brain areas are implicated in schizophrenia? A large body of evidence indicates that the disturbance of cerebral function is widespread. In particular, association cortex of frontal, temporal and parietal lobes, and related subcortical nuclei, are involved. Relevant to the issue of clinical heterogeneity of schizophrenia is the observation that different clusters of symptoms are associated with aberrant cerebral activity in different cerebral regions. For example, the characteristic symptoms of schizophrenia cluster into three syndromes: reality distortion, disorganization and psychomotor poverty (core negative features) [2]. Each of these syndromes is associated with aberrant activity in a particular set of sites located in association cortex and subcortical nuclei [3]. This observation confirms the evidence from many other studies implicating diverse cerebral areas, and provides external validation for subdividing the characteristic symptoms of the illness into these three syndromes. It should be noted that these syndromes are not separate illnesses but tend to coexist within an individual patient; each individual might have some degree of malfunction at all of the cerebral sites involved.

Secondly, what is the nature of the functional disorder? Functional imaging studies suggest that the essential problem is a disorder of coordination of cerebral activity. Much of the evidence indicates abnormal fronto-temporal connectivity [4]. There is also evidence that connections involving other areas of association cortex and subcortical nuclei are abnormal [5]. If the problem is a disorder of connectivity, the prospects for treating the essential defect in function are potentially better than if the central problem was a focal loss of neurons. The nature of the molecular abnormality responsible for the putative disordered connectivity remains to be ascertained.

Third, when does the pathophysiological process begin? There is now convincing evidence that schizophrenia is associated with subtle abnormalities of early neuronal development [6]. This association might indicate either that disordered development creates a non-specific vulnerability to schizophrenia, or that disordered neurodevelopment is an essential feature of the illness.

In conclusion, there has been encouraging progress in the quest to identify the cardinal pathophysiological process that defines schizophrenia. Once this has been achieved, definitive answers to questions such as the differentiation of schizophrenia from other psychotic disorders, time course and prognosis, will be possible.

REFERENCES

1. Watt D.C., Katz K., Shepherd M. (1983) The natural history of schizophrenia: a five-year prospective follow-up of a representative sample of schizophrenics by means of a standardized clinical and social assessment. *Psychol. Med.*, **13**: 663–670.
2. Liddle P.F. (1987) The symptoms of chronic schizophrenia: a re-examination of the positive–negative dichotomy. *Br. J. Psychiatry*, **151**: 145–151.
3. Liddle P.F., Friston K.J., Frith C.D., Hirsch S.R., Jones T., Frackowiak R.S.J. (1992) Patterns of cerebral blood flow in schizophrenia. *Br. J. Psychiatry*, **160**: 179–186.
4. McGuire P.K., Frith C.D. (1997) Disordered functional connectivity in schizophrenia. *Psychol. Med.*, **26**: 663–667.
5. Liddle P.F., Passmore M., Friston K.J., Frith C.D. (1997) Functional connectivity during word generation in schizophrenia. *Schizophr. Res.*, **24**: 168.
6. Waddington J.L., Buckley P.F. (1995) *The Neurodevelopmental Basis of Schizophrenia*. Landes, Austin.

1.5
The Significance of Intuition for the Diagnosis of Schizophrenia

Alfred Kraus[1]

The current classification and diagnosis in psychiatry, as presented in the diagnostic manuals of DSM-IV and ICD-10, are based on operational criteria

[1]*Department of Psychiatry, University of Heidelberg, Vosstrasse 4, 69115 Heidelberg, Germany*

and specific rules for use (so-called algorithms). To a large extent intuition is excluded from the diagnostic process. What is lost with the exclusion of intuition? Can we afford this loss [1]?

The intuition of the schizophrenic element is mainly identified with the praecox-feeling. Minkowski's [2] "diagnostique par penetration" and Tellenbach's [3] "atmospheric diagnosis" are also intuitive approaches to the essence of the schizophrenic element. After Rümke [4] described the praecox-feeling referring to dementia praecox, Wyrsch [5] further analysed this intuitive recognition of the schizophrenic person. He recognized that it is based neither only on signs such as facial or gestural expressions or a bad emotional contact, nor only on an impairment of understanding other people's motives. According to Wyrsch, the praecox-feeling has nothing to do with symptoms or other single features, but rather with a certain modality of being ("Eine Daseinsweise"), a certain way of "being in the world and taking part in it". What Wyrsch explicitly asserted, that this intuitive recognition is no "guessing and presuming" but "really recognition", is decisive in this context. Also according to Müller-Suur [6] the intuitive perception of the schizophrenic element is not the perception of something vague, but of a "definite incomprehensibility" ("ein bestimmtes Unverständliches"). It is in our opinion a relatively definite changed form of being-in-the-world ("In-der-Welt-sein") with an order of its own. What is incomprehensible, but intuitively perceived as something well defined, are certain basic structures of our being which have changed, as for instance the temporality and spatiality of being, the being with others, etc. — in short the ontological status of the person. Because these structures are not concrete, but are constituting objectivity (*Gegenständlichkeit*), they are called prepredicative structures.

We want to show this first with the hallucinations of schizophrenic patients. The schizophrenic patient does not experience hallucination as a normal perception: (a) his hallucination is like an event on another stage, not in the world, but in front of it [7], that means not participating in the field of normal perception; (b) the person concerned is at the mercy of this perception not only because the hallucinated voice is coming from everywhere, but also because his body scheme [8] has changed (the perceived voice reaches the centre of the person, while the activity of the ego is blocked, and it is really impossible to objectify it); (c) schizophrenic hallucination is like a revelation, stirring up the whole being of the person. The intuitive diagnosis of hallucination is not made because this kind of perception has no real object, as the operational definition of the "Arbeitsgemeinschaft fur Methodik und dokumentation in der Psychiatrie" (AMDP) says, but because the quality of this kind of perception is, as we have shown, different and cannot be compared with normal perception. Therefore,

Steffens and Graham [9] recently proposed not to conceive schizophrenic hallucination as a perceptive disturbance at all, but as a disturbance of active self-consciousness.

Delusion is another example showing the significance of intuition in the diagnostics of schizophrenia, intuition here also recognizing a change of prepredicative structures. As to DSM-IV, delusions are erroneous beliefs. The difference between delusion and strongly held ideas is seen only in the degree of conviction with which the belief is held, despite clear contradictory evidence. But can superstitious and fanatical people not also keep up erroneous beliefs with a similar strong opposition against contradictory evidence? What really enables us to diagnose a delusion is not only the assessment of lack of insight, abnormality of certainty and incorrectibility [10] in connection with a wrong judgement of reality, not statements of the patient about facts, but his totally different kind of relationship to reality and to others. What the intuition of delusion recognizes, is not an alteration of cognitive function, but a change of the personality of the patient and his relationship to the world, as Jaspers already stated [10]. The whole ontological status of the patient has changed. Thus, it is this intuitively grasped, changed self of the patient and his changed relationship to the world which gives his abnormal certainty or lack of insight a special quality, and makes it a real criterion of delusion.

REFERENCES

1. Kraus A. (1994) Phenomenological and criteriological diagnosis: different or complementary? In *Philosophical Perspectives on Psychiatric Diagnosis and Classification* (Eds J. Sadler, O.P. Wiggins, M. Schwartz), pp. 148–162. Johns Hopkins University Press, Baltimore.
2. Minkowski E. (1827) *Psychopathologie des schizoides et des schizophrènes*. Payot, Paris.
3. Tellenbach H. (1968) *Geschmack und Atmosphäre*. Müller, Salzburg.
4. Rümke H.C. (1958) Die klinische Differenzierung innerhalb der Gruppe der Schizophrenien. *Nervenarzt*, **29**: 40–53.
5. Wyrsch J. (1946) Über die Intuition bei der Erkennung des Schizophrenen. *Schweiz Med. Wochenschr.*, **46**: 1173–1176.
6. Müller-Suur H. (1958) Das sogenannte Praecoxgefühl. *Fortschr. Neurol. Psychiatrie*, **29**: 145–152.
7. Merleau-Ponty M. (1945) *Phénomenologie de la Perception*. Gallimard, Paris.
8. van den Berg J.H. (1982) On hallucinating: critical-historical overview and guidelines for further study. In *Phenomenology and Psychiatry* (Eds A.J.J. de Koning, F.A. Jenner), pp. 97–110. Academic Press, London.
9. Steffens G.L., Graham G. (1994) Voices and selves. In *Philosophical Perspectives on Psychiatric Diagnosis and Classification* (Eds J. Sadler, O.P. Wiggins, M. Schwartz), pp. 178–192. Johns Hopkins University Press, Baltimore.
10. Jaspers K. (1965) *Allgemeine Psychopathologie*. Springer, Berlin.

1.6
Heterogeneity vs. Homogeneity in Operationally-diagnosed Schizophrenia

John L. Waddington[1] and Paul J. Scully[1]

It is surely correct to conclude that schizophrenia, even when diagnosed according to contemporary, operationalized criteria (DSM-III-R/IV; ICD-10), is a disorder characterized by diversity in phenomenology and long-term outcome, and that no known biological or psychological index is pathognomonic of the disease. However, the affirmation that schizophrenia is therefore a heterogeneous group of disorders requires further consideration in relation to the available data and how they should be analysed to address directly this fundamental issue [1]. For example, the proposition that a certain proportion of patients with the disorder evidence a given abnormality while a lesser proportion of controls do so, is not informative. More specifically, to say that $X\%$ of patients evidence a given abnormality in comparison with only $Y\%$ of controls $(X > Y)$ cannot be interpreted fully when the presence or absence of that abnormality is defined using some arbitrary value along the continuous or categorical scale used in the measure thereof; such an arbitrary definition of abnormality inherently dichotomizes patients (and controls) into two (or more) groups independent of whether the underlying distribution of the measured variable actually indicates the presence of such (sub)groups.

Consider the "core", most widely replicated and accepted biological finding in the brains of individuals with schizophrenia, namely ventricular enlargement [1]. There is now a substantial body of evidence to contradict the (widely held) assertion that such enlargement is present in some but not all patients with the disease; on the contrary, ventricular size in patients with schizophrenia is distributed unimodally in a manner similar to that of normal individuals, the difference being that in patients the mean of this distribution is shifted significantly to the right (greater ventricular size) [2, 3].

Several conclusions follow from these analyses [1]: (a) ventricular enlargement appears to be a population phenomenon in essentially *all* patients with schizophrenia; (b) overlap between the distributions of ventricular size in patients and controls, with only a proportion of patients having ventricular size outside of the control range or 2 SDs above the control mean, affirm that this measure has limited diagnostic utility, but should not be misinterpreted as indicating any subgroup(s) or heterogeneity, for which there is no evidence; (c) for *each* patient, even those having "small" ventricles well within the control range, ventricular size appears greater than would have

[1]*Department of Clinical Pharmacology, Royal College of Surgeons in Ireland, 23 St Stephen's Green, Dublin 2, Ireland*

been the case had schizophrenia not emerged in that person. Whether this generic increase in ventricular size does or does not progress over the course of chronic illness has been a contentious issue [1]; a recent prospective study [4] has indicated progression therein, with the distribution of enlargement not deviating from unimodality in a manner consistent with a homogeneous process. Similarly, neuronal size in layer III of the prefrontal cortex in schizophrenia evidences a unimodal distributional shift in mean to the left (reduced neuronal size) relative to controls [5]; though a large number of neurons were examined in only a limited number of cases, the data indicate a homogeneous effect.

This analytical approach has been applied to other aspects of schizophrenia in comparison with control populations, within a developmental model of the disorder [1], as follows: reduced premorbid IQ in the late teens [6], reduced educational test score in childhood [7], increased craniofacial dysmorphogenesis over the first half of pregnancy [8]. When each of these diverse experimental findings along a lifetime trajectory of disease [1] is analysed in this manner, the data appear to be characterized consistently by a unimodal distributional shift in mean value among patients, and thus a homogeneous process, at each time-point and for each level of enquiry.

In summary, while this and alternative analytical approaches need be applied to additional levels of enquiry at a wider range of time-points along this dynamic, lifetime trajectory [1], the evidence to date suggests that when schizophrenia is diagnosed in accordance with contemporary, operationalized criteria, diversity in a range of biological and psychosocial measures may reflect normal variation within an unexpectedly homogeneous process. The extent to which these notions might generalize to other operationally-defined disorders, particularly schizophrenia spectrum conditions, other non-affective and affective psychoses and bipolar illness, is unknown.

ACKNOWLEDGEMENT

The authors' studies are supported by the Stanley Foundation.

REFERENCES

1. Waddington J.L., Lanc A., Scully P.J., Larkin C., O'Callaghan E. (1998) Neurodevelopmental and neuroprogressive features in schizophrenia: antithetical or complementary over a lifetime trajectory of disease? *Psychiatr. Clin. N. Am.*, **21**: 123–149.
2. Harvey I., McGuffin P., Williams M., Toone B.K. (1990) The ventricle–brain ratio (VBR) in functional psychoses: an admixture analysis. *Psychiatry Res. (Neuroimaging)*, **35**: 61–69.

3. Daniel D.G., Goldberg T.E., Gibbons R.D., Weinberger D.R. (1991) Lack of a bimodal distribution of ventricular size in schizophrenia: a Gaussian mixture analysis of 1056 cases and controls. *Biol. Psychiatry*, **30**: 887–903.
4. Davis K.L., Buchsbaum M.S., Shihabuddin L., Cohen J.S., Metzger M., Frecska E., Keefe R.S., Powchik P. (1998) Ventricular enlargement in poor-outcome schizophrenia. *Biol. Psychiatry*, **43**: 783–793.
5. Rajkowska G., Selemon L.D., Goldman-Rakic P.C. (1998) Neuronal and glial somal size in the prefrontal cortex: a postmortem morphometric study of schizophrenia and Huntington disease. *Arch. Gen. Psychiatry*, **55**: 215–224.
6. David A.S., Malmberg A., Brandt L., Allebeck P., Lewis G. (1997) IQ and risk for schizophrenia: a population-based cohort study. *Psychol. Med.*, **27**: 1311–1323.
7. Jones P.B., Rodgers B., Murray R.M., Marmot M. (1994) Child developmental risk factors for adult schizophrenia in the British 1946 birth cohort. *Lancet*, **344**: 1398–1402.
8. Lane A., Kinsella A., Murphy P., Byrne M., Keenan J., Colgan K., Cassidy B., Sheppard N., Horgan R., Waddington J.L. *et al* (1997) The anthropometric assessment of dysmorphic features in schizophrenia as an index of its developmental origins. *Psychol. Med.*, **27**: 1155–1164.

1.7
Diagnosis of Schizophrenia: Arguments for a Narrowing of the Concept

Peter Berner[1]

The explicit criteria for schizophrenia provided by the DSM-IV and the ICD-10 certainly allow us to establish the diagnosis more reliably, but they have apparently not increased its prognostic and aetiopathogenetic validity. This failure can be attributed to the fact — especially stressed by Maj [1] with regard to DSM-IV — that both consensus classifications lack an underlying paradigm. They combine elements of the diagnostic proposals of Kraepelin, Bleuler, and Schneider, but without taking into account the different concepts from which they were derived. Thus, the DSM-IV and ICD-10 symptomatological criteria for schizophrenia incorporate not only some fundamental and first rank symptoms but also some features belonging to either Bleuler's accessory or Schneider's second rank symptoms. Since the consensus classifications consider all these phenomena only as characteristic, they add, referring to Kraepelin, a chronological criterion in order to counterbalance their lack of specificity. The arbitrary definition of the required continuity raises, however, doubts about the usefulness of this strategy: the persistence of symptoms over a certain time may increase the probability of a chronic course but does not predict it.

The fact that the consensus definitions of schizophrenia establish a heterogeneous group of disorders calls into question the maintenance of

[1] *14, Rue Mayet, Paris, France*

this category. A more promising strategy would be to restrict the diagnosis to the presence of features which can be linked to a concept of their genesis. In this regard Bleuler's approach may still serve as a guideline.

Bleuler presumed that schizophrenic disorders were caused by a particular basic dysfunction, which may have different aetiologies. He assumed that nearly all clinically seizable schizophrenic symptoms are secondary elaborations, but that some of them are particularly linked with the basic dysfunction and occur in no other conditions. He considered therefore these "fundamental symptoms" decisive for the diagnosis and opposed them to "accessory symptoms", also supposed to appear on the basis of other disturbances.

A revival of Bleuler's concept should focus on the identification of features which may be linked with a high probability to a particular basic dysfunction. This selection must start with the elimination of symptoms the unspecificity of which has already become obvious.

Janzarik [2] has convincingly shown that first-rank symptoms, as well as some of the features considered by Bleuler as fundamental—such as ambivalence, depersonalization and derealization—emerge on the basis of rapid alterations of the mood–drive state. Janzarik's observation that this "dynamic instability" may occur in abnormal conditions of various origins raises doubts as to the specificity of these phenomena. This is supported by many studies demonstrating that they can be observed in organic, affective and neurotic disorders, as well as in character disturbances [3–7].

Several studies suggest that formal thought disorders as well as affective blunting occur in schizophrenia and sometimes in organic diseases, but not in affective or psychogenetic disorders [8–10]. This led to the conclusion that the diagnosis of schizophrenia should be based on these features. This proposal has been contradicted with regard to formal thought disorders in view of the claim that these phenomena can also be observed in mood disorders [11, 12]. The validity of this argument must, however, be relativized: recent neuropsychological research indicates that in schizophrenics a disinhibition of the associative network deviates the thinking toward removed or unrelated thoughts, whereas manic flight of ideas only speeds up the access to nearby associations [13]. If the distinction between these two different associative processes is not clearly evaluated—which is often difficult—a manic acceleration of association can erroneously be qualified as derailment. Negative thought disorders can apparently not be distinguished from similar phenomena occurring in depression. They can, therefore, only be used as a diagnostic criterion for schizophrenia in the absence of a depressive mood. If clearly seizable positive thought disorders are combined with affective states, allowing the diagnosis of a mood disorder, the condition can be classified as schizoaffective disorder. This diagnosis becomes in this perspective more restrictive and allows the assumption that such narrowly defined schizoaffective states rely on the coincidence of two different vulnerabilities.

The diagnostic value of the components of the "negative factor" can also be called into question because they may be the result of different basic disturbances; their occurrence in schizophrenia has been hypothetically attributed to the same primary deficiency which causes formal thought disorders [14]. But if negative symptoms are not combined with disorganized thought their diagnostic validity must remain on the level of probability.

The review of the various features proposed up to now for the diagnosis of schizophrenia suggests that formal thought disorders should be considered as the most pertinent ones. In this perspective we have developed the Vienna research criteria for schizophrenic psychoses, on the basis of follow-up studies of paranoic patients [15]. These criteria, called "endogenomorphic-schizophrenic axial syndrome" exclude Schneider's first rank symptoms as well as Bleuler's accessory symptoms and some of his fundamental symptoms, because they are deemed to be expressions of a dynamic instability devoid of any specificity. Thus, only formal thought disorders and affective blunting were included. If the latter is not accompanied by thought disorders the diagnosis is only qualified as probable. The application of these criteria in genetic and follow-up studies demonstrates that they have a highly significant predictive value for the occurrence of schizophrenic disorders among first-degree relatives as well as for a chronic illness course.

Basing the diagnosis of schizophrenia on the presence of thought blocking and derailments, muddled speech and kryptic neologisms has two disadvantages. The first concerns the fact that the required formal thought disorders may often not be present for long periods. Second, the attribution to schizophrenia may also be missed in patients presenting permanently solely negative symptoms or only very discrete thought disorders. But are these risks not much less important than the danger of labelling subjects as schizophrenics whose disorder may be based on very heterogeneous origins? In this perspective it seems preferable to attribute patients not manifesting clearly seizable thought disorders to categories referring only to the surface symptomatology. Such patients can then, for instance, be given the diagnosis of a "paranoid" or "paranoid-hallucinatory syndrome" or a "deficit syndrome". This narrowing of the diagnosis of schizophrenia may not only be beneficial for research, but may also preserve the patient and his relatives from developing the pessimistic expectations with regard to their prognosis, which are commonly linked with the term schizophrenia in public opinion [16, 17].

REFERENCES

1. Maj M. (1998) Critique of the DSM-IV operational criteria for schizophrenia. *Br. J. Psychiatry*, **172**: 458–460.
2. Janzarik W. (1988) *Strukturdynamische Grundlagen der Psychiatrie*. Enke, Stuttgart.

3. Mentzos Z. (1967) *Mischzustände und Mischbildhafte Phasische Psychosen*. Enke, Stuttgart.
4. Carlson G.A., Goodwin F.K. (1973) The stage of mania. A longitudinal analysis of the manic episode. *Arch. Gen. Psychiatry*, **28**: 221–222.
5. Nunn C.M.H. (1979) Mixed affective states and natural history of manic-depressive psychosis. *Br. J. Psychiatry*, **134**: 153–160.
6. Mellor C.S. (1982) The present status of first rank symptoms. *Br. J. Psychiatry*, **140**: 423–424.
7. Crichton P. (1996) First rank symptoms or rank-and-file symptoms? *Br. J. Psychiatry*, **169**: 537–540.
8. Abrams R., Taylor M.A. (1978) A rating scale for emotional blunting. *Am. J. Psychiatry*, **135**: 226–229.
9. Taylor M.A., Abrams R. (1978) The prevalence of schizophrenia. A reassessment using modern criteria. *Am. J. Psychiatry*, **135**: 945–948.
10. Berner P. (1981) The demarcation between schizophrenia and cyclothymia. *Encephal. Arch. Neurol. Psychiatry*, **18**: 147–159.
11. Andreasen N.C. (1979) Thought language and communication disorders. *Arch. Gen. Psychiatry*, **36**: 1315–1330.
12. Spitzer M.A. (1997) A cognitive neuroscience view of schizophrenic thought disorder. *Schizophr. Bull.*, **23**: 29–50.
13. Davis K.L., Kahu R.S., Ko G., Davidson M. (1991) Dopamine in schizophrenia. A review and reconceptualization. *Am. J. Psychiatry*, **148**: 1474–1486.
14. Berner P. (1967) Der Lebensabend der paranoiker. *Wien Z. Nervenheilkunde*, **27**: 176–184.
15. Schanda H., Berner P., Gabriel E., Kronberger M.L. Küfferle B. (1983) The genetics of delusional psychoses. *Schizophr. Bull.*, **9**: 563–570.
16. Schanda H., Thau K., Küfferle K., Kieffer W., Berner P. (1984) Heterogeneity of delusional syndromes: diagnostic criteria and course prognosis. *Psychopathology*, **17**: 280–289.
17. Berner P., Gabriel E., Kronberger M.L. Küfferle B., Schanda H., Trappl R. (1984) Course and outcome of delusional psychoses. *Psychopathology*, **17**: 28–36.

1.8
Schizophrenia: A Provisional Diagnostic Convention

Gisela Gross[1] and Gerd Huber[1]

Due to the lack of pathognomonic somatic findings, every diagnostic concept of schizophrenia can only be a provisional convention. If, for example, first rank symptoms (FRS) are present and a brain disease is excluded, "we speak in all modesty of schizophrenia" [1]. Here, to assert "right" or "wrong" diagnoses is not justified. We can only state that the disorder may be called schizophrenia according to the criteria, for example, of Kraepelin, Bleuler, Schneider, Leonhard, ICD-10 or DSM-IV. The crucial question is not whether

[1] *Department of Psychiatry, University of Bonn, D-53105 Bonn (Venusberg), Germany*

the state *is* schizophrenia, but "does it fit with what I am accustomed to call schizophrenia" [1]? The frequency of FRS depends on the duration of observation. In the long courses, FRS occur in 79% of cases, in the first 6 months after onset in 52% [2]. The most frequent among FRS and second rank symptoms (SRS) are delusional ideas (86%) and auditory hallucinations (75%), followed by schizophrenic ego-experiences (51%), delusional perception (42%), and bodily (39%), visual (33%), olfactory (13%) and gustatory (11%) hallucinations [2]. In 21% of cases the diagnosis has to rely merely on SRS and expression symptoms [2]. Of the latter, formal thought disorders have — because of their infrequency (e.g. blocking 22%) and little specificity — less diagnostic value, except incoherence (54%). Catatonic initial syndromes (4.7%) occur more rarely than in the past [2]. In the whole course, catatonic hyper- and hypophenomena are found in 55% of cases. Also disturbances of affect and initiative and the negative symptoms (NS) affective flattening, avolition, alogia and anhedonia, occurring in a variety of disorders, are of little diagnostic value, even if blunted and inappropriate affect are differentiated from "feeling of unfeelingness", present mainly in endogenous depressions [1], but also in pure residues of schizophrenia [2, 3]. "Anhedonia" is a much too all-inclusive term. Cognitive deficits in neuropsychological tests must be distinguished from cognitive thought disorders, a frequent (75%) basic symptom (BS) in basic stages, partly correlated with cognitive deficits [2, 4]. The BS's diminution of emotional responsiveness, drive, initiative and thought intentionality [3] are the subjective pendants of the NS affective flattening, avolition and alogia.

As to the "prodromal or residual symptoms" (PRS), essential empirical data of the BS research [5, 6] are neglected in DSM-IV and ICD-10. As the pure residues [7], prodromes and outpost syndromes [8], preceding the first psychotic episode 3.3 or 10 years respectively [2], are determined by BS, which are, unlike NS and the PRS of DSM, experiential and not behavioural in kind, typically only recognizable by the self-reports of the patients, who have no lack of insight and are able to develop coping strategies [3, 5, 6]. The BS are rateable by the Bonn Scale for the Assessment of BS [3] and can be differentiated in non-characteristic level-1 and rather characteristic level-2-BS; out of distinct level-2 cognitive thought, perception and action BS, distinct FRS develop, as has been shown in the first prospective early recognition study in schizophrenia [9, 10], the transition rows study [11] and earlier inquiries [5, 6, 12]. Early treatment including the prodromes improves the long-term prognosis [2, 13]. BS, positive symptoms (PS) and NS must be differentiated and develop in this chronological sequence: first BS, followed only years later by PS and finally NS [3, 5, 9, 10].

The data regarding the outcome depend on the diagnostic concept. The results of the European long-term studies, using Schneiderian and/or Bleulerian criteria, represent — according to Zubin — a revolution in the knowledge of schizophrenia [13]. Besides 22% with complete remissions, 40% of the cases remit with mainly slight "pure residues", determined by BS as the prodromal stages; 56% are fully employed, even if only 38% at the premorbid level [2]. The long-term studies have also shown the huge heterogeneity of outcome, with social remission ranging in the 12 course types from 100% to 2% [2, 14]. The prognostically favourable factors of the Bonn study, for example, acute onset, depressive syndromes, psychoreactive precipitation, normal primary personality, are identical to criteria used to classify schizoaffective or cycloid psychoses [6, 14]. As to the subtypes, the cenaesthetic schizophrenia [15, 16] became by its very long (7 years in average) prodromes a prototype for the early recognition research. This type is still today less known, as is the case with the "pure defect" (7), corresponding partly to Crow's type II, that is, correlated with ventricular enlargement, but determined by BS and not by NS [2, 5, 17]. We found in schizophrenics an enlargement of lateral and, preferentially, third ventricles, associated with the "pure defect" and partly progressing parallel to the psychopathological deficit [7, 12, 17]. The first episode of schizophrenia begins before age 20 in females in 18% of cases and in males in 32% of cases, while late-onset schizophrenia is seen in females in 22.4% of cases and in males in 10.6% of cases [2].

REFERENCES

1. Schneider K. (1992) *Klinische Psychopathologie*, 14th edn. Thieme, Stuttgart.
2. Huber G., Gross G., Schüttler R. (1979) *Schizophrenie. Eine verlaufs- und sozialpsychiatrische Langzeitstudie*. Springer, Berlin.
3. Gross G., Huber G., Klosterkötter J., Linz M. (1987) *BSABS. Bonn Scale for the Assessment of Basic Symptoms*. Springer, Berlin.
4. Hasse-Sander I., Gross G., Huber G., Peters S., Schüttler R. (1982) Testpsychologische Untersuchungen in Basisstadien und reinen Residual-zuständen schizophrener Erkrankungen. *Arch. Psychiat. Nervenkr.*, **231**: 235–249.
5. Süllwold L., Huber G. (1986) *Schizophrene Basisstörungen*. Springer, Berlin.
6. Huber G. (1999) *Psychiatrie*, 6th edn. Schattauer, Stuttgart.
7. Huber G. (1966) Reine Defektsyndrome und Basisstadien endogener Psychosen. *Fortschr. Neurol. Psychiatrie*, **34**: 409–426.
8. Gross G. (1969) Prodrome und Vorpostensyndrome schizophrener Erkrankungen. In *Zyklothymie und Schizophrenie* (Ed. G. Huber), pp. 177–187. Thieme, Stuttgart.
9. Gross G., Huber G., Klosterkötter J. (1992) Early diagnosis of schizophrenia. *Neurol. Psychiatry Brain Res.*, **1**: 17–22.
10. Gross G., Huber G. (1998) Prodromes and primary prevention of schizophrenic psychoses. *Neurol. Psychiatry Brain Res.*, **6**: 51–58.
11. Klosterkötter J. (1988) *Basissymptome und Endphänomene der Schizophrenie*. Springer, Berlin.
12. Huber G. (1957) *Pneumencephalographische und psychopathologische Bilder bei endogenen Psychosen*. Springer, Berlin.
13. Gross G., Huber G. (1995) Psychopathology and biological-psychiatric research. *Neurol. Psychiatry Brain Res.*, **3**: 161–165.

14. Gross G., Huber G. (1986) Classification and prognosis of schizophrenic disorders in light of the Bonn follow-up studies. *Psychopathology*, **19**: 50–59.
15. Huber G. (1957) Die coenästhetische Schizophrenie. *Fortschr. Neurol. Psychiatrie*, **25**: 491–520.
16. Huber G. (1992) "Cenesthetic schizophrenia" — a subtype of schizophrenic disease. *Neurol. Psychiatry Brain Res.*, **1**: 54–60.
17. Gross G., Huber G., Schüttler R. (1982) Computerized tomography studies on schizophrenic diseases. *Arch. Psychiatr. Nervenkr.*, **231**: 519–526.

1.9
Diagnosing Schizophrenia: A Personal View

Assen Jablensky[1]

In reviewing the "state-of-the-art" of diagnosing schizophrenia, one hundred years after the concept of dementia praecox became established, we cannot escape addressing the question *what is the entity that we wish to diagnose?* Is schizophrenia a disease, a syndrome arising as a "final common pathway" for a variety of pathological processes, or a loose collection of poorly interrelated symptoms and syndromes of multiple underlying causes, held together by nosographic convention or lack of a better alternative?

By lumping together hebephrenia, catatonic insanity and dementia paranoides into "one illness process", Kraepelin initiated a project for world psychiatry that remains unfinished: to validate schizophrenia as a disease entity by emulating the great nineteenth-century medical and neuropathological precedents, best illustrated by general paresis. The process of discovery was to proceed in stages: clinical (grouping the variable symptoms on the basis of a common outcome and thus describing a provisional disease entity that could be delineated from other entities); epidemiological (mapping its incidence and distribution across populations and cultures); and laboratory (describing its neuropathology, pathophysiology and neuropsychology, ultimately narrowing down the search for causes). As it were by default, this design is still providing a conceptual framework for schizophrenia research, in spite of recurring doubts on the validity of its assumptions. Kraepelin was among the first to realize the flaws, and to anticipate the critique, of the disease entity theory, when he wrote, late in his life, that "our formulation of the problem may be incorrect ... the affective and schizophrenic forms of mental disorder do not represent the expression of particular pathological processes, but rather indicate the areas of our personality in which these processes unfold"[1]. Yet we continue to rely almost exclusively on

[1]*Department of Psychiatry, University of Western Australia, 50 Murray Street, Perth, WA 6000, Australia*

symptoms and history in diagnosing schizophrenia, thereby inferring an underlying pathological process.

What is the value of symptoms in defining schizophrenia and in leading us to where its causes might be? Much of the current research into the causes of schizophrenia is predicated on a genetic paradigm, while the clinical diagnosis is predicated on its symptoms. However, neither the symptoms, nor the course of schizophrenia (including age at onset) appear to be under tight genetic control. A telling example is provided by the Genain monozygotic quadruplets, concordant for schizophrenia [2]. Although sharing a virtually identical genome, the four sisters display very different clinical types of illnesses and outcomes. The high heritability of the phenotype of schizophrenia (defined by symptoms) does not necessarily imply a simple direct pathway from genes to symptoms and behaviour. Complex intermediary mechanisms and feedback loops are likely to be involved, and the search for endophenotypes is a strategy of rising importance [3]. Promising leads include abnormalities in the P50 event-related potential, the control of antisaccadic eye movements and sustained attention, all present in the majority of patients, in a high proportion of their asymptomatic relatives, and in a low proportion of controls drawn from the general population. While the functional relationship of such endophenotypes to the clinical symptoms remains yet to be understood, their genetic basis may be simpler to dissect than that of schizophrenia. Other, novel candidate markers and phenotypes are likely to emerge from functional brain imaging and neurochemistry. It is this kind of empirical systematic research, abreast with advances in basic neuroscience, that will eventually bring us to a state of knowledge from which attempts to define the nature of schizophrenia will be more than speculation. Until then, efforts to reduce schizophrenia to linear causal models are likely to be defeated by the complexity of the disorder and the persisting gaps in fundamental knowledge about the organization of brain functioning.

This suggests a medium-term research agenda that involves a two-track approach. On one track, clinical description should be further refined using comprehensive, semi-standardized phenomenological interviewing schedules such as the Schedules for Clinical Assessment in Neuropsychiatry (SCAN) [4] rather than rating scales as short cuts. Alternative typologies, like Leonhard's system of subtyping the disorder [5] are probably worth exploring more systematically. On the other track, the search and testing of endophenotypes and the exploration of their associations with segments of the schizophrenic syndrome, as well as with candidate genes and regions, must transcend the conventional diagnostic boundaries and extend into neighbouring territories (affective and personality disorders) and general population samples.

Up to this point I deliberately avoided any mention of the current diagnostic criteria of ICD-10 and DSM-IV. They are, beyond doubt, extremely useful for several different purposes, but research into the aetiology of schizophrenia need not be subordinated to their dictate. Their role has been aptly described as "gatekeeping" [6]. It is important to reiterate that such criteria do not *define* schizophrenia but rather provide a common frame of reference enabling clinicians and researchers to index their diagnostic formulations for retrieval and comparisons.

REFERENCES

1. Kraepelin E. (1920) Die Erscheinungsformen des Irreseins. *Zeit. Gesam. Neurol. Psychiatrie*, **62**: 1–29.
2. Rosenthal D. (1963) *The Genain Quadruplets*. Basic Books, New York.
3. Wickham H., Murray R.M. (1997) Can biological markers identify endophenotypes predisposing to schizophrenia? *Int. Rev. Psychiatry*, **9**: 355–364.
4. Wing J.K., Sartorius N., Üstün T.B. (1998) *Diagnostic and Clinical Measurement in Psychiatry. A Reference Manual for SCAN*. Cambridge University Press, Cambridge.
5. Leonhard K. (1995) *Aufteilung der Endogenen Psychosen und ihre Differenzierte Ätiologie*. 7 Auflage. Thieme, Stuttgart.
6. Andreasen N.C. (1998) Understanding schizophrenia: a silent spring? *Am. J. Psychiatry*, **155**: 1657–1659.

1.10

Comments on the Diagnosis of the Schizophrenic Syndrome

Aksel Bertelsen[1]

The introduction of a non-aetiological criteria-based diagnostic classification in ICD-10 and DSM-III/IV has represented a major advantage in psychiatric research and clinical psychiatry. This applies particularly to the schizophrenic syndrome, which previously was diagnosed in widely different ways in various countries even within the frame of ICD-8 and ICD-9 [1]. The diagnostic approach based upon operationally defined criteria ensures a high reliability of the schizophrenic syndrome in schizophrenia, schizoaffective disorder, DSM-IV schizophreniform disorder and ICD-10 acute schizophrenia-like psychotic disorder. Reliability, however, does not guarantee validity, but all the same is an indispensable prerequisite for obtaining a diagnosis of useful validity. How does it help to have a definition of schizophrenia of high validity, if other psychiatrists are unable to reproduce the diagnosis because of lack of explicit criteria, which could be operationalized? Previously, "autism" or "schizophrenie-gefühl" have been

[1]*Aarhus Psychiatric Hospital, DK-8240 Risskov, Denmark*

suggested as nuclear phenomena for the schizophrenia diagnosis, but both have so far resisted attempts to be operationalized in order to be used as diagnostic criteria, probably because of the inherent subjective component on the part of the observer with poor inter-observer reliability.

The Schneider's first-rank symptoms have proved to be particularly useful because they are purely descriptive and operationalizable, and they are therefore applied in both the ICD-10 and DSM-III/IV criteria, although with different emphasis. Schneider claimed that the first-rank symptoms were highly characteristic for schizophrenia, but not pathognomonic, because they also appear in psychotic disorders with organic aetiology, which therefore has to be excluded. It has been stated that first-rank symptoms appear quite frequently in affective disorders [2]. This probably has been caused by inappropriate understanding of the proper definitions of these symptoms, which have to be assessed very carefully following the explicit description by Schneider to avoid false-positive assessments [3]. The first-rank symptoms of hallucinatory commenting and discussing voices thus have to be in the third person, assessed by two or three cited examples of their verbatim content. Subjective disorders of thoughts and control are not only delusions, but also and foremost experiences of thought insertion, withdrawal or broadcasting, or of foreign control of actions, feelings or will. But to avoid false-positive assessments, Schneider required explanatory delusions to accompany the experiences to ensure their presence [4]. The same applies to passivity or influence phenomena, which are combinations of somatic hallucinations and explanatory delusions, which both have to be present. This is, however, not made sufficiently explicit in the ICD-10 and DSM criteria for schizophrenia and the schizophrenia-related disorders, but has been taken into consideration in the Present State Examination included in the Schedules for Clinical Assessment in Neuropsychiatry (SCAN) Version 2.1, for diagnostic assessment according to both ICD-10 and DSM-IV [5].

Unfortunately, the ICD-10 and DSM-IV criteria differ, particularly for schizoaffective disorders. ICD-10 and DSM-IV both require concurrent affective and schizophrenic syndromes. DSM-IV further requires at least 2 weeks with delusions and hallucinations in the absence of prominent mood symptoms. In contrast to ICD-10, DSM-IV allows schizophrenia-characteristic symptoms to appear during mood disorders. The ICD-10 definition of schizoaffective disorder, therefore, is much broader, including many cases of DSM-IV mood disorders with psychotic symptoms. The "new" diagnosis, "schizoaffective disorder", introduced with ICD-10 and DSM-III-R/IV, therefore, is in particular need of validation to see which of the concepts is the more valid. External validation by genetic research as the most promising has so far pointed to a strong genetic aetiological factor with morbid risk figures higher than for mood disorders or schizophrenia, but with no indication of a separate independent disorder. A combination of mood disorder and schizophrenia genes seems the most probable explanation, with secondary cases of mood disorder and to a lesser degree schizophrenia among the first-degree relatives, and only a minor risk of schizoaffective disorder [6].

For schizophrenia, the genetic aetiological factors are well demonstrated. That "schizophrenia is a disorder of unknown aetiology" is correct only in the sense that the aetiology and pathogenesis is not completely clarified and fully demonstrated. We do indeed know much about aetiology with dominating genetic factors in a multifactorial aetiological model, which also has been clearly demonstrated for DSM and ICD-10 schizophrenia [7]. Identification of one or more of the schizophrenia genes is, however, still awaiting the results from intensive research in molecular genetics. This would allow elucidation of the pathogenetic development of the schizophrenic syndrome, establishing schizophrenia as a truly nosological entity or, probably, entities, a group of schizophrenias as Bleuler suggested when he introduced the term.

REFERENCES

1. Cooper J.E., Kendell R.E., Gurland B.J., Skarpe L., Copeland J.R.M., Simon R. (1972) *Psychiatric Diagnosis in New York and London.* Oxford University Press, London.
2. Carpenter W.T., Strauss J.S., Muleh S. (1973) Are there pathognomonic symptoms in schizophrenia? *Arch. Gen. Psychiatry*, **131**: 682–687.
3. World Health Organization (1973) *The International Pilot Study of Schizophrenia*, Ch. 11. World Health Organization, Geneva.
4. Schneider K. (1967) *Klinischer Psychopathologie. Achte, ergänzte Auflage.* Thieme Verlag, Stuttgart.
5. World Health Organization (1999) *Schedules for Clinical Assessment in Neuropsychiatry*. Version 2.1. Cambridge University Press, Cambridge.
6. Bertelsen A., Gottesman I.I. (1995) Schizoaffective psychoses. Genetical clues to classification. *Am. J. Med. Genet.*, **60**: 7–11.
7. Gottesman I.I. (1991) *Schizophrenia Genesis. The origins of Madness.* Freemann, New York.

1.11
The Schizophrenic Syndrome: A Warning and a Conjecture
John E. Cooper[1]

This commentary is limited to two topics: first, how best to avoid some drawbacks of "diagnostic criteria", and second, a conjecture that some of

[1]*Meadow Cottage, 25 Ireton Grove, Attenborough, Nottingham NG9 6BJ, UK*

the effects of the schizophrenic syndrome can be usefully interpreted at the conceptual level of a reduction of some of the ordinary social rituals of everyday life.

ICD-10 and DSM-IV share two problems in the way that they present the necessary names and criteria by which the subject matter of this review is identified. They both use the term "schizophrenia" as if one illness is being described, and they both give a list of symptoms under the title of "diagnostic criteria". But experienced psychiatrists know that even Bleuler described "the group of schizophrenias", and they know that the heading "diagnostic criteria" should be replaced by "criteria for identifying the disorder", since there are no implications about underlying processes or knowledge of causes.

Until these defects are put right in future versions of the classifications, psychiatric teachers and researchers should take care to make it clear that to identify a disorder is not the same as making a diagnosis. Reference should always be to "the schizophrenic syndrome" or the "schizophrenic disorder", and the single misleading term "schizophrenia" should be avoided.

One of the most persistent impressions I have formed about patients with long-standing schizophrenic syndromes can be interpreted as a remarkable indifference to their immediate environment, both social and physical. This is an interpretation, since when asked about the points noted below, the patients themselves seem to be unaware of any problem, and have no specific complaints. This indifference shows as an apparent unawareness of minor discomforts in their immediate physical environment, but it is the indifference to the immediate social environment that I should like to examine, that is, their indifference to other persons. This is manifest as a lack of the normal social rituals, such as greetings, farewells and the general niceties of trivial but polite conversation.

To have a diminished ability to engage in the social rituals of everyday life can be a very serious problem; "friendship exists through ritual" is a well-known maxim in some schools of social anthropology. Most social roles cannot be performed satisfactorily in any society without accompanying social rituals, such as greetings, thanks and farewells. These exchanges allow a person to establish and re-affirm an identity and a position in the social group; this in turn facilitates performance of work or family duties.

The successful performance of a social ritual requires the brain and mind to be functioning at the very highest levels. It requires the awareness, monitoring and coordination of internal emotional and motor states, and the perception of and responses to similar states in the other person concerned. A variety of complicated motor and sensory processes are involved, such as the recognition of facial expressions, the appreciation of subtle variations of tone of voice, the performance of gestures, and the adoption of appropriate postures.

All animals have a repertoire of social rituals, by which they express both their own individual identity and the identity of their species. We are being most typically human when these social rituals are performed, and it would not be surprising if the performance of these very human activities requires that part of the brain that is most typically human — in other words, the prefrontal cortex. A comment by Andreasen [1] implies this, although without direct mention of the concept of social rituals, "the negative symptoms of schizophrenia may represent a loss of functions that are generally thought to reside in the frontal lobes".

There are some studies on patients with schizophrenic syndromes that can be regarded as underpinning this suggestion. Their authors do not mention the concept of social rituals directly, but often come very close. For instance, Brown [2] reports marked loss of politeness in persons with schizophrenic syndromes, and Davison *et al* [3] conclude that "schizophrenics showed a generalised decrease in all facial behaviours measured". The efforts of Frith, Done and others [4] to establish "a neuropsychology of schizophrenia" are also relevant, in that a theme of "faulty self-monitoring" runs through the conclusions of several of their studies.

The point of this conjecture is that, if even partially correct, it has implications for social treatments of some of the things lost (or perhaps never present) in persons with long-standing schizophrenic syndromes. Social skills training, as carried out in many centres at present, often includes some aspects of what we are here calling social rituals, but, without doing a systematic survey, my impression is that this is usually an incidental part rather than a main focus. Perhaps what is needed is a purposeful and concentrated programme that first assesses whatever social rituals are appropriate for the individual in question, and then tries to instil or regain any that are missing. Since social rituals are heavily dependent upon culture, there are all kinds of interesting opportunities to compare and contrast across different cultures both the states of ritual defect, and attempts to find remedies.

REFERENCES

1. Andreasen N. (1989) Neural mechanisms of negative symptoms. *Br. J. Psychiatry*, **155** (Suppl. 7), 93–98.
2. Brown R. (1996) Politeness in schizophrenia. In *Psychopathology: Evolving a Science of Mental Disorder* (Eds S. Matthysse, F. Benes, D. Levy, J. Kagan), pp. 336–351. Cambridge University Press, Cambridge.
3. Davison P.S., Frith C.D., Harrison-Read P.E., Johnstone E.C. (1996) Facial and other non-verbal communicative behaviour in chronic schizophrenia. *Psychol. Med.*, **26**: 707–713.
4. Frith C.D., Done D.J. (1989) Experiences of alien control in schizophrenia reflect a disorder in the central monitoring of action. *Psychol. Med.*, **19**: 359–363.

1.12
A Century of Schizophrenia is Enough
Jane Kelly[1] and Robin M. Murray[1]

As Charles Pull's comprehensive review indicates, after a hundred years of investigation, schizophrenia remains a chronically unsatisfactory disease. Even as he outlines the supposed strengths of the concept, Prof. Pull reminds us that there are no pathognomonic symptoms of schizophrenia and that those individuals who receive the diagnosis have very different characteristics and widely varying outcome. Although Prof. Pull indicates that the use of standardized interviews and operational definitions enables trained clinicians to make the diagnosis reliably, there now exists a "Tower of Babel" of different operational definitions, some of which, such as the DSM criteria, are modified with confusing regularity. Consequently, the number of individuals diagnosed as schizophrenic varies by a factor of three depending on which definition is used [1]. The borders of some definitions are quite arbitrary; for example, according to ICD-10, if an illness lasts for 29 days, it is not schizophrenia, if it lasts for 32 days then it is schizophrenia. Most importantly, there is no sharp boundary between the phenomena of schizophrenia and manic-depressive psychosis; indeed, so many patients fall between the two psychotic categories, that an intermediate form, the so-called schizoaffective psychosis, had to be invented.

It has become increasingly clear that there is overlap in genetic predisposition to schizophrenia and affective psychosis [2–4]. Pull also notes that abnormalities in biological markers such as eye tracking and event-related potentials are found in other psychotic conditions. Furthermore, the meta-analysis of Elkis et al [5] has shown that lateral ventricular enlargement, the most consistent abnormality in those diagnosed as schizophrenic, is also found in affective psychosis. The fact that neither genetic predisposition nor biological abnormalities are specific for schizophrenia undermines the Kraepelinian concept of schizophrenia as a discrete disease entity.

In our view, therefore, 100 years of schizophrenia is enough. But what should we replace it with? Murray et al [6] pointed to the evidence that a number of developmental risk factors have been established for early-onset psychosis. These include obstetric complications and late winter/spring birth [7], as well as psychomotor and speech delay, inability to play and poorer cognitive performance [8]. Other patients, conventionally diagnosed as schizophrenic, have no developmental risk factors, often have symptoms of, or relatives with, affective disorder, and many become ill following social adversity. Murray et al [6] sought to divide the traditional category of schizophrenia into neurodevelopmental (or congenital) and adult-onset

[1] Institute of Psychiatry, Maudsley Hospital, De Crespigny Park, Denmark Hill, London SE5 8AF, UK

cases; the latter had much in common with affective psychosis. This proposal deliberately harks back to views which were commonplace 100 years ago [9], but were displaced by the stultifying disease concept of dementia praecox/schizophrenia.

The existence of a neurodevelopmental form of psychosis received further support from latent class analyses [10, 11], and from a twin study [12]. However, the neurodevelopmental adult-onset distinction has similar/difficulty to the Kraepelinian system in dealing with cases on the borders between the categories; that is, some psychotic patients appear to have both neurodevelopmental impairment and socially reactive/affective characteristics. Furthermore, it has become clear that neurodevelopmental risk factors are not specific to schizophrenia. Thus, obstetric complications [7], childhood impairments [13] and cerebral ventricle enlargement [5] are also risk factors for affective psychosis, although the effect size is not so great as for schizophrenia.

A more plausible "dimensional" version of this idea is that there exists a spectrum of psychosis which is under the influence of two major aetiological effects. The first, "neurodevelopmental impairment", operates across psychosis but has maximal effect in chronic cases with an early onset and poor outcome. Such cases tend to be male and have a history of obstetric complications or of a family member with a similar illness; they are likely to have shown poor childhood function and to have structural brain abnormalities. The second effect arises when "social adversity" acts on genetic predisposition to affective psychosis to produce an acute psychosis. The effect of this factor is maximal at the acute onset—good outcome pole of psychosis; such cases tend to have good premorbid function and to be female, and generally show less evidence of structural brain abnormality. Thus, at the extreme poles of a continuum of psychosis, neurodevelopmental and social/affective aetiologies predominate respectively; however, in many of the intervening cases, both aetiological factors are operating.

Might a classification based on such dimensional concepts have more biological validity than the Kraepelinian system? A number of factor analytical studies of the symptoms shown by psychotic patients have produced three psychotic dimensions or syndromes (positive, negative, and disorganization) and two affective syndromes (mania and depression). Sham *et al* [14] showed that the positive and negative syndromes had pronounced, but different, developmental antecedents, while mania and depression did not; disorganization appeared to be a hybrid, being predicted by the combination of low IQ and a family history of mania.

One of the main purposes of classification is to predict outcome. How would a dimensional classification system work in this regard? Van Os *et al* [15], who studied the clinical characteristics of some 700 chronic psychotic patients, found that a four-dimensional model (positive, negative, manic and depressive dimensions) best fitted the data. They then compared the ability of dimensional and categorical representations of the patients' psychopathology to predict outcome; the dimensional approach had greater predictive power than conventional diagnostic categories.

In summary, we agree with Charles Pull that neither symptoms nor biological markers are specific to schizophrenia. While Pull looks to a day when more specific markers for schizophrenia will validate the concept and facilitate its diagnosis, we consider that this is an illusion. We are more impressed by the evidence that not only biological markers but also risk factors for psychosis operate across diagnostic categories. Indeed, not only are dimensions more closely related to risk factors than categories, but dimensions are also more useful in predicting outcome of psychosis. In short, psychotic patients should be distinguished by differences of degree rather than of kind, as a function of overlapping dimensions of psychopathology [16]. Professor Pull's article is a valiant eulogy for a concept which should be buried with the twentieth century.

REFERENCES

1. Castle D., Wessely S., Der G., Murray R.M. (1991) The incidence of operationally defined schizophrenia in Camberwell, 1965 to 1984. *Br. J. Psychiatry*, **159**: 790–794.
2. Taylor M. (1992) Are schizophrenia and affective disorder related? A selective literature review. *Am. J. Psychiatry*, **149**: 22–32.
3. Kendler K., McGuire M., Gruenberg A., O'Hare A., Spellman M., Walsh D. (1993) The Roscommon family study. 1. Methods, diagnosis of probands, and risk of schizophrenia in relatives. *Arch. Gen. Psychiatry*, **50**: 527–540.
4. Cardno A.G., Marshall E.J., Coid B., Macdonald A.M., Ribchester T.R., Davies N.J., Venturi P., Jones L.A., Lewis S.W., Sham P.C. *et al* (1999) Heritability estimates for psychotic disorders: the Maudsley Twin Psychosis Series. *Arch. Gen. Psychiatry*, **56**: 162–168.
5. Elkis H., Friedman L., Wise A., Meltzer H. (1995) Meta-analyses of studies of ventricular enlargement and cortical sulcal prominence in mood disorders. *Arch. Gen. Psychiatry*, **52**: 735–746.
6. Murray R.M., O'Callaghan E., Castle D.J., Lewis S.W. (1992) A neurodevelopmental approach to the classification of schizophrenia. *Schizophr. Bull.*, **18**: 319–332.
7. Hultman C., Sparen P., Takei N., Murray R., Cnattingus S. (1999) Prenatal and perinatal risk factors for schizophrenia, affective psychosis, and reactive psychosis of early onset: case-control study. *Br. Med. J.*, **318**: 421–426.
8. Jones P., Rodgers B., Murray R., Marmot M. (1994) Child developmental risk factors for adult schizophrenia in the British 1946 birth cohort. *Lancet*, **344**: 1398–1402.
9. Clouston T.S. (1891) *The Neuroses of Development*. Oliver and Boyd, Edinburgh.
10. Castle D.J., Sham P.C., Wessely S., Murray R.M. (1994) The subtyping of schizophrenia in men and women: a latent class analysis. *Psychol. Med.*, **24**: 41–51.
11. Sham P.C., Castle D.J., Wessely S., Farmer A.E., Murray R.M. (1998) Further exploration of a latent class typology of schizophrenia. *Schizophr. Res.*, **20**: 105–115.

12. Corrigall R.J., Murray R.M. (1994) Twin concordance for congenital and adult onset psychosis: the validity of a novel classification of schizophrenia. *Acta Psychiatr. Scand.*, **89**: 142–145.
13. Van Os J., Jones P., Lewis, G., Murray R. (1997) Developmental precursors of affective illness in a general population birth cohort. *Arch. Gen. Psychiatry*, **54**: 625–632.
14. Sham P., Guerra A., Jones P., Lewis S., Mata I., Murray R. (1999) Do premorbid risk factors have a pathoplastic effect on the clinical symptom profile in psychosis? Submitted for publication.
15. Van Os J., Gilvarry C., van Horn E., Tattan T., White I., Murray R.M. on behalf of the UK 700 Group (1999) A comparison of the utility of dimensional and categorical representations of psychosis. *Psychol. Med.*, **29**: 595–606.
16. Van Os J., Jones P., Sham P., Bebbington P., Murray R.M. (1998) Risk factors for onset and persistence of psychosis. *Soc. Psychiatry Psychiatr. Epidemiol.*, **33**: 596–605.

1.13
Diagnosis of Schizophrenia: A View from Developing Countries

Narendra N. Wig[1]

This commentary deals with the question of diagnosis of schizophrenia in the context of developing countries of Asia and Africa, where incidentally more than half of the world's population lives. It is only recently that scientifically reliable observations are becoming available from these countries, which at times significantly differ from those made in Western countries. Before we consider data regarding the diagnosis of schizophrenia from developing countries, it may be pertinent to list some of the important differences that exist in the psychiatric setting of developing countries as compared to developed countries:

- Mental hospital beds are relatively few in developing countries. As a result, most of the psychiatric patients are seen in general hospitals or in outpatient clinics. Thus, while in Europe or the USA psychiatric observations have been made largely on long-stay schizophrenic patients admitted to mental hospitals, in developing countries these observations have been made mostly in general hospitals and in outpatient settings.
- Social setting in developing countries is also significantly different from Western countries. In a recent comparative follow-up study of schizophrenic patients in Liverpool (England) and Bangalore (India) it was found that while over 98.3% of schizophrenic patients in Bangalore lived with their families, this was the case for only 48.6% of patients with schizophrenia in Liverpool [1].

[1] *Postgraduate Institute of Medical Education and Research, Chandigarh, India*

Though it is well recognized now that schizophrenia occurs in all cultures, it is important to note that significant differences exist in symptomatology in developing countries as compared to the industrially developed countries:

- Catatonic symptoms which have become rare in Western countries are still commonly seen in Asian and African countries. Both auditory and visual hallucinations are more commonly seen in developing countries.
- Schneider's first-rank symptoms of schizophrenia are seen less frequently in developing countries as compared to the developed countries. This is particularly true for symptoms representing subjectively experienced thought disorder, for example, thought insertion or thought broadcast or primary delusions [2].

In Prof. Pull's review, in the section on course and outcome, there are two areas where the findings from developing countries are significantly different from those from developed countries and should be taken note of. Firstly, in developing countries psychiatrists see a large number of cases of acute psychosis which resemble schizophrenia but have a shorter course and good recovery. Secondly, judged by any criteria, outcome of schizophrenia, in general, is better in developing countries as compared to developed ones.

In the Collaborative Study on Determinants of Outcome of Severe Mental Disorders (DOSMD), the largest diagnostic subtype of schizophrenia in developing countries was acute schizophrenic episode (as per ICD-9) and it constituted 40.3% of the total cases from these countries. In developed countries this subtype represented only 10.9% of cases [2]. With the current available information in the literature it is difficult to say whether acute transient psychosis as frequently seen in developing countries is a distinct disorder or a valid subgroup of schizophrenia. Cooper et al [3], while reviewing the diagnostic data from the multinational World Health Organization (WHO) study on acute psychosis, found that typical schizophrenic symptoms were present in nearly half the cases of acute psychotic states from various centres.

In the final summary of his review, Prof. Pull concludes that outcome of schizophrenia is "usually poor". The evidence from developing countries does not support this conclusion. In fact, the outcome has usually been reported favourable in the majority of cases, with complete or partial remission. The difference between developing and developed countries in terms of outcome is well documented now in the WHO International Pilot Study on Schizophrenia (IPSS) and DOSMD studies with a follow-up of 2 to 5 years. These findings have also been confirmed by a number of independent studies. That this finding is not dependent on the duration of illness or acuteness of onset is confirmed by the study of Kulhara and Chandiramani [4], in which more than one diagnostic criterion was used for outcome. With the available evidence from developing countries, it seems that chronicity of schizophrenia may partly be culturally determined. Hence, it may not be justified to assume chronicity as an essential criterion for the diagnosis of schizophrenia.

REFERENCES

1. Sharma V., Srinivasa Murthy R., Kishore Kumar K.V.R., Agarwal M., Wilkinson G. (1998) Comparison of patients with schizophrenia from Liverpool, England and Sakalwara-Bangalore, India. *Int. J. Soc. Psychiatry*, **44**: 225–230.
2. Jablensky A., Sartorius N., Ernberg G., Anker M., Korten A., Cooper J.E., Day R., Bertelsen A. (1992) Schizophrenia: manifestations, incidence and course in different cultures. A World Health Organization study. *Psychol. Med.*, (Suppl. 20).
3. Cooper J.E., Jablensky A., Sartorius N. (1990) WHO collaborative study on acute psychosis using the SCAAPS schedule. In *Psychiatry: A World Perspective*, Vol. 1 (Eds C.N. Stefanis, A.D. Rabavilas, C.R. Soldatos), pp. 185–192. Elsevier, Amsterdam.
4. Kulhara P., Chandiramani K. (1988) Outcome of schizophrenia in India using various diagnostic systems. *Schizophr. Res.*, **1**: 339–349.

1.14
Studies on Schizophrenic Symptomatology in Peru
Alberto Perales[1]

There is nothing new under the sun. Once more, Prof. Pull reveals, in his thorough review, that psychiatrists of past decades exhaustively described the clinical manifestations of schizophrenia. They had to develop semiologic abilities to describe their clinical observations, and time has proven that they were privileged to develop those skills. Unfortunately, today, the stress of psychiatric training on semiology has considerably diminished in medical schools and postgraduate courses and, as a result, clinical skills of new specialists have been negatively affected. The exact recognition of symptoms, on which diagnostic process is scientifically grounded, is nowadays superficially treated. Thus, a sound semiologic training is a compulsory precondition for exact symptom recognition. Not only will this prevent diagnostic confusion in the recognition of the different manifestations of the disorder, but it will also be essential for clinical therapeutic decisions and for avoiding misleading paths for research.

Although international classification systems aim to harmonize the concept of schizophrenia, we should not forget, until proven wrong, that schizophrenia seems to be not a single entity but a group of disorders with a common core syndrome. It is for this reason that students of psychiatry

[1] *Av. Javier Prado oeste 445, Dpto. 101, Lima 27, Peru*

should be taught to use diagnostic criteria of present classifications not as absolute and indisputable truths, but as points of reference to correctly identify the disorder, always remembering that the concept of schizophrenia is still based on conventions.

Due to the short space available, I will only mention some of the contributions made by Peruvian psychiatry in clinical research on schizophrenia. For many decades, several observations of outstanding Peruvian psychiatrists [1–5] established almost a dictum: among Peruvian schizophrenic patients, those native to the highlands would show a less florid clinical picture and a more frequent depressive symptomatology in comparison to those native to the coast (born at sea level). A research study was carried out [6] to test this hypothesis. Schizophrenics (diagnosed by DSM-III criteria) from the coast were those who grew up and lived in cities located between 0 and 500 m above sea level, during their first 16 years at least, while the highlanders were those who grew up and lived in cities located at 1800 m above sea level during their first 16 years at least. Then, two groups of patients, one from the coast (mean age 26.7 years) and one from the highlands (mean age 30.8 years), consisting of 20 males and 10 females each, were compared. The Brief Psychiatric Rating Scale and the Hamilton Depression Scale were used. The Mann–Whitney statistical test was applied. The data showed no significant differences between the groups. In another study carried out in Peru, Ponce [7] applied a phenomenological and statistical approach to evaluate the delusional content of 100 paranoid schizophrenics. He found 66 types of delusional themes. Comparing Ponce's results with those published by Andreasen and Black [8], we noticed that the three most frequent types of delusions were those of persecution (81%), reference (49%) and mind reading (48%) in the latter sample, and those of reference (65%), persecution (59%) and harm (34%) in the former. Delusions of harm involved the patient's conviction that someone had affected his health by using either witchcraft or sorcery. Delgado [9] pointed out that although the mechanisms of the delusional symptom are related to the specific schizophrenic brain disorder (pathogenic factor), the content is strongly influenced by culture (pathoplastic factor).

REFERENCES

1. Valdizán H. (1915) La alienación mental entre los primitivos peruanos. Tesis Doctoral. Universidad Nacional Mayor de San Marcos, Lima.
2. Gutiérrez Noriega C. (1937) Observaciones Biotipológicas y Psicopatológicas en los enfermos mentales Peruanos con referencia a factores raciales y geográficos. *Actualidad Médica Peruana*, 2: 408–431.
3. Gutiérrez Noriega C. (1937) Biotipologia del Perú Antiguo. *Actualidad Médica Peruana*, 2: 118–130.

4. Gutiérrez Noriega C. (1937) Diseño de un estudio Psicológico y Antropológico de la Raza Amerindia. *Actualidad Médica Peruana*, **3**: 159–195.
5. Gutiérrez Noriega C. (1944–1947) Las enfermedades mentales en la raza india. *Revista Peruanidad*, **5**: 1674–1679.
6. Perales A. (1986) Estudio sintomatológico comparativo entre esquizofrénicos oriundos de la Costa y de la Sierra del Perú. Tesis de Bachiller. Universidad Nacional Mayor de San Marcos, Lima.
7. Ponce M. (1961) El contenido delusional en la esquizofrenia paranoide (Estudio estadístico y fenomenológico). Tesis de Bachiller No. 5320. Universidad Nacional Mayor de San Marcos, Lima.
8. Andreasen N.C., Black D.W. (1995) *Introductory Textbook of Psychiatry*. American Psychiatric Association Press, Washington, DC.
9. Delgado H. (1955) *Curso de Psiquiatría*, 2nd edn. Imprenta Santa María, Lima.

1.15
Neuropsychological and Psychophysiological Contributions to the Diagnosis of Schizophrenia

Allan F. Mirsky[1] and Connie C. Duncan[2]

Although impaired attention in schizophrenia was described more than a hundred years ago by Kraepelin (cited by Hoch [1]), it was not assessed systematically until the 1930s and 1940s, with reaction time paradigms (summarized in [2]). Following publication of the Continuous Performance Test (CPT) of sustained attention as a test of brain damage [3], investigators employed it to study schizophrenia. Stammeyer [4] reported that many patients could perform the test as well as controls; however, when the CPT was accompanied by distraction, patients' performance deteriorated significantly. Little change occurred in the controls' performance. This was the first demonstration of the principle that increased attentional demands in patients could reveal a deficit that might otherwise escape detection. This finding was confirmed by Wohlberg and Kornetsky [5] in a study of remitted patients, and by a number of other investigators cited by Pull. Currently, researchers make the CPT more demanding by degrading the task stimuli [6, 7].

The attentional deficits in schizophrenia vary according to task stimulus modality. Patients and their relatives perform worse on an auditory than a visual CPT [6]. Possible explanations include compromise of structures in the auditory brain stem and/or left temporal lobe [7].

[1]*Section on Clinical and Experimental Neuropsychology, Laboratory of Brain and Cognition, National Institute of Mental Health, 15 North Drive, Bethesda, MD 20982-2668, USA*

[2]*Clinical Psychophysiology and Pharmacology Laboratory, Department of Psychiatry, Uniformed Services University of the Health Sciences, 4301 Jones Bridge Road, Bethesda, MD 20814, USA*

Thus, the impairment shown on the CPT, proposed initially as a test of brain damage, emphasizes the role of brain dysfunction in schizophrenia. Moreover, the similarity of the deficits on the CPT in patients with schizophrenia and with idiopathic generalized seizures (including greater difficulty with auditory than visual tasks), suggest a shared pathophysiology in the two disorders [8–10].

Pull's review emphasizes the sensitivity of sustained attention tests, such as the CPT, as markers of vulnerability to schizophrenia. However, such sensitivity is also seen in other tests of attention. In a study in Ireland, tests assessing the capacity to focus and to shift attention were also found to show impairment in the patients and in their relatives [6]. In the Israeli High-Risk Study, children at genetic risk for schizophrenia showed impairment at ages 11 and 17 on a number of tests measuring aspects of attention [11, 12]. Moreover, poor performance on a cancellation task at ages 11 and 17 (especially under conditions of distraction) predicted which children at risk would develop a schizophrenia spectrum disorder at age 25 [11].

Differences between auditory and visual processing are also reflected in the P300 component of the event-related brain potentials. Patients show substantial reductions in the amplitude of P300 elicited by auditory stimuli as well as a less reliable reduction in the visual P300. Moreover, there is some evidence that visual but not auditory P300 increases in proportion to favourable response to medication [13]. These data, as well as the neuropsychological findings, support the view of the greater vulnerability of auditory than visual information processing in schizophrenia.

In conclusion, vulnerable persons may be identified by a number of different attentional capacities, including sustained attention, focused attention and the ability to shift attentional focus. Moreover, sensitivity is increased by using more demanding attention tasks, as well as those employing stimuli in the auditory modality. Although the basis of these findings is not well understood, they suggest that brain systems involved in the regulation of attention are compromised in persons with schizophrenia and their relatives.

REFERENCES

1. Hoch A. (1896) Kraepelin on psychological experimentation in psychiatry. *Am. J. Insanity*, **52**: 387–396.
2. Shakow D. (1979) *Adaptation in Schizophrenia: The Theory of Segmental Set*. John Wiley, New York.
3. Rosvold H.E., Mirsky A.F., Sarason I., Bransome E.D. Jr., Beck L.H. (1956) A continuous performance test of brain damage. *J. Consult. Psychol.*, **20**: 343–350.
4. Stammeyer E.C. (1961) The effects of distraction on performance in schizophrenic, psychoneurotic, and normal individuals. Unpublished doctoral dissertation. Catholic University, Washington, DC.

5. Wohlberg G.W., Kornetsky C. (1973) Sustained attention in remitted schizophrenics. *Arch. Gen. Psychiatry*, **28**: 533–537.
6. Mirsky A.F., Yardley S.J., Jones B.P., Walsh D., Kendler K.S. (1995) Analysis of the attention deficit in schizophrenia — a study of patients and their relatives in Ireland. *Psychiatry Res.*, **29**: 23–42.
7. Mirsky A.F. (1996) Familial factors in the impairment of attention in schizophrenia: Data from Ireland, Israel and the district of Columbia. In *Psychopathology — The Emerging Science of Mental Disorder* (Eds S. Matthysse, D.F. Benes, D. Levy, J. Kagan), pp. 364–406. Cambridge University Press, Cambridge.
8. Mirsky A.F., Anthony B.J., Duncan C.C., Ahearn M.B., Kellam S.G. (1991) Analysis of the elements of attention: a neuropsychological approach. *Neuropsychol. Rev.*, **2**: 109–145.
9. Mirsky A.F., Duncan C.C. (1986) Etiology and expression of schizophrenia: neurobiological and psychosocial factors. *Ann. Rev. Psychol.*, **37**: 291–319.
10. Duncan C.C. (1988) Application of event-related brain potentials to the analysis of interictal attention in absence epilepsy. In *Elements of Petit Mal Epilepsy* (Eds M.S. Myslobodsky, A.F. Mirsky), pp. 341–364. Lang, New York.
11. Mirsky A.F., Ingraham L.J., Kugelmass S. (1995) Neuropsychological assessment of attention and its pathology in the Israeli cohort. *Schizophr. Bull.*, **21**: 193–204.
12. Mirsky A.F., Silberman E.K. (Eds) (1985) The Israeli high-risk study. *Schizophr. Bull.*, **11**: 19–154.
13. Duncan C.C. (1990) Current issues in the application of P300 to research on schizophrenia. In *Schizophrenia: Concepts, Vulnerability, and Intervention* (Eds E.R. Straube, K. Hahlweg), pp. 117–134. Springer, New York.

2

Pharmacological Treatment of Schizophrenia: A Review

W. Wolfgang Fleischhacker

Department of Psychiatry, Innsbruck University Clinics, Innsbruck, Austria

INTRODUCTION

Ever since antipsychotic drug treatment was introduced into clinical psychiatry almost half a century ago, establishing a breakthrough in the management of schizophrenic disorders, this new therapeutic area is characterized by a continuing attempt to optimize the results of treatment efforts for these patients. A plethora of medications, called neuroleptics in classical terminology, a term that is increasingly replaced by the indication driven word antipsychotics, has been synthesized and tested to this end. Molecules of different chemical structures, ranging from tricyclic phenothiazines to thioxanthenes, butyrophenones, dibenzoxazepines, substituted benzamides and benzisoxazole derivatives are used in the treatment of schizophrenia today. The development of clozapine was clearly a quantum leap in these efforts. This drug, available in some European countries since the early 1970s and introduced in the USA in the 1990s, was the first antipsychotic that effectively treated the symptoms of schizophrenia with only a minimal risk to induce extrapyramidal motor side effects (EPS) [1, 2]. Next to changing the mindset concerning clinical efficacy and adverse drug effects, the success of clozapine has also strikingly influenced preclinical development strategies for new antipsychotics. By and large this was fuelled by the recognition that clozapine has excellent antipsychotic efficacy without blocking nigrostriatal dopamine (D_2) receptors at a similar extent as classical neuroleptics [3]. Up to this point, powerful D_2-blockade was seen as a prerequisite for an antipsychotic effect. Eventually, clozapine's differing pharmacologic profile had as a consequence that a number of new points are now considered in the preclinical screening of putative antipsychotic drugs. These include dopamine blockade in extrastriatal, mesofrontal and mesolimbic dopaminergic pathways, which have been studied using

Schizophrenia, Second Edition. Edited by Mario Maj and Norman Sartorius.
© 2002 John Wiley & Sons Ltd.

a host of different procedures, ranging from single neuron action potential recordings [4] to the expression of neuropeptides [5] and immediate early genes [6]. Phases I and II in clinical psychopharmacology have also experienced a methodological boost, including modern neuroimaging techniques such as positron emission tomography (PET) and single photon emission computed tomography (SPECT), which have been shown helpful to characterize the action of new drugs both qualitatively and quantitatively [7–11]. These strategies are complemented by experiments evaluating non-dopaminergic systems, such as the serotonergic [12] and the glutamatergic [13] pathways. Thus, clinical psychopharmacology, just as after the introduction of chlorpromazine, has catalysed new research in the neurobiology of schizophrenia.

Clozapine has also helped change the demands on the clinical management of schizophrenia. While there used to be a strong emphasis on positive symptom reduction in the early days of pharmacologic treatment, new therapeutic targets have been identified. Next to treating delusions and hallucinations, the field of negative symptoms and cognitive dysfunction, as well as the dimensions of suicide prevention, quality of life and psychosocial reintegration, are now very much in the foreground of our considerations. Safety research has also become a new major focus.

The following review is restricted to pharmacologic interventions. Clearly, modern concepts of schizophrenia management include psychosocial and rehabilitative measures. Even though pharmacotherapy is still very much the backbone of our treatment efforts, it should always be embedded into integrative treatment procedures, which include all levels of intervention.

In the following we will draw an artificial line between short-term and long-term management, well aware that these cannot always be clearly differentiated. When discussing short-term treatment we focus on symptom control and crisis intervention, while making maintenance of therapeutic effects and relapse prevention main topics in the long-term treatment section, together with aspects of quality of life and psychosocial reintegration.

SHORT-TERM TREATMENT (ACUTE TREATMENT)

Early Intervention Strategies

Following the seminal work of the late Richard Jed Wyatt (14), who was the first to point out, based on his own work and the reports of others, that a long course of untreated symptoms may have a negative impact on the treatability and outcome of schizophrenia patients, efforts to shorten the duration of untreated psychosis (DUP) have skyrocketed. Many centres in the world have established early intervention clinics. As this concept is often misunderstood or presented in different ways, it needs to be clarified that such programmes may have different foci: while some attempt to identify and treat young people while they are still in a prodromal phase of the illness, others have the goal to establish comprehensive treatment plans for young patients that already have a confirmed diagnosis of a first episode of schizophrenia. Clearly, the former interventions are still very much at an experimental stage, and many open questions (type and duration of intervention, "stigmatizing" patients by such interventions, prophylactic effect on developing a true diagnosis of schizophrenia, etc.) remain to be answered. On the other hand, every bit of knowledge that we have about the course and outcome of schizophrenia certainly supports to intervene as early as possible in patients with a confirmed diagnosis. This is independent of the assumption that an ongoing psychotic episode may be neurotoxic. As with every other disease, it is imperative to reduce the suffering of patients and their significant others as effectively and quickly as possible.

Choice of Drug

Before the launch of clozapine, it was generally taken for granted, and backed up by many comparative trials, that the available neuroleptics differed in terms of tolerability but not regarding their efficacy. As a rule of thumb, high potency drugs were associated with a greater risk for extrapyramidal motor side effects, while low potency medications were said to have more autonomic adverse events. The latter have also been said to be more sedative, even though this was never formally studied in clinical trials [15]. These differences in safety profile made the choice of drug mainly side-effect-guided.

Other criteria of choice include the potential for plasma level measurements, which will be discussed in a separate section, as well as the availability of depot preparations. In patients who have been pre-exposed to antipsychotics, it will be advisable to fall back on medication that has shown a beneficial benefit–risk profile during the treatment of previous episodes. It must also be mentioned in this context that the choice of drug is of particular importance when treating patients for the first time, as a dysphoric response to an antipsychotic drug is known to influence the attitude towards further pharmacologic treatments [16]. Especially stressful side effects may lead to a long-lasting negative attitude towards medication, which is unfavourable given the fact that many patients will eventually require long-term treatment.

Clozapine was the first drug for which qualitative and quantitative differences to traditional antipsychotics could be convincingly demonstrated [17–20]. Not only is clozapine more efficacious in patients suffering from treatment-resistant schizophrenia, but it has also been shown to have advantages in terms of the treatment of negative symptoms [17, 21] as well as in various psychosocial domains including quality of life [22] and prevention of suicidal behaviour [23].

The fact that clozapine has good antipsychotic efficacy and a minimal risk to induce extrapyramidal symptoms (EPS) has triggered the term "atypical" neuroleptic. This classification was originally designed to differentiate clozapine from the older, traditional neuroleptics, which have sometimes been referred to as "typical". Unfortunately, neither preclinical nor clinical psychopharmacology offers a succinct definition for "atypicality". As a categorical distinction between "typical" and "atypical" antipsychotic drugs is not possible, some psychopharmacologists have fallen back on a dimensional point of view in which various antipsychotics with more or less "atypical" [24] properties can be found. These properties include a low incidence of EPS, a reduced tendency to increase prolactin levels, as well as greater improvements against the negative symptoms of schizophrenia than traditional drugs. This is where clozapine and other new drugs, which will be described in more detail at a later stage, show advantages over traditional neuroleptics. As the term "atypical antipsychotic" does not describe a homogeneous group of medications, it is really of very limited use. Antipsychotics that show more or less similarities to clozapine should more correctly be classified as antipsychotics of the second generation [25].

Since clozapine cannot be used as a first-choice drug, given worldwide legal restrictions that arise from the drug's high risk to induce agranulocytosis [26], there was a strong urge to develop antipsychotics without the propensity to induce blood dyscrasias. This led to the development and consequent registration of amisulpride, olanzapine, quetiapine, risperidone, sertindole, ziprasidone and zotepine. Much can be said in favour of the use of these agents as first-line drugs. Merely the fact that they have a significantly lower EPS risk than traditional neuroleptics [27] would be argument enough. One of the disadvantages of many of these novel antipsychotics, however, is the lack of parenteral formulations, including depot preparations. As most of the published data on the novel drugs provide results from pre-registration phase II and III clinical trials performed in a highly selected group of schizophrenic patients, one would be well advised to await more extensive phase IV data and experiences made under routine treatment conditions before giving definitive recommendations for the use of these drugs [25]. Lastly, pharmacoeconomic aspects need to be acknowledged, as the new drugs are substantially more expensive than their predecessors. However, these high drug costs have been shown to be counterbalanced by a reduction in overall treatment costs, through lower relapse rates and less subsequent rehospitalizations, as has been shown in various long-term studies [28].

In conclusion, it appears to be justified to recommend novel antipsychotics as first-line treatment especially in patients with first manifestations of schizophrenic disorders. It is still unclear whether these new drugs will eventually replace the traditional antipsychotics which at this time and date still play an important role, especially in the treatment of multi-episode patients who have shown a good response to these drugs and have tolerated them well in the past.

Dose, Plasma Level and Route of Administration in Acute Treatment

Ever since neuroleptics were introduced into clinical practice, dose recommendations have varied up to 100-fold. On the basis of a meta-analysis of studies using traditional drugs, Baldessarini et al [29] state that 100–700 mg of chlorpromazine equivalents per day represent an adequate dose range for most psychotic patients. This was confirmed in various more recent dose finding studies. These showed that doses in excess of 20 mg haloperidol [30, 31] or fluphenazine [32], or 6 mg of risperidone [33] daily do not provide substantial additional therapeutic benefit. The lower end of the dose spectrum is less well defined. While McEvoy et al [34], for instance, reported that most of their patients responded well to a mean of 3.4 mg haloperidol daily, Van Putten et al [31] found improvement in only 6% of their patients treated with less than 5 mg of haloperidol. This discrepancy can at least in part be explained by different patient selections in the respective studies: in the first trial almost half of the patients were either first-episode schizophrenics or patients suffering from schizoaffective disorders, while the second team studied mainly chronically ill schizophrenic patients, who most likely differ from the first group of patients in terms of treatment response.

Various authors have also reported that the incidence of side effects increases with dose [29, 31, 32, 35]. This is especially well documented for EPS, and implies that a potential efficacy advantage of a higher dose may by nullified by reduced tolerability. It has also been substantiated in two independent studies that first-episode patients are especially sensitive to EPS induced by risperidone. In such cases, doses of 1–3 mg/day have been found equally effective and much better tolerated than higher doses (36, 37). Clearly, the dose should be adjusted to the needs of individual patients within a certain frame of reference. Doses will therefore also be dependent on target syndromes, meaning that higher doses will be used in more agitated patients, while lower doses are given to patients with prevailingly negative symptoms, although these recommendations come from a clinical empirical background rather than from controlled trials.

For clozapine there is a distinct discrepancy between the United States and Europe. The doses used in clinical trials as well as in everyday practice in many centres of the US are about double the 200–300 mg daily that represent the mean dose in many European countries [35]. The reasons for this are not entirely clear. A possible explanation is that clozapine is used more restrictively in the US and is therefore mainly given to patients who are more severely ill. These differences in dose are of high clinical relevance, as at least some of the side effects of clozapine, such as seizures or confusion, are dose- and plasma-level dependent [35, 38]. It seems strange that more than 20 years after the registration of clozapine we still lack a sound dose finding study.

Some antipsychotics can also be administered parenterally. In principle, this route of administration should be confined to emergency situations, where lack of insight or acute psychopathology lead to a high risk of harming oneself or others. Next to that, parenteral application may be necessary in the select patients whose well-documented pharmacokinetic problems render reaching adequate drug plasma levels on oral medication difficult.

There are no well-documented plasma level/efficacy correlation studies for most of the traditional antipsychotics, with the exception of fluphenazine and haloperidol. A haloperidol plasma level of around 15 ng/ml has been described as optimal by various independent groups [39–41]. Research also suggests that no additional therapeutic benefit is to be expected at fluphenazine plasma levels beyond 1.5–2 ng/ml [42].

Judging effective clozapine plasma levels is much more difficult and has to be seen in the light of the dosing discrepancies discussed above. Consequently US authors recommend considerably higher plasma levels [43, 44] than those that have been documented in successfully treated European patients [45, 46]. It must be noted, though, that American data stem from prospectively designed plasma level response studies, while European authors have reported clozapine plasma concentrations derived from naturalistic study designs. In the most recent American report, VanderZwaag et al [47] suggest that optimal plasma levels range between 200 and 250 ng/ml and submit that quite a few patients have also responded well to levels below this range. These numbers come closer to those found by European groups. VanderZwaag et al [47] also stress that the time of venipuncture and the distribution of clozapine doses over the day have a considerable impact on clozapine plasma levels. Giving the full daily dose in the evening before blood for plasma levels is drawn, for instance, results in higher levels than if patients are treated with divided daily doses.

Even though plasma level monitoring of antipsychotics cannot yet be recommended as a routine procedure, it may be of help in certain instances. These include non-response to an adequate antipsychotic dose, the suspicion of compliance problems, the use of pharmacologic combination treatment which may lead to pharmacokinetic interactions, such as combinations between certain antipsychotics and specific serotonin re-uptake inhibitors. Clinically significant elevations of clozapine plasma levels have been found for instance when this drug was combined with fluvoxamine [48]. The possi- bility of monitoring plasma levels should also be entertained in very young or old patients and in such patients that suffer from relevant concomitant medical diseases. Unusual side effects, especially if they occur at low doses, may also justify checking antipsychotic plasma levels.

Duration of Acute Treatment

As there generally is a lot of inter-individual variation in the response to the acute treatment of schizophrenia, the question of when to expect first signs of this response or, alternatively, at which time the response may be judged to be insufficient and a treatment change should be initiated, is commonly asked. Respective recommendations range between 1 and 2 weeks up to half a year. Some answers may be found in reports such as that by Levinson *et al* [49], which documents that patients who ultimately respond to antipsychotic treatment have shown an amelioration of various non-specific symptoms, such as sleep disturbance or anxiety and agitation, but also of positive symptoms within the first two treatment weeks. One may cautiously conclude from such studies that ongoing treatment needs to be re-evaluated if patients show no response whatsoever within the first treatment weeks.

There are some suggestions from clozapine trials that one needs to have more patience in treatment-resistant patients [50, 51]. Treatment trials of up to 3 months have been recommended.

Insufficient Treatment Response

The concept of treatment-resistant schizophrenia is not a homogeneous one. Only the rare patient does not respond at all to psychopharmacologic interventions. Most patients show at least a partial response in one or the other symptom of their disorder. It is not uncommon, for instance, that delusions or hallucinations remit, while negative symptoms remain unchanged. Sometimes, the definition of treatment-resistant schizophrenia also includes patients who do respond to antipsychotic treatment but do not tolerate it due to significant side effects [52].

The definition of treatment-resistant or treatment-refractory schizophrenia usually follows two different lines of thought: one is based on the necessity of reproducible research; the other is built upon the needs of everyday clinical practice.

Research calls for well-defined criteria that allow study of the issue in different research centres and ultimately make a comparison of different studies possible. Next to obtaining an exact drug history, patients in such studies usually undergo at least one prospective antipsychotic treatment trial [17]. Only if the history of the patient and the well-documented results of this treatment attempt yield no adequate response is such a patient classified as treatment resistant.

In routine clinical care, the treating physician usually cannot fall back on all of this sophisticated information. Judgement must often rely on an incomplete history provided either by the patient or his/her significant others and on far from perfect case notes. This information is then amalgamated with the clinical impression that usually regards overall social functioning and quality of life next to psychopathology.

It is not uncommon that the researcher's and the clinician's judgements differ quantitatively. Many patients in whom the clinician is not satisfied with treatment response will not fulfil strict research criteria, while on the other hand patients entering research studies may represent a select population and results provided by the studies of such patients are sometimes difficult to generalize for a more clinical population.

It used to be common practice to switch patients who have not adequately responded to a neuroleptic to another drug of a different chemical class. Similarly, this was recommended for patients who did not tolerate certain medications. Research on this issue has produced controversial findings [52–54]. So far clozapine is the only drug for which this procedure is scientifically justified [17]. Other second generation antipsychotics studied in this indication have led to either dissappointing [55] or difficult to interpret results, due to methodological inadequacies [52]. For more information please refer to the section in which the respective drugs are briefly reviewed.

Taking all the published evidence into account, we recommend the following in the case of inadequate treatment response: if patients have not shown at least partial response to an adequate dose of a traditional antipsychotic after 2 to 3 weeks, compliance and plasma levels should be checked. This may lead to additional supportive psychosocial measures or to an adaptation of dose. If these modifications do not yield relevant results within the next 2 to 3 weeks, switching to a second-generation drug or clozapine is indicated. This recommendation is based on solid evidence considering clozapine. On the other hand, it is clinically prudent to try one of the newer antipsychotics first, although the evidence that these have advantages over traditional neuroleptics in such instances is indirect at best, in order to avoid the necessity of white blood count monitoring obligatory with clozapine treatment. Patients who are switched to one of the novel agents should be evaluated for treatment response within the 4–6 weeks; in the case of clozapine treatment, a new treatment trial should last at least 2–3 months. If response remains unsatisfactory, various options should be considered. These include concomitant administration of lithium [56–58] or carbamazepine [59], as well as, alternatively, the use of benzodiazepines [60], specific serotonin re-uptake inhibitors [61–63] or serotonin antagonists [64]. Electroconvulsive therapy also still has its place in these last resort treatment trials [65]. All of these options result from clinical experience rather than from controlled double-blind prospective treatment trials.

Novel antipsychotics are increasingly used as drugs of first choice. What to do if patients do not respond to these agents is still an open question. Increasing the dose, sometimes beyond the levels recommended by the manufacturers, switching to other novel antipsychotics or to traditional neuroleptics, but also combining novel and classical drugs [66], appear to be the most commonly chosen alternatives.

It has to be made very clear that the treatment of patients suffering from treatment-resistant schizophrenia represents a highly complex clinical problem that needs to be taken care of by the experienced and well-trained specialist.

Adverse Effects During the Acute Treatment with Antipsychotics

Table 2.1 gives an overview of antipsychotic-induced adverse events. This table deliberately omits prevalence or incidence rates as, given huge methodologic differences between the available studies, unjustified comparisons of

TABLE 2.1 Adverse effects of antipsychotic drugs

Extrapyramidal	*Antiadrenergic*
acute dystonia	orthostatic hypotension
dyskinesia	ECG alterations
akathisia	→ tachycardia
parkinsonism	→ tachyarrhythmia
tardive dyskinesia	→ depressed ST segments
dystonia	→ flattened U waves
(akathisia)	→ prolonged QT intervals
Anticholinergic	sexual dysfunctions
dry mouth	*Haematologic*
constipation	eosinophilia
blurred vision	leucocytosis
urinary retention	leucopenia
sexual dysfunctions	agranulocytosis
Ophthalmologic	*Dermatologic*
lenticular changes	photosensitivity
pigmentary retinopathy	seborrhoeic dermatitis
Endocrine and metabolic	*Sexual*
increased prolactin	diminished libido
gynaecomastia	orgasmic dysfunctions
galactorrhoea	erectile dysfunction incl. priapism
weight gain	ejaculatory dysfunction
sexual dysfunctions	reduced volume
lipid and glucose metabolism	delayed ejaculation
dysfunctions	
EEG alterations and seizures	*Neuroleptic malignant syndrome*

relative risks may lead to misinterpretation. For the classical drugs, the main focus has traditionally been on EPS [67]. As the novel antipsychotics induce EPS to a significantly lesser extent [27], non-EPS associated side effects have gained interest following their introduction into clinical practice.

Many side effects can successfully be managed by dose reduction or switching from one drug to another [68]. So far specific pharmacologic interventions are only successful against EPS. Even though the efficacy of anticholinergics against acute dystonia or parkinsonism [69] and that of beta-blockers in treating akathisia [70] are impressive, these drugs should be used cautiously. Anticholinergics are potent psychotropic drugs [71] that may lead to memory deficits [72], substance abuse [73], as well as to a worsening of psychotic symptoms [74]. Therefore, the general prophylactic use of anticholinergic drugs is discouraged, a position also fortified by a World Health Organization (WHO) recommendation [75]. The exception to this rule are patients with a high risk for EPS such as young male patients or patients with a history of significant EPS.

Concerning many of the non-EPS associated adverse events, individual tolerance levels have to be discussed with the patients. This follows the general rule that there is increasing emphasis on the subjective attitude of patients and their relatives to pharmacotherapy, as this has been found to be a crucial factor for compliance [76]. Consequently, drug-induced side effects must be an ongoing topic even during the acute treatment phase.

The use of the novel antipsychotics as first-line drugs is an important prophylactic measure to reduce the EPS risk. Next to that, a slow increase of dose and using lower doses altogether prevent some of the acute side effects. Naturally this approach is limited in very acutely, severely ill patients.

LONG-TERM TREATMENT

Next to maintaining the effects of acute treatment and relapse prevention, an improvement in quality of life and psychosocial integration are the goals of long-term treatment of patients suffering from schizophrenic disorders.

There is increasing evidence that the long-term outcome of schizophrenia is correlated to early pharmacological interventions and successful relapse prevention [77–79]. It is one of the best documented and most reproduced results in psychiatric outcome research that the long-term treatment with antipsychotics is the major factor in preventing relapses and recurrences of the disorder [67, 80]. The relapse risk is reduced by about two-thirds if long-term antipsychotic medication is sustained [81]. In order to optimize treatment response, pharmacological measures have to be complemented by psychosocial interventions. As discussed in the introductory section, the latter are not the topic of this review and will be summarized elsewhere.

Even given optimal treatment conditions, about 20% of all schizophrenic patients will experience a relapse despite antipsychotic prophylaxis [82]. On the other hand, another 20% will suffer from a single episode of schizophrenia only, no matter whether they are treated or not [83]. Unfortunately, we have yet no way to predict the outcome of schizophrenia in individual patients. Therefore, all patients suffering from schizophrenia, including those with first episodes, are advised to continue medication on a long-term basis [84–87]. The rare patient with brief psychotic episodes without negative psychosocial consequences may be an exception to this rule as would be a patient with an intolerance to all existing antipsychotics.

Choice of the Antipsychotic

The choice of the antipsychotic will follow similar considerations to those outlined in the acute treatment section. One has to keep is mind that switching from one antipsychotic to another may pose problems, as the efficacy and tolerability of the respective antipsychotics show significant intra-individual variation. It is therefore preferable to plan long-term treatment already when initiating acute treatment, in order not to have to change drugs between treatment phases.

Unfortunately, pharmacoeconomic considerations play an increasing role in the choice of antipsychotics in many countries. As the novel drugs are considerably more expensive than traditional neuroleptics, clinicians and patients are increasingly confronted with restrictive reimbursement policies. This is especially disturbing when taking into account that pharmacoeconomic studies have convincingly shown that higher drug costs are outweighed by savings in other areas of treatment such as reduced rehospitalization and relapse rates [28, 88].

Next to efficacy, tolerability and subjective acceptance of a drug by the patient are important factors in long-term treatment. The benefit–risk profile of an antipsychotic has to be a regular topic in treatment sessions with patients and their significant others.

Duration of Treatment

Two types of studies give direct or indirect information on the length of treatment issue: prospective placebo-controlled long-term trials and discontinuation studies. In the latter, antipsychotics are discontinued under controlled conditions in patients who had been prophylactically treated for varying amounts of time. While prospective studies usually extend over time periods from 1 to 2 years, discontinuation studies often provide information about considerably longer courses of treatment. Both study options unanimously document a high relapse risk without antipsychotic prophylaxis [80, 89].

A 1- to 2-year maintenance treatment is usually recommended for patients suffering from first episodes of schizophrenia. Multi-episode patients should be in remission for at least 5 years until the discontinuation of antipsychotic treatment is discussed [84–87].

The time frames recommended above must be seen in the light of the fact that there are no prospective relapse prevention studies which cover a time period of more than 2 years and that all discontinuation trials have shown high relapse rates, even if patients had been in remission for many years before stopping antipsychotics. Therefore, these recommendations must be considered a minimal standard. Especially in first-episode patients they are also influenced by practical considerations, in so far as it is unrealistic to suggest life-long pharmacologic relapse prevention, even though, when judging the available evidence, this would not appear unreasonable. It is also evident that such recommendations, although commonplace in various chronic somatic diseases, are still met by much irrational criticism when applied to the psychiatrically ill.

In the last decade, five independent research groups have evaluated the effects of so-called intermittent pharmacologic treatment [90–94]. These studies were based on the assumption that it should be possible to educate patients and their significant others about early warning signs of an impending relapse. In such patients, antipsychotics could be stopped after successful acute treatment and reinitiated in the case of impending relapse, detected by the advent of early warning signs. This was hypothesized to lead to a reduced use of antipsychotics, thereby minimizing the risk for long-term side effects such as tardive dyskinesia (TD).

Patients randomized to this type of management showed significantly higher relapse rates than patients on continuous antipsychotic treatment. Even though patients on intermittent treatment received significantly fewer cumulative antipsychotic doses, there were no differences in the incidence of TD between groups. In summarizing the available evidence, it can be concluded that intermittent treatment has not been shown to be a generally practical alternative to the current recommendation of continuous antipsychotic administration, especially when considering a separate study in which an increased TD risk was found in patients with interruptions of neuroleptic treatment [95]. First-episode patients may be an exception to this rule [96].

The strategic goal of the long-term treatment of patients suffering from schizophrenic disorders remains to minimize the risk of a psychotic relapse in order to avoid all its negative biological and psychosocial consequences.

Dose, Plasma Levels and Route of Administration in Long-term Treatment

In general, the same doses of antipsychotic that have been efficacious during the acute and the stabilization phases are also recommended at the beginning of relapse prevention. For most patients these doses range between 5 and 15 mg daily of oral haloperidol or a respective equivalent dose of another antipsychotic [84]. Dose–response relationships of the novel antipsychotics have not yet been sufficiently studied; the few available double-blind, long-term trials [97–99] indicate that the principle of maintaining patients on the dose that had been used in the acute treatment is also helpful with these drugs.

If a dose reduction is indicated, it should not be performed in steps larger than 20% of the previous dose. The intervals between these steps should be between 3 and 6 months, as it is well known that relapses following insufficient neuroleptic doses may appear with a significant time lag [80, 100]. Naturally, it should be attempted to treat patients with a minimal effective dose. In clinical practice this is not always easy and may, while trying to reach this dose, lead to a risk of underdosing and subsequent relapse.

The administration of depot antipsychotics is an important treatment option during long-term management. These injectable preparations produce relatively constant plasma levels of the neuroleptics over a period of several weeks [91]. The disadvantages of this type of treatment include the fact that some patients refuse intramuscular injections or develop pain or irritations at the injection site. Another problem is that the dose of a depot antipsychotic cannot be reduced once administered. Advantages include the facilitation of management through a certainty concerning compliance and the fact that the patients do not need to take medication every day. Various expert groups have therefore promoted the use of depot antipsychotics [84, 101, 102].

If a treatment with these drugs is anticipated, patients should first be treated with the oral form of the antipsychotic, in order to gather information about dose requirements and the benefit–risk profile of the drug. Ideally, patients should be switched from the oral to the depot route after successful stabilization has been achieved. This should be done in an overlapping fashion, as depot medications reach steady state plasma levels only after a certain period of time [103].

Dose finding studies are available for haloperidol and fluphenazine. They are the basis of the following recommendations: 50–200 mg haloperidol decanoate every 4 weeks [104] or 12.5–50 mg fluphenazine decanoate in bi-weekly intervals [101] represent an optimal dose range for many patients.

Adverse Effects of Long-term Treatment with Antipsychotics

Most acute antipsychotic-induced side effects can become chronic. Clearly, clinicians will do the best to avoid this, although in some instances compromises may be necessary, especially when clear benefits of medication outweigh the relevance of certain side effects. As discussed previously, this benefit–risk determination must be an integral component of all treatment strategies.

Some side effects may already be apparent during acute treatment but become relevant only during long-term management. These include sedation, weight gain and sexual dysfunctions [105]. As these adverse events are thought to have a negative impact on compliance, they warrant special consideration.

Tardive dyskinesia is a specific long-term side effect that is relatively common with traditional antipsychotics [106]. The annual cumulative incidence rate is around 5% [107]. Given the increased attention to tardive dyskinesia and the implementation of prophylactic measures, severe and irreversible manifestations have become considerably less frequent. It is important to acknowledge that tardive dyskinesia is not necessarily irreversible. Observations over long time periods have shown that this motor side effect remits spontaneously in about half of the afflicted patients despite continuous antipsychotic treatment [108].

While no well-documented case of clozapine-induced tardive dyskinesia has been published so far, it is important to note that this does not hold true for the other novel compounds. Even if these drugs have a certain risk for tardive dyskinesia, this is still significantly lower than that found with traditional antipsychotics [109, 110].

The management of chronic side effects of antipsychotics, with the exception of tardive dyskinesia, follows the same principles as have been described in the acute treatment section. Treating manifest tardive dyskinesia is still unsatisfactory; prophylactic measures are therefore of utmost importance. Patients have to be examined regularly with regard to incipient tardive dyskinesia. As soon as such symptoms are found, if continuous antipsychotic treatment is considered necessary, an attempt to reduce the dose should be the first step. If tardive dyskinesia progresses despite this, treatment must be changed to clozapine or another compound with a low TD risk. Patients with a shorter duration of TD may also profit from an addition of tocopherol (vitamin E) [111]. As the risk to induce weight gain and disturbances of glucose and lipid metabolism differs significantly between antipsychotics, these complications are discussed below, when the specific drugs are reviewed.

SECOND-GENERATION ANTIPSYCHOTICS

The problem of artificially categorizing all novel antipsychotics as "atypical" has been alluded to earlier in this review. A critical review of these drugs clarifies that they are pharmacologically heterogeneous substances [27]. This most likely results in diverging clinical profiles, although these are not yet fully understood.

New developments are briefly summarized below. As this is currently a very prosperous field of research, the interested reader is referred to the most recent publications in scientific journals. Table 2.2 summarizes receptor affinities and dose recommendations for the novel antipsychotics. As some of the features of clozapine are mentioned elsewhere in the review, they are not discussed in this section.

Amisulpride

Amisulpride is a substituted benzamide and a specific dopamine D2 and D3 antagonist [112–114]. The terminal elimination half-life is approximately 12 hours [115].

In patients with positive symptoms, higher doses (400–800 mg/day) of amisulpride led to reductions in mean Brief Psychiatric Rating Scale (BPRS) scores similar to those achieved with haloperidol [116, 117] or flupenthixol [118]. In studies of patients with predominantly negative symptoms of schizophrenia, 50–300 mg were more effective than placebo [119–122]. EPS induced by amisulpride are dose related and lower than those caused by haloperidol,

TABLE 2.2 Novel antipsychotics

Drug	Receptor profile*	Recommended dose (mg/day)†
Amisulpride	D	300–800 (50–1200)
Clozapine	5HT, D, α, M, H	200–450 (50–900)
Olanzapine	5HT, D, M, α, H	10 (5–20)
Quetiapine	H, 5HT, α, D	150–750
Risperidone	5HT, D, α, H	4–6 (1–16)
Sertindole	5HT, D, α	12–20 (4–24)
Ziprasidone	5HT, D	40–160
Zotepine	5HT, D, α, H, M	100–300 (50–450)

D, Dopamine; α, α-adrenergic; M, muscarinic; H, histamine; 5HT, serotonin.
*Listed in order of descending affinity.
†Doses in general correspond to the recommendations of the manufacturer. Doses listed in parentheses represent extremes sometimes justified in individual patients.

flupenthixol or fluphenazine in comparative trials. Amisulpride induced less tardive dyskinesia than haloperidol in patients with schizophrenia [123].

Amisulpride provoked higher prolactin increases than did haloperidol or flupenthixol [124]. However, no differences were found in the incidence of clinical endocrine adverse events. Amisulpride was associated with lower weight gain than risperidone in a trial comparing the two drugs [125].

Olanzapine

Olanzapine is similar to clozapine both in its chemical structure and in its pharmacologic properties [126]. It has a plasma half-life of about 30 hours [127]; the manufacturer recommends doses between 5 and 20 mg daily. An acute i.m. formulation of olanzapine should soon become available.

Before registration, olanzapine was compared to placebo and haloperidol in clinical trials [128, 129]. It was shown to be superior to placebo [128] and at least equal to haloperidol [128, 129] when treating patients with schizophrenic or schizoaffective disorder. It was more effective than haloperidol in treating depressive [130] and negative symptoms [131] in schizophrenic patients. The problems in interpreting these findings will be discussed at the end of this review.

All therapeutic effects of olanzapine are maintained over longer periods of time as 1-year extension studies against placebo and haloperidol have shown [98, 132]. In a study with similar design as the classic clozapine trial [17], olanzapine was compared to chlorpromazine in patients suffering from treatment-resistant schizophrenia. The drugs did not differ from each other and showed disappointing response rates [55]. In contrast, a more recent study comparing olanzapine to clozapine found both drugs to be comparably effective in treatment resistant patients, with olanzapine showing a tolerability advantage [131].

In all clinical trials and at all dose levels olanzapine induced extrapyramidal symptoms that, with the exception of akathisia, were not higher than those found in patients randomized to placebo [133]. Olanzapine was shown to be associated with a significantly lower tardive dyskinesia risk than haloperidol [109]. As with most other antipsychotics with strong antiserotonergic effects, the treatment with olanzapine leads to a significant weight gain in a considerable number of patients [128, 129, 134]. Disturbances of glucose and lipid metabolism [135, 136], as well as de novo diabetes mellitus type II, have been reported following olanzapine treatment. Whether or not this is linked to the weight gain induced by the drug is as yet unclear. Despite its similarities to clozapine, no indications for any relevant adverse effects to white blood cells have been reported. With the exception of a small sample of young first-episode patients [137], olanzapine has not been reported to induce a sustained increase in prolactin levels.

Quetiapine

While quetiapine also structurally resembles clozapine, its preclinical pharmacology is different, especially with respect to a lack of anticholinergic
effects [138]. It has a short half-life (about three hours) [139]. Dose recommendations range between 150 and 750 mg daily.

In phase II and III studies, quetiapine was found to be superior to placebo
and comparable to haloperidol [140–142] and chlorpromazine [143].

The risk to induce acute EPS was not higher than that of placebo, and
data concerning TD are available from elderly populations which show a
considerably lower risk than one would expect when treating such patients
with traditional neuroleptics. The fact that quetiapine has also been shown
effective in treating L-dopa-induced psychosis in Parkinson's disease patients
without worsening motor functions also speaks [144] to the good EPS
tolerability of this drug. Transient elevations of liver enzymes, dizziness
and orthostatic hypotension, especially in the first days of treatment, have
led to the recommendation of a slow dose increase during the initiation
of treatment. The evidence concerning quetiapine-induced weight gain is
equivocal: while weight gain has been found in short-term studies [145],
other authors [146, 147] have not found this to be a problem in longer term
trials. Quetiapine does not lead to a clinically relevant prolactin increase.

Risperidone

Risperidone is a new molecule. Its elimination half-life has been reported
to be between 3.2 and 24 hours [148]. Recent dose recommendations are
2–6 mg daily. Risperidone has also been tested against placebo [33] and
haloperidol [149]. As with the other drugs, its therapeutic effect was found to
be better than placebo and similar to haloperidol. Risperidone has been found
superior to haloperidol in a relapse prevention study, following patients for
at least 1 year [99]. It has also been shown to be equally efficacious in
treatment resistant schizophrenia patients, although this trial has been much
criticized [52]. The main points of critique were that the sample size may
have been too small, the doses of clozapine too low, and that there was
no differentiation between patients who had not responded to previous
treatments and patients who had not tolerated previous neuroleptics. For
negative symptoms, advantages like those of olanzapine have been found
when comparing the drug to haloperidol [150]. Preliminary results have also
shown positive effects when treating children and adolescents [151, 152],
although this group of patients may have a higher risk to gain weight on
risperidone than adults [153, 154].

Risperidone also has a lesser risk to induce acute EPS than traditional
neuroleptics. In contrast to the other drugs, the EPS risk of risperidone

is dose dependent. Higher doses start to resemble traditional antipsychotics; above 12 mg daily, the EPS rate is similar to that of haloperidol [33, 149]. As amisulpride, risperidone appears to have a higher propensity to increase serum prolactin levels than traditional neuroleptics like haloperidol [155, 156].

As for quetiapine, a slow dose increase is recommended to prevent disturbing sedation and/or hypotension.

Sertindole

Sertindole has the longest half-life of all the novel drugs (close to 3 days) [157]. Doses between 4 and 24 mg daily are used to treat patients with schizophrenia. Pre-registration clinical trials comparing sertindole to placebo [158] and haloperidol [158, 159] have yielded similar results as for the previously mentioned novel antipsychotics. A long-term study found significantly lower rehospitalization rates with sertindole compared to haloperidol [97]. The same holds true for its EPS profile. An unusual side effect reported for sertindole is a reduction of the ejaculatory volume. Next to that, weight gain has been found.

Sertindole leads to a prolongation of the QTC interval in the ECG [158–160]. This effect is not only more common but also more pronounced than with any other of the novel antipsychotics and is still discussed with respect to its clinical relevance. While this book was being printed, the European regulatory agency was re-evaluating the safety profile of this drug.

Ziprasidone

Ziprasidone differs pharmacologically from the previously described drugs by its potent $5-HT_{1A}$ agonistic effect and by the inhibition of serotonin and noradrenaline re-uptake [161, 162]. The half-life is reported to be between 3.2 and 10 hours [161]; the dose range is 80–160 mg daily. Ziprasidone is also available as an acute i.m. formulation. 10–20 mg have been reported to be effective single doses.

These doses were also evaluated in clinical trials in which ziprasidone was compared to placebo [163] and/or haloperidol [163, 164]. Again, positive and negative symptoms (at higher doses) were improved similar to other novel antipsychotics. In a placebo-controlled 1-year trial, in which stable patients were switched to either ziprasidone or placebo, the former had a significantly higher efficacy than placebo to reduce the risk of impending relapse [165]. A recent study available on the FDA website has produced evidence that ziprasidone induces a mean prolongation of the QTc interval of 20.3 msec. This was a larger increase than the one induced by haloperidol, risperidone, olanzapine and quetiapine. Only 2 out of 2988 patients (0.06%)

having received ziprasidone in placebo controlled clinical trials showed QTc intervals above 500 msec. While so far none of the published studies or the post-marketing experiences have revealed increases of cardiac arrhythmias or excess risk for unexplained sudden death following ziprasidone treatment, the clinical consequences of the drugs' propensity to increase QTc interval are still under investigation.

EPS risk is comparable to the other new medications. The most commonly found side effect is sedation. Interestingly, and in contrast to all the drugs discussed above and below, ziprasidone has not been found to induce weight gain.

Zotepine

Zotepine is also structurally related to clozapine [166]. Similar to ziprasidone, it inhibits the re-uptake of noradrenaline with a potency comparable to tricyclic antidepressants [167]. The recommended dose is 50–450 mg daily.

Again, results of clinical trials resemble those found with other novel antipsychotics [168–171]. It was also used successfully in a small study treating patients with prevailingly negative symptoms [172]. When patients with stable symptoms were switched to either placebo or zotepine and followed for 6 months, the risk of relapse was significantly higher in the placebo group [173].

Zotepine has fewer side effects on the extrapyramidal motor system than haloperidol. Dose-dependent adverse effects include sedation, transient elevations of liver enzymes, and seizures.

Methodological Considerations of Treatment Trials with Antipsychotic Drugs

When analysing the clinical trials initiated by various pharmaceutical companies over the last decade in order to license new antipsychotics, it needs to be considered that all of these studies were performed in a highly selected group of patients. These were usually in their late 30s and two-thirds were of male gender. The average duration of illness was over 10 years in many cases and frequent hospitalizations preceded the clinical trial. Little is known about the pretreatment of these patients and wash-out phases were generally short. In almost all studies, about 20% of the population suffered from schizoaffective disorder.

When looking at response rates of these 6–8 week clinical trials, it becomes evident that the scores of the rating scales used to measure psychopathology (the Brief Psychiatric Rating Scale, BPRS, or the Positive and Negative Symptom Scale, PANSS were used) were reduced by 20–40% at the most.

This holds true for the experimental as well as for the comparator drugs (mostly haloperidol or chlorpromazine).

As stated at the outset, this brief summary of recent clinical trials exemplifies that the investigated sample was a highly selected one. Chronically ill, frequently hospitalized male schizophrenic patients, who probably responded only insufficiently to previous treatment attempts and were usually far from reaching full remission during the course of the clinical trial, constituted the core group, on which the benefit–risk evaluation of the test substance was based.

The attempt to generalize results obtained from studying this group of patients to the whole population of schizophrenic patients appears problematic, to say the least. The spectrum of schizophrenia includes many patients, who hardly ever make it into phase II and III clinical trials. These range from early-onset female patients with suicidal ideation all the way to hostile and agitated treatment-refractory patients. One must not be surprised, therefore, if the results from clinical trials cannot always be translated into clinical practice.

Many clinicians are disappointed with the efficacy of the novel compounds in treating acutely psychotic patients, which may be related to the fact that many of the new drugs have less sedative effects than their traditional counterparts. This often calls for additional sedative medication in the early stages of treatment. A lack of sedation must not be confused with a lack of antipsychotic efficacy, which always, also with the older drugs, takes days to weeks to kick in.

Most of the novel antipsychotics have been reported to be more efficacious in treating negative symptoms than traditional neuroleptics. These findings have to be interpreted with a grain of salt, as this effect is only documented for patients suffering from positive and negative symptoms concomitantly for most antipsychotics. It is accepted knowledge that negative symptoms in this group of patients respond to treatment considerably better than primary enduring negative symptoms as seen in patients with deficit states of schizophrenia [174]. *Post-hoc* path analyses have been performed for olanzapine [175] and risperidone [150] to analyse how much the improvement of negative symptoms has been influenced by intervening variables. It has been reported that at least a part of the therapeutic efficacy is independent of an improvement in positive symptoms or a reduction of EPS [83, 175]. As path analysis is not a confirmatory, inferential statistical method, these results need to be replicated using other study designs. Amisulpride [122], ritanserin [64] and zotepine [172] have been studied in patients with prevailingly negative symptoms and have been documented to lead to an amelioration of deficit states. Ritanserin was used as an add-on to an ongoing neuroleptic treatment; amisulpride and zotepine were shown to be beneficial as monotherapy in low doses. Clozapine [176] has been found to be superior to haloperidol in treating positive but not negative symptoms, and to be associated with long-term improvements in social and occupational functioning for patients with and without the deficit syndrome.

The evaluation of the tolerability of novel antipsychotics contains some potential pitfalls as well. Side effect assessment is performed in different ways in different studies: while some trials include specific side effect rating scales, others rely on spontaneous reporting of patients and/or clinicians. These two methods will understandably yield different incidence rates. A reliable comparison of antipsychotics is only possible if drugs are compared within the same clinical trial.

EPS present a specific problem. All published controlled clinical trials with the novel antipsychotics find an EPS risk that corresponds to that found in the placebo group. In this context, it needs to be noted that patients in the placebo group generally develop EPS at a rate of about 20%. This seemingly paradox finding can be explained in different ways: as clinical trials tend to have brief wash-out periods, EPS resulting from pretreatment often carry over into the comparative part of the study. If these effects occur, they may be misinterpreted as induced by whatever drug these patients are being treated with in the clinical trial. Withdrawal dyskinesias, which occur frequently if tardive dyskinesia is masked by traditional antipsychotics [177, 178], can be an alternative explanation. Next to that, problems in differential diagnoses, such as the delineation of acute akathisia from agitation in acutely psychotic patients, can lead to a misdiagnosis of motor symptoms [179]. Kraepelin [180] has already described that schizophrenia may be accompanied by motor symptoms. Phenomenologically, these are very similar to drug-induced dyskinesias. Several reports in recent years have also found movement disorders in drug-naïve schizophrenic patients [181, 182]. Lastly, a true placebo effect, as it may be expected in neuroleptic experienced patients, as well as the tendency of patients abusing anticholinergics to feign EPS in order to receive the desired prescription, may be seen as possible reasons for the surprisingly high EPS incidence in the placebo groups of clinical trials. One must keep in mind that the fact that the EPS rate of a new drug corresponds to that found with placebo must not lead to the false assumption that the novel compound has no EPS risk at all.

In conclusion, it is emphasized that efficacy and tolerability data from phase III clinical trials should be converted into everyday clinical practice with all due caution and with regard to the potential sources of error discussed above, in order to prevent unrealistic expectations.

SPECIAL ASPECTS OF THE PHARMACOTHERAPY OF SCHIZOPHRENIA

Negative and Depressive Symptoms; Suicidality

Various methodological issues impede the interpretation of clinical trials in patients suffering from negative and/or depressive symptoms in the course of schizophrenia. Differential diagnosis is one of them: negative symptoms, depression and akinesia share many common features. This makes diagnosis difficult, especially in a cross-sectional evaluation. Negative symptoms can be of secondary nature, for instance as a result of EPS or as sequelae of positive symptoms or psychosocial deprivation [174]. Depressive syndromes in schizophrenia are commonly seen as an inherent feature of the illness; they can also occur as a psychological reaction to the diagnosis [183–185]. Problems of clinical trials evaluating negative symptoms have been dealt with in the previous section.

Imipramine has a positive effect against depressive syndromes in schizophrenic patients [183]. Recently serotonin re-uptake inhibitors have also been shown to exert beneficial effects in this indication as well as against negative symptoms [186]. For a review of potential treatment strategies for these symptoms complicating the clinical picture of schizophrenia see [187]. Before pharmacologic treatment is initiated, it is important to come to a reliable diagnosis. The fact that negative and depressive syndromes are difficult to manage must not lead to therapeutic nihilism. This is especially important in light of the fact that patients suffering from schizophrenia have a high suicide risk [188]. Preliminary results on the suicide prophylactic effect of clozapine are very encouraging [23, 189].

Cognitive Functions

Cognitive disturbances have been described ever since the first systematic research in schizophrenia. They include a general intellectual deficit that has a special emphasis in memory and executive functions [190, 191]. These dysfunctions hinder the rehabilitation of schizophrenic patients independently of the other psychopathological symptoms [192]. They constitute a negative predictor for the course of the illness [193, 194]. Classical neuroleptics have little influence on cognitive dysfunctions, if at all, and may lead to a deterioration of cognitive abilities [190]. This seems to be different with novel antipsychotics. Clozapine, for instance, has been shown to ameliorate various cognitive functions, especially attention and verbal fluidity [195]. An improvement of working memory has been found after treatment with risperidone [196], while olanzapine has been shown to enhance selective attention [197]. In general, effect sizes in studies evaluating the effects of second generation antipsychotics on cognitive impairment tend to be modest and a number of methodologically problems still limit the conclusions drawn from the available studies [198–200]. All evidence taken together does indicate, though, that second generation antipsychotics might also have advantages over the traditional drugs in this important facet of the schizophrenia syndrome.

Compliance

As in any other illness in which a long-term intake of medication is necessary, compliance is also of high clinical relevance in patients suffering from schizophrenic disorders. This is also documented by the fact that less than 50% of the schizophrenic patients in long-term treatment take their medication according to the physician's recommendations [201]. Non-compliance has implications that go beyond mere patient management. It may distort the results of psychopharmacological trials, especially of placebo-controlled studies in which the experimental drug has more side effects than placebo. In this case, non-compliance can be expected to be more prominent in the active treatment group than in the placebo-treated patients. Consequently, these non-compliant patients will show a lower rate of treatment response, whereby the difference between placebo and active compound may be artificially diminished. This may lead to an underestimation of potential therapeutic advantages of the experimental drug. Similar problems can occur in a comparison of two active drugs that show different side effect profiles.

Compliance is influenced by a host of different variables. These are usually grouped into patient-related, clinician-related, treatment-related and environment-related factors [202]. Patient-related factors include demographic characteristics such as age [203], sex [204, 205] and social status, but also illness-associated characteristics such as type of disorder and psychopathological symptoms [206–208].

Various aspects of the clinician–patient relationship [209, 210] as well as the information accessible to patients are also part of the influences on compliance [211].

The psychosocial environment of patients also determines attitudes towards treatment and health belief concepts [212, 213].

Adverse effects of drugs are the best studied treatment-related factor [201]. These include EPS, in particular akathisia [16], as well as weight gain and sexual dysfunctions [214–216]. In contrast, several authors have reported that side effects do not have a negative effect on compliance [202, 217]; even a positive influence has been found [218]. These paradoxical findings can easily be explained by an indirect improvement of the clinician–patient relationship and the information about treatment in the case of the advent of drug-induced adverse events. Both appear to have a positive influence on compliance that outweighs the negative consequences of side effects. Another important treatment-related factor is the complexity of treatment. Polypharmacy and multiple therapists with poorly defined roles impede the cooperation between the patient and the treatment team.

Interventions to enhance compliance can be targeted to all of these levels. Ideally, they should be implemented at the beginning of treatment. The success of compliance-enhancing measures is well documented [219, 220]. On the basis of a working doctor–patient relationship, concise and relevant information provided to patients and their significant others must be an integral part of these efforts. Information must also include illness concepts, as these are often unrealistic. Next to that, the prevention and/or rapid management of adverse effects play a crucial role.

Lastly, compliance of clinicians with rational, scientifically determined treatment guidelines and recommendations will optimize treatment efforts and reduce the uncertainty of patients and/or relatives confronted with different treatment concepts suggested by different doctors.

SUMMARY

Pharmacotherapy is the basis of the management of patients suffering from schizophrenic disorders. There is no doubt that the novel antipsychotics enhance the spectrum of acute and long-term treatment options. It is to be expected that the better tolerability of these agents, especially in terms of a reduced EPS risk, will also facilitate rehabilitative measures. An improvement in cognitive functions should contribute to that. On the other hand, it must be emphasized that antipsychotics may induce non-extrapyramidal side effects which in turn can have a negative influence on compliance and psychosocial treatment. The prescriber will therefore still be charged with establishing a sound risk–benefit profile of medication, which is not yet available for the novel antipsychotics. More post-marketing research data are necessary to establish such profiles.

New findings in the field of psychopharmacology, together with advances in psychosocial treatment strategies, have given rise to a new optimism in the treatment of this severe psychiatric disorder. The continuous process of scientific evaluation of new treatment options is a prerequisite for an optimal integration of these into the treatment of schizophrenia. The following paragraphs highlight the current state of research in the clinical psychopharmacology of schizophrenia.

Consistent Evidence

Many clinical trials from throughout the world have consistently shown that neuroleptics/antipsychotics are effective drugs in the management of the acute symptoms of schizophrenia. It is also beyond doubt that novel antipsychotics have clear advantages over the older medications in terms of a substantially lower risk to induce extrapyramidal motor side effects.

The fact that continuing antipsychotic medication maintains its beneficial effects over many years and prevents relapse in most schizophrenic patients is also based on findings from numerous studies. Unfortunately, these positive aspects are overshadowed by a considerable reluctance of patients to stay on long-term medication. Effective doses are known for many of the available drugs, although optimal doses still need to be established for many of them. Clozapine is still the only antipsychotic for which efficacy advantages over traditional neuroleptics have been documented in a number of independently conducted studies.

Incomplete Evidence

Of the many clinical issues for which the research base is incomplete only a few will be outlined in the following.

- There are some indications that a delay in initiating pharmacologic treatment worsens the outcome of patients suffering from schizophrenia. Whether early intervention strategies even in the prodromal phase can remediate this problem is a pressing question.
- For many drugs, including clozapine, optimal dose levels have yet to be established. For long-term treatment, although many authors agree to treat with "minimally effective doses", these are yet to be determined. The same applies for plasma levels of antipsychotic medication, where evidence for acute treatment is available for some drugs but the knowledge about long-term plasma level requirements is scant.
- Most of the evidence available to date about the benefit–risk profiles of the second-generation antipsychotics stem from industry sponsored, preregistration clinical trials. The field badly needs supplementary information based on results from independent, large scale post-marketing studies, reflecting everyday clinical practice as much as possible. In such studies the new antipsychotics should also be compared to each other and ideally, to lower doses of traditional neuroleptics (other than haloperidol or chlorpromazine). Results from such trials will undoubthfully provide helpful guidance concerning differential indications of antipsychotics.
- More research needs to be done to improve treatment recommendations for symptoms outside the positive spectrum. These include: negative symptoms, especially primary negative symptoms, where there is still debate whether or not antipsychotic treatment helps; depressive symptoms, where we know surprisingly little about potential effects of non-tricyclic antidepressants; as well as cognitive dysfunctions. We also

need to learn more about the interactions between pharmacotherapy and psychosocial measures.
• More information on clinically relevant long-term side effects of the second-generation antipsychotics is eagerly awaited. This pertains especially to the critical areas of glucose and lipid metabolism and aberrations of cardiac conductivity.

Areas Still Open to Research

Several aspects of the pharmacotherapy of schizophrenia are in dire need of future research:

• We still have no way of predicting which patient will eventually respond to what antipsychotic and whether or not he/she will tolerate the drug chosen. We continue to have no answer to the important question of which patients are or are not at risk for relapse. This is, of course, a crucial question, when planning long-term treatment strategies.
• We also have no reliable clue as to what to do with a patient not responding to one of the novel antipsychotics. Although many empirically based treatment attempts for these patients exist, none of them has been the subject of larger scale, controlled clinical trials.
• Lastly, we still do not know the real neurobiological mechanism of action determining the efficacy of antipsychotic drugs, more specifically which neurotransmitter system is involved in what type of therapeutic or adverse response.

REFERENCES

1. Fitton A., Heel R. (1990) Clozapine. A review of its pharmacological properties, and therapeutic use in schizophrenia. *Drugs*, **40**: 722–747.
2. Kurz M., Hummer M., Oberbauer H., Fleischhacker W.W. (1995) Extrapyramidal side effects of clozapine and haloperidol. *Psychopharmacology*, **118**: 52–56.
3. Farde L., Nordström A.L., Wiesel F.A., Pauli S., Halldin C., Sedvall G. (1992) PET analysis of central D_1 and D_2 dopamine receptor occupancy in patients treated with classic neuroleptics and clozapine—relationship to extrapyramidal side effects. *Arch. Gen. Psychiatry*, **49**: 538–544.
4. Skarsfeldt T. (1995) Differential effects of repeated administration of novel antipsychotic drugs on the activity of midbrain dopamine neurons in the rat. *Eur. J. Pharmacol.*, **281**, 289–294.
5. Bissette G., Nemeroff C.B. (1995) The neurobiology of neurotensin. In *Psychopharmacology: The Fourth Generation of Progress* (Eds F.E. Bloom, D.J. Kupfer), pp. 573–583. Raven Press, New York.

6. Deutch A.Y., Duman R.S. (1996) The effects of antipsychotic drugs on Fos protein expression in the prefrontal cortex: cellular localization and pharmacological characterization. *Neuroscience*, **70**: 377–389.

7. Nordström A., Farde L., Nyberg S., Karlsson P., Halldin C., Sedvall G. (1995) D_1, D_2, and 5-HT$_2$ receptor occupancy in relation to clozapine serum concentration: a PET study of schizophrenic patients. *Am. J. Psychiatry*, **152**: 1444–1449.

8. Nyberg S., Farde L., Halldin C. (1997) A PET study of 5-HT$_2$ and D_2 dopamine receptor occupancy induced by olanzapine in healthy subjects. *Neuropsychopharmacology*, **16**: 1–7.

9. Pilowsky L.S., O'Connell P., Davies N., Busatto G.F., Costa D.C., Murray P.J., Kerwin R.W. (1997) In vivo effects on striatal dopamine D_2 receptor binding by the novel atypical antipsychotic drug sertindole — a ^{123}I IBZM single photon emission tomography (SPET) study. *Psychopharmacology*, **130**: 152–158.

10. Travis M.J., Busatto G.F., Pilowsky L.S., Mulligan R., Acton P.D., Gacinovic S., Mertens J., Terrière D., Costa D.C., Ell P.J. *et al* (1998) 5-HT$_{2A}$ receptor blockade in patients with schizophrenia treated with risperidone or clozapine: a SPET study using the novel 5-HT$_{2A}$ ligand ^{123}I-5-I-R-91150. *Br. J. Psychiatry*, **173**: 236–241.

11. Farde L., Nyberg S. (1998) Dosing determination for novel antipsychotics — a PET-based approach. *Int. J. Psychiatr. Clin. Pract.*, **2** (Suppl. 1): 39–42.

12. Roth B.L., Meltzer H.Y. (1995) The role of serotonin in schizophrenia. In *Psychopharmacology: The Fourth Generation of Progress* (Eds F.E. Bloom, D.J. Kupfer), pp. 1215–1227. Raven Press, New York.

13. Bunney B.G., Bunney W.E., Carlsson A. (1995) Schizophrenia and glutamate. In *Psychopharmacology: The Fourth Generation of Progress* (Eds F.E. Bloom, D.J. Kupfer), pp. 1205–1214. Raven Press, New York.

14. Wyatt R.J., Henter I. (2001) Rationale for the study of early intervention. *Schizophr. Res.*, **51**: 69–76.

15. Wirshing W.C., Marder S.R., Van Putten T., Ames D. (1995) Acute treatment of schizophrenia. In *Psychopharmacology: The Fourth Generation of Progress* (Eds F.E. Bloom, D.J. Kupfer), pp. 1259–1266. Raven Press, New York.

16. Van Putten T. (1974) Why do schizophrenic patients refuse to take their drugs? *Arch. Gen. Psychiatry*, **31**: 67 72.

17. Kane J., Honigfeld G., Singer J., Meltzer H.Y. (1988) Clozapine for the treatment-resistant schizophrenic. *Arch. Gen. Psychiatry*, **45**: 789–796.

18. Fischer-Cornelssen K.A., Ferner V.J. (1976) An example of European multicenter trials: multispectral analysis of clozapine. *Psychopharmacol. Bull.*, **2**: 34–39.

19. Gerlach I., Koppelhus P., Helweg E., Monrad A. (1974) Clozapine and haloperidol in a single-blind cross-over trial: therapeutic and biochemical aspects in the treatment of schizophrenia. *Acta Psychiatr. Scand.*, **50**: 410–424.

20. Fleischhacker W.W. (1999) Clozapine: a comparison with other novel antipsychotics. *J. Clin. Psychiatry*, **60** (Suppl. 12): 30–34.

21. Claghorn J., Honigfeld G., Abuzzahab F.S., Wang R., Steinbook R., Tuason V., Klerman G.L. (1987) The risks and benefits of clozapine versus chlorpromazine. *J. Clin. Psychopharmacol.*, **7**: 377–384.

22. Meltzer H.Y., Burnett S., Bastani B., Ramirez L.F. (1990) Effects of six months of clozapine treatment on the quality of life of chronic schizophrenic patients. *Hosp. Comm. Psychiatry*, **41**: 892–897.

23. Meltzer H.Y. (2001) Treatment of suicidality in schizophrenia. *Ann. N.Y. Acad. Sci.*, **932**: 44–60.

24. Fleischhacker W.W. (2002) Second generation antipsychotics. *Psychopharmacology*, **162**: 90–91.
25. Sartorius N., Fleischhacker W.W., Gjerris A., Kern U., Knapp M., Leonard B.E., Lieberman J.A., Lopez-Ibor J.J., van Raay B., Twomey E. (2002) The usefulness and use of second-generation antipsychotic medication. *Curr. Opin. Psychiatry*, **15** (Suppl. 1): S1–S51.
26. Alvir J.M.J., Lieberman J.A., Safferman A.Z., Schwimmer J.L., Schaaf J.A. (1993) Clozapine-induced agranulocytosis: incidence and risk factors in the United States. *N. Engl. J. Med.*, **329**: 162–167.
27. Fleischhacker W., Hummer M. (1997) Drug treatment of schizophrenia in the 1990s: achievements and future possibilities in optimising outcomes. *Drugs*, **53**: 915–929.
28. Glazer W.M., Johnstone B.M. (1997) Pharmacoeconomic evaluation of antipsychotic therapy for schizophrenia. *J. Clin. Psychiatry*, **58** (Suppl. 10): 50–54.
29. Baldessarini R.J., Cohen B.M., Teicher M.H. (1988) Significance of neuroleptic dose and plasma level in the pharmacological treatment of psychoses. *Arch. Gen. Psychiatry*, **45**: 79–91.
30. Rifkin A., Doddi S., Karagi B. (1991) Dosage of haloperidol for schizophrenia. *Arch. Gen. Psychiatry*, **48**: 166–170.
31. Van Putten T., Marder S.R., Mintz J., Poland R.E. (1992) Haloperidol plasma levels and clinical response: a therapeutic window relationship. *Am. J. Psychiatry*, **149**: 500–505.
32. Levinson D.F., Simpson G.M., Singh H., Yadalam K., Jain A., Stephanos M.J., Silver P. (1990) Fluphenazine dose, clinical response, and extrapyramidal symptoms during acute treatment. *Arch. Gen. Psychiatry*, **47**: 761–768.
33. Marder S.R., Meibach R.C. (1994) Risperidone in the treatment of schizophrenia. *Am. J. Psychiatry*, **151**: 825–835.
34. McEvoy J.P., Hogarty G.E., Steingard S. (1991) Optimal dose of neuroleptic in acute schizophrenia. *Arch. Gen. Psychiatry*, **48**: 739–745.
35. Fleischhacker W.W., Hummer M., Kurz M., Kurzthaler I., Lieberman J., Pollack S., Safferman A., Kane J. (1994) Clozapine dose in the US and Europe: implications for therapeutic and adverse effects. *J. Clin. Psychiatry*, **55** (Suppl. B): 78–81.
36. Emsley R.A., Risperidone Working Group (1999) Risperidone in the treatment of first episode psychotic patients: a double-blind multi-center study. *Schizophr. Bull.*, **25**: 721–729.
37. Kopala L.C., Good K.P., Honer W.G. (1997) Extrapyramidal signs and clinical symptoms in first-episode schizophrenia: response to low-dose risperidone. *J. Clin. Psychopharmacol.*, **17**: 308–313.
38. Haring C., Neudorfer C., Schwitzer J., Hummer M., Saria A., Hinterhuber H., Fleischhacker W.W. (1994) EEG alterations in patients treated with clozapine in relation to plasma levels. *Psychopharmacology*, **114**: 97–100.
39. Volavka J., Cooper T., Czobor P., Bitter I., Meisner M., Laska E., Gastanaga P., Krakowski M., Chou S.C.Y., Crowner M. *et al* (1992) Haloperidol blood levels and clinical effects. *Arch. Gen. Psychiatry*, **49**: 354–361.
40. Janicak P.G., Javaid J.I., Sharma R.P., Leach A., Dowd S., Davis J.M. (1997) A two-phase, double-blind randomized study of three haloperidol plasma levels for acute psychosis with reassignment of initial non-responders. *Acta Psychiatr. Scand.*, **95**: 343–350.

41. Coryell W., Miller D.D., Perry P.J. (1998) Haloperidol plasma levels and dose optimization. *Am. J. Psychiatry*, **155**: 48–53.
42. Levinson D.F., Simpson G.M., Lo E.S., Cooper T.B., Singh H., Yadalam K., Stephanos M.J. (1995) Fluphenazine plasma levels, dosage, efficacy, and side effects. *Am. J. Psychiatry*, **152**: 765–771.
43. Potkin S.G., Bera R., Gulasekaram B., Jin Y., Costa J., Gerber B., Richmond G., Ploszaj D., Carreon D., Cooper T., Sitanggan K. (1994) Plasma clozapine concentrations predict clinical response in treatment-resistant schizophrenia. *J. Clin. Psychiatry*, **55** (Suppl. B): 133–136.
44. Miller D.D., Fleming F., Holman T.L., Perry P.J. (1994) Plasma clozapine concentrations as a predictor of clinical response: a follow-up study. *J. Clin. Psychiatry*, **55** (Suppl. B): 117–121.
45. Kurz M., Hummer M., Kurzthaler I., Oberbauer H., Fleischhacker W.W. (1995) Efficacy of medium-dose clozapine for treatment resistant schizophrenia. *Am. J. Psychiatry*, **152**: 1690–1691.
46. Haring C., Fleischhacker W.W., Schett P., Humpel C., Barnas C., Saria A. (1990) Influence of patient-related variables on clozapine plasma levels. *Am. J. Psychiatry*, **147**: 1471–1475.
47. VanderZwaag C., McGee M., McEvoy J.P., Freudenreich O., Wilson W.H., Copper T.B. (1996) Response of patients with treatment-refractory schizophrenia to clozapine within three serum level ranges. *Am. J. Psychiatry*, **153**: 1579–1584.
48. Hiemke C., Weigmann H., Härtter S., Dahmen N., Wetzel H., Müller H. (1994) Elevated serum levels of clozapine after addition of fluvoxamine. *J. Clin. Psychopharmacol.*, **14**: 279–281.
49. Levinson D.F., Singh H., Simpson G.M. (1992) Timing of acute clinical response to fluphenazine. *Br. J. Psychiatry*, **160**: 365–371.
50. Meltzer H.Y. (1989) Duration of a clozapine trial in neuroleptic-resistant schizophrenia. *Arch. Gen. Psychiatry*, **46**: 672.
51. Kane J.M., Marder S.R., Schooler N.R., Wirshing W.C., Umbricht D., Baker R.W., Wirshing D.A., Safferman A., Ganguli R., McMeniman M. *et al* (2001) Clozapine and haloperidol in moderately refractory schizophrenia. *Arch. Gen. Psychiatry*, **58**: 965–972.
52. Bondolfi G., Dufour H., Patris M., May J.P., Billeter U., Eap C.B., Baumann P., for the Risperidone Study Group (1998) Risperidone vs. clozapine in treatment-resistant chronic schizophrenia: a randomized double-blind study. *Am. J. Psychiatry*, **155**: 499–504.
53. Kinon B.J., Kane J.M., Johns C., Perovich R., Ismi M., Koreen A.R., Weiden P.J. (1993) Treatment of neuroleptic-resistant schizophrenic relapse. *Psychopharmacol. Bull.*, **29**: 309–314.
54. Shalev A., Hermesh H., Rothberg J., Munitz H. (1993) Poor neuroleptic response in acutely exacerbated schizophrenic patients. *Acta Psychiatr. Scand.*, **87**: 86–91.
55. Conley R.R., Tamminga C.A., Bartko J.J., Richardson C., Peszke M., Lingle J., Hegerty J., Love R., Gounaris C., Zaremba S. (1998) Olanzapine compared with chlorpromazine in treatment-resistant schizophrenia. *Am. J. Psychiatry*, **155**: 914–920.
56. Growe G.A., Crayton J.A., Klass D.B. (1979) Lithium in chronic schizophrenia. *Am. J. Psychiatry*, **136**: 454–455.

57. Wilson W.H. (1993) Addition of lithium to haloperidol in non-affective, antipsychotic non-responsive schizophrenia: a double blind, placebo controlled, parallel design clinical trial. *Psychopharmacology*, **111**: 359–366.

58. Collins P.J., Larkin E.P., Shubsachs A.P.W. (1991) Lithium carbonate in chronic schizophrenia—a brief trial of lithium carbonate added to neuroleptics for treatment of resistant schizophrenic patients. *Acta Psychiatr. Scand.*, **84**: 150–154.

59. Schulz S.C., Kahn E.M., Baker R.W., Conley R.R. (1990) Lithium and carbamazepine augmentation in treatment refractory schizophrenia. In *The Neuroleptic Nonresponsive Patient: Characterization and Treatment* (Eds B. Angrist, S.C. Schulz), pp. 109–136. American Psychiatric Association, Washington, DC.

60. Wolkowitz O.M., Rapoport M.H., Pickar D. (1990) Benzodiazepine augmentation of neuroleptics. In *The Neuroleptic Nonresponsive Patient: Characterization and Treatment* (Eds B. Angrist, S.C. Schulz), pp. 87–108. American Psychiatric Association, Washington, DC.

61. Decina P., Mukherjee S., Bocola V., Saraceni F., Hadjichristos C., Scapicchio P. (1994) Adjunctive trazodone in the treatment of negative symptoms of schizophrenia. *Hosp. Comm. Psychiatry*, **45**: 1220–1223.

62. Goff D.C., Brotman A.W., Waites M., McCormick S. (1990) Trial of fluoxetine added to neuroleptics for treatment-resistant schizophrenic patients. *Am. J. Psychiatry*, **47**: 492–494.

63. Silver H., Kushnir M., Kaplan A. (1996) Fluvoxamine augmentation in clozapine-resistant schizophrenia: an open pilot study. *Biol. Psychiatry*, **40**: 671–674.

64. Duinkerke S.J., Botter P.A., Jansen A.A.I., Van Dongen P.A.M., Van Haaften A.J., Boom A.J., Van Laarhoven J.H.M., Busard H.L.S.M. (1993) Ritanserin, a selective 5-HT$_{2/1C}$ antagonist, and negative symptoms in schizophrenia: A placebo-controlled double-blind trial. *Br. J. Psychiatry*, **163**: 451–455.

65. Krueger R.B., Sackeim H.A. (1995) Electroconvulsive therapy and schizophrenia. In *Schizophrenia* (Eds S.R. Hirsch, D.R. Weinberger), pp. 503–545. Blackwell Science, Oxford.

66. Shiloh R., Zemishlany Z., Aizenberg D., Radwan M., Schwartz B., Dorfman-Etrog P., Modai I., Khaikin M., Weizman A. (1997) Sulpiride augmentation in people with schizophrenia partially responsive to clozapine: a double-blind, placebo-controlled study. *Br. J. Psychiatry*, **171**: 569–573.

67. Casey D.E. (1996) Extrapyramidal syndromes: epidemiology, pathophysiology and the diagnostic dilemma. *CNS Drugs*, **5** (Suppl. 1): 1–12.

68. Csernansky J.G., Newcomer J.G. (1995) Maintenance drug treatment for schizophrenia. In *Psychopharmacology: The Fourth Generation of Progress* (Eds F.E. Bloom, D.J. Kupfer), pp. 1267–1275. Raven Press, New York.

69. Remington G., Bezchlibnyk-Butler K. (1996) Management of acute antipsychotic-induced extrapyramidal syndromes. *CNS Drugs*, **5** (Suppl. 1): 21–35.

70. Fleischhacker W.W., Roth S.D., Kane J.M. (1990) The pharmacologic treatment of neuroleptic-induced akathisia. *J. Clin. Psychopharmacol.*, **10**: 12–21.

71. Fleischhacker W.W., Barnas C., Günther V., Meise U., Stuppäck C.H., Unterweger B. (1987) Mood-altering effects of biperiden in healthy volunteers. *J. Affect. Disord.*, **12**: 153–157.

72. Fayen M., Goldman M.B., Moulthrop M.A., Luchins D.J. (1988) Differential memory function with dopaminergic versus anticholinergic treatment of drug induced extrapyramidal symptoms. *Am. J. Psychiatry*, **145**: 483–486.

73. Smith J.M. (1980) Abuse of antiparkinsonian drugs—a review of the literature. *J. Clin. Psychiatry*, **41**: 351–354.

74. Tandon R., Mann N.A., Eisner W.H., Coppard N. (1990) Effect of anticholinergic medication on positive and negative symptoms in medication-free schizophrenic patients. *Psychiatry Res.*, **31**: 235–241.
75. World Health Organization (1990) Prophylactic use of anticholinergics in patients on long-term neuroleptic treatment. *Br. J. Psychiatry*, **156**: 412–414.
76. Marder S.R. (1998) Facilitating compliance with antipsychotic medication. *J. Clin. Psychiatry*, **59** (Suppl. 3): 21–25.
77. Crow T.J., McMillan J.F., Johnson A.L., Johnstone E.C. (1986) The Northwick Park study of first episodes of schizophrenia: II. A randomized controlled trial of prophylactic neuroleptic treatment. *Br. J. Psychiatry*, **148**: 120–127.
78. Loebel A., Lieberman J., Alvir J., Geisler J., Koreen A., Chakos M. (1995) Time to treatment response in successive episodes of early onset schizophrenia. *Schizophr. Res.*, **15**: 158.
79. Wyatt R.J. (1992) Neuroleptics and the natural course of schizophrenia. *Schizophr. Bull.*, **17**: 325–351.
80. Kane J.M., Lieberman J.A. (1987) Maintenance pharmacotherapy in schizophrenia. In *Psychopharmacology — The Third Generation of Progress* (Ed. H.Y. Meltzer), pp. 1103–1109. Raven Press, New York.
81. Kissling W. (1991) Duration of neuroleptic maintenance treatment. In *Guidelines for Neuroleptic Relapse Prevention in Schizophrenia* (Ed. W. Kissling), pp. 94–112. Springer, Berlin.
82. Steingard S., Allen M., Schooler N.R. (1994) A study of the pharmacologic treatment of medication-compliant schizophrenics who relapse. *J. Clin. Psychiatry*, **55**: 470–472.
83. Möller H.J., Van Zerssen D. (1995) Course and outcome of schizophrenia. In *Schizophrenia* (Eds S.R. Hirsch, D.R. Weinberger), pp. 106–127. Blackwell Science, Oxford.
84. Kissling W., Kane J.M., Barnes T.R.E., Dencker S.J., Fleischhacker W.W., Goldstein J.M., Johnson D.A.W., Marder S.R., Müller-Spahn F., Tegeler J. *et al* (1991) Guidelines for neuroleptic relapse prevention in schizophrenia: towards a consensus view. In *Guidelines for Neuroleptic Relapse Prevention in Schizophrenia* (Ed. W. Kissling), pp. 155–163. Springer, Berlin.
85. American Psychiatric Association (1997) Practice guideline for the treatment of patients with schizophrenia. *Am. J. Psychiatry*, **54** (Suppl.).
86. Lehmann A.F., Steinwachs D.M., Co-investigators of the PORT project (1998) At issue: translating research into practice: the schizophrenia patient outcomes research team (PORT) treatment recommendations. *Schizophr. Bull.*, **24**: 1–10.
87. Gaebel W., Falkai P. (1998) *Praxisleitlinien in Psychiatrie und Psychotherapie, Band 1: Behandlungsleitlinie Schizophrenie* (Ed. Deutsche Gesellschaft für Psychiatrie, Psychotherapie und Nervenheilkunde). Steinkopff, Darmstadt.
88. Rosenheck R., Cramer J., Xu W., Thomas J., Henderson W., Frisman L., Fye C., Charney D. (1997) A comparison of clozapine and haloperidol in hospitalized patients with refractory schizophrenia. *N. Engl. J. Med.*, **337**: 809–815.
89. Gilbert P.L., Harris M.J., McAdams L.A., Jeste D.V. (1995) Neuroleptic withdrawal in schizophrenic patients. *Arch. Gen. Psychiatry*, **52**: 173–188.
90. Pietzcker A., Gaebel W., Köpcke W., Linden M., Müller P., Müller-Spahn F., Tegeler J. (1993) Intermittent versus maintenance neuroleptic long-term treatment in schizophrenia — 2-year results of a German multicenter study. *J. Psychiatr. Res.*, **27**: 321–339.
91. Carpenter W.T., Hanlon T.E., Heinrichs D.W., Summerfelt A.T., Kirkpatrick B., Levine J., Buchanan R.W. (1990) Continuous versus targeted medication in schizophrenic outpatients: outcome results. *Am. J. Psychiatry*, **147**: 1138–1148.

92. Herz M.I., Glazer W.M., Mostert M.A., Sheard M.A., Szymanski H.V. (1991) Intermittent vs. maintenance medication in schizophrenia: two-year results. *Arch. Gen. Psychiatry*, **48**: 333–339.

93. Jolley A.G., Hirsch S.R., McRink A., Manchanda R. (1989) Trial of brief intermittent neuroleptic prophylaxis for selected schizophrenic outpatients: clinical outcome at one year. *Br. Med. J.*, **298**: 985–990.

94. Schooler N.R., Keith S.J., Severe J.B., Matthews S.M., Bellack A.S., Glick I.D., Hargreaves W.A., Kane J.M., Ninan P.T., Frances A. *et al* (1997) Relapse and rehospitalization during maintenance treatment of schizophrenia: the effects of dose reduction and family treatment. *Arch. Gen. Psychiatry*, **54**: 453–463.

95. Van Harten P.N., Hoek H.W., Matroos G.E., Koeter M., Kahn R.S. (1998) Intermittent neuroleptic treatment and risk for tardive dyskinesia: Curacao extrapyramidal syndromes study III. *Am. J. Psychiatry*, **155**: 565–567.

96. Gaebel W., Janner M., Frommann N., Pietzcker A., Kopcke W., Linden M., Muller P., Müller-Spahn F., Tegeler J. (2002) First vs. multiple episode schizophrenia: two-year outcome of intermittent and maintenance medication strategies. *Schizophr. Res.*, **53**: 145–159.

97. Daniel D.G., Wozniak P., Mack R.J., McCarthy B.G., Sertindole Study Group (1998) Long-term efficacy and safety comparison of sertindole and haloperidol in the treatment of schizophrenia. *Psychopharmacol. Bull.*, **34**: 61–69.

98. Tran P.V., Dellva M.A., Tollefson G.D., Wentley A.L., Beasley C.M. (1998) Oral olanzapine versus oral haloperidol in the maintenance treatment of schizophrenia and related psychoses. *Br. J. Psychiatry*, **172**: 499–505.

99. Csernansky J.G., Mahmoud R., Brenner R. The Risperidone-USA-79 Study Group (2002) A comparison of risperidone and haloperidol for the prevention of relapse in patients with schizophrenia. *N. Engl. J. Med.*, **346**: 16–22.

100. Johnson D.A.W. (1979) Further observations on the duration of depot neuroleptic maintenance therapy in schizophrenia. *Br. J. Psychiatry*, **135**: 524–530.

101. Davis J.M., Matalon L., Watanabe M.D., Blake L.M. (1994) Depot antipsychotic drugs: place in therapy. *Drugs*, **47**: 741–773.

102. Kane J.M., Aguglia E., Altamura A.C., Ayuso Gutierrez J.L., Brunello N., Fleischhacker W.W., Gaebel W., Gerlach J., Guolfi J.D., Kissling W. *et al* (1998) Guidelines for depot antipsychotic treatment in schizophrenia. European Neuropsychopharmacology Consensus Conference in Siena, Italy. *Eur. Neuropsychopharmacol.*, **8**: 55–66.

103. Altamura C.A., Colacurcio F., Mauri M.C., Moro A.R., DeNovellis F. (1989) Haloperidol decanoate in chronic schizophrenia: a study of 12 months with plasma levels. *Prog. Neuropsychopharmacol. Biol. Psychiatry*, **14**: 25–35.

104. Davis J.M., Kane J.M., Marder S., Brauzer B., Gierl B., Schooler N.R., Casey D.E., Hassan M. (1993) Dose response of prophylactic antipsychotics. *J. Clin. Psychiatry*, **54** (Suppl. 3): 24–30.

105. Whitworth A.B., Fleischhacker W.W. (1995) Adverse effects of antipsychotic drugs. *Int. Clin. Psychopharmacol.* **9** (Suppl. 5): 21–27.

106. American Psychiatric Association (1992) *Tardive Dyskinesia: A Task Force Report of the American Psychiatric Association*. American Psychiatric Press, Washington, DC.

107. Kane J.M., Woerner M., Lieberman J. (1988) Tardive dyskinesia: prevalence, incidence and risk factors. *J. Clin. Psychopharmacol.*, **8**: 52S–56S.

108. Gardes G., Casey D.E., Cole J.O., Pezenyi A., Kocsis E., Azato M., Samson J., Conley C. (1994) Ten-year outcome of tardive dyskinesia. *Am. J. Psychiatry*, **151**: 836–841.

109. Tollefson G.D., Beasley C.M., Tamura R.N., Tran P.V., Potvin J.H. (1997) Blind, controlled, long-term study of the comparative incidence of treatment-emergent tardive dyskinesia with olanzapine or haloperidol. *Am. J. Psychiatry*, **154**: 1248–1254.

110. Lemmens P., Brecher M., Van Baelen B. (1999) A combined analysis of double-blind studies with risperidone vs. placebo and other antipsychotic agents: factors associated with extrapyramidal symptoms. *Acta Psychiatr. Scand.*, **99**: 160–170.

111. Adler L.A., Edson R., Lavori P., Peselow E., Duncan E., Rosenthal M., Rotrosen J. (1998) Long-term treatment effects of vitamin E for tardive dyskinesia. *Biol. Psychiatry*, **43**: 868–872.

112. Coukell A.J., Spencer C.M., Benfield P. (1996) Amisulpride: a review of its pharmacodynamic and pharmacokinetic properties and therapeutic efficacy in the management of schizophrenia. *CNS Drugs*, **6**: 237–256.

113. Schoemaker H., Claustre Y., Fage D., Rouquier L., Chergui K., Curet O., Oblin A., Gonon F., Carter C., Benavides J., Scatton B. (1997) Neurochemical characteristics of amisulpride, an atypical dopamine D2/D3 receptor antagonist with both presynaptic and limbic selectivity. *J. Pharmacol. Exp. Ther.*, **280**: 83–97.

114. Sokoloff P., Andrieux M., Besancon R., Pilon C., Martres M.P., Giros B., Schwartz J.C. (1992) Pharmacology of human dopamine D3 receptor expressed in a mammalian cell line: comparison with D2 receptor. *Eur. J. Pharmacol.*, **225**: 331–337.

115. Dufour A., Desanti C. (1988) Pharmacokinetics and metabolism of amisulpride. *Ann. Psychiatry*, **3**: 298–305.

116. Möller H.J., Boyer P., Fleurot O., Rein W. (1997) Improvement of acute exacerbation of schizophrenia with amisulpride: a comparison with haloperidol. *Psychopharmacology*, **132**: 396–401.

117. Delcker A., Schoon M.L., Oczkowski B., Gaertner H.J. (1990) Amisulpride versus haloperidol in treatment of schizophrenic patients: results of a double-blind study. *Pharmacopsychiatry*, **23**: 125–130.

118. Wetzel H., Grunder G., Hillert A., Philipp M., Gattaz W.F., Sauer H., Adler G., Schroder J., Rein W., Benkert O. (1998) Amisulpride versus flupentixol in schizophrenia with predominantly positive symptomatology: a double-blind controlled study comparing a selective D2-like antagonist to a mixed D1-/D2-like antagonist. *Psychopharmacology*, **137**: 223–232.

119. Paillere-Martinot M.L., Lecrubier Y., Martinot J.L., Aubin F. (1995) Improvement of some schizophrenic deficit symptoms with low doses of amisulpride. *Am. J. Psychiatry*, **152**: 130–133.

120. Boyer P., Lecrubier Y., Puech A.J. (1995) Treatment of negative symptoms in schizophrenia with amisulpride. *Br. J. Psychiatry*, **166**: 68–72.

121. Danion J.M., Rein W., Fleurot O. (1999) Improvement of schizophrenic patients with primary negative symptoms treated with amisulpride. *Am. J. Psychiatry*, **156**: 610–616.

122. Loo H., Poirier-Littre M.-F., Theron M., Rein W., Fleurot O. (1997) Amisulpride versus placebo in the medium-term treatment of the negative symptoms of schizophrenia. *Br. J. Psychiatry*, **170**: 18–22.

123. Colonna L., Saleem P., Dondey-Nouvel L., Rein W. and the Amisulpride Study Group (2000) Long-term safety and efficacy of amisulpride in subchronic or chronic schizophrenia. *Int. Clin. Psychopharmacol.*, **15**: 13–22.

124. Wetzel H., Grunder G., Hillert A., Philip M., Gattaz W.F., Sauer H., Adler G., Schroder J., ReW W., Benkert O. (1998) Amisulpride versus flupenthixol in

schizophrenia with predominantly positive symptomatology: a double-blind controlled study comparing a selective D20-like antagonist to a mixed D1-/D2-like antagonist. *Psychopharmacology*, 137: 223–232.

125. Peuskens J., Bech P., Möller H.J., Bale R., Fleurot O., Rein W. (1999) Amisulpride vs. risperidone in the treatment of acute exacerbations of schizophrenia. *Psychiatry Res.*, 88: 107–117.

126. Bymaster F.P., Calligaro D.O., Falcone J.F., Marsh R.D., Moore N.A., Tye N.C., Seeman P., Wong D.T. (1996) Radioreceptor binding profile of the atypical antipsychotic olanzapine. *Neuropsychopharmacology*, 14: 87–96.

127. Eli Lilly and Company, data on file.

128. Beasley C.M., Tollefson G., Tran P., Satterlee W., Sanger T., Hamilton S. (1996) Olanzapine versus placebo and haloperidol. *Neuropsychopharmacology*, 14: 111–123.

129. Tollefson G.D., Beasley C.M., Tran P.V., Street J.S., Krueger J.A., Tamura R.N., Graffeo K.A., Thieme M.E. (1997) Olanzapine versus haloperidol in the treatment of schizophrenia and schizoaffective and schizophreniform disorders: results of an international collaborative trial. *Am. J. Psychiatry*, 154: 457–465.

130. Tollefson G.D., Sanger T.M., Thieme M.E. (1998) Depressive signs and symptoms in schizophrenia: a prospective blinded trial of olanzapine and haloperidol. *Arch. Gen. Psychiatry*, 55: 250–258.

131. Tollefson G.D., Birkett M.A., Kiesler G.M., Wood A.J., the Lilly Resistant Schizophrenia Study Group (2001) Double-blind comparison of olanzapine versus clozapine in schizophrenic patients clinically eligible for treatment with clozapine. *Biol. Psychiatry*, 49: 52–63.

132. Hamilton S.H., Revicki D.A., Genduso L.A., Beasley C.M. Jr. (1998) Olanzapine versus placebo and haloperidol: quality of life and efficacy results of the North American double-blind trial. *Neuropsychopharmacology*, 18: 41–49.

133. Tran P.V., Dellva M.A., Tollefson G.D., Beasley C.M., Potvin J.H., Kiesler G.M. (1997) Extrapyramidal symptoms and tolerability of olanzapine versus haloperidol in the acute treatment of schizophrenia. *J. Clin. Psychiatry*, 58: 205–211.

134. Weiss F., Danzl C., Hummer M., Kemmler G., Lindner C., Reinstadler K., Fleischhacker W.W. (1998) Weight gain induced by olanzapine. *Schizophr. Res.*, 29 (special issue 1/2): 179.

135. Meyer J.M. (2001) Novel antipsychotics and severe hyperlipidemia. *J. Clin. Psychopharmacol.*, 21: 369–374.

136. Liebzeit K.A., Markowitz J.S., Caley C.F. (2001) New onset diabetes and atypical antipsychotics. *Eur. Neuropsychopharmacol.*, 11: 25–32.

137. Wudarsky M., Nicolson R., Hamburger S.D., Spechler L., Gochman P., Bedwell J., Lenane M.C., Rapaport J.L. (1999) Elevated prolactin in pediatric patients on typical and atypical antipsychotics. *J. Child Adolesc. Psychopharmacol.*, 9: 239–245.

138. Saller F.C., Salama A.I. (1993) Seroquel: biochemical profile of a potential atypical antipsychotic. *Psychopharmacology*, 112: 285–292.

139. Fulton B., Goa K.L. (1995) ICI-204,636. An initial appraisal of its pharmacological properties and clinical potential in the treatment of schizophrenia. *CNS Drugs*, 4: 68–78.

140. Small J.G., Hirsch S.R., Arvanitis L.A., Miller B.G., Link C.G.G., Seroquel Study Group (1997) Quetiapine in patients with schizophrenia: a high- and

low-dose double-blind comparison with placebo. *Arch. Gen. Psychiatry*, **54**: 549–557.

141. Arvanitis L.A., Miller B.G., Seroquel Trial 13 Study Group (1997) Multiple fixed doses of "Seroquel" (quetiapine) in patients with acute exacerbation of schizophrenia: a comparison with haloperidol and placebo. *Biol. Psychiatry*, **42**: 233–246.

142. Borison R.L., Arvanitis L.A., Miller B.G., Seroquel Study Group (1996) ICI 204.636. An atypical antipsychotic: efficacy and safety in a multicenter, placebo-controlled trial in patients with schizophrenia. *J. Clin. Psychopharmacol.*, **16**: 158–169.

143. Hirsch S., Link C.G., Goldstein J.M., Arvanitis L.A. (1996) ICI 204.636. A new atypical antipsychotic drug. *Br. J. Psychiatry*, **168** (Suppl. 29): 45–56.

144. Anonymous (2001) Quetiapine offers promise for difficult-to-treat psychosis complicating Parkinson's disease. *Drugs Ther. Perspect.*, **17**: 1–5.

145. Wetterling T. (2001) Body weight gain with atypical antipsychotics. A comparative review. *Drug Saf.*, **24**: 59–73.

146. Mullen J., Jibson M.D., Sweitzer D. (2001) A comparison of the relative safety, efficacy, and tolerability of quetiapine and risperidone in outpatients with schizophrenia and other psychotic disorders: the Quetiapine Experience with Safety and Tolerability (QUEST) Study. *Clin. Ther.*, **23**: 1839–1854.

147. Brecher M., Rak I.W., Melvin K., Jones A.M. (2000) The long-term effect of quetiapine (Seroquel) monotherapy on weight in patients with schizophrenia. *Int. J. Psychiatry Clin. Pract.*, **4**: 287–291.

148. Byerly M.J., DeVane C.L. (1996) Pharmacokinetics of clozapine and risperidone: a review of recent literature. *J. Clin. Psychopharmacol.*, **16**: 177–187.

149. Peuskens J. (1995) Risperidone in the treatment of patients with chronic schizophrenia: a multi-national, multi-centre, double-blind, parallel-group study versus haloperidol. *Br. J. Psychiatry*, **166**: 712–726.

150. Möller H.J. (1995) The negative component in schizophrenia. *Acta Psychiatr. Scand.*, **91** (Suppl. 388): 11–14.

151. Mandoki M.W. (1995) Risperidone treatment of children and adolescents: increased risk of extrapyramidal side effects? *J. Child Adolesc. Psychopharmacol.*, **5**: 49–67.

152. Sternlicht H.C., Wells S.R. (1995) Risperidone in childhood schizophrenia. *J. Am. Acad. Child. Adolesc. Psychiatry*, **34**: 5.

153. Hellings J.A., Zarcone J.R., Crandall K., Wallace D., Schroeder S.R. (2001) Weight gain in a controlled study of risperidone in children, adolescents and adults with mental retardation and autism. *J. Child Adolesc. Psychopharmacol.*, **11**: 229–238.

154. Martin A., Landau J., Leebens P., Ulizio P., Cicchetti D., Scahill L., Leckman J.F. (2000) Risperidone-associated weight gain in children and adolescents: a retrospective chart review. *J. Child Adolesc. Psychopharmacol.*, **10**: 259–268.

155. Kleinberg D.L., Davis J.M., de Coster R., Van Baelen B., Brecher M. (1999) Prolactin levels and adverse events in patients treated with risperidone. *J. Clin. Psychopharmacol.*, **19**: 57–61.

156. Markianos M., Hatzimanolis J., Lykouas L. (2001) Neuroendocrine responsivities of the pituitary dopamine system in male schizophrenic patients during treatment with clozapine, olanzapine, risperidone, sulpiride, or haloperidol. *Eur. Arch. Psychiatry Clin. Neurosci.*, **251**: 141–146.

157. Dunn C.J., Fitton A. (1996) Sertindole. *CNS Drugs*, **5**: 224–230.
158. Zimbroff D.L., Kane J.M., Tamminga C.A., Daniel D.G., Mack R.J., Wozniak T.J., Sebree T.B., Wallin B.A., Kashkin K.B., Sertindole Study Group (1997) Controlled, dose–response study of sertindole and haloperidol in the treatment of schizophrenia. *Am. J. Psychiatry*, **154**: 782–791.
159. Van Kammen D.P., McEvoy J.P., Targum S.D., Kardatzke D., Sebree T., Sertindole Study Group (1996) A randomized, controlled, dose-ranging trial of sertindole in patients with schizophrenia. *Psychopharmacology*, **124**: 168–175.
160. Hale A., Van der Burght M., Wehnert A., Friberg H.H. (1996) A European dose-range study comparing the efficacy, tolerability and safety of four doses of sertindole and one dose of haloperidol in schizophrenic patients. Poster presented at the 20th CINP Congress, Melbourne, 23–27 June.
161. Davis R., Markham A. (1997) Ziprasidone. *CNS Drugs*, **8**: 153–159.
162. Tandon R., Harrigan E., Zorn S.H. (1997) Ziprasidone: a novel antipsychotic with unique pharmacology and therapeutic potential. *J. Serotonin Res.*, **4**: 159–177.
163. Keck P. Jr., Buffenstein A., Ferguson J., Feighner J., Jaffe W., Harrigan E.P., Morrissey M.R., Ziprasidone Study Group (1998) Ziprasidone 40 and 120 mg/day in the acute exacerbation of schizophrenia and schizoaffective disorder: a 4-week placebo-controlled trial. *Psychopharmacology*, **140**: 173–184.
164. Goff D.C., Posever T., Herz L., Simmons J., Kletti N., Lapierre K., Wilner K.D., Law C.G., Ko G.N. (1998) An exploratory haloperidol-controlled dose-finding study of ziprasidone in hospitalized patients with schizophrenia or schizoaffective disorder. *J. Clin. Psychopharmacol.*, **18**: 296–304.
165. Arato M., O'Connor R., Meltzer H., Bradbury J. (1997) Ziprasidone: efficacy in the prevention of relapse and in the long-term treatment of negative symptoms of chronic schizophrenia. *Eur. Neuropsychopharmacol.*, 7 (Suppl. 2): 214.
166. Prakash A., Lamb H.M. (1998) Zotepine: a review of its pharmacodynamic and pharmacokinetic properties and therapeutic efficacy in the management of schizophrenia. *CNS Drugs*, **9**: 154–175.
167. Rowley H., Kilpatrick I., Needham P., Heal D. (1998) Elevation of extracellular cortical noradrenaline may contribute to the antidepressant activity of zotepine: an in vivo microdialysis study in freely moving rats. *Neuropharmacology*, **37**: 937–944.
168. Fleischhacker W.W., Barnas C., Stuppäck C.H., Unterweger B., Miller C.H., Hinterhuber H. (1989) Zotepine vs. haloperidol in paranoid schizophrenia: a double-blind trial. *Psychopharmacol. Bull.*, **25**: 97–100.
169. Petit M., Raniwalla J., Tweed J., Leutenegger E., Dollfus S., Kelly F. (1996) A comparison of an atypical and typical antipsychotic, zotepine versus haloperidol in patients with acute exacerbation of schizophrenia: a parallel-group double-blind trial. *Psychopharmacol. Bull.*, **32**: 81–87.
170. Dieterle D.M., Müller-Spahn F., Ackenheil M. (1991) Efficacy and tolerance of zotepine in a double-blind comparison with perazine in schizophrenics. *Fortschr. Neurol. Psychiatrie*, **59** (Suppl. 4): 18–22.
171. Klieser E., Lehmann E., Tegeler J. (1991) Double-blind comparison of 3×75 mg zotepine and 3×4 mg haloperidol in acute schizophrenics. *Fortschr. Neurol. Psychiatrie*, **59** (Suppl. 1): 14–17.
172. Barnas C., Stuppäck C., Miller C., Haring C., Sperner-Unterweger B., Fleischhacker W.W. (1992) Zotepine in the treatment of schizophrenic patients with prevailingly negative symptoms: a double blind trial vs. haloperidol. *Int. Clin. Psychopharmacol.*, **7**: 23–27.

173. Cooper S.L., Butler A., Tweed J., Raniwalla J., Welch C.P. (1997) Zotepine in the prevention of relapse. Poster presented at 6th World Congress of Biological Psychiatry, Nice, 22–27 June.

174. Carpenter W.T. (1996) The treatment of negative symptoms: pharmacological and methodological issues. *Br. J. Psychiatry*, **168** (Suppl. 29): 17–22.

175. Tollefson G.D., Sanger T.M., Beasley C.M. (1997) Negative symptoms: a path analytic approach to a double-blind, placebo- and haloperidol-controlled clinical trial with olanzapine. *Am. J. Psychiatry*, **154**: 466–474.

176. Buchanan R.W., Breier A., Kirkpatrick B., Ball P., Carpenter W.T. Jr. (1998) Positive and negative symptom response to clozapine in schizophrenic patients with and without the deficit syndrome. *Am. J. Psychiatry*, **155**: 751–760.

177. Gardos G., Cole J.O. (1995) The treatment of tardive dyskinesia. In *Psychopharmacology: The Fourth Generation of Progress* (Ed. F. Bloom), pp. 1503–1511. Raven Press, New York.

178. Schultz S.K., Miller D.D., Arndt S., Ziebell S., Gupta S., Andreasen N.C. (1995) Withdrawal-emergent dyskinesia in patients with schizophrenia during antipsychotic discontinuation. *Biol. Psychiatry*, **38**: 713–719.

179. Miller C.H., Fleischhacker W.W. (2000) Managing antipsychotic induced acute and chronic akathisia. *Drug Safety*, **22**: 73–81.

180. Kraepelin E. (1919) *Dementia Praecox and Paraphrenia*. Livingstone, Edinburgh.

181. Caligiuri M.P., Lohr J.B., Jeste D.V. (1993) Parkinsonism in neuroleptic-naïve schizophrenic patients. *Am. J. Psychiatry*, **150**: 1343–1348.

182. Chatterjee A., Chakos M., Koreen A.R., Geisler S., Sheitman B., Woerner M., Kane J.M., Alvir J.M.J., Lieberman M.A. (1995) Prevalence and clinical correlates of extrapyramidal signs and spontaneous dyskinesia in never-medicated schizophrenic patients. *Am. J. Psychiatry*, **152**: 1724–1729.

183. Siris S.G. (1995) Depression and schizophrenia. In *Schizophrenia* (Eds S.R. Hirsch, D.R. Weinberger), pp. 128–145. Blackwell Science, Oxford.

184. Liddle P.F., Barnes T.R.E., Curson D.A., Patel M. (1993) Depression and the experience of psychological deficits in schizophrenia. *Acta Psychiatr. Scand.*, **88**: 243–247.

185. Hausmann A., Fleischhacker W.W. (2002) Differential diagnosis of depressed mood in patients with schizophrenia: a review. *Acta Psychiatr. Scand.*, in press.

186. Goff D.C., Kamal K.M., Sarid-Segal O., Hubbard J.W., Amico E. (1995) A placebo-controlled trial of fluoxetine added to neuroleptics in patients with schizophrenia. *Psychopharmacology*, **117**: 417–423.

187. Hausmann A., Fleischhacker W.W. (2000) Diagnosis and management of depression in schizophrenia. *CNS Drugs*, **14**: 289–299.

188. Roy A. (1990) Relationship between depression and suicidal behaviour in schizophrenia. In *Depression in Schizophrenia* (Ed. L.E. DeLisi). American Psychiatric Press, Washington, DC.

189. Meltzer H.Y., Okayli G. (1995) The reduction of suicidality during clozapine treatment in neuroleptic-resistant schizophrenia: impact on risk–benefit assessment. *Am. J. Psychiatry*, **152**: 183–190.

190. Mortimer A. (1997) Cognitive function in schizophrenia — do neuroleptics make a difference? *Pharmacol. Biochem. Behav.*, **56**: 789–795.

191. Sharma T., Mockler D. (1998) The cognitive efficacy of atypical antipsychotics in schizophrenia. *J. Clin. Psychopharmacol.*, **18** (Suppl. 1): 12S–19S.

192. Goldberg T.E., Gold J.M. (1995) Neurocognitive deficits in schizophrenia. In *Schizophrenia* (Eds S.R. Hirsch, D.R. Weinberger), pp. 146–162. Blackwell, Oxford.

193. Kolakowska T., Williams A.O., Ardern M., Reveley M.A., Jambor K., Gelder M.G., Mandelbrote B.M. (1985) Schizophrenia with good and poor outcome. I. Early clinical features, response to neuroleptics and signs of organic dysfunction. *Br. J. Psychiatry*, **146**: 229–246.
194. Perlick D., Mattis S., Stasny P., Teresi J. (1992) Neuropsychological discriminators of long-term inpatient or outpatient status in chronic schizophrenia. *J. Neuropsychiat. Clin. Neurosci.*, **4**: 428–434.
195. Schall U., Catts S., Chaturvedi S., Liebert B., Redenbach J., Karayanidis F., Ward P. (1998) The effect of clozapine therapy on frontal lobe dysfunction in schizophrenia: neuropsychology and event-related potential measures. *Int. J. Neuropsychopharmacol.*, **1**: 19–29.
196. Green M., Marshall B., Wirshing W., Ames D., Marder S., McGurk S., Kern R.S., Mintz J. (1997) Does risperidone improve verbal working memory in treatment-resistant schizophrenia? *Am. J. Psychiatry*, **154**: 799–804.
197. Cuesta M.J., Peralta V., Zarzuela A. (2001) Effects of olanzapine and other antipsychotics on cognitive function in chronic schizophrenia: a longitudinal study. *Schizophr. Res.*, **48**: 17–28.
198. Harvey P.D., Keefe R.S. (2001) Studies of cognitive change in patients with schizophrenia following novel antipsychotic treatment. *Am. J. Psychiatry*, **158**: 176–1984.
199. Sachs G., Katschnig H. (2001) Kognitive Funktionsstörungen bei schizophrenen Patienten. *Psychiat. Prax.*, **28**: 60–68.
200. Weiss E., Kemmler G., Fleischhacker W.W. (2002) Improvement of cognitive dysfunction after treatment with second-generation antipsychotics. *Arch. Gen. Psychiatry*, **59**: 572–573.
201. Fenton W.S., Blyler C.R., Heinssen R.K. (1997) Determinants of medication compliance in schizophrenia: empirical and clinical findings. *Schizophr. Res.*, **23**: 637–651.
202. Oehl M., Hummer M., Fleischhacker W.W. (2000) Compliance with antipsychotic treatment. *Acta Psychiatr. Scand.*, **102** (Suppl. 407): 83–86.
203. Schwartz D., Wang W., Zeitz L., Goss M.E. (1962) Medication errors made by elderly, chronically ill patients. *Am. J. Public Health*, **52**: 2018–2029.
204. Danion J.M., Neunruther C., Krieger-Finance F., Imbs J.L., Singer L. (1987) Compliance with long-term lithium treatment in major affective disorders. *Pharmacopsychiatry*, **20**: 230–231.
205. Swett J., Noones J. (1989) Factors associated with premature termination from outpatient treatment. *Hosp. Comm. Psychiatry*, **40**: 947–951.
206. Schou M. (1997) The combat of non-compliance during prophylactic lithium treatment. *Acta Psychiatr. Scand.*, **95**: 361–363.
207. Pan P.C., Tantam D. (1989) Clinical characteristics, health beliefs and compliance with maintenance treatment: a comparison between regular and irregular attenders at a depot clinic. *Acta Psychiatr. Scand.*, **79**: 564–570.
208. Drake R.E., Osher F.C., Wallach M.A. (1989) Alcohol use and abuse in schizophrenia. *J. Nerv. Ment. Dis.*, **177**: 408–414.
209. Meise U., Günther V., Gritsch S. (1992) Die Bedeutung der Arzt-Patienten-Beziehung für die Patientencompliance. *Wien Klin Wochenschr*, **104**: 267–271.
210. Ley P., Spelman M.S. (1965) Communication in an outpatient setting. *Br. J. Soc. Clin. Psychol.*, **4**: 114–116.
211. Bäuml J., Kissling W., Buttner P., Pitschell-Walz G., Mayer C., Boerner R., Engel R., Peuker I., Welschehold M. (1993) Informationszentrierte Patienten- und Angehörigengruppen zur Complianceverbesserung bei schizophrenen Psychosen. *Verhaltenstherapie*, **3** (Suppl. 1): 1–96.

212. Blackwell B. (1973) Drug therapy. *N. Engl. J. Med.*, **2**: 249–252.
213. Hoge S.K., Appelbaum P.S., Lawlor T., Beck J.C., Litman R., Greer A., Gutheil T.G., Kaplan E. (1990) A prospective, multicenter study of patients' refusal of antipsychotic medication. *Arch. Gen. Psychiatry*, **47**: 949–956.
214. Silverstone T., Smith G., Goodall E. (1988) Prevalence of obesity in patients receiving depot antipsychotics. *Br. J. Psychiatry*, **153**: 214–217.
215. Pfeiffer W., Kockott G., Fischl B., Schleuning G. (1991) Unerwünschte Wirkungen psychopharmakologischer Langzeittherapie auf die sexuellen Funktionen. *Psychiatr. Prax.*, **18**: 92–98.
216. Buchanan A. (1992) A two-year prospective study of treatment compliance in patients with schizophrenia. *Psychol. Med.*, **22**: 787–797.
217. Hummer M., Kemmler G., Kurz M., Kurzthaler I., Oberbauer H., Fleischhacker W.W. (1999) Sexual disturbances during clozapine and haloperidol treatment. *Am. J. Psychiatry*, **156**: 631–633.
218. Willcox D.R.C., Gillan R., Hare E.H. (1965) Do psychiatric outpatients take their drugs? *Br. Med. J.*, **2**: 790–792.
219. Kemp R., Kirov G., Everitt B., Hayward P., David A. (1998) Randomised controlled trial of compliance therapy. *Br. J. Psychiatry*, **172**: 413–419.
220. Eckman T.A., Liberman R.P., Phipps C.C., Blair K.E. (1990) Teaching medication management skills to schizophrenic patients. *J. Clin. Psychopharmacol.*, **10**: 33–38.

Commentaries

2.1
Pharmacotherapy of Psychotic Disorders: A Perspective on Current Developments

Ross J. Baldessarini[1]

The broad and compelling clinical utility of antipsychotic agents led to revolutionary changes in modern psychiatry [1]. They are highly effective, though essentially palliative, across virtually the entire spectrum of syndromes marked by severe agitation with psychotic features, including organic mental disorders and major affective syndromes as well as schizophrenia and other delusional, brief, and other idiopathic psychotic syndromes [2, 3]. Over 95% of short-term, controlled efficacy trials of antipsychotics show statistical superiority to placebos, though response rates and levels of individual improvement are more limited than such results may suggest [2, 3]. Moreover, most trials of standard neuroleptics involved patients diagnosed with schizophrenia by broad criteria, further encouraging exaggerated expectations of putative "antischizophrenia" drugs [3, 4].

Antipsychotic effectiveness is clearest in acute syndromes marked by agitation with psychotic abnormalities of thought and perception. Lack of motivation and capacity for independent living remain unsolved challenges in schizophrenia, even with newer treatments [3–5]. Only a minority of patients meeting contemporary diagnostic criteria for schizophrenia attain full early remission or virtual absence of psychotic symptoms, and later functional recovery [3–5]. Since affective psychotic disorders are more prevalent than schizophrenia, and other psychotic conditions are common, the actual and potential utility of antipsychotic therapy is arguably much greater in conditions other than schizophrenia [5, 6].

As antipsychotic experimental therapeutics grows in complexity [3], it is increasingly left to the pharmaceutical industry, whose licensing–marketing aims are much narrower than the field requires for adequate judgements about long-term cost–benefit relationships. Contemporary trials include too many unrepresentative samples of poorly treatment-responsive, chronic

[1]Mailman Research Center, McLean Hospital, 115 Mill Street, Belmont, MA 02178-9106, USA

TABLE 1 Characteristics of modern antipsychotic agents

Agent	Doses (mg/day)			Advantages	Disadvantages
	Typical	Extreme	Injectable		
Clozapine	150–450	12.5–900	No	Very low EPS and TD risk	Agranulocytosis (even with monitoring)
				Superior efficacy	Severe weight gain and secondary health risks
				Antiaggressive	New-onset diabetes mellitus
				Probably antisuicidal	Seizures (dose-dependent risk)
				Improves cognition	Anticholinergic (risk of delirium)
				May be mood-stabilizing	Oral only; short-acting
				Sedating	Excessive sedation, hypotension
				Close monitoring required	WBC costly, inconvenient
				Probably cost-effective	Very expensive
				Tolerated in Parkinson's disease	May worsen obsessions/compulsions
					High risk of withdrawal relapse
Olanzapine	5–15	2.5–30	Experimental	Low EPS and TD risk	Severe weight gain
				Probably antimanic	May induce mania
				Sedating	Excessive sedation
					Possible new-onset diabetes mellitus
					Some EPS and TD risk
					Limited tolerability in Parkinson's disease
					Oral only
					Very limited dose range
					Relatively expensive
					Long-term data limited

continues overleaf

TABLE 1 (continued)

Agent	Doses (mg/day)			Advantages	Disadvantages
	Typical	Extreme	Injectable		
Quetiapine	250–500	50–750	No	Very low EPS and TD risk Sedating Possibly antimanic	Cataract risk Excessive sedation Relatively expensive Long-term data very limited
Risperidone	2–8	0.25–16	Proposed	Moderate EPS risk Probably antimanic	Dose-dependent EPS; some TD risk May induce mania NMS, rhabdomyolysis Potentially severe hyperprolactinaemia Contraindicated with breast cancer Poorly tolerated in Parkinson's disease Hypotension with rapid dosing Need for slow dosing Limited dose range Oral only Relatively expensive Long-term data limited

EPS, extrapyramidal symptoms; NMS, neuroleptic malignant syndrome; TD, tardive dyskinesia; WBC, white blood cell count. Short-term intramuscular injections of olanzapine have been used experimentally, and it may be possible to develop long-acting fatty-acid ester prodrug derivatives of pharmacologically active 9-hydroxy-risperidone. Clinical development of sertindole and ziprasidone was recently suspended due to their association with cardiac depressant effects (with prolonged QT interval in the electrocardiogram), with presumed risk of tachyarrhythmias.

patients followed at specialized clinics. Long-term assessments of clinically meaningful outcomes and functional recovery in broader clinical samples are uncommon, as are controlled evaluations of synergistic interactions of antipsychotic medication with cost-effective rehabilitation [3, 5]. Under-appreciated drug carryover, and discontinuation-associated effects of interrupting ongoing treatment now routinely confound studies of psychosis [7, 8]. Most "schizophrenic" patients tolerating 6 months without medication (c. 50%) have remained stable thereafter, suggesting high levels of diagnostic or clinical heterogeneity that further obscure requirements for long-term treatment [8]. Hopes that newer antipsychotics may be superior in effectiveness as well as better tolerated than older neuroleptics are yet unproved, with the notable exception of clozapine [9].

Finally, psychiatry is now strongly influenced by aggressive marketing of newer antipsychotics, and much more independent research is required to assess their long-term cost–benefit relationships. Such drugs (Table 1) have convincing short-term efficacy over a placebo and comparable average benefits to standard neuroleptics. Clozapine, olanzapine, quetiapine and risperidone have reduced (but not eliminated) risks of acute extrapyramidal symptoms and tardive dyskinesia, with apparently improved acceptance by both patients and clinicians. However, they may be insufficient alone in acute psychoses, are often supplemented with standard neuroleptics or potent sedatives, currently lack injectable or long-acting forms, and are expensive. They also vary in risks of producing untoward metabolic effects, including hyperprolactinaemia, new-onset diabetes, and sometimes severe weight gain, presumably with increased risks of long-term adverse health consequences. Finally, the putative superior safety and tolerability of newer antipsychotics against conservative, carefully individualized use of standard neuroleptics remains to be proved [10].

ACKNOWLEDGEMENTS

Supported, in part, by NIH career investigator award MH-47370, a grant from the Bruce J. Anderson Foundation, and by the Mailman Research Center Private Donors Neuropharmacology Research Fund.

REFERENCES

1. Baldessarini R.J. (1999) Fifty years of biomedical psychiatry and psychopharmacology in America. In *50 Years of American Psychiatry: Celebrating the 150th Anniversary of the Founding of the American Psychiatric Association.* (Eds R. Menninger, J. Nemiah). American Psychiatric Press, Washington, DC.
2. Baldessarini R.J., Fleischhacker W., Sperk G. (1991) *Pharmakotherapie in der Psychiatrie.* Thieme, Stuttgart.

3. Baldessarini R.J. (1996) Drugs and the treatment of psychiatric disorders. In *Goodman and Gilman's The Pharmacological Basis of Therapeutics* (Eds J.G. Hardman, L.E. Limbird, P.B. Molinoff, R.W. Ruddon, A.G. Gilman), pp. 399–459. McGraw-Hill, New York.

4. Hegarty J.D., Baldessarini R.J., Tohen M., Waternaux C.M., Oepen G. (1994) One hundred years of schizophrenia: a meta-analysis of the outcome literature. *Am. J. Psychiatry*, **151**: 1409–1416.

5. Tohen M., Hennen J., Zarate C.M. Jr, Baldessarini R.J., Strakowski S.M., Stoll A.L., Faedda G.L., Suppes T., Gebre-Medhin P., Cohen B.M. (2000) Two-year syndromal and functional recovery in 219 cases of first-episode major affective disorders with psychotic features. *Am. J. Psychiatry*, **157**: 220–228.

6. Kessler R.C., McGonagle K.A., Zhao S., Nelson C.B., Hughes M., Eshelman S., Wittchen H.-U., Kendler K.S. (1994) Lifetime and 12-month prevalence of DSM-III-R psychiatric disorders in the US: results from the National Comorbidity Study. *Arch. Gen. Psychiatry*, **51**: 8–19.

7. Cohen B.M., Tsuneizumi T., Baldessarini R.J., Campbell A., Babb S. (1992) Differences between antipsychotic drugs in persistence of brain levels and behavioral effects. *Psychopharmacology*, **108**: 338–344.

8. Viguera A.C., Baldessarini R.J., Hegarty J.M., Van Kammen D., Tohen M. (1997) Risk of discontinuing maintenance medication in schizophrenia. *Arch. Gen. Psychiatry*, **54**: 49–55.

9. Baldessarini R.J., Frankenburg F.R. (1991) Clozapine—a novel antipsychotic agent. *N. Engl. J. Med.*, **324**: 746–754.

10. Baldessarini R.J., Cohen B.M., Teicher M.H. (1988) Significance of neuroleptic dose and plasma level in the pharmacological treatment of psychoses. *Arch. Gen. Psychiatry*, **45**: 79–91.

2.2

Pharmacotherapy of Schizophrenia: Gaps in our Knowledge

John Kane[1]

The introduction of a new generation of antipsychotic medications is a very welcome development in the treatment of schizophrenia (and other psychotic disorders). I agree with Prof. Fleischhacker that the term "atypical" has outlived its usefulness [1]. The criteria which have generally been used to define atypicality (e.g. less frequent extrapyramidal side effects (EPS) and/or superior efficacy for positive and/or negative symptoms) are so far quantitative rather than qualitative. The term atypical has no real scientific relevance as the mechanism(s) responsible for the various differences have not been established.

The new generation drugs do have important advantages in terms of reduced adverse reactions, particularly neurologic side effects such as akathisia and parkinsonism. So far the results are encouraging with respect to

[1]*Long Island Jewish Medical Center, Hillside Hospital, Glen Oaks, NY 11004, USA*

tardive dyskinesia (TD), but those data are still limited. We have been impressed by the relationship between early occurring EPS and the subsequent development of TD [2]. Therefore, the clear reduction in EPS seen with the new generation drugs should hopefully bode well for a reduction in TD.

There are a number of areas where the new drugs have yet to be fully tested which will ultimately determine or clarify their potential advantages. It is hoped that a reduction in adverse effects will lead to enhanced compliance, but as Fleischhacker points out this has not been consistently established and certainly needs to be studied with the new generation drugs. The problem of weight gain could prove to be an important factor in long-term compliance. Clearly, rates of non-compliance contribute to high rates of relapse among persons with schizophrenia. A substantial proportion of patients (approximately 20% in one year) relapse even when receiving long-acting, depot injections [3]. This would suggest that antipsychotic prophylaxis (at least with conventional medications) is far from 100% effective. Whether or not the new generation drugs can improve outcome in this respect remains to be seen. One important gap in our knowledge, even with conventional drugs, is what are the best strategies for managing patients who "break through" maintenance medication? Many clinicians will increase dosage in such individuals, but there are no data supporting the value of this approach. Another critical gap in our knowledge is in the context of acute treatment. When and by what criteria should an initial trial be abandoned or modified, and to what other medication(s) should patients be switched? We now require a whole new generation of studies involving dosage escalation, adjunctive treatments and switching to various other medications to inform clinical practice. Ironically, none of these issues were well studied even after many years of use of conventional antipsychotic medications.

Considerable appropriate attention is being focused on cognitive functioning in schizophrenia. Clearly this aspect of the illness does contribute considerably to the functional deficits and disability associated with this disease. However, will the effects of new generation antipsychotic drugs be of sufficient magnitude to impact functional outcome? Ultimately the question regarding cognitive functioning is but one dimension of the larger issue as to how far have we advanced treatment across the full range of substantive measures of outcome.

As new treatments emerge and advantages are documented, a continuing challenge will be the application of this new knowledge in clinical practice. Increasingly, obstacles in this context are being studied with the realization that public health issues are far more complex than proving the value of a specific treatment in a clinical trial.

Currently in our field there are striking examples of the underutilization of specific treatments with clear advantages. As Fleischhacker points out, clozapine is the only drug so far with established efficacy in treatment of refractory patients, yet in many countries around the world (including the USA) clozapine is significantly underutilized.

Similarly, despite proven advantages for depot drugs in preventing non-compliance (or at least making detection straightforward) [4], these medications are also used far less than they should be. Though now there is a dilemma in choosing between a conventional depot drug and a new generation oral medication, hopefully long-acting preparations of the newer drugs will become available soon.

We all face an enormous challenge of ensuring that treatment advances can be applied on the broadest possible scale.

REFERENCES

1. Kane J.M. (1997) What makes an antipsychotic atypical? CNS Drugs, 7: 347–348.
2. Saltz B.L., Woerner M.G., Kane J.M., Lieberman J.A., Alfir J.A., Bergman K.J., Blank K., Koblenzer J., Kahamer K. (1991) Prospective study of tardive dyskinesia incidence in the elderly. JAMA, 266: 2402–2406.
3. Kane J.M. (1996) Schizophrenia. N. Engl. J. Med., 334: 34–41.
4. Glazer W.M., Kane J.M. (1992) Depot neuroleptic therapy: an underutilized treatment option. J. Clin. Psychiatry, 53: 426–433.

2.3
Atypical Antipsychotic Drugs and Schizophrenia

Herbert Y. Meltzer[1]

Professor Fleischhacker provides an excellent overview of the current approach to the use of antipsychotic drugs in the treatment of schizophrenia. We agree that clozapine, risperidone, olanzapine and quetiapine have sparked a multifaceted revolution in current thinking and practice with regard to the treatment of this illness as well as other disorders in which antipsychotic drugs have an important role. There is, however, disagreement between Fleischhacker and me as to whether to refer to the drugs listed above as "atypical" antipsychotics, which Fleischhacker feels has no clear definition and therefore he suggests "novel" or "second generation" as alternatives. As discussed in detail elsewhere [1], there has been a very clear definition of atypicality from its first introduction by Hippius and Angst to describe the lack of extrapyramidal side effects (EPS) of clozapine in animal models and man. Preclinical pharmacologists have adhered to this definition, while clinical

[1]Department of Psychiatry, Vanderbilt University School of Medicine, 1601 23rd Avenue South, Nashville, TN 37212, USA

investigators have generally confused the issue by introducing other criteria of atypicality such as improvement in negative symptoms. Terms like novel or new as alternatives are unsatisfactory, because they are quickly outdated by the latest additions to the armamentarium. In which generation(s) of antipsychotic drugs should clozapine and ziprasidone, which are 30 years apart in their introduction, be considered? I also suggest that the term "typical" rather than "traditional" be retained for haloperidol-type agents. I am concerned that conservative clinicians may be overly reluctant to break with tradition! I would settle for "old-fashioned" or tardive-dyskinesia-producing antipsychotics as an alternative, to get the appropriate message across.

I am generally in agreement with the precepts and practice of the algorithm for treatment choices which Fleischhacker recommends, with some important differences. The issue of whether patients who have a "good response" to typical neuroleptics should be switched to an atypical antipsychotic rests on what is a good response. All too many clinicians think a good response is control of positive symptoms and a modicum of social function, ignoring cognitive deficits, poor work and sexual function, significant negative symptoms, and increasing risk of tardive dyskinesia with ageing. Only patients with the equivalent of Global Assessment of Functioning Scale (GAFS) scores ±70 might be considered for continuation with the typical neuroleptics in my view, and only after the risk of tardive dyskinesia has been evaluated. The chances of doing better with one or more of the atypicals is sufficiently high that substitution of the latter in these "good responders" should be recommended.

The recommendations that are made for patients who do not respond adequately to typical antipsychotics or to one of the non-clozapine atypicals are confusing. It is suggested that after a single trial of a typical neuroleptic, patients should be treated with clozapine or perhaps one of the other atypical antipsychotic drugs. Most commonly, it is recommended that one, but no more than one, of the non-clozapine atypicals be tried before clozapine [2]. It would have been useful to discuss explicitly what happens when there is a failure to respond adequately to one of the atypical antipsychotic drugs. I strongly recommend that the next agent be clozapine rather than another kind of atypical, unless the issue has been tolerability.

This raises the issue of the perception of clozapine by clinicians — a perception that may be transmitted to patients — that the drug is sufficiently dangerous to be withheld until all other steps have been exhausted. The risk of clozapine is in fact minimal, with about 1 in 10000 dying from agranulocytosis [3]. At the time of writing, it appears that clozapine, and only clozapine, reduces the risk of suicide in schizophrenia, which is as high as 10% lifetime [4]. The other risks of clozapine are not trivial, but the chances of recovery to a meaningful extent would seem to most rational observers to warrant risking agranulocytosis [5]. The proportion of patients who are highly resistant to typical neuroleptic drugs is about 30%, but only about 5% are receiving clozapine treatment.

My view of the discrepancy between dosage of clozapine in Europe and the USA is that a higher proportion of more recent onset, non-treatment-resistant schizophrenic patients are being treated with clozapine in Europe. Both factors lead to lower dosage of clozapine in my experience. This means even fewer of the more genuinely treatment-resistant patients are receiving clozapine or even any other of the atypical agents.

Although we have made great strides in the pharmacotherapy of schizophrenia in recent years and enabled perhaps as many as 15% of patients to achieve levels of recovery that were unimaginable with typical neuroleptic drugs, the majority of patients with schizophrenia remain moderately-severely disabled. To go beyond this requires at least the following: optimal utilization of current therapies from the first episode on; possible identification of patients in the prodrome, and initiation of treatment with these agents before psychosis and cognitive deterioration emerges; and development of more effective antischizophrenic, as differentiated from antipsychotic, agents.

REFERENCES

1. Meltzer H.Y. (1995) The concept of atypical antipsychotics. In *Advances in the Neurobiology of Schizophrenia* (Eds J.A. den Boer, H.G.M. Westenberg, H.M. van Praag), pp. 265–273. Wiley, Chichester.
2. Collaborative Working Group (1998) Measuring outcome in schizophrenia: differences among the atypical antipsychotics. *J. Clin. Psychiatry*, **59** (Suppl. 12): 3–9.
3. Alvir J.M.J., Lieberman J.A., Saffererman A.Z., Schwimmer K.L., Schaaaf H.A. (1993) Clozapine-induced agranulocytosis: incidence and risk factors in the United States. *N. Engl. J. Med.*, **329**: 161–167.
4. Meltzer H.Y., Okayli G. (1995) The reduction of suicidality during clozapine treatment in neuroleptic-resistant schizophrenia: impact on risk–benefit assessment. *Am. J. Psychiatry*, **152**: 183–190.
5. Meltzer H.Y. (1997) Treatment-resistant schizophrenia: the role of clozapine. *Curr. Med. Res. Opinion*, **14**: 1–20.

2.4

Compliance Issues and the New Antipsychotics

Thomas R. E. Barnes[1]

In his comprehensive review of the pharmacotherapy of schizophrenic disorders, Prof. Fleischhacker refers to the increasingly robust association between early pharmacological intervention and long-term outcome. Delay

[1] *Department of Clinical Psychiatry, Imperial College School of Medicine, London W6 8RP, UK*

in initiating antipsychotic treatment, such that there is a relatively prolonged period of unchecked psychosis, has been related to poor response to medication, and a poorer long-term outcome in terms of negative symptoms, social functioning and likelihood of relapse [1]. Whatever the explanation for this association, it raises the importance of several of the other issues addressed in the review related to ensuring adherence to maintenance drug treatment. Specifically, one implication is that, even after starting medication, extended episodes of active psychosis related to partial or complete non-compliance with medication might also augur a poor outcome. If this were so, then it becomes critical that prescribing clinicians choose an appropriate and well-tolerated antipsychotic drug to treat schizophrenia during the first episode, and in the early stages of the illness, in order to minimize compliance problems. Prof. Fleischhacker argues for the novel antipsychotics to be first-line treatment in such patients (excepting clozapine, because of its restricted licensed indications). Nevertheless, it should be borne in mind that while a better side-effect profile has been claimed for these newer drugs (such as clozapine, risperidone, olanzapine, amisulpride, ziprasidone and zotepine) compared with conventional drugs, significantly improved compliance in the long term has yet to be convincingly demonstrated.

Compliance is a complex phenomenon, and it may be simplistic to assume that the lower incidence of extrapyramidal side effects (as well as the associated reduction in the requirement for antiparkinsonian agents), clearly established for the newer drugs, will necessarily translate into better adherence to the medication regime. Studies examining the association between extrapyramidal side effects and compliance have yielded discrepant findings, which may partly reflect whether an attempt was made to measure the subjective burden of these side effects. For example, Fleischhacker et al [2] reported a lack of concordance between objectively-rated extrapyramidal symptoms and compliance with antipsychotic medication. However, the presence of akathisia and subjective dysphoria, side effects diagnosed by eliciting patients' subjective experience, has been found to predict future non-compliance [3–5]. Further, the influence of non-neurological problems on compliance may have been underestimated. Side effects such as sedation and weight gain, both of which are not uncommon with some of the newer drugs, have been shown to adversely affect medication compliance [6].

Speculating further, compliance may also be a relevant variable when considering the evidence for a lower risk of tardive dyskinesia in patients taking particular atypical antipsychotics [7, 8], particularly in those clinical trials directly comparing a newer drug with a conventional antipsychotic [9]. If tablet taking were more erratic in the patients taking the conventional drug, then there would be a greater likelihood of withdrawal dyskinesia being observed in that group at some point during the study period. Also, interruptions in treatment have emerged as a possible risk factor for the development of tardive dyskinesia [10].

Ultimately, superiority for the newer antipsychotics needs to be demonstrated in terms of enhanced compliance and greater relapse prevention than the conventional drugs. Further, prescribing clinicians want to know the relative liability for a range of non-neurological side effects across all the new drugs. This information can only be provided by direct comparisons between the newer drugs in so-called "head-to-head" clinical studies. Currently, knowledge about such side effects with the new antipsychotics comes predominantly from trials that have tested only one new drug, often against a conventional antipsychotic. That the conventional comparator has most commonly been haloperidol in relatively high doses, often up to 20 mg a day, makes the apparent superiority of the side effect profile with the newer drugs difficult to interpret. Further, the reported incidence of any individual side effect with a particular drug tends to vary between studies, depending on the nature of the rating instrument and stringency of the criteria used to identify it, as well as the characteristics of the patient sample.

While the full clinical impact of these newer drugs awaits evaluation, clinicians may sometimes find it difficult to decide whether or not to recommend to a relatively stable patient a change from depot antipsychotic medication to a newer drug because of a disappointing clinical response or some intolerance of adverse effects. The advantage of avoiding covert non-compliance with the depot injection will be lost by switching to the newer, oral drug. Thus, there is the possibility that unreliable tablet-taking will go unnoticed, and lead to an increased risk of psychotic relapse. However, this concern needs to be balanced against the possibility of a better therapeutic response and improved tolerability.

Professor Fleischhacker notes that the patients entering clinical trials are highly selected, which limits the generalizability of the findings to clinical practice. This may be particularly true in respect of compliance with pharmacotherapy. Bowen and Barnes [11] studied a sample of patients with schizophrenia who were identified as eligible for a placebo-controlled study of an antipsychotic preparation. Those consenting to participate in the study had a history of a significantly greater number of psychiatric hospital admissions, were receiving higher doses of antipsychotic medication and exhibited more neurological side effects than those who declined to participate, although there was no difference in the overall severity of illness between the two groups. Perhaps most critically, over the subsequent 9 months, those not consenting to take part in the study were significantly less compliant with medication and general treatment plans, as well as less likely to consent to further research participation. This suggests a relatively consistent link between consent to research and compliance with treatment.

REFERENCES

1. McGlashan T. (1996) Early detection and intervention of schizophrenia: research. *Schizophr. Bull.*, **22**: 327–345.
2. Fleischhacker W.W., Meise U., Gunther V., Kurz M. (1994) Compliance with antipsychotic drug treatment: influence of side effects. *Acta Psychiatr. Scand.*, **89** (Suppl. 382): 11–15.
3. Van Putten T. (1974) Why do schizophrenic patients refuse to take their drugs? *Arch. Gen. Psychiatry*, **31**: 67–72.
4. Van Putten T., May P.R.A., Marder S.R., Wittmann L.A. (1981) Subjective response to antipsychotic drugs. *Arch. Gen. Psychiatry*, **38**: 187–190.
5. Awad A.G., Hogan T.P. (1994) Subjective response to neuroleptics and the quality of life: implications for treatment outcome. *Acta Psychiatr. Scand.*, **89** (Suppl. 380): 27–32.
6. Goff D.C., Shader R.J. (1995) Non-neurological side effects of antipsychotic agents. In *Schizophrenia* (Eds S.R. Hirsch, D.R. Weinberger), pp. 566–584. Blackwell, Oxford.
7. Umbricht D., Kane J.M. (1996) Medical complications of new antipsychotic drugs. *Schizophr. Bull.*, **22**: 475–483.
8. Gutierrez-Esteinou R., Grebb J.A. (1997) Risperidone: an analysis of the first three years in general use. *Int. J. Clin. Psychopharmacol.*, **12** (Suppl. 4): 3–10.
9. Tollefson G.D., Beasley C.M., Tamura R.N., Tran P.V., Potvine J.H. (1997) Blind, controlled trial long-term study of the comparative incidence of treatment emergent tardive dyskinesia with olanzapine or haloperidol. *Am. J. Psychiatry*, **154**: 1248–1254.
10. Van Harten P.N., Hoek H.W., Matroos G.E., Koeter M., Kahn R.S. (1998) Intermittent neuroleptic treatment and risk for tardive dyskinesia: Curacao Extrapyramidal Syndromes Study III. *Am. J. Psychiatry*, **155**: 565–567.
11. Bowen J.T., Barnes T.R.E. (1994) The clinical characteristics of schizophrenic patients consenting or not consenting to a placebo controlled trial of antipsychotic medication. *Hum. Psychopharmacol.*, **9**: 423–433.

2.5

Schizophrenia and Second-generation Antipsychotics: Mechanistic Implications and Potential for Early Intervention

John L. Waddington[1] and John F. Quinn[1]

There is little doubt as to how the renaissance of clozapine has impacted on our perspectives of antipsychotic medication: its influence has been profound at multiple levels, from mechanistic underpinnings at the neuronal level, through concepts of efficacy and adverse effects, to broader considerations of antipsychotic drug use.

[1]*Department of Clinical Pharmacology, Royal College of Surgeons in Ireland, 123 St Stephen's Green, Dublin 2, Ireland*

At a mechanistic level, clozapine has so extensive a range of pharmacological actions, at multiple levels of neuronal function, as to seriously confound isolation of its essential properties; hence this breadth to its range of actions can be considered either as a rich reservoir for theorizing on or, alternatively, extremely muddy waters in which to fish for the substrate(s) of its advantageous profile [1]. In terms of the classical D_2 dopamine receptor blockade hypothesis of neuroleptic drug action, attention now extends to antagonism of a broader family of D_2-like ($D_{2/3/4}$) receptors in antipsychotic activity. While it has been proposed that clozapine occupies a lower percentage of brain D_2 receptors than do typical antipsychotics, there are counter-arguments that higher, more typical occupancies are attained empirically and theoretically [2] or that D_2 occupancy in important extrastriatal regions such as the temporal cortex may materially exceed that evident in more conventional basal ganglia estimates [3]. However, several of these counter-arguments require experimental replication or empirical support. The extent to which the modest preference of clozapine for D_4 over D_2 receptors might be relevant is not yet clear [2, 3]. While an initial study of the selective D_4 antagonist L-745 870 indicates a lack of antipsychotic activity, the ongoing development of a range of additional D_4 antagonists (e.g. CP-293 019; PD-172 760; PNU-101 387; RO61-6270) should provide further insight into these critical issues.

It is not yet clear whether a common action or profile of actions is shared by clozapine and subsequent novel antipsychotics (amisulpride, olanzapine, quetiapine, risperidone, sertindole, ziprasidone, zotepine), or whether diverse actions can underpin similar therapeutic profiles [1]. One of the most widely considered unifying models for such agents is variable D_2 antagonism combined with more prominent 5-HT$_{2A}$ antagonist activity. However, it should be noted that chlorpromazine is capable of giving almost complete occupancy of cortical 5-HT$_{2A}$ receptors, like clozapine, olanzapine and risperidone, with high occupancy of basal ganglia D_2 receptors, like olanzapine and risperidone; conversely, amisulpride occupies D_2 receptors in the absence of 5-HT$_{2A}$ receptor occupancy [4]. On this basis, it is difficult to equate combined D_2/5-HT$_2$ antagonism with any particular therapeutic profile. However, initial clinical studies with the selective 5-HT$_{2A}$ antagonist MDL 100 907 appear provocative.

The descriptor "atypical" is widely applied to clozapine and subsequent novel antipsychotics, but such terminology may not be helpful. While it has at its core reduced liability to induce extrapyramidal side effects (EPS), clozapine confirms that it is now realistic to have yet higher aspirations for new agents; these include broader domains of superior efficacy, improved adverse effect profiles beyond EPS liability, and pharmacoeconomic considerations [1, 5]. The balance between these various advantages (and liabilities) in their overall profiles appears to differ among individual agents; hence the descriptor "second generation" antipsychotics, with specification of individual profiles, may be more appropriate [6]. Availability of depot and other parenteral preparations would be a further advantage, particularly in the context of non-compliant and hostile/aggressive patients where the absence of acute sedative effects might pose management problems. The optimal mode of transition between conventional and novel antipsychotics remains to be defined.

There is an increasing body of evidence that intervention with antipsychotics at the earliest signs of psychotic disturbance can lead to improved long-term outcome; a fundamental challenge is the extent to which "second generation" antipsychotics might reduce physician concerns over possible consequences of early intervention and favour improved patient compliance over this crucial phase of illness [1, 7]. Additionally, might they allow safer intervention with medication at a yet earlier, prodromal phase of the illness, given the increased likelihood of then treating behavioural states which do not prove to be the harbingers of a psychotic process?

ACKNOWLEDGEMENTS

The authors' studies are supported by the Stanley Foundation.

REFERENCES

1. Waddington J.L., Scully P.J., O'Callaghan E. (1997) The new antipsychotics and their potential for early intervention in schizophrenia. *Schizophr. Res.*, **28**: 207–222.
2. Seeman P., Tallerico T. (1998) Antipsychotic drugs which elicit little or no Parkinsonism bind more loosely than dopamine to brain D2 receptors, yet occupy high levels of these receptors. *Mol. Psychiatry*, **3**: 123–134.
3. Pilowsky L.S., Mulligan R.S., Acton P.D., Ell P.J., Costa D.C., Kerwin R.W. (1997) Limbic selectivity of clozapine. *Lancet*, **350**: 490–491.
4. Trichard C., Palliere-Martinot M.-L., Attar-Levy D., Recassens C., Monnet F., Martinot J.-L. (1998) Binding of antipsychotic drugs to cortical 5-HT$_{2A}$ receptors; a PET study of chlorpromazine, clozapine and amisulpride in schizophrenic patients. *Am. J. Psychiatry*, **155**: 505–508.
5. Waddington J.L., O'Callaghan E. (1997) What makes an antipsychotic "atypical"? Conserving the definition. *CNS Drugs*, **7**: 341–346.
6. Kane J.M. (1997) Commentary on "What makes an antipsychotic atypical?" *CNS Drugs*, **7**: 347–348.
7. Waddington J.L., Buckley P.F., Scully P.J., Lane A., O'Callaghan E., Larkin C, (1998) Course of psychopathology, cognition and neurological abnormality in schizophrenia: developmental origins and amelioration by antipsychotics? *J. Psychiatr. Res.*, **32**: 179–189.

2.6
Dose and Duration of Antipsychotic Treatment: Key Variables, Critical Uncertainties
Guy M. Goodwin[1]

The classical antipsychotics have traditionally imposed such severe side effects on patients that their use was always accompanied by the suspicion that the benefits were close to being outweighed by the costs. By offering us new choices that reduce the burden of side effects, the recent rush to market of a whole range of new antipsychotics must be welcomed. At the same time, the evaluation of the relative efficacy and effectiveness of these novel drugs poses new problems and sharpens the focus on older ones.

Atypical antipsychotics are defined from animal screens as less likely dose for dose to produce catalepsy, believed to be the animal equivalent of extrapyramidal motor side effects (EPS), while retaining activity against, for example, amphetamine actions that may model psychosis. This desirable pharmacology has translated into claims that newer compounds offer acute antipsychotic action without EPS. Indeed, the adjective "atypical" implies a qualitative advance. The proper quantitative question of any antipsychotic is "how large is the therapeutic ratio between antipsychotic action and unacceptable motor side effects?"

There is a supplementary question. Have the classical neuroleptics been used at doses unnecessarily high to produce antipsychotic action? A quantitative review of 22 published trials demonstrated that no clinical improvement was found above doses equivalent to 375 mg of chlorpromazine, while a significant increase in adverse reactions was noticed [1]. It appears that psychiatrists tend to use antipsychotics at too high a dose [2]. Often this may be the consequence of trying to use one drug to achieve two acute ends: antipsychotic action and sedation. The older term "major tranquillizer" enshrined the concept, in fact. There is now an increasing practice based on anecdotal clinical experience, rather than clinical trials, to use lower doses of classical antipsychotic drugs in combination with selectively sedative compounds like benzodiazepines. The critical question is whether the advantages of the new drugs can to some extent be obtained by sticking to lower doses of classical neuroleptics. On this view, instead of immediately declaring "novel atypicals" to be first line, a rational pharmacology could start with low doses of classical antipsychotics and escalate to more expensive options when increases in dose, required to produce antipsychotic action, produce unacceptable side effects [3].

Acute treatment has uncertain short-term objectives. What we usually know about any intervention is how fast a rating scale score changes (with the

[1]University of Oxford, Department of Psychiatry, The Warneford Hospital, Oxford, OX3 7JX, UK

confound of "last observations carried forward"). However, the complexity of the psychotic syndrome, the possibility that we should be targeting individual symptoms or symptom dimensions, perhaps with different drugs, and more empirical questions relating to broader objectives of clinical management, are largely unaddressed by the existing evidence. Ultimately one wishes to see resolution of psychosis and return to a range of activities of daily living. Conventional measures fail to address outcomes the patient and carers may prioritize for the effectiveness of treatment. In an era when evidence-based patient choice may be increasingly important, this is unacceptable. Furthermore, the clinician does not know when the patient can be expected to leave hospital, require reduced nursing or profit from rehabilitation.

Schizophrenia is, par excellence, a chronic disease and we should be clear how long to offer treatment and which treatment to offer. The evidence favouring an effect of neuroleptics on relapse and recurrence of illness over a 1–2 year interval is persuasive. Nevertheless, some of this evidence is related to the rapid relapse seen on drug withdrawal. A parallel example in the treatment of bipolar disorder may be instructive. There, mania after lithium withdrawal has inflated the apparent efficacy of the drug in discontinuation designs, and presents particular clinical dangers in poorly compliant clinic populations [4]. The same considerations may well apply in schizophrenia. So, there is real uncertainty about the best duration of treatment to advise. Currently, we are stuck with the formula that what gets you well may keep you well and how long we should be treating for is left vague. We should be initiating really large trials, randomizing patients to different duration of intended treatment and incorporating simple outcomes as endpoints, following the precedent from general medicine [5].

We remain even more uncertain about the relative effectiveness of different drugs to influence the course of the illness. The apparently greater efficacy of clozapine, in particular, ought eventually to prompt a long-term pragmatic trial to establish the fact either for clozapine or a safer alternative.

REFERENCES

1. Bollini P., Pampallona S., Orza M.J., Adams M.E., Chalmers T.C. (1994) The antipsychotic drugs: is more worse? A meta-analysis of the published randomized control trials. *Psychol. Med.*, **24**: 307–316.
2. Baldessarini R.J., Cohen B.M., Teicher M.H. (1988) Significance of neuroleptic dose and plasma level in the pharmacological treatment of psychoses. *Arch. Gen. Psychiatry*, **45**: 79–91.
3. Royal College of Psychiatrists. (2000) Management of Schizophrenia, Part I: Pharmacological Treatments.

4.   Goodwin G.M. (1994) Recurrence of mania after lithium withdrawal: implications for the use of lithium in the treatment of bipolar affective disorder. *Br. J. Psychiatry*, **164**: 149–152.
5.   Peto R., Collins R., Gray R. (1995) Large-scale randomized evidence: large, simple trials and overviews of trials. *J. Clin. Epidemiol.*, **48**: 23–40.

2.7
Dosing Problems of Classical Neuroleptics and the Relevance of Novel/Atypical Antipsychotics in the Pharmacotherapy of Schizophrenic Disorders

Hans-Jürgen Möller[1]

While there is growing consensus that a high dose approach, applying about 10-fold the standard dose, does not seem to be beneficial, even in most cases of therapy-resistant schizophrenics, the question of whether a comparatively low dose approach is preferable to a medium range of dosing in the therapy of acute schizophrenic episodes does not seem to be definitely answered. Especially the frequently hypothesized problem of more extrapyramidal side effects at a medium compared to a low dose range needs to be questioned based on recent studies. The study from McEvoy *et al* [1] is often quoted as proof for sufficient efficacy of a low dose approach in acute therapy. However, the study seems to contain severe methodological pitfalls. The authors compared the treatment results of an individually titrated low dose of haloperidol (3.7 ± 2.3 mg/day), which induced only very mild parkinsonian symptoms, with a medium dose range (11.6 ± 4.7 mg/day). They did not find better efficacy in those patients who were switched to the medium dose. However, a pitfall of this study might be the inadequate duration (14 days) of the control-group design and a possibly too small sample size to find differences [2]. Of special interest in this context is the seven-arm sertindole–haloperidol study, as part of which three different doses of haloperidol—4, 8, 16 mg/day—were compared in the treatment of acute schizophrenia, under double-blind conditions [3]. There were no distinct differences in extrapyramidal side effects between the various haloperidol dosage groups. Frequencies for administration of anticholinergics were between 40% and 50% for all three doses.

With respect to prophylactic long-term treatment, the low dose approach should also not be overdone, as we learn from the relevant studies in this field. The "low dose strategy" appears to be efficacious only when the dosage is not lowered too much (not more than about one-fifth of

[1]*Psychiatric Hospital, Nussbaumstrasse 7, D-80336 Munich, Germany*

the standard dosage) and only when selected patients (e.g. history of neuroleptic stabilization with relatively small dosages, no destabilization during change to these low dose treatments) are treated [4, 5]. According to clinical experience and data available from controlled studies, the optimal dosage has to be individually determined for each patient. The minimal effective dosage seems to be 6.5–12.5 mg every 2 weeks for fluphenazine decanoate, 20 mg every 2 weeks for flupenthixol decanoate, 50–60 mg every 4 weeks for haloperidol decanoate, 2.5 mg daily for oral haloperidol and 2.5 mg daily for oral fluphenazine hydrochloride [6].

The introduction of the novel/atypical antipsychotics gives the chance to overcome these dosing problems, given the fact that these drugs have no or only a very low risk of extrapyramidal side effects and in most cases no dose-related increase of these side effects. They also have to be seen as a major step forward as regards a richer efficacy profile (negative symptoms, affective symptoms). The better extrapyramidal tolerability results in improved compliance. Nevertheless, these drugs are also not free of problems which may interfere with compliance, such as weight gain.

The term atypical antipsychotics has been discussed controversially, however it seems meaningful when used not in a classificatory but in a dimensional sense. There should be no doubt that the available atypical antipsychotics differ from traditional ones as far as their pharmacological profile, clinical efficacy (especially with regard to negative symptoms), tolerability and the state of evaluation of these parameters are concerned. Similar to the case with traditional neuroleptics, we are dealing with a heterogeneous group in which one specific drug cannot easily be substituted by another. The indications for each atypical antipsychotic have to be reviewed in each individual patient, as is the case for classical neuroleptics. However, comparing this new generation of atypical antipsychotics to the family of typical neuroleptics, their overall advantages should be highlighted.

The superior efficacy of novel/atypical antipsychotics on negative symptoms should be especially focused upon. The data from recent empirical studies, most of which were performed according to a more sophisticated design for the evaluation of drug effects on negative symptoms, show that these drugs are more useful for treating negative symptoms in acute schizophrenic patients than the classical neuroleptics such as haloperidol and chlorpromazine. Apparently, the greater efficacy in negative symptoms can only partially be explained by indirect effects via better extrapyramidal tolerability, better effects on productive psychotic symptoms, etc., and is to a certain degree due to a direct effect of the atypical antipsychotic on negative symptoms, as has been shown using a path analytical approach [7]. This view is confirmed by the results from one trial studying the efficacy of an atypical antipsychotic in patients suffering from chronic schizophrenia with stable, predominantly negative, symptoms [8].

The usefulness of the novel/atypical antipsychotics seems of relevance not only for acute treatment but especially for prophylactic long-term treatment of schizophrenic patients. The better acceptance of novel antipsychotics by patients might lead to a generally more widespread use of oral long-term treatment in the future. In this respect, the recently published "guidelines for depot-antipsychotic treatment in schizophrenia" [9] might assess the situation too conservatively in favour of depot neuroleptics. However, the need for depot antipsychotics will remain in those patients who are non-compliant due to lack of insight or who have a very unstable, fluctuating disease course which reduces their capacity for a close and continuous patient–doctor relationship [10].

REFERENCES

1. McEvoy J.P., Hogarty G.E., Steingard S. (1991) Optimal dose of neuroleptic in acute schizophrenia. A controlled study of the neuroleptic threshold and higher haloperidol dose. *Arch. Gen. Psychiatry*, **48**: 739–745.
2. Möller H.-J. (1996) Treatment of schizophrenia: state of the art. *Eur. Arch. Psychiatry Clin. Neurosci.*, **246**: 229–234.
3. Zimbroff D.L., Kane J.M., Tamminga C.A., Daniel D.G., Mack R.J., Wozniak P.J., Sebree T.B., Wallin B.A., Kashkin K.B. (1997) Controlled, dose–response study of sertindole and haloperidol in the treatment of schizophrenia. Sertindole study group. *Am. J. Psychiatry*, **154**: 782–791.
4. Kane J.M., Rifkin A., Woerner M., Reardon G., Sarantakos S., Schiebel D., Ramos Lorenzi J. (1983) Low-dose neuroleptic treatment of outpatient schizophrenics. I. Preliminary results for relapse rates. *Arch. Gen. Psychiatry*, **40**: 893–896.
5. Marder S.R., Van Putten T., Mintz J., Lebell M., McKenzie J., May P.R. (1987) Low- and conventional-dose maintenance therapy with fluphenazine. Two-year outcome. *Arch. Gen. Psychiatry*, **44**: 518–521.
6. Kissling W. (1994) Compliance, quality assurance and standards for relapse prevention in schizophrenia. *Acta Psychiatr. Scand.*, **89** (Suppl. 382): 16–24.
7. Möller H.-J., Müller H., Borison R.L., Schooler N.R., Chouinard G. (1995) A path-analytical approach to differentiate between direct and indirect drug effects on negative symptoms in schizophrenic patients. A re-evaluation of the North American risperidone study. *Eur. Arch. Psychiatr. Clin. Neurosci.*, **245**: 45–49.
8. Möller H.-J. (1999) Atypical neuroleptics: a new approach in the treatment of negative symptoms. *Eur. Arch. Psychiatry Clin. Neurosci.*, **249** (Suppl. 4): 99–107.
9. Kane J.M., Aguglia E., Altamura A.C., Gutierrez J.L.A., Brunello N., Fleisch-hacker W.W., Gaebel W., Gerlach J., Guelfi D., Kissling W. *et al* (1998) Guidelines for depot antipsychotic treatment in schizophrenia. *Eur. Neuropsychopharmacol.*, **8**: 55–66.
10. Möller H.-J. Long-term management of schizophrenia. Submitted for publication.

2.8
Can We Use Pharmacotherapy More Logically in Schizophrenia and Other Psychoses?

Patrick McGorry[1]

In the past decade we have begun to emerge from something of a dark age in which antipsychotics have been widely used in the treatment of psychotic illnesses in seriously excessive doses. There has been little regard by many for the subjective experiences of patients and evidence on dosages which has been available for some time. During the early years of antipsychotic use, there were serious attempts to define the lower limits of treatment effectiveness in relation to the threshold for distressing neurological side effects [1]. Subsequently, rapid neuroleptization inflicted a range of acute and chronic iatrogenic effects upon a generation of psychotic patients. Many found themselves marooned on excessive doses which produced distressing and disabling side effects. Even after the waning of enthusiasm for this damaging approach, impatient dosing in the acute phase and a lack of knowledge of the time course of action of the antipsychotic effects [2], plus a willingness to use the adverse effects — sedation and extrapyramidal side effects (EPS) — of the antipsychotics to deal with acute agitation and insomnia, rather than the safer and gentler benzodiazepines, has perpetuated the problem. This has created a huge backlog of problems, some of which can be addressed by careful dose reduction strategies and switching to novel antipsychotics, as described in Fleischhacker's comprehensive review. Such a salvage operation for those who unfortunately failed to receive the benefits of the novel antipsychotics and the low dose approach seems feasible [3]. However, we need to identify this large cohort of patients as conceptually separate from those with emerging psychosis, who, with the benefit of better evidence and a rational approach, can be treated more effectively with many fewer adverse effects in a phase specific way.

At present, the earliest evidence-based use of pharmacotherapy is as soon as clear-cut positive symptoms have emerged and a diagnosis of a DSM-IV or ICD-10 psychotic disorder can be made. The recognition of first-episode psychosis in contrast to first-episode schizophrenia (a more complex task) is an important practical distinction, since drug treatment within first-episode psychosis is syndromal [4]. Low-dose antipsychotics in the 2–4 mg haloperidol equivalent range are empirically highly effective, not only in research samples [2] but in real-world clinical settings too [4]. Furthermore, these dosing levels are supported by positron emission tomography (PET) data which show the clinical feasibility of treating

---

[1]*Department of Psychiatry, University of Melbourne, Locked Bag 40 Parkville Victoria 3052, Australia*

most treatment-responsive cases without causing significant EPS [5]. This requires longer intervals in the acute phase between dose increments. In our own service, over 60% of a sample of 96 first-episode cases responded by 3–4 weeks to 2 mg of risperidone as a first-line treatment. By around 12 weeks 80–90% have achieved remission, some requiring a change in therapy. While the novel antipsychotics do seem to confer additional advantages, there would be substantially less difference in tolerability and efficacy between them and the typicals if the latter were used in doses below or at the neuroleptic threshold in the first episode and beyond. Even for new multiepisode patients, especially treatment-responsive cases, it seems that only a slightly higher dose of around 4 mg may be required for most patients [2]. In our experience, this low-dose acute strategy requires a commitment to a combination of acute benzodiazepine use (often in high doses for a brief period) and supportive nursing interventions, to avoid the use of sedating antipsychotics for management of the behavioural, dysphoric and sleep disturbances which commonly occur.

Beyond the first episode, it is critical to identify early treatment resistance. Once two novel antipsychotics have been given an adequate trial without remission of positive symptoms, after considering adherence issues, substance use and the psychosocial environment, we would offer clozapine as the next logical step. There seems little point withholding this until entrenched treatment resistance has developed, when it may be less effective and more psychosocial damage will have occurred. On the other hand, clozapine is not and should not be considered the "last resort", since other strategies (typical neuroleptics, emerging novel antipsychotics and cognitive behavioural treatments) may yet prove to be effective. Relapse prevention is a key part of management, as identified by Fleischhacker; however, it is not an end in itself, and it is important to win the war rather than merely the battle. A flexible attitude and a comprehensive community-based psychosocial programme is essential for this to be possible. The ultimate goal is for patients to accept responsibility for illness self-management where the vulnerability to illness persists. More studies are required to determine who needs longer term protection and for how long.

With the above caveats, I believe Fleischhacker's careful review condenses much of the evidence required for enhancing the psychopharmacological treatment of patients with schizophrenia and related psychoses. This in turn provides a sound basis for a more enlightened future era.

REFERENCES

1. Haase H.J., Janssen P.A.J. (1985) *The Action of Neuroleptic Drugs*, 2nd edn. Elsevier, New York.

2. McEvoy J.P., Hogarty G.E., Steingard S. (1991) Optimal dose of neuroleptic in acute schizophrenia: a controlled study of the neuroleptic threshold and higher haloperidol dose. *Arch. Gen. Psychiatry*, **48**: 739–745.
3. Schooler N.R., Keith S.J., Severe J.B., Matthews S.M., Bellack A.S., Glick I.D., Hargreaves W.A., Kane J.M., Ninan P.T., Frances A. *et al* (1997) Relapse and rehospitalization during maintenance treatment of schizophrenia: the effects of dose reduction and family treatment. *Arch. Gen. Psychiatry*, **54**: 453–463.
4. McGorry P.D., Edwards J., Mihalopoulos C., Harrigan S.M., Jackson H.J. (1996) EPPIC: an evolving system of early detection and optimal management. *Schizophr. Bull.*, **22**: 305–326.
5. Farde L., Nyberg S. (1998) Dosing determination for novel antipsychotics — a PET-based approach. *Int. J. Psychiatr. Clin. Pract.*, **2** (Suppl. 1): 39–42.

2.9

Long-term Treatment in Schizophrenia: For Whom and How Long?

Wolfgang Gaebel[1]

Pharmacological treatment in schizophrenia should be illness-phase orientated [1]. However, as Fleischhacker states, the line between acute and long-term treatment is an artificial one, which cannot be clearly drawn. Primary prevention is an ambitious goal, and there are now increasing research activities on this issue, raising a number of conceptual, ethical, and methodological questions [2]. Secondary prevention of re-exacerbation, however, is still the main treatment goal in manifest schizophrenia — but for whom and how long? Current treatment guidelines give clear recommendations [1], but evidence is based on selected patients — the rate of non-response and placebo-response amounting to 20–30%.

The florid acute episode in most cases resolves and transits into a stable phase of remission and recovery [3]. Obviously, the risk of relapse and recurrence is not constant during the illness course. According to the vulnerability-stress-coping model, the probability of relapse/recurrence depends on the interaction between vulnerability factors, stressors and protectors [4]. Imbalance — possibly reflected by prodromal symptoms — moves the psychobiological system from a stable state of remission/recovery to a destabilized state of psychotic exacerbation. Identification of the underlying processes could provide better understanding of the developing psychopathology and psychophysiology of schizophrenia, and could also be of predictive value in order to initiate therapeutic actions [5].

[1]*Department of Psychiatry, Heinrich-Heine-University, Rheinische Kliniken Düsseldorf, Bergische Landstrasse 2, D-40629 Düsseldorf, Germany*

Since demographic, clinical and biological variables are of only limited usefulness as predictors of illness course [6], the concept of prodromal symptoms as predictors of psychotic (re-)manifestation has been put forward [7]. However, research findings are not consistent and there are a number of still unresolved conceptual and methodological issues [8]. The relapse predictive validity of prodromal symptoms has been assessed in a number of studies [9]. Sensitivity rates range from 8% to 81%, and specificity rates range from 70% to 93%, our own findings [10] being at the extremes of the range (sensitivity 10%, specificity 93%). With a corresponding positive predictive value of 43%, relapse prediction by early warning signs is obviously no better than by chance.

The rationale of intermittent treatment was based on the assumptions that relapse is an episodic phenomenon in stabilized schizophrenics, that prodromal symptoms are valid predictors of relapse, and that impending relapse can be prevented by early neuroleptic intervention. According to Fleischhacker, all controlled 2-year studies on early intervention treatment have not confirmed this strategy to be as effective as maintenance treatment in preventing relapse. A recent reanalysis of our own data [11] demonstrates, however, that first-episode patients seem to profit more from early intervention, intermittent, targeted medication than multiple episode patients. These findings need replication given the guideline recommendation that remitted first-episode patients may be slowly withdrawn from drug treatment after 1 to 2 years of maintenance treatment [1].

In accordance with Fleischhacker's conclusion, the application of intermittent treatment based on early warning signs cannot be generally recommended. Overall poorer results, restricted feasibility, greater burden on the patients and their families, as well as greater demands on treatment facilities contribute to this conclusion. Moreover, the neuropharmacological rationale of intermittent treatment is far from clear, and an increased risk of tardive dyskinesia may be associated. On the other hand, stepwise drug withdrawal under monitoring of early warning signs may be the only possible way to identify patients who do not need continuous treatment — and to manage patients not accepting maintenance medication. In accordance with clinical experience [12], recovery from an acute episode seems to be the most important prerequisite, that is, patients stable without medication and — if at all — at risk for recurrence, not for relapse. Fully recovered first-episode patients, in particular, might be candidates for an intermittent prodrome-guided early intervention strategy. A controlled study on this issue is now underway [13].

REFERENCES

1. American Psychiatric Association (1997) *Practice Guideline for the Treatment of Patients with Schizophrenia*. American Psychiatric Association, Washington, DC.

2. McGlashan T.H. (1998) Early detection and intervention of schizophrenia: ratio-nale and research. *Br. J. Psychiatry*, **172** (Suppl. 33): 3–6.
3. Wyatt R.J., Damiani M., Henter I. (1998) First episode schizophrenia: early inter-vention and medication discontinuation in the context of course and treatment. *Br. J. Psychiatry*, **172** (Suppl. 33): 77–83.
4. Zubin J., Steinhauer S.R., Condray R. (1992) Vulnerability to relapse in schizo-phrenia. *Br. J. Psychiatry*, **161** (Suppl. 18): 13–18.
5. Herz M.I., Lamberti J.S. (1995) Prodromal symptoms and relapse prevention in schizophrenia. *Schizophr. Bull.*, **21**: 541–551.
6. Gaebel W., Awad A.G. (Eds) (1994) *Prediction of Neuroleptic Treatment Outcome in Schizophrenia*. Springer, Wien.
7. Herz M.I., Melville C. (1980) Relapse in schizophrenia. *Am. J. Psychiatry*, **137**: 801–805.
8. Gaebel W., Jänner M., Frommann N., Pietzcker A., Köpcke W., Linden M., Mül-ler P., Müller-Spahn F., Tegeler J. (1999) Prodromal states in schizophrenia. *Compr. Psychiatry*, **41** (Suppl. 1): 76–85.
9. Jørgensen J.M. (1998) Early signs of psychotic relapse in schizophrenia. *Br. J. Psychiatry*, **172**: 327–330.
10. Gaebel W., Frick U., Köpcke W., Linden M., Müller P., Müller-Spahn F., Piet-zcker A., Tegeler J. (1993) Early neuroleptic intervention in schizophrenia: are prodromal symptoms valid predictors of relapse? *Br. J. Psychiatry*, **163** (Suppl. 21): 8–12.
11. Pietzcker A., Gaebel W., Köpcke W., Linden M., Müller P., Müller-Spahn F., Tegeler J. (1993) Continuous vs. intermittent neuroleptic longterm treatment in schizophrenia — results of a German multicenter study. *J. Psychiatry Res.*, **27**: 321–339.
12. Chiles J.A., Sterchi D., Hyde T., Herz M.I. (1989) Intermittent medication for schizophrenic outpatients: who is eligible? *Schizophr. Bull.*, **15**: 117–121.
13. Gaebel W., Möller H.J. (1999) Kompetenznetzwerk Schizophrenie. Research grant, German Ministry of Research, Bonn.

2.10
Novel Antipsychotics in Schizophrenia and Related Disorders: Preliminary Findings from a First-episode Study

Stein Opjordsmoen[1]

Recent literature indicates that reduction of the duration of untreated psychosis (DUP) may improve the prognosis of schizophrenia [1]. However, there is still a lack of empirical evidence, since studies have not been able to rule out that poor prognosis in "long DUP patients" might be due to sampling bias.

The TIPS project [2] aims at answering this question by comparing the outcome of consecutively admitted first-onset patients from a catchment area

[1]*Clinic for Psychiatry, University of Oslo, Ullevaal Sykehus, N-0407 Oslo, Norway*

with an early detection programme for reducing DUP (Rogaland County, Norway, population 320 000) with that of patients from two catchment areas with "usual detection" (Ullevaal Sector, Oslo, Norway, population 190 000 and Roskilde, Denmark, population 95 000). All patients receive the same 2-year treatment programme including medication, multi-family group intervention and individual supportive psychotherapy. Course and outcome are studied by using a wide range of assessments, including psychopathology and neuropsychology. Extrapyramidal side effects (EPS) are recorded according to the St. Hans Rating Scale [3]. The study was planned in 1995–96 to include patients from 1997 through 2000 with subsequent follow-ups. It was decided to use perphenazine as the first drug of choice. If there are persistent negative or positive symptoms or side effects, the medication should be changed to risperidone, with clozapine as the third drug.

In schizophrenia (DSM-IV), maintenance medication for 2 years was recommended, while 1 year was recommended in schizophreniform disorder, 1–2 years in schizoaffective disorder and 6 months in brief psychosis. During 1997 new research data on novel antipsychotics, especially concerning compliance and side effects, made us revise the protocol, with olanzapine as the first drug, followed by risperidone, any other novel antipsychotic or perphenazine, and clozapine as the fourth choice. This allows us to compare the results from a traditional neuroleptic with a novel antipsychotic as the first choice. Preliminary data from the Ullevaal site [4] are the following: 32 patients were recruited (13 male and 19 female, median age 29 years). Their diagnosis was schizophrenia ($n = 11$), schizophreniform disorder ($n = 8$), schizoaffective disorder ($n = 3$), delusional disorder ($n = 3$), brief psychosis ($n = 1$), major depressive disorder with mood-incongruent psychotic features ($n = 4$), psychotic disorder NOS ($n = 2$).

Fifteen patients were included in 1997 (group 1) and 17 in 1998 (group 2); the follow-up period was 1 month–2 years. At follow-up, only one patient from group 1 was still on perphenazine (8 mg), while two were on risperidone (2 mg and 6 mg respectively), six on olanzapine (10 mg $n = 5$, 5 mg $n = 1$). Additionally, one of these received valproate and two selective serotonin reuptake inhibitors (SSRIs), one was on valproate only (mood disorder, with severe EPS on antipsychotics), and five patients had no medication (in agreement with the therapist in three cases — two of these had used perphenazine successfully, one had to change to risperidone, two patients had stopped the medication against advice, out of whom one was still psychotic).

Change of medication in group 1 was undertaken because of EPS in five instances, dysphoria in three, impotence in one and lack of treatment response in one.

In group 2, thirteen patients still used olanzapine (mean dose 10.4 mg), one of these with additionally an antiparkinsonian drug (akathisia), and three with SSRIs (one had akathisia on this combination). One patient used an SSRI only (mood disorder), one received perphenazine depot (compliance problem, had akathisia at follow-up and received an antiparkinsonian drug as well), and two patients had stopped the medication against advice (one of them was still psychotic). In two of the patients on olanzapine weight gain was reported. No other side effects were recorded.

Only three patients (20%) who received a traditional neuroleptic (perphenazine) could be treated successfully without persistent side effects. Therefore, a frequent change of medication to a novel drug was found in this group. In none of the cases treated initially with a novel drug (olanzapine), has change of medication been undertaken because of lack of treatment response or side effects, but the effect is reported to be insufficient in one case. The observation period is 1 year longer in the first group, and it remains to be seen if the tendency will be confirmed with follow-up periods of similar length in the groups. Some of the patients who started with perphenazine in 1997 received olanzapine as the second drug during 1998 without trying risperidone. The data as regards risperidone, therefore, are too scarce at this point.

The findings are preliminary and must be interpreted with caution. Nevertheless, they support the use of novel antipsychotics as first-line treatment in first-episode patients with schizophrenia and related disorders. In our sample the doses could be kept relatively low. Reasons might be that it included first-onset patients, with female preponderance. The study is performed under naturalistic conditions. The findings are therefore relevant for everyday clinical practice. These data will be extended and reported with standardized measures from all three sites later.

REFERENCES

1. McGlashan T.H., Johannessen J.O. (1996) Early detection and intervention with schizophrenia: rationale. *Schizophr. Bull.*, **22**: 201–222.
2. Vaglum P., McGlashan T.H., Simonsen E., Johannessen J.O., Opjordsmoen S., Friis S. (1998) The TIPS project: an international multicenter site for early detection. Presented at the APA Annual Meeting, Toronto, 30 May–4 June.
3. Gerlach J., Korsgaard S., Clemmesen P., Lund Lauersen A.-M., Magelund G., Noring U., Povlsen U.J., Bech P., Casey D.E. (1993) The St. Hans Rating Scale for extrapyramidal syndromes: reliability and validity. *Acta Psychiatr. Scand.*, **87**: 244–252.
4. Melle I., Friis S., Sortland E., Opjordsmoen S., Ellefsen E., Tvedt K.S. (1998) TIPS: the Norwegian comparison site, Ullevaal Hospital. Presented at the APA Annual Meeting, Toronto, 30 May–4 June.

2.11
The Pharmacotherapy of Schizophrenia in Clinical Practice
René S. Kahn and Jan M. Van Ree[1]

The article of Prof. Fleischhacker provides a comprehensive and inclusive review on the treatment of schizophrenia. Several points may require some comments, more for emphasis than elaboration. Prof. Fleischhacker mentions that the treatment of schizophrenia has changed since the introduction of non-sedative newer antipsychotics. However, clinicians are used to administer antipsychotics as sedatives or to combat agitation and aggression initially in the treatment of schizophrenia and other psychotic disorders. The antipsychotic effects may not be immediately evident, although it has been described that antipsychotics may reduce psychotic symptoms very early — in a matter of days — in the treatment of schizophrenia [1, 2]. Psychiatrists still increase doses of typical and also atypical antipsychotics. Indeed, the average dose of olanzapine appears to be 17.5 mg/day, although efficacy has been demonstrated with doses as low as 10 mg/day. It may be that psychiatrists in clinical practice focus more on the "absence" of sedative effects of the new antipsychotics than on the antipsychotic effects of these compounds. Sedation should be induced by sedatives, such as the benzodiazepines. After a few days, they can be tapered when the initial agitation has decreased.

Although long-term efficacy (up to a year) of the atypical antipsychotics has been convincingly demonstrated, Prof. Fleischhacker points out that phase IV studies are needed until definitive conclusions can be made on the applicability of atypical antipsychotics. Moreover, it should be cautioned that the fact that the atypical antipsychotics do not induce extrapyramidal side effects (EPS) more than placebo, does not suggest that these drugs do not induce any EPS. It is evident that these compounds do induce akathisia, and in some cases it may be just as pronounced as it was with the classical antipsychotic drugs. We should remain vigilant in detecting EPS, including tardive dyskinesia and akathisia. Furthermore, it is clear that the newer drugs are not free from side effects, as weight gain and sexual side effects can be pronounced.

The treatment of negative symptomatology in schizophrenia still remains an important issue. So far, there is little, if any, convincing evidence that the currently available antipsychotics affect the core negative symptoms. There may be a decrease of these symptoms during treatment, but in most cases this can also be explained in the context of the improvement of the condition of the patient. We urgently need antipsychotics that are

[1]*Departments of Psychiatry and Pharmacology, Rudolf Magnus Institute for Neurosciences and Academic Hospital Utrecht, Utrecht University, Heidelberglaan 100, 3584 CX Utrecht, The Netherlands*

effective in decreasing negative symptomatology of schizophrenic patients. This effectiveness should be established in patients in whom these symptoms are not secondary to other symptomatology.

All in all, the newer antipsychotics appear to have opened a new chapter in the treatment of schizophrenia. Their main advantage may be that they humanize the treatment of some of these patients and hopefully may eventually improve their course of illness.

REFERENCES

1. Stern R.G., Kahn R.S., Harvey P.D., Amin F., Apter S., Hirschowitz J. (1993) Early response to haloperidol treatment in chronic schizophrenia. *Schizophr. Res.*, **10**: 165–171.
2. Stern R.G., Kahn R.S., Davidson M., Nora R.M., Davis K.L. (1994) Early response to clozapine in schizophrenia. *Am. J. Psychiatry*, **151**: 1817–1818.

2.12
A New Era of Hope in Treating Persons with Schizophrenia

Anthony F. Lehman[1]

As documented by Prof. Fleischhacker's excellent review of pharmacotherapy for persons with schizophrenia, we have entered what may be a new era in the treatment of persons with psychotic disorders. The review raises several important points to ponder as we move forward into this new era of hope. Despite the advances represented by new antipsychotic medications, there is a great deal that we do not know about how to optimize pharmacotherapies. The review raises questions about optimal dosing, and notes significant differences in dosing between Europe and the United States that we do not understand. Such variations in practice also occur within much smaller geographic areas and are a point of great concern regarding inappropriate practice variations that impact on the quality of care [1]. The paper also points to the importance of attending to outcomes other than psychotic symptoms, especially functional status and quality of life. We must pay more attention to strategies that improve negative symptoms and that address comorbid depression, which can prove so lethal among young persons with schizophrenia. The importance of combined pharmacologic and psychosocial therapies is also emphasized. For example, it is important to acknowledge that research indicates that adding family

[1]*Department of Psychiatry, University of Maryland School of Medicine, 645 West Redwood St., Baltimore, MD 21201, USA*

education and support to a good regimen of pharmacotherapy can further reduce relapse rates by about 50% [2]. Finally, we must improve the processes of delivering treatments, in particular the therapist–patient relationship, that can substantially influence the course of care. Our research agenda must be expanded beyond the traditional randomized clinical trial to answer many of the questions raised in Prof. Fleischhacker's review.

This new era of hope in treatment of schizophrenia is shaped by at least three forces. First of all, recent and ongoing advances in the neurosciences are yielding a better understanding of how the brain functions and are offering many new opportunities to design treatments for psychosis and other disorders of the brain. These scientific advances instil renewed interest and hope for treatment of patients who have lived with disability for many years and spur a new activism in efforts to intervene early with patients at the beginning of these disorders to try to avert disabilities. The most visible manifestation of these new treatment efforts are the new antipsychotic agents, but with them has come renewed interest in psychosocial programmes that enable patients to take advantage of the clinical gains made with new medications.

A second phenomenon contributing to this emerging era of renewed hope is the dramatic growth of family and consumer advocacy. Once disempowered by treatment systems that viewed patients as incompetent and families as part of the problem, patients and families have developed strong voices in the shaping of public images and policy towards mental illness. In the United States, the National Alliance for the Mentally Ill has grown to over 185 000 members and about 1200 chapters in all 50 states and is a powerful lobby for programmes to treat severe mental illnesses at the national, state and local levels. Hence we have not only new opportunities for better treatments afforded by science, but demand for better treatments from consumers and their advocates.

The third phenomenon driving this new era is managed care. While not always a positive force in improving the quality of care to date, managed care does espouse principles of providing care that have been demonstrated effective, so-called evidence-based practice, and offers the tools to promote more sound practice. If used appropriately, managed care could insist that effective treatments are made available to patients and that resources be used to support the best care.

One visible product of this new era is the introduction of several sets of criteria to define quality care. These include the American Psychiatric Association's Guidelines for Treatment of Schizophrenia [3], the Schizophrenia Patient Outcomes Research Team (PORT) Treatment Recommendations [4], the Veterans Affairs Practice Guidelines for Psychosis Treatment [5], and the Expert Consensus Guidelines for Treatment of Schizophrenia [6]. Most important about these is that they provide explicit guidelines for treating persons with schizophrenia and other psychoses and establish expectations about quality care. They constitute some common tools that can be used by patients and families to evaluate the care they are receiving, by providers to assess the quality of care they offer, by insurance companies and other payers to make decisions about what to purchase, and by advocates to guide advocacy agendas. In order to maximize advantages afforded by new developments in pharmacotherapies and psychosocial treatments, strategies that disseminate knowledge about and appropriate use of these new technologies must be promoted.

REFERENCES

1. Lehman A.F., Carpenter W.T., Goldman H.H., Steinwachs D.S. (1995) Treatment outcomes in schizophrenia: implications for practice, policy, and research. *Schizophr. Bull.*, **21**: 669–676.
2. Dixon L.B., Scott J.E. (1995) Family interventions for schizophrenia. *Schizophr. Bull.*, **21**: 631–644.
3. American Psychiatric Association (1997) *Practice Guideline for the Treatment of Patients with Schizophrenia.* American Psychiatric Association, Washington, DC.
4. Lehman A.F., Steinwachs D.S., Co-investigators of the PORT Project (1998) Translating research into practice: the Schizophrenia Patient Outcomes Research Team (PORT) Treatment Recommendations. *Schizophr. Bull.*, **24**: 1–10.
5. Veterans Health Administration (1998) *Clinical Practice Guidelines for the Management of Persons with Psychoses.*
6. Frances A., Docherty J.P., Kahn D.A. (1996) The Expert Consensus Guideline Series: Treatment of schizophrenia. *J. Clin. Psychiatry*, **57** (Suppl. 12B): 1–58.

2.13

New Perspectives in Antipsychotic Pharmacotherapy

Joseph Peuskens[1]

Neuroleptics were the first effective antipsychotic treatment: reducing positive symptoms at the acute psychotic episode, neuroleptic therapy enables patients to be discharged from the hospital and, by preventing psychotic relapses, the psychosocial integration can be maintained. Soon neuroleptics were considered to be the cornerstone of the treatment of psychotic disorders in general and of schizophrenia more specifically. However, neuroleptics only partly fulfilled the promises, the prognosis of schizophrenia still remains poor, and different aspects of antipsychotic therapy were considered to improve treatment outcome.

With the introduction of neuroleptics, in the early 1950s, the number of institutionalized patients rapidly decreased. Unfortunately, severely disabled

[1] *University Centre St Jozef, Leuvensesteenweg 517, B 3070 Kortenberg, Belgium*

patients were often dumped in society without adequate provisions, unprepared to cope with the demands of social and professional integration. Antipsychotic pharmacotherapy should be part of a large and comprehensive therapeutic approach aiming at the psychosocial rehabilitation of the patient. While neuroleptic medication can reduce positive symptoms and prevent psychotic relapses, psychotherapeutic support and training of coping strategies help the patient to adapt to the environment and to cope with stress, and familial and socioprofessional interventions modify environmental factors to the capacities of the patient. This multidimensional approach is continuously offered, assessed and coordinated over time and over different settings and adapted to each individual patient and his specific needs. In this way, the risk of provoking exacerbation of psychotic symptoms by overstimulation and inducing regression and deficit by understimulation may be avoided [1].

Furthermore, the importance of early treatment with antipsychotic medication at the beginning of the psychotic process has been stressed. The earlier antipsychotic treatment is started, the better the short- and long-term outcomes will be [2]. Partly this may be attributed to the fact that at the acute psychotic episode a pathological process is reactivated or superimposed on a pre-existing deficit, but also the longer the normal psychosocial development is disturbed and interrupted during adolescence the poorer the patient will be prepared and the lower are his chances to establish a successful social and professional integration [3].

Recently, more careful and lower dosing of classical neuroleptics has been advocated to improve efficacy and to reduce side effects. Clinical studies show that high dosing does not induce a higher or more rapid antipsychotic effect. Neuroimaging research showed that neuroleptics at low doses (3–5 mg haloperidol) result in an occupancy of cerebral dopamine D_2 receptors of about 70%, sufficient to obtain an antipsychotic effect, while at a higher occupancy extrapyramidal symptoms (EPS) are provoked, indicating also that antipsychotic effects and EPS are not inextricably linked [4].

Prevention of psychotic relapses is essential, but the incidence of relapse is very high due to poor compliance with maintenance antipsychotic treatment. Although avoiding side effects is important for the adherence to maintenance treatment, it has been shown that systematic and repeated psychoeducation of the patient, the family and health care professionals is necessary. Informing patient, family and health care workers on the pathophysiological mechanisms in schizophrenia, the relapse risks and on the importance of prophylactic therapy has proven to be effective, and several systematic educational modules have been developed [5, 6].

Nevertheless, 10–20% of schizophrenic patients do not respond to antipsychotic treatment, while many (up to 50%) patients continue to suffer from residual psychotic symptoms. Furthermore, negative symptoms as well as cognitive deficits are either not improved or only marginally improved by classical antipsychotics and have an important impact on rehabilitation. Depressive episodes are frequent, and the incidence of suicide attempts and of suicide in schizophrenia is high. Side effects, especially EPS and tardive dyskinesia, reduce the acceptability of neuroleptic treatment for the patient and the health care professional and as such antipsychotic treatment is postponed and maintenance treatment is not prescribed or interrupted too soon.

Certainly important progress is being made with the development of the new antipsychotics. At least as effective in reducing positive symptoms, the new antipsychotics also reduce negative symptoms and affective symptoms and improve cognitive functioning. Inducing few or no extrapyramidal symptoms, treatment with new antipsychotics is more acceptable to patients and professionals, offering perspectives for better compliance with acute and prophylactic treatment. Having an antipsychotic effect without inducing important side effects, new antipsychotics may offer the possibility of prevention of the first psychotic episode, by treating patients at the appearance of the first premorbid signs [7], while for first-episode patients, often being particularly vulnerable to side effects, treatment with new antipsychotics is indicated. Also the protection offered by lifelong prophylaxis with new antipsychotics will certainly outweigh the disadvantages of the few side effects.

New antipsychotics are valuable alternatives to classical neuroleptics, particularly in the treatment of patients sensitive to EPS (elderly patients, patients with psychotic mood disorders), and as such they are an important step in the treatment of psychotic syndromes in general. Treatment with new antipsychotics will not only reduce symptomatology but also support and promote the participation of patients in the psychosocial rehabilitation and result in a better overall quality of life.

REFERENCES

1. Peuskens J. (1996) Proper psychosocial rehabilitation for stabilised patients with schizophrenia: the role of new therapies. *Eur. Neuropsychopharmacol.*, 6: 7–12.
2. Wyatt R. (1991) Neuroleptics and natural course of schizophrenia. *Schizophr. Bull.*, 17: 325–351.
3. Lieberman J.A. (1998) Pathophysiology in the clinical course of schizophrenia. *Int. Clin. Psychopharmacol.*, 13: 3–6.
4. Farde L., Wiesel F.A., Halldin C., Sedvall G. (1988) Central D2-dopamine receptor occupancy in schizophrenic patients treated with antipsychotic drugs. *Arch. Gen. Psychiatry*, 45: 71–76.
5. Kissling W. (1994) Duration of neuroleptic maintenance treatment. In *Guideline for Neuroleptic Relapse Prevention in Schizophrenia* (Ed. W. Kissling), pp. 94–112. Springer, Berlin.

6. Liberman R. (1986) Social and Independent Living Skills. Medication-Management Module. Camarillo State Hospital, UCLA Department of Psychiatry, McNeil Pharmaceutical.
7. McGorry P., Edwards J., Michalopoulos C., Harrigan S., Jackson H. (1996) EPPIC: an evolving system of early detection and optimal management. *Schizophr. Bull.*, **22**: 305–326.

2.14
Some Aspects of the Maintenance Treatment of Schizophrenia

Carlo L. Cazzullo[1]

I would like to focus on some aspects of the current pharmacological management of schizophrenic disorders, which have not been specifically examined in Fleischhacker's review.

The first point concerns the period of time between the acute schizophrenic episode and the implementation of long-term therapy. This period is defined as the "stabilization phase". It usually starts after an acute schizophrenic episode (with the patient's hospital discharge) and lasts from 3 to 6 months, being characterized by a continuous neuroleptic treatment. Surprisingly, the "stabilization" process has received little attention in the literature, in contrast to the acute and maintenance phases of antipsychotic therapy in schizophrenia. Such a knowledge gap, at least partly, can explain the high rates of complications occurring after the hospital discharge.

During this period, psychotic symptoms can further improve, albeit at a slower pace, and this is particularly evident in patients with a shorter duration of illness compared to those with a more lasting (chronic) schizophrenic disorder. In patients treated with haloperidol decanoate (HL-D), the ratio between the plasma levels of HL and the administered doses tends to increase progressively in the first 4–5 months, thus indicating that patients can be undertreated in the period after implementation of a therapy with HL-D, following an acute treatment with conventional HL ("shifting phase"). This finding is particularly relevant if plasma levels of HL during hospitalization period and after discharge are compared [1]. Thus, schizophrenic patients during the "stabilization" phase of treatment with neuroleptics are particularly susceptible to relapse for various clinical and pharmacological reasons, particularly if receiving HL-D.

A second issue I would like to cover is the treatment of more vulnerable populations, such as elderly or adolescents, which has become more and more important in recent years and deserves a special featuring of the use of typical antipsychotics compared to adult population. Treatment of adolescents poses

[1] *Association Ricerche sulla Schizophrenia, Via Tamagno 5, 20124 Milano, Italy*

three main problems: the higher metabolic rate; the proneness to develop extrapyramidal reactions; and the hormonal fragility [2]. Because of the first of these problems, the dosage should be the same or higher, but because of the other two conditions it should be reduced and strictly monitored, in our experience, to avoid severe disruption of hormone functioning (e.g. prolactin, oestrogens, growth hormone, etc.).

Concerning the use of atypical compounds, in children and adolescents there are few data on a better tolerability profile of clozapine and risperidone.

The use of antipsychotics in the elderly is another important issue, which involves drug tolerability, the dose and modality of administration, and the comparison between typical and atypical compounds [3]. Elderly patients suffering from basal subclinical dysfunctioning of subcortical nuclei are more prone to develop parkinsonian symptoms. Another point is represented by the frequent anergic or residual patterns encountered in the elderly, which may require some combination antidepressive therapy. In general, due to tolerability problems and impaired hepatic metabolism, the average dosage of typical compounds should be reduced; more recent preliminary data on the use of atypical compounds are promising [4], especially since they have been used for treating psychotic symptoms occurring in senile dementia and Parkinson's disease dementia.

A last point I would like to stress is the importance of psychosocial treatments, which are now increasingly available [5, 6]. It is already well known [7] that the presence of high expressed emotions (EE) in the family may facilitate relapse also in the presence of pharmacological treatment. Psychoeducational intervention, also at its first level (information group), has shown the capacity of increasing the adherence to pharmacological treatment [8]. On the other hand, the second level (support group, psychoeducational family intervention) is able to reduce both the familial EE level and the rate of relapse in chronic schizophrenic patients [9].

REFERENCES

1. Altamura C.A., Colacurcio F., Mauri M.C., Moro A.R., DeNovellis F. (1989) Haloperidol decanoate in chronic schizophrenia: a study of 12 months with plasma levels. *Progr. Neuropsychopharmacol. Biol. Psychiatry*, **14**: 25–35.
2. Green W.H. (1995) *Child and Adolescent Clinical Psychopharmacology. Antipsychotic Drugs*. Williams and Wilkins, Baltimore.
3. Altamura A.C., Curreli R. (1998) Antipsychotics in the elderly. The use of "typical" vs. "atypical" compounds. In *Mental Disorders in the Elderly: New Therapeutic Approaches* (Eds N. Brunello, S. Langer, G. Racagni), pp. 125–138. Karger, Basel.
4. Cazzullo C.L., Altamura A.C. (1985) Bioavailability of some atypical antidepressants and therapeutic management of late life depressive states. *Integr. Psychiatry*, **3**: 50S–54S.

5. Cazzullo C.L., Bertrando P., Clerici M., Bressi C., Da Ponte C., Albertini E. (1989) The efficacy of information group intervention on relatives of schizophrenics. *Int. J. Soc. Psychiatry*, **35**: 313–323.
6. Cazzullo C.L., Clerici M., Bertrando P. (1994) Future strategies in family research and intervention. *Integr. Psychiatry*, **10**: 20–23.
7. Bebbington P., Kuipers L. (1994) The predictive utility of expressed emotion in schizophrenia: an aggregate analysis. *Psychol. Med.*, **24**: 707–718.
8. Lam D.H. (1991) Psychosocial family intervention in schizophrenia: a review of empirical studies. *Psychol. Med.*, **21**: 423–441.
9. Hogarty G.E., Anderson C.M., Reiss D.J., Kornblith S.J., Greenwald D.P., Ulrich R.F., Carter M. (1991) Family psychoeducation, social skills training and maintenance chemotherapy in the aftercare treatment of schizophrenia. II. Two year effects of a controlled study on relapse and adjustment. *Arch. Gen. Psychiatry*, **48**: 340–347.

2.15

Highlights on the Management of Schizophrenia

Ahmed Okasha[1]

Our goals in the short-term management of schizophrenia are symptom control and crisis intervention. Long-term management is targeted to maintenance of therapeutic effect, relapse prevention, social reintegration and promoting quality of life. Although the management of schizophrenia encompasses psychosocial intervention, rehabilitative measures and pharmacological treatment, the paper by Fleischhacker focuses on drug treatment. We all agree that there is no scientific evidence that newer antipsychotics (NAPs) are superior to classical neuroleptics (CNLs), at least regarding positive symptoms. Antipsychotics, whether atypical or classical, may differ in tolerability rather than efficacy. The argument against the high cost of NAPs can be buffered by the lower relapse rate and reduced rehospitalization. The dose required for the treatment of schizophrenia, either in the acute or maintenance phase, should be adjusted to the needs of the individual, taking into consideration the ethnic and transcultural variables in the pharmacokinetics and pharmacodynamics. While Americans and Europeans use clozapine in doses ranging from 300 to 800 mg/day, in our clinical experience in the Arab World, patients can be controlled by 150–300 mg/day and even agranulocytosis is very rarely recorded [1].

Fleischhacker points out that, if there is partial response to CNLs after 2 or 3 weeks, we should augment the dose and have supportive psychosocial intervention for a further 2 weeks, then use NAPs for 2 or 3 months and, if there is unsatisfactory response, add lithium, or benzodiazepines, or

[1]*Institute of Psychiatry, Ain Shams University, 3 Shawarby Street, Kasr El Nil, Cairo, Egypt*

selective serotonin re-uptake inhibitors (SSRIs) and, lastly, electroconvulsive therapy (ECT). In developing countries, the onset of schizophrenia is usually managed, primarily, with ECT and neuroleptics. If there is no response in 3 weeks, we initiate increased dosages, augmentative therapy or change of medication. If there is a partial response in 4–5 weeks, we follow the same steps as no response. It is customary, in our culture, to start with CNLs, if the patient is young, fit and can tolerate some side effects; otherwise, we can start with NAPs. We agree that treatment of the first episode should continue from 9 months to 1 year. We should be aware that, in developing countries, we encounter more acute transient psychotic episodes than schizophrenia.

We are in complete agreement that multi-episodic schizophrenia requires, at least, 3–5 years of maintenance therapy. The challenge we face with NAPs is that there is not enough data on how long we should continue maintenance therapy especially in view of the high cost. Is it possible to shift to CNLs after remission for 1 year on NAPs? In this case, is there a possibility that the patient is sensitized against side effects through exposure to NAPs?

It was mentioned that compliance is influenced by diverse variables grouped into patient-related, clinician-related, treatment-related and environment-related factors. Compliance in traditional societies, where the physicians' image is still high and respectable, is mainly dependent on doctor–patient relationship. I have met hundreds of patients who adhered to CNLs, in spite of many side effects, because of the trust in the physician's recommendations. Non-compliance will be mainly due to economic reasons, as still the majority of mental patients in developing countries are not medically insured and they have to buy their medications, especially the NAPs.

All the new drugs are launched after extensive drug trials, which have a lot of exclusion and inclusion criteria. The majority of these trials prefer not to include females in their fertile period. So, in clinical settings, we may face many problems, indications and contraindications that are not included in drug trials. This requires that the psychiatrist should be abreast of scientific knowledge and pharmacological understanding and independent of the industry's advice. The proper use of antipsychotics is an art depending on good clinical experience.

Ambulatory patients and those who require an active social life will be unable to tolerate the side effects, especially the extrapyramidal, anticholinergic and cognitive complications of CNLs, and we are better to start with the novel antipsychotics.

A study of tardive dyskinesia in an Egyptian sample [2] detected a prevalence of only 1.7% as compared to the international figures of 5% [3]. This can be attributed to the lower doses used, the non-compliance because of the cost and lack of family education, and the absence of supply of medications from mental health state services, because of exhaustion of the state subsidies.

There are three further points worthy of comment. First, there are some claims that the effect of NAPs on cognitive functions is unrelated to positive and negative symptoms or the severity of psychosis. Second, the effect of NAPs on negative symptoms can be secondary to improvement of the depression which is an integral part of the clinical picture of schizophrenia. Third, there have not been enough follow-ups on NAPs to know the long-term sequelae, especially with some NAPs that, when you increase the dose, become typical antipsychotics.

The improved tolerability associated with NAPs has swung the risk–benefit balance in favour of early and aggressive treatment. By intervening early and providing long-term maintenance treatment, the course of schizophrenic disorder may be altered, with overall decreased deterioration and chronicity and improved functioning and quality of life resulting in lower societal costs [4].

REFERENCES

1. Okasha A. (1998) The Impact of Culture and Ethnicity on Psychopharmacology. Presented at the APA Annual Meeting, 30 May–4 June.
2. Okasha A., El Dawla A.S., Khalil A.H., Saad A. (1993) Presentation of acute psychosis in an Egyptian sample: a transcultural comparison. *Compr. Psychiatry*, **34**: 4.
3. Kane J., Honigfeld G., Singer J., Meltzer H.Y. (1998) Clozapine for the treatment-resistant schizophrenic. *Arch. Gen. Psychiatry*, **45**: 789–796.
4. De-Quardo J. (1998) Pharmacological treatment of first episode schizophrenia: early intervention is key to outcome. *J. Clin. Psychiatry*, **59** (Suppl. 19): 9–17.

2.16

Pharmacotherapy of Schizophrenia: The Case of Developing Countries

Driss Moussaoui[1]

Eighty per cent of schizophrenic patients of the world live in developing countries. However, very few studies are conducted to detect potential specificities of the management of schizophrenia in these countries, as compared to what happens in the industrialized ones. The current state of knowledge is that there are more similarities than differences in the management of schizophrenic disorders. For example, it is clear that neuroleptics represent

[1] *University Psychiatric Center Ibn Rushd, Bd. Tarik Ibn Ziad, Casablanca, Morocco*

an essential tool in the treatment of this group of diseases worldwide. Among the differences, however, it seems that in developing countries the outcome of schizophrenia is better than in industrialized ones. There are many reasons for such differences. Among others, one can mention the solidarity of the extended family towards schizophrenic patients, as well as the lesser social pressure to obtain professional achievement. This explains why the number of psychiatric beds in developing countries can be small, and still an acceptable service can be delivered to the patients and their families through community-based institutions. A city like Casablanca, Morocco, for example, with 5 million inhabitants, has 200 beds only. On the other hand, more than 40 000 psychiatric patients consult in outpatient clinics every year, about half of them having a schizophrenic disorder. Without family solidarity, it would have been impossible to satisfy most of the urgent needs of mental health in the city with that small number of beds.

Part of this solidarity is passive tolerance, which also has a downside. It is a fact in developing countries that many families do not seek medical help for schizophrenic patients who do not disrupt their social life with violent acts or acute delusional states. It is not unusual to see patients having their very first contact with a medical institution 20 years after the beginning of the illness. Meanwhile, a number of them have consulted one or many traditional healers. As time goes by, we see a progressive decrease in this solidarity/tolerance phenomenon. More and more families are in a burn-out situation towards their patient, and sometimes even towards a father or a mother suffering from a schizophrenic disorder.

This cultural change is counterbalanced by the tools of modern psychiatry. What would have been the situation of these patients in developing countries if neuroleptics did not exist? The only alternative would have been to build larger and larger asylums at an unbearable cost, representing the worst possible scenario from every point of view. Fortunately, no developing country considers this as a viable strategy for the future. That is why community-based services are easier to initiate in developing countries, where services are often built from scratch.

The problem is with budget. The institutions of the public sector can buy only neuroleptics of the first generation, which are very effective in reducing positive symptoms, but which have little effect on negative ones. Many patients need antipsychotics of the second generation, but cannot afford them.

A special type of neuroleptics is particularly precious and affordable: long-acting neuroleptics. They are not only useful for schizophrenic patients with little insight and reluctance to comply with the medical prescription, but also for patients who live in remote areas, where neuroleptics are not easy to get.

In the pharmacotherapy of schizophrenia, there are some clinical aspects which are of a cultural nature. For example, tremor is perceived by some traditional families in Maghrebian countries as a symptom of an illness which could lead to the death of the patient. This has to do with the past history of various epidemic or endemic infectious diseases in these countries, especially malaria. That is why such a common side effect as tremor can produce a lot of anxiety in the patient and in his/her family. If such cultural perception is not addressed, the result would be non-compliance and subsequent relapses.

Finally, what could be the contribution of psychiatrists from developing countries to research on pharmacotherapy of schizophrenia? One of the characteristics of these countries is the availability of large numbers of never medicated schizophrenic patients. We can therefore observe situations similar to the one prevailing during the pre-neuroleptic era. That is how, for example, we found a prevalence of abnormal involuntary movements in schizophrenic patients who never received neuroleptics which is higher than the one existing in already treated patients. Some of these movements were not very different from those seen in patients with tardive dyskinesia [1].

Another field of research, which is still neglected, is the one of transethnic psychopharmacology. As a matter of fact, it has been shown that there are some differences in the pharmacokinetics in patients from various ethnic origin, explaining, to some extent, differences in side effects. It is clear that one of the future challenges of pharmacotherapy of schizophrenia is the necessity of taking into account the pharmacogenetic differences in various regions of the world. This could have a direct impact on the clinical aspects of the prescription of psychotropic medications to schizophrenic patients.

REFERENCE

1. Kadri N., Fenn D., Moussaoui D., Green C., Tilane A., Bentounsi B., Casey D., Hoffman W. (1997) Abnormal involuntary movements in never medicated schizophrenic patients. *Biol. Psychiatry*, **42**: 135 S.

3

Psychotherapies for Schizophrenia: A Review

Max Birchwood and Elizabeth Spencer
Northern Birmingham Mental Health NHS Trust, Aston, Birmingham, UK

INTRODUCTION

Historical Overview of the Psychotherapies for Schizophrenia

Prior to the 1970s, individual and group psychotherapies for schizophrenia were generally based on psychodynamic theories, or theories that conceived of schizophrenia as being caused by the behaviour or communication patterns of the sufferer's family [1]. As well as being ineffective in terms of the core psychotic symptoms [2, 3], these treatment methods stigmatized sufferers' families, often their main support system. Thus, following the introduction of effective antipsychotic medication in the 1960s, there was a shift of focus away from psychological interventions for schizophrenia.

Gradually, there was dissatisfaction with the over-reliance on pharmacological treatments for schizophrenia, as it emerged that a high proportion of individuals with schizophrenia continue to experience positive symptoms of psychosis despite taking antipsychotic medication [4, 5]. Similarly, the usefulness of this medication in remediating the social and cognitive deficits associated with the illness was found to be limited [6, 7]. Furthermore, in a series of now classic studies, Brown, Vaughn and their colleagues demonstrated that the nature of the family environment to which the schizophrenia sufferer returns after hospital discharge is strongly predictive of psychotic relapses over the ensuing 9 months [8, 9]. Thus, controlled trials of psychological interventions designed to promote acquisition of social skills and reduce relapse by improving family atmosphere emerged in the 1980s [10–12]. Their positive results were well received and promoted increased interest in psychological therapies in this population.

Schizophrenia, Second Edition. Edited by Mario Maj and Norman Sartorius.
© 2002 John Wiley & Sons Ltd.

Concurrent with these developments, the usefulness of cognitive therapy for the symptoms of depression [13] encouraged clinicians and researchers to extend its techniques to the treatment of medication-resistant positive symptoms of psychosis. The use of a cognitive intervention for psychotic symptoms in schizophrenia had been reported as early as 1952 by Beck. He used a variety of cognitive techniques (such as the careful examination of the antecedents of the symptoms, reality-testing, and homework exercises) in the treatment of a patient with paranoid schizophrenia [14]. Such techniques form the basis of the cognitive behavioural approach to the individual treatment of psychotic symptoms today. Psychological interventions moved away from concentrating on traditional psychiatric diagnostic classes to a detailed focus on the experiential and behavioural phenomena associated with schizophrenia. Single symptom interventions have been woven into global treatment strategies as part of the development of cognitive behavioural therapy. This was accompanied by a need for increased precision in the measurement of individual symptoms in order to plan treatment. Promising results initially appeared in case reports and uncontrolled trials. However, in the last few years, several randomized controlled trials have been published (e.g. [15, 16]). Recently also, attention has been focused on the treatment of depression in schizophrenia in its own right [17].

Rationale for the Use of Psychotherapies in Schizophrenia

The stress–vulnerability model [18] conceives of the symptoms of schizophrenia as resulting from the actions of environmental stresses on the vulnerable individual. Possible individual vulnerability factors include basic information processing deficits and other, as yet unspecified, biological factors, poor adherence to prescribed medication, and social skill deficits that may increase the occurrence of an environmental stressor or amplify its effects. Environmental stressors may include drug use and various social stressors, such as disruptive life events or a hostile or critical family environment [19]. Psychotherapies are ideally suited to address a number of stress and vulnerability factors. For example: family interventions attempt to change adverse family environments; social skills training aims at buffering the individual's coping skills; psychoeducation may address adherence to medication; and individual cognitive psychotherapies focus on improving coping skills and intervening in information processing.

There now exists a body of literature, including a number of methodologically sound randomized controlled trials covering four types of psychotherapy of schizophrenia which can be implemented in the general clinical setting: family interventions; cognitive behavioural psychotherapy; social skills training; and psychoeducation. Data on effectiveness from these trials can be used to guide clinical practice.

Planning Psychotherapies for Schizophrenia: What Are the Dependent Variables?

While most research attention has focused on the prevention of psychotic relapse and the reduction of persistent (generally positive) psychotic symptoms, schizophrenia can be a chronic disorder that involves multiple handicaps. It may affect all aspects of functioning, begins in adolescence or young adulthood and often derails critical educational and social milestones. Its psychotic symptoms are fearful and demoralizing, and it is associated with a high rate of depression and feelings of hopelessness and a high rate of suicide [20]. Caring for a person with schizophrenia can lead to high levels of burden and, consequently, the sufferer's social network may become overtaxed. If the sufferer has lost or failed to develop appropriate social skills, this social network may become permanently depleted. Furthermore, problems experienced by sufferers may vary with the stage of their illness or with their developmental stage and age.

Consequently, in planning and implementing psychotherapies for schizophrenia, any or all of a range of outcome variables, including relapse rates, level of positive and negative psychotic symptoms, depressed mood, family burden, and social and occupational functioning, can legitimately be the focus of therapeutic endeavour. Functional outcomes may require assessment with broad based instruments such as the Quality of Life Scale [21]. Conversely, intensive cognitive treatment of an individual positive symptom will require assessment instruments, such as the Beliefs about Voices Scale [22], which provide detailed multidimensional assessment of psychotic symptomatology.

Thus, in choosing an appropriate psychotherapy for schizophrenia, not only its overall effectiveness but also its effectiveness on the outcome variable of interest and with the patient population group being treated is important. In this paper we review evidence for the effectiveness of family interventions, cognitive behavioural psychotherapy, social skills training and psychoeducation for schizophrenia in the light of these considerations.

FAMILY INTERVENTIONS FOR SCHIZOPHRENIA

The interest in family interventions for schizophrenia grew out of observations that 30–40% of patients with schizophrenia who take medication as prescribed continue to relapse [4, 5] and that those discharged to live with families characterized by high levels of criticism, hostility and emotional overinvolvement (collectively termed "Expressed Emotion"(EE)) are at high risk of psychotic relapse [8, 9].

Since the early 1980s there have been numerous trials, of increasing methodological rigour, investigating the effectiveness of family interventions, primarily in decreasing rates of psychotic relapse, and to a certain extent in improving social functioning in people with schizophrenia, through reducing families' EE.

Most such family interventions share a common set of assumptions:

1. Schizophrenia is regarded as an illness, the course of which is influenced by a variety of psychosocial factors (the "stress–vulnerability" model).
2. The family is seen as an invaluable ally in the rehabilitation of the patient, and the formation of a therapeutic alliance with family members is seen as crucial [23].
3. While the family is not implicated in the aetiology of the illness, it is presumed that attempts to positively alter the emotional climate of the family will favourably alter the outcome of the illness for the individual patient.
4. Family interventions are seen as complementary to, not alternatives for, drug treatments of schizophrenia, and are usually delivered in the context of a comprehensive psychosocial care package.

Some studies have investigated the effects of brief educational interventions (generally less than ten sessions) on knowledge and attitudes among families of schizophrenia sufferers [24–31]. These interventions are generally short, the patient is usually not present during the sessions, and they focus solely or mainly on the delivery of information about schizophrenia, rather than on explicit skills training.

Most of these studies have found significant increases in knowledge about schizophrenia following the intervention [24–26, 29, 30, 32]. Furthermore, knowledge gains were maintained to a certain extent after 6 to 9 months [23, 24, 30, 32]. Some studies [23, 25, 28], but not all [31], have also found significant short-term improvements in measures of carer distress and sense of burden. However, it appears that there is some recurrence in distress and pessimism over the 6 months following the intervention [23, 32]. Also, none of these interventions has resulted in robust changes in measures of family atmosphere [23, 27, 28, 30]. Importantly also, studies involving European or American samples have found no evidence of a reduction in the rates of psychotic relapse following family interventions involving education alone [30, 33].

Studies which have evaluated different methods of information delivery have determined that face-to-face family educational sessions and educational printed or video material can all result in significant increases in knowledge about schizophrenia and short-term decreases in carer distress. No method, however, has been found to be superior in maintaining reductions in career distress at 6 months [23, 32]. Nevertheless, these modest positive results are of relevance to services with limited resources which may be unable to conduct face-to-face family educational programmes.

Despite these limited treatment effects, attention has been drawn to the other positive aspects of family education, in providing a non-threatening medium for family engagement [25], as a consumer right, and as a basis for problem solving [34]. Birchwood *et al* [32] found that improvements in measures of family distress were positively correlated with knowledge gains, and carer optimism that they had a positive role to play, suggesting that the provision of accurate information is, in itself, helpful.

Thus, more recent family interventions have incorporated family education as merely one aspect of a comprehensive treatment package. Since most of these interventions have as their theoretical framework the EE literature, their aim is usually to improve family atmosphere, and so reduce the patient's relapse rate, by increasing the family's ability to cope with problems and communicate in a positive fashion, with appropriate expectations and boundaries.

Most of the comprehensive family intervention packages evaluated in controlled trials to date comprise psychoeducational and skills training components. Virtually all include formal education, usually in the form of lectures, often supported by printed or audiovisual material, delivered either in the clinic or in the family home. Most utilize either didactic instruction in coping techniques and problem solving, usually accompanied by homework exercises, or the modelling of successful coping strategies used by other families met through relatives' groups. Some include explicit training in communication skills. Packages differ, however, in the site of treatment, whether the intervention is provided in a single or multifamily setting and whether the patient is included in the family sessions. Only a small minority of family interventions have not used this approach but have, rather, borrowed from psychodynamic or other schools of family therapy.

Table 3.1 displays the results of the major randomized controlled trials of comprehensive family interventions. These can be divided into: those evaluating brief behavioural family interventions either in the inpatient or outpatient setting [35–38]; those evaluating care packages including longer behavioural family interventions against standard care control [11, 39–46]; those investigating the effectiveness of alternative models of behavioural family interventions [33, 47–55]; those evaluating family interventions in a non-Western setting, among minority groups or among special populations [46, 56–59]; and, finally, those evaluating family interventions which are not based on a behavioural model [60–62].

The Effectiveness of Family Interventions for Schizophrenia in Postponing Psychotic Relapse

There is now little doubt that family interventions in schizophrenia are effective in postponing psychotic relapse over periods of up to 2 years.

TABLE 3.1 Randomized controlled trials of family interventions

Study	Importance	Conditions	N	Subjects	Components of family intervention	Results
Goldstein *et al*, 1978 [35]	Early study of brief family intervention	Family intervention/moderate dose neuroleptics	25	Patients with first or second episode schizophrenia	Six weekly sessions of crisis-oriented family intervention conducted as outpatients, aimed at acceptance of psychosis and crisis-management (identification of precipitating stressors and formulation of plan to deal with future stressors)	*6-week relapse rates*: 0% moderate dose/family intervention condition; 24% low dose/no family intervention condition (significant). No significant difference between relapse rates of other groups
		Family intervention/low dose neuroleptics	27			*6-month relapse rates*: Similar pattern
		Moderate dose neuroleptics only	28			*Other results*: Significant main effect of family intervention on total BPRS scores at discharge
		Low dose neuroleptics only	24			
Glick *et al*, 1985 [36] Haas *et al*, 1988 [37]	Study of brief family intervention in inpatient setting	Inpatient family intervention	92	Inpatients with schizophrenia, schizophreniform or schizoaffective disorders or major affective disorders	Minimum of six sessions over hospital stay of average 5 weeks, encouraging acceptance of illness, crisis management, and acceptance of the need for continued treatment	*Results at discharge*: Significant benefits of family intervention on global outcome only in some patients with schizophrenia (females with good prehospital functioning)
		Standard hospital care	94			

			N	Patients	Intervention	Results
Vaughan et al, 1992 [38]	Study of brief family intervention	Relatives' counselling	18	Patients with schizophrenia living in high EE households	Ten weekly counselling sessions without patient present. Focus on education, problem and communication skills	Significant positive effect on family attitude toward treatment and support _9-month relapse rates:_ 41% family intervention; 65% control (not significant) _Other 9-month results:_ No significant difference in readmission rates (50% in both groups). No significant between-group differences in mean symptom scores 83% relatives satisfied with counselling
		Standard care	18			
Leff et al, 1982, 1985 [39, 40]	Compares family intervention against individual care	Social intervention package	12	Patients with schizophrenia in high contact with high EE relative	Four home-based educational lectures, a fortnightly relatives' group for 9 months and between one and 25 home-based family sessions	_9-month relapse rates:_ 9% family intervention; 50% control (significant) _2-year relapse rates (including suicides):_ 40% family intervention; 78% control (not significant)
		Standard care	12			

continues overleaf

TABLE 3.1 (continued)

Study	Importance	Conditions	N	Subjects	Components of family intervention	Results
Falloon et al, 1982, 1985, 1987 [41–44]	Compares family intervention against individual care	Family management Individual case management	18 18	Patients with schizophrenia or paranoid psychosis, living with or in close contact with at least one parent, and whose families showed high EE or stress	Wide range of strategies based on social learning theory, aiming to teach structured problem solving and communication skills. Sessions were home-based for first 9 months and initially weekly, reducing gradually to monthly for 2 years.	*9-month relapse rates*: 6% family intervention; 44% control (significant) *2-year relapse rates*: 17% family intervention; 83% control (significant) *Other 9-month results*: Improvements in specific symptoms and remission and hospitalization rates all significantly favouring family intervention group. Consistent and significant differences in a variety of measures of social functioning favouring family intervention group. Significantly less relative distress and subjective global burden and greater levels of coping in family intervention group

Hogarty et al, 1986, 1991 [11, 45]	Compares family intervention and social skills training against standard individual care	Family treatment and medication	22	Patients with schizophrenia or schizoaffective disorder living in a high EE household	Provision of information, instruction in coping strategies, communication skills and problems solving, initially weekly, then reducing to monthly for 2 years.	*Other 24-month results:* Significantly lower hospitalization rates throughout 24 months. Many significant differences in social functioning preserved at 2 years
		Social skills training and medication	23			*1-year relapse rates:* 23% family intervention group; 49% medication only control (significant)
		Family treatment, social skills treatment and medication	23			*2-year relapse rates:* 34% family intervention; 66.7% medication only control (significant)
		Medication only	35			*Other 9-month results:* No clear benefit of family intervention on adjustment among non-relapsed patients
						Other 2-year results: Minor and inconsistent effects of measures of adjustment among non-relapsed patients. Significant effect on employment

continues overleaf

TABLE 3.1 (*continued*)

Study	Importance	Conditions	N	Subjects	Components of family intervention	Results
Linszen et al, 1996 [46]	Compares family intervention against individual care in patients with recent-onset schizophrenia	Individual intervention (IPI), high EE group	26	Patients with schizophrenia, schizoaffective disorder, schizophreniform disorder or other psychosis, aged 16 to 25	18 clinic-based family therapy sessions, based on Falloon model	*12-month relapse rates:* 23% IPI, high EE; 18% IPFI, high EE; 0% IPI, low EE; 13% IPFI, low EE. No significant interaction between EE and treatment condition. No main effect of treatment condition or EE on relapse
		IPI plus behavioural family intervention (IPFI), high EE group	22			
		IPI, low EE group	13			
		IPFI, low EE group	15			
Tarrier et al, 1988, 1989 [33, 47] Barrowclough and Tarrier, 1990 [48]	Compares effectiveness of different models of family intervention	Behavioural intervention — enactive (high EE subjects)	16	Patients with schizophrenia living in high and low EE homes	Both behavioural intervention conditions: two family education sessions, three stress management sessions and eight sessions of goal setting over 9 months with option to continue thereafter. Enactive condition used participative methods of instruction; Symbolic used discussion	*9-month relapse rates:* 12% behavioural intervention groups combined; 53% control (high EE sample) (significant) 17% enactive group, 8% symbolic group in high EE sample (not significant). No significant effect of the educational programme on relapse rates in high or low EE samples Significant improvements
		Behavioural intervention — symbolic (high EE subjects)	16			
		Education only (high EE subjects)	16			
		Routine treatment (high EE subjects)	16			
		Education only (low EE subjects)	9			
		Routine treatment (low EE subjects)	10			

in behavioural intervention groups combined in overall measure of social functioning and four subscales. No consistent improvement in control (high EE sample)

2-year relapse rates: 33% behavioural intervention groups combined; 59% control (high EE sample) (significant)

5-year relapse rates: 62% behavioural intervention groups combined; 83% control (high EE sample) (significant)

8-year relapse rates: 67% behavioural intervention groups combined; 88% control (high EE sample) (significant)

continues overleaf

TABLE 3.1 (continued)

Study	Importance	Conditions	N	Subjects	Components of family intervention	Results
Leff et al, 1989, 1990 [49, 50]	Compares effectiveness of different models of family intervention	Education plus relatives' group Education plus family sessions	11 12	Patients with schizophrenia in high face-to-face contact with a high EE relative	Two home-based education sessions in both conditions Relative's group condition: fortnightly meetings for 9 months; patient not present Family sessions condition: home-based sessions up to once a fortnight for 9 months, then less frequently up to 2 to 3 years if desired; patient present	*9-month relapse rates:* 33% relatives' group; 8% family therapy (not significant). Small, statistically non-significant social and occupational changes in both intervention groups. Five of eleven families in relatives' group condition attended no groups *2-year relapse rates:* 36% relatives' group; 33% family therapy group (not significant). 17% relatives' group attenders; 60% non-attenders
Zastowny et al, 1992 [51]	Compares effectiveness of different models of family intervention in an inpatient setting	Behavioural family management (BFM) Supportive family management (SFM)	13 17	Inpatients with schizophrenia aged 18 to 35	Weekly sessions for 16 weeks during inpatient stay with monthly sessions for 12 months after discharge. Behavioural family management: psychoeducation,	*16-month relapse rates:* 53% BMF; 47% SFM (not significant) *Other 16-month results:* Significant improvements in measures of overall social functioning for both treatments combined

| Randolph 1994 [52] | Examines effectiveness of a different site of delivery of family intervention | Behavioural family management Standard care | 21 20 | Patients with schizophrenia or schizoaffective disorder | problem solving and communication skills training Supportive family management: provision of information and advice about difficulties, utilization of brief family therapy techniques 25 clinic-based sessions of education and instruction in problem solving and communication skills over 12 months | Significant reductions in family conflict and family burden, improvements in knowledge about mental illness for both treatments combined *12-month relapse rates:* 14.3% family intervention; 55% control (significant) *Other 12-month results:* No difference in BPRS scores; 3% family intervention group hospitalized versus 50% controls Attrition minimal No significant treatment by EE interaction in predicting exacerbations |

continues overleaf

TABLE 3.1 (continued)

Study	Importance	Conditions	N	Subjects	Components of family intervention	Results
McFarlane et al, 1995 [53]	Compares effectiveness of different models of family intervention	Multiple family group treatment (MFG)	83	Patients with schizophrenia, schizoaffective disorder or schizophreniform disorder	Three engagement sessions, followed by biweekly meetings for 2 years involving psychoeducation, instruction in problem solving and coping skills. SFT involved single families meeting with single clinician; MFG involved six families (patient present) and two clinicians	*2-year relapse rates*: 16% MFG; 27% SFT (not significant). Relapse rates for subgroup completing treatment 32% MFG; 48% control (significant) *Other 2-year results*: Significant interaction between treatment effect and level of positive symptoms at discharge
		Single family treatment (SFG)	89			
McFarlane et al, 1996 [54]	Compares multiple family group treatment against individual assertive community treatment	Multiple family group treatment (MFG)/assertive outreach	37	Patients with schizophrenia, schizoaffective disorder or schizophreniform disorder and complicating factors	Initial psychoeducational workshop for families only followed by biweekly problem-solving meetings of six families including patients	*2-year results*: No significant difference in hospitalization rates between experimental and control conditions. No significant differences in changes in positive, negative or total symptoms. Mean rate 18% MFG; 6% control group in sheltered employment (significant)
		Standard assertive outreach care	31			

Study	Focus	Condition	N	Patients	Intervention	Results
Schooler et al, 1997 [55]	Compares effectiveness of different models of family intervention and their interaction with antipsychotic medication dose reduction	Applied family management (AFM)/standard dose medication	52	Patients with schizophrenia, schizoaffective disorder or schizophreniform disorder	Applied family management: psychoeducational workshop, educational booklets, home-based psychoeducational, problem solving and communication skills sessions weekly, then monthly for 2 years. Supportive family management: psychoeducational workshop, then monthly family group meetings for 2 years	Mean rate 10% in both conditions in non-sheltered employment (not significant). *2-year relapse rates:* No significant difference between family intervention conditions within medication conditions. *Other 2-year results:* No significant differences between rehospitalization rates between family intervention conditions overall or within medication conditions
		AFM/low dose medication	54			
		AFM/targeted dose medication	51			
		Supportive family management (SFM)/standard dose medication	55			
		SFM/low dose medication	52			
		SFM/targeted medication	49			
Xiong et al, 1994 [56]	Extends family intervention to non-Western setting (China)	Family intervention	34	Patients with schizophrenia living with at least one adult family member	2–3 month introduction and 1–2 years of clinic-based family counselling sessions, initially every	*12-month relapse rates:* 33.3% family intervention group; 60.7% controls (significant)
		Standard care	29			

continues overleaf

TABLE 3.1 (*continued*)

Study	Importance	Conditions	N	Subjects	Components of family intervention	Results
					2 to 4 weeks plus monthly family group. Strategies involved printed educational information, home and work visits, discussion about problems and coping strategies.	*12-month rehospitalization rates:* 12.5% family intervention group; 35.7% controls (significant) *Other 12-month results:* significantly greater improvements in measures of total symptoms and psychosocial functioning in family intervention group versus controls *18-month results:* significant differences in percentage employed and family burden favouring family intervention group No significant differences between groups in medication use

Study		Intervention	N	Patients		Results
Xiang et al, 1994 [57]	Extends family intervention to non-Western setting (China)	Family intervention Standard care	36 41	Patients with schizophrenia and affective psychosis	Aimed to educate family and help them identify and solve problems. Family psychoeducation using family visits, workshops and monthly supervision over 4 months	*4-month results:* significant differences in treatment compliance, rate of symptomatic improvement, percentage in full-time work, and social functioning favouring family group condition. Significant decrease in percentage of families who gave poor care or mistreated patient in experimental but not in control group.
Zhang et al, 1994 [58]	Extends family intervention to non-Western setting (China) and a first episode schizophrenia sample	Family intervention Standard care	42 41	Patients with schizophrenia	Initial educational session followed either by 3 monthly multiple family groups (with patient) or single family sessions depending on clinical need. Focus of psychoeducation facilitating compliance and reduction of hostility and overprotectiveness	*18-month readmission rates:* 15.4% family intervention; 53.8% control (significant even after adjusting for medication compliance) *Other 18-month results:* Significantly greater improvements in BPRS scores and global functioning favouring family

continues overleaf

TABLE 3.1 (continued)

Study	Importance	Conditions	N	Subjects	Components of family intervention	Results
						intervention group. More outpatient visits in family intervention group than control
Telles et al, 1995 [59]	Investigates the cross-cultural applicability of the Falloon intervention among Hispanic Americans	Behavioural family management Individual case management	42 to-tal	Patients of Mexican, Guatemalan or Salvado-ran descent with schizo-phrenia living with family member	Clinic-based intervention, initially weekly, reducing to monthly over 1 year, involving education and problem solving and communication skills training	Only 9% of families classified as high EE *1-year results:* Among unacculturated patients risk of exacerbation significantly greater with family treat-ment (p < 0.004). No significant effect for acculturated patients. Similar pattern of effects for BPRS total scores, GAS and some BPRS subscales
Kottgen et al, 1984 [60]	Examines effectiveness of an uncon-ventional model of family therapy	Family intervention Standard care, high EE group Standard care, low EE group	16 14 20	Patients with schizo-phrenia from high EE homes	Patients and families had separate groups. Two conditions of varying frequency of groups for 2 years. Interpretative and supportive focus	*9-month relapse rates:* 33% family intervention; 47% high and low EE control combined (not significant)

						Results
Levene et al, 1989 [61]	Examines effectiveness of an unconventional model of family therapy	Focal family therapy Supportive management counselling	5 5	Patients with schizophrenia and poor response to medication	Weekly sessions for up to 6 months post-discharge Focal family therapy condition: isolates and identifies unhelpful "focal" interactions. Borrows from brief therapy. Supportive management counselling: psychoeducation, crisis management, problem solving and communication skills	*Results at termination of therapy:* No significant difference in functional improvement between conditions. Significant improvement in symptomatology in focal family therapy group. No significant change in measures of family relationships for either group
De Giacomo et al, 1997 [62]	Examines the effectiveness of an unconventional model of family therapy	Elementary pragmatic model of family therapy plus psychoactive drug treatment Standard pharmacotherapy	19 19	Patients with schizophrenia, a duration of illness less than 3 years and living parents or spouse	10 weekly family sessions. No psychoeducational sessions but answers to questions provided. Emphasis on paradoxical interventions. Medication provided by family therapy team	*1-year results:* Significantly greater decreases in BPRS scores and scores on a measure of social improvement in the elementary pragmatic model group relative to the control

The magnitude of the treatment effect was recently quantified by Marie and Streiner [63], who performed a methodologically strict meta-analysis of 12 randomized controlled studies of family interventions for schizophrenia. They concluded that there is robust evidence that family interventions decrease relapse rates at 12, 18 and 24 months, although the data for longer follow-up periods had a high level of imprecision. Similarly, family interventions reduce hospital admission over follow-up periods up to 18 months. The magnitude of the treatment effect is reflected in the fact that between six and seven families must be treated to prevent one relapse of schizophrenia at about 1 year, and between five and six families to prevent one hospitalization.

Examination of the individual studies in Table 3.1 supports this conclusion. With the exception of the study by Linszen et al [46], all evaluations of long-term (9 months to 2 years) behavioural family interventions conducted in Western samples have shown significant reductions in psychotic relapse rates at 9 months to 1 year compared with standard care controls. Relapse rates for patients in the family intervention condition have ranged from 6% [41, 42] to 19% [11, 45], with corresponding control relapse rates of 44% [41, 42] and 35% [11, 45]. Hospitalization rates have also been found to be reduced [41].

In contrast, a study by Linszen et al [46], conducted in a sample of patients with recent-onset schizophrenia who were unselected for family level of EE, found no significant reduction in 12-month relapse rates attributable to the family intervention and no significant interaction of level of Expressed Emotion with treatment condition when predicting relapse rates. It is notable in this study, however, that overall relapse rates were relatively low, the individual intervention received by the control group was of very high quality, and patients in both conditions had received some family intervention during their hospitalizations prior to randomization. Similarly, the patients, all of whom had relatively short durations of illness, may have responded well to standard treatment. Thus, a ceiling for treatment effects may have existed.

The effects of the three studies involving brief courses of family interventions on patient relapse and symptomatology [35–38] were weaker. In the study by Goldstein et al [35], six weekly sessions of crisis-oriented family therapy were administered in the outpatient setting. Within medication conditions there were no significant decreases in relapse rates attributable to family therapy, although there was a significant main effect of family intervention on total scores of the Brief Psychiatric Rating Scale (BPRS). A similar brief family intervention performed in an inpatient setting [36, 37] also found post-treatment effects on global functioning to be limited to a small subgroup of the subjects with schizophrenia. The 10-week intervention studied by Vaughan et al [38] also failed to significantly reduce relapse rates of psychotic symptomatology among patients relative to controls, despite being well received by the families. Thus, short courses of family therapy, like brief education-only interventions, appear of limited usefulness.

The effect of long-term ongoing family interventions in preventing relapse has been generally preserved into the second year, although relapse rates are invariably higher than in the first year, ranging from 17% [42] to 40% [39, 40]. In all of these studies the frequency of contact between clinicians and families declined in the second year. However, in the single intervention that failed to preserve a significant treatment effect into the second year [40], clinician and family contact in the second intervention year was minimal, each family attending an average of 1.1 groups and 1.1 family sessions between months 9 and 24.

Hogarty et al [45] interpret these findings as indicating that family interventions postpone rather than prevent relapse in schizophrenia. They suggest that maintenance of the family intervention effect requires the continued availability of clinicians to family members, possibly throughout the patient's age of risk. They underscore this by the uncontrolled results of the follow-up of their 1986 subjects to the seventh post-study year, which showed that at least 83% had sustained a psychotic relapse or rehospitalization during that period. In contrast, Tarrier et al [64] report controlled data indicating a significantly lower rate of relapse at all follow-up points (9 months and 2, 5 and 8 years) in the group who had received family intervention in their earlier study [33, 47] compared with the control group, although there was a clear trend for an increasing rate of relapse in the family intervention group as time progressed.

Thus, in summary, comprehensive family interventions do postpone psychotic relapse and rehospitalization among patients with schizophrenia, but those that have proved consistently effective have been of at least 9 months' duration. Most treatment benefits are gained during the period of active intervention and there is insufficient evidence at the moment to say for how long these benefits are maintained.

The Effectiveness of Family Interventions for Schizophrenia in Improving Patient Psychosocial Functioning

Relatively few studies have examined the impact of family interventions for schizophrenia on broad measures of patient functioning.

Methodological and conceptual problems complicate the investigation of psychosocial functioning in family intervention studies. Hogarty et al [45] point out that analysis of entire samples with inclusion of end-point assessments made at the time of relapse will confound the well-documented success of family interventions in decreasing relapse, with their effects in improving functioning in the unrelapsed patient. However, the use of only unrelapsed patients will lead to an unrepresentative sample of possibly hardy individuals where it may be difficult to detect a treatment effect.

Falloon *et al* [44] chose to include their entire sample in the analysis and found widespread and consistent positive results. They found that, at the end of the 9-month period of intensive intervention, the family management group had significantly more favourable scores on a wide variety of self-report, clinical and observer rated measures of social functioning, including measures of overall social impairment, the performance of household tasks, and of work or study activity and friendships. At 24 months, the difference between the groups was still significant in some aspects of social functioning, including overall social impairment and family dissatisfaction with the patient's role performance. Falloon *et al* [44] comment on the fact that this was achieved without a specific emphasis on social rehabilitation and hypothesize that it was obtained through reduction of the florid symptoms of schizophrenia and enhancement of the family's general problem-solving abilities. Barrowclough and Tarrier [48] also reported a significant improvement in an overall measure of social adjustment as well as in subscales measuring withdrawal, interpersonal functioning and prosocial activities at 9-month follow-up in patients in their combined Behavioural Intervention groups, with little improvement in similar measures among controls. Since the information was gained from relative reports, however, the fact that the apparent improvement in social functioning resulted from a decrease in hostile or critical attitudes of relatives due to the intervention cannot be excluded.

Hogarty *et al* [45], on the other hand, considering only unrelapsed patients, did not find any consistent significant differences in measures of role performance or overall adjustment to favour the family intervention group at either 9-month or 2-year follow-up, although they did find that more patients from the family intervention group were working at 2 years. Similarly, Leff *et al* [49] found only small and non-significant changes in the social and occupational functioning of patients after 9 months of family intervention. These data were for their two family treatments combined, however, and the rate of non-attendance was high. Other studies which have found significant positive social effects in the family intervention condition are difficult to interpret, due to culturally ungeneralizable settings [56, 57] or incomparable or absent standard care control groups [51, 56, 57, 61].

Thus, while there is suggestive evidence that family interventions improve patient functioning, whether this effect is independent of their effects in preventing relapse is yet to be demonstrated.

The Effectiveness of Family Interventions for Schizophrenia in Reducing Family Distress and Burden of Care

Given the theoretical underpinnings of most family interventions in schizophrenia, it is not surprising that most evaluations of their effectiveness have also examined changes in family Expressed Emotion. Overall, significant positive changes in one or more of its components have generally been found [11, 33, 39, 40, 47]. However, surprisingly few studies have examined whether the relatives who attend these family interventions gain any benefit from them in terms of reduction of distress or burden of care.

Even following interventions that were ineffective in altering patient variables [38, 60], families reported satisfaction with the intervention, suggesting that they find the opportunity for support itself beneficial. Zastowny et al [51] found a significant decline in family conflict and burden after participation in both of their family invervention conditions, but this cannot be attributed to the intervention in the absence of a standard care control group.

The only study which has systematically investigated the effects of family intervention on relative distress is that of Falloon and Pederson [43]. After the first 9 months of treatment, the relatives who had been involved in the family intervention had significantly better scores on a global measure of subjective burden and were significantly less distressed about the patient's behavioural disturbance and social performance deficits than were the control relatives. Unlike the control relatives, they showed a significant decline in minor psychiatric symptoms over the 9 months, but due to baseline differences this may have been due to regression towards the mean. Relatives from the family intervention group also showed significantly higher scores on ratings of the effectiveness of coping over 9 months of the intervention, although there were some methodological problems in calculating a baseline measure.

Thus, more research is needed on the effects of comprehensive family interventions on the well-being of relatives. One problem here is that many families who are low in Expressed Emotion also report high burden [32]. Family interventions that are burden-focused should be blind to Expressed Emotion [65]. Overall, they have been successful in reducing Expressed Emotion in families and, presumably, this is experienced positively by relatives. There is suggestive evidence that they also reduce subjective burden and distress and increase coping, but this conclusion is based on only one study and requires replication.

The Most Effective Model of Family Intervention in Schizophrenia

Recent studies [33, 49, 51–55] have gone beyond the now answered question of the overall effectiveness of family interventions in schizophrenia to investigate the relative effectiveness of variations on the method and site of delivery.

Randolph [52] and Tarrier *et al* [33, 47] addressed straightforward questions about the best site of delivery and method of instruction for classical psychoeducational and skills-based family interventions conducted with single family units, including the patients.

Randolph [52] found that the significantly lower rates of psychotic relapse in the family intervention condition versus standard care were preserved when an intervention based on that of Falloon [41] was delivered in the clinic rather than family home setting. While the 1-year relapse rate in the family intervention group of 14.3% is higher than that obtained by Falloon [41], it is comparable to that achieved in other home-based family interventions [11, 33]. Rates of hospitalization were particularly low (3%) in the family intervention group, and, while treatment condition had no effect on BPRS scores, this may have been because all patients were relatively well at baseline. Despite the clinic-based nature of the intervention, attrition rate was minimal, possibly due to the fact that the investigators made one or two home visits to engage families, usually early in the programme.

Tarrier *et al* [33, 47] also made straightforward modifications to a home-based family intervention including the classic techniques of education, stress management and goal setting. They found that, in terms of reducing the rate of psychotic relapse at 9 months to 2 years, there was no significant advantage in including elaborate activities such as role playing, guided practice and record keeping in preference to simple discussion and instruction, into the family session. They confirmed, however, that education alone has no effect on psychotic relapse rates. Similarly, Zastowny *et al* [51] found that family sessions involving education, advice and discussion about problems were as effective in reducing rates of relapse as those involving more structured problem-solving methods, although the rates of relapse in both groups were relatively high.

Four main recent studies have examined whether effective behavioural family interventions can be delivered in a group setting [49–55]. Clearly, such a question is relevant to services with limited resources.

In the intervention conducted by Leff *et al* [49, 50], individual families were either given family sessions in their own home (with the patient present), or invited to attend a relatives' group where no patients attended. There was no significant difference in relapse rates between the two family intervention conditions at either 9 months or 2 years. The results of this study are difficult to interpret, however, as five of the eleven families recruited to attend the relatives' group did not attend any groups at all, and the small sample size reduces the statistical power of the analysis. It appears that attendance at the relatives' group was helpful, since, among the six families who attended the group, the 2-year relapse rate was only 17%. The highest rate of relapse in the study was 60%, found among the patients whose families failed to attend the group. However, given the methodological limitations of this study, no conclusions about the relative effectiveness of the two interventions can be drawn. It is important to note, however, that, as in some other studies which have failed to show a treatment effect from family intervention [38, 60], the schizophrenia sufferers did not attend the family sessions.

In contrast, McFarlane *et al* [53, 54] have examined the effectiveness of "multiple family groups", an intervention involving the meeting of a small number of families for education, support and problem solving, with the schizophrenia sufferers present for all sessions. In their first study [53], they evaluated the multiple family groups condition relative to a classic hospital-based single family intervention programme. While overall rates of relapse were not statistically significantly different between the conditions, if the subgroup of families and patients who completed treatment only were considered, the relapse rate associated with the multiple family groups condition (32%) was significantly lower than that associated with the single family intervention condition (48%). There was a significant interaction between treatment condition and baseline symptomatology, in that the beneficial effect of the multiple family group condition in reducing relapse was most pronounced in those patients who were most symptomatic at baseline. Unlike the Leff *et al* [49, 50] study, the attrition rates for the two conditions over the 2-year period were comparable and moderate (25% for the single family condition and 29% for the multiple family condition), probably due to the use of several initial single family engagement sessions.

The authors attribute the greater relative treatment effectiveness of the multiple family group condition to the larger numbers of individuals involved in problem solving and to the development of a social support network. However, the essentially negative results of their next study [54] must temper enthusiasm about this approach. They found that the multiple family group condition was not associated with lower rates of relapse, hospitalization or symptoms, compared with a standard control in a group of difficult patients with schizophrenia being treated within an assertive outreach framework. The only significant result was in the area of employment, where significantly more patients from the family intervention condition than from the control group were in sheltered employment after 2 years of intervention. The authors suggest that, since in both cohorts, patients showed significant improvements in measures of relapse and psychotic symptoms over the study period, the functional domain was left to indicate the relative effectiveness of the family intervention condition. The alternative explanation, that the multiple family group intervention had a relatively weak treatment effect in this difficult patient group, requires more research on this mode of treatment.

Schooler *et al* [55] also compared the effectiveness of an individual and a group family intervention within the context of neuroleptic dose reduction. Three dose levels were manipulated using fluphenazine decanoate under double-blind conditions: standard (12.5 to 50 mg biweekly), low dose (2.5 to 10 mg biweekly) or early targeted intervention (medication free but given fluphenazine at the onset of any psychotic prodrome). Participants were randomized to one of two family strategies: the traditional psychoeducational skills-based family interventions developed by Ian Falloon, who trained the team (Applied Family Management); or a supportive family approach involving group meetings, case management and consultation for family problems (Supportive Family Management). There was no significant effect of type of family intervention on relapse-free time nor any interaction between type of family intervention and dose condition. Patients receiving targeted treatment had a shorter relapse-free period and community tenure. Interestingly, there was no difference between low and standard dose regimes in time to (or risk of) relapse or hospitalization, although "rescue medication" was used more often in the low dose than in the standard group.

The Supportive Family Management group received an impressive level of therapeutic input. The authors point out the difficulty of maintaining fidelity of family intervention across five sites, and also note that eliminating many patients who failed to meet criteria for clinical stability reduces the opportunity to show a differential effect of family treatment, since the most severe and persisting symptomatic patients were excluded. However, they conclude that the study definitively shows that family support and encouragement is essential, but that the specialized inputs inherent in Applied Family Management are not. The caveats and limitations discussed here do not support such a confident assertion.

Thus, there is suggestive evidence from single studies that behavioural skills-based family interventions offered to individual families in a clinic setting are as effective as similar interventions conducted in the family home, and that discussion about problems might be as effective as more active methods of instruction. The relative effectiveness of multiple family groups compared with family interventions conducted among single families is unclear. It appears that to be effective the patient must be present in the family sessions and the main problem in conducting interventions with groups of families is engaging them and encouraging them to attend.

The Effectiveness of Family Interventions for Schizophrenia in Patient Subgroups

Table 3.1 shows that samples of patients from families who are low in Expressed Emotion are under-represented in studies of family interventions in schizophrenia. Strictly speaking, the effectiveness of these behavioural family interventions against a standard care control in the Western setting have only repeatedly been demonstrated in samples of patients from high Expressed Emotion homes [39, 41, 11, 49]. The single study which compared a comprehensive behavioural family intervention against a control in a sample unselected for Expressed Emotion [46] found no beneficial effect on relapse rates attributable to the family intervention.

There is suggestive evidence that patients from low Expressed Emotion homes may benefit from family interventions, however.

Randolph [52] found, for example, that there was no significant treatment by Expressed Emotion interaction in predicting psychotic exacerbations in their sample. Leff *et al* [50] also did not find a significant relationship between reduction in Expressed Emotion and relapse rate. Furthermore, McFarlane *et al* [53] enrolled a population unselected for Expressed Emotion and showed positive overall results. There is also evidence that up to 40% of low expressed emotion families experience problems of burden, stress or coping, suggesting that they may benefit from interventions [32].

An excessive restriction of family interventions to high expressed emotion families ignores the influence that untreated psychosis in a patient may have on the emotional atmosphere of the family. Tarrier *et al* [33, 47], for example, showed that some of their low expressed emotion relatives who received standard care only changed to high expressed emotion during the intervention. Furthermore, the choice to focus on high expressed emotion relatives comes from the association of measures of this concept with psychotic relapse. As we have indicated, if carer burden is chosen as a legitimate outcome variable in its own right, the justification for excluding low expressed emotion relatives from intervention may disappear.

Family interventions are now increasingly being conducted in non-Western settings. There has recently been a series of reports about family interventions performed in China [56–58]. All of these have shown beneficial effects of the family intervention condition on a wide variety of outcome variables, including rates of relapse and rehospitalization and level of psychotic symptoms. However, the extent to which their research findings can be generalized to a Western population is unclear. For example, the control condition against which all of these family interventions are compared involves haphazard attendance at an outpatient clinic (standard care). In general, attendance at follow-up and compliance with medication [56, 57] were increased in patients in the family intervention condition, and the extent to which the treatment effects were a function of this is unclear. Perhaps the most interesting aspect of these investigations, however, is that they demonstrate that family interventions can be conducted in services that are not rich in resources and that it is possible to adjust them to the needs of differing cultural groups [56].

Whether behavioural family interventions can be successfully applied in ethnic or cultural minorities in a Western setting is still unknown. The study by Telles *et al* [59], which found that, among unacculturated Hispanic Americans, family intervention actually significantly increased the risk of psychotic exacerbation, suggests that the answer may be no. Further research is needed in this area. Similarly, it is unclear whether family interventions are useful in patients suffering from recent-onset schizophrenia, since one of the two studies conducted in this population [46] failed to demonstrate a beneficial effect attributable to the family intervention and detected an increase in distress in the low Expressed Emotion families, and the other study [58], conducted in China, is difficult to generalize from.

The Effectiveness of "Unconventional" Family Interventions for Schizophrenia

Only three studies have investigated the usefulness of family interventions for schizophrenia which are not based on an educational and behavioural skills training model. Much of this work is difficult to interpret due to method-ological problems in the research. Kottgen *et al* [60] used a family intervention based on psychodynamic principles and found that it did not reduce rates of psychotic relapse relative to control. Conversely, Levene *et al* [61] found that Focal Family Therapy, a technique related to Brief Therapy, resulted in signifi-cant improvements in psychotic symptomatology while a behavioural family therapy intervention did not. Since subjects in the Focal Therapy condition had higher baseline symptomatology scores, however, it is possible that their improvement with time was a result of regression towards the mean rather than an effect of the family therapy. Finally, De Giacomo *et al* [62] evaluated a family therapy model in which there was no formal psychoeducation and which relied heavily on paradoxical interventions. Furthermore, medication management was the responsibility of the family therapy team, while in the standard care control condition it was conducted by pharmacothera-pists. Although the investigators found significant advantages for the family therapy condition in terms of improvements in symptoms and functioning, the medication regimes were quite different between the conditions and it is unclear to what extent this contributed to the significant difference.

Thus, consistent evidence for the effectiveness of family therapy interven-tions in schizophrenia only exists for those based on a psychoeducational and skills training model. Research on other types of family therapy is limited and has methodological drawbacks.

INDIVIDUAL COGNITIVE BEHAVIOURAL THERAPY FOR SCHIZOPHRENIA

The Cognitive Behavioural Therapy (CBT) approach to psychosis and psychotic symptoms is a relatively recent development. There was in fact a brief flirtation by the radical behaviourists in the late 1960s and early 1970s, based on the operant conditioning paradigm, but this focused exclusively on the behavioural concomitants of psychotic thinking and not on their phenomenological underpinnings [66]. Recent interest in CBT originated in the UK and was influenced by the work of Carlo Perris in Sweden. The CBT approach which has emerged in fact comprises two different strands, each with its own theoretical substrate, although of late these two approaches have become conjoined in practice.

The first approach is inspired by the stress-vulnerability model of schizophrenia. Vulnerability here is viewed as a "black box" drawing mainly from the biomedical tradition. The focus is upon symptoms (e.g. voices) or clusters of symptoms (e.g. a psychotic episode). It is assumed here that stressors capable of triggering or exacerbating symptoms may be generated or modulated by the individual and thus the focus is on how the individual deals with these putative stressors and triggers of symptoms. One class of stressors emanates from the immediate social environment, for example, close friends or relatives high in expressed emotion, and these are assumed to be modulated by the patient's own appraisal of their stressfulness and his/her coping strategies. The work of Gerard Hogarty on "Personal Therapy", which we will review, operates entirely within this framework.

Another class of stressors are the symptoms themselves — the distress they cause is assumed to be linked to the patient's own ways of coping with them. Thus Falloon and Talbot [67] documented the coping strategies used by voice hearers and concluded that those who had multiple strategies available to them were more able to cope with their voices. Tarrier [68], on the other hand, focusing on a wider range of psychotic symptoms, concluded that those who applied strategies consistently tended to fare the best. These were conventionally divided into affective strategies (e.g. relaxation, sleep, etc.), behavioural strategies (being active, drinking alcohol, etc.) and cognitive (distraction, challenging voices, switching attention away from voices, etc.). It is assumed that certain strategies are unhelpful and generate stress in the individual, which impinges reciprocally on the symptoms themselves, thus exacerbating them. This underpins the approach known as Coping Strategy Enhancement (CSE) [16], in which patients are offered a range of strategies which are implemented in an empirical fashion to determine their effectiveness in symptom control. This approach suffers some implementation difficulties, however. For example, if a delusional belief is formulated as the stressor, then the implementation of a strategy can only occur in the context of the individual's belief, for example that he or she is being persecuted. Thus distraction and other similar strategies cannot be offered if they are seen by the individual as exacerbating the supposed threat. Coping strategies in relation to voices, for example, are not randomly assigned to hallucinators but are almost entirely driven by the beliefs (delusions) that patients have about their voices; offering coping strategies incompatible with these beliefs are commonly rejected [69]. Nevertheless, although without empirical validation, it seems likely that certain strategies may indeed exacerbate distress and problem behaviour (e.g. where a patient may decide to confront a supposed persecutor). The CSE approach views the individual as an active agent who attempts to reduce the threat or distress posed by psychotic symptoms, but does not concern itself with the content or meaning that psychotic symptoms may have to the individual. There is also in this approach assumed to be a fundamental discontinuity between normal and abnormal functioning, which comes about once the biological vulnerability is "on-line".

The second CBT strand draws its theoretical strength from the cognitive therapy (CT) approach [70]. Here the emphasis is on the similarity between normal (but strongly held) beliefs and delusional beliefs in terms of psychological processes at play in their maintenance. Thus Brett-Jones *et al* [71] showed that delusional beliefs, like everyday beliefs, lead the individual to recruit evidence to support them and to de-emphasize or dismiss contradictory ones.

This supports one of the strategies in cognitive therapy, which is to encourage the individual to weigh evidence which contradicts a delusion. While it is possible that there are biases in the thinking of people with psychosis, CT acts to compensate for this rather than correcting the basic information-processing abnormality resulting in psychotic experience [72]. Some delusions in psychosis are closely linked to primary psychotic experiences, such as hallucinations. Birchwood and Chadwick [73] argue that certain beliefs about voices' power may be considered as a quasi-rational response to anomalous experience, and the meaning attributed to them in terms of identity, power and the consequence of disobedience has been shown to determine distress and behaviour in relation to the voice. This is inherent in the CT approach which focuses on the "evidence" of voices as support for a delusion (e.g. that a voice is that of the devil).

The CT approach in depression emphasizes the importance of evaluative beliefs about the self (e.g. self-worth) in the genesis and maintenance of depressed mood, and such beliefs are addressed during therapy. The application of this school of CT to psychosis also embraces an emphasis on evaluative beliefs about the self. The precise relationship between self-evaluative beliefs and delusional thinking is a much debated issue of the present time. It has been argued, for example, that delusions may serve the function of defending the individual from the full impact of low self-worth through blaming others for negative events rather than the self—the so-called "paranoid defence" [74]. The content of psychotic thinking often reflects such personal issues; for example, for the patient who has been sexually abused, this theme tends to crop up in the content of voice activity or in the supposed identity of the voice [73].

While these two approaches to CBT in psychosis have led to very different therapeutic strategies, they do share much in common:

1. They each place heavy emphasis on the formulation of a supportive and trusting relationship. In CT this is essential, if the client is to feel safe in order to examine directly the veracity of a belief.
2. In many ways both approaches are not strictly a "treatment" in the conventional sense. They each place the individual at the centre of therapy and encourage him/her to take responsibility for and control of his/her psychotic experiences. Thus in the CT approach it is acknowledged that a change in a delusional belief might not occur, but that a satisfactory outcome might ensue: for example, a patient might decide that a persecutor is in fact unable to harm him/her, and feel relief.
3. It follows therefore that both approaches are collaborative in spirit and not prescriptive, and that the intervention is individualized for each patient depending on the nature and content of the beliefs, the presence of other evaluative beliefs, and so on.
4. Both approaches emphasize the scientific method as inherent in the process of therapy. In the CT strand, for example, a patient may be invited to consider, in a collaborative manner, alternative constructions and meanings of a particular piece of "evidence", paving the way for an empirical (reality) test. This is sometimes known as "collaborative empiricism".
5. There is a common focus on symptoms rather than syndromes; this is not necessarily ideological, but a pragmatic issue. In one study, for example, CT was applied to the syndromes of acute psychosis, but did so by addressing three core delusional beliefs [76].

Randomized Controlled Trials of Cognitive Behavioural Therapy for Schizophrenia

Most data on this type of intervention come from case reports and uncontrolled trials. However, six controlled trials exist and are summarized in Table 3.2.

While four of these trials [15, 16, 76, 79] involved random assignment of subjects to experimental and control groups, the study by Garety *et al* [72] involved sequential allocation of subjects to cognitive therapy and waiting-list control groups. It is included in this review due to its importance as an early controlled trial in the area and as the pilot study to the larger London–East Anglia Study. The study by Tarrier *et al* [75] was also not totally randomized, in that their waiting list control group was drawn from

TABLE 3.2 Randomized trials of cognitive therapy for schizophrenia

Study	Importance	Conditions	N	Subjects	Components of cognitive intervention	Results
Tarrier et al, 1993 [75]	First randomized controlled trial of cognitive therapy in schizophrenia	Coping strategy enhancement (CSE) Problem solving (PS)	15 12	Patients with schizophrenia, with medication-resistant psychotic symptoms and on stable medication	Ten sessions over 5 weeks involving assessment of symptoms and associated antecedents, coping and consequences. Patient taught to monitor symptoms and institute coping strategies	*Immediate post-intervention*: Significantly greater decrease in total symptom severity scores in CSE group compared to PS after adjusting for baseline scores (p < 0.025). Significantly greater decrease in CSE group relative to PS only evident in delusion subscale. 60% CSE, 36% PS patients had achieved a 50% reduction in total symptom severity scores from baseline (p < 0.06) *9-month results*: 42% of CSE group still had a 50% reduction in total symptom severity scores from baseline

| Garety *et al*, 1994 [72] | Pilot study for London–East Anglia Study | Cognitive behavioural therapy | 13 | Patients with schizophrenia or schizoaffective disorder and distressing medication-resistant psychotic symptoms | Weekly or fortnightly sessions over 6 months involving enhancement of coping strategies, relabelling and psychoeducation, goal setting, challenging delusions and modification of dysfunctional assumptions | *6-month results*: Significantly greater decrease in total BPRS scores in CBT group compared with PS ($p < 0.01$). Improvements in measure of delusional conviction and some measures of delusional distress and interference significantly favouring CBT group. No significant between-group difference in changes in measures of social avoidance or hallucinations. Decrease in scores on Beck Depression Inventory in CBT group small, but significantly greater than that in PS group ($p < 0.05$) |
| | | Waiting list control receiving standard care | 7 | | | |

continues overleaf

TABLE 3.2 (continued)

Study	Importance	Conditions	N	Subjects	Components of cognitive intervention	Results
Drury et al, 1996 [76, 77]	First randomized controlled trial of cognitive therapy in acute phase of psychosis	Cognitive therapy Recreational therapy and informal support	20 20	Inpatients with acute non-affective psychosis	Sessions for 8 hours per week during inpatient stay involving challenging of delusions, testing of key beliefs and encouragement of coping strategies	*12-week results*: Significantly greater decrease in measure of positive symptoms in CT group compared with control (p < 0.0001). No significant difference in measure of positive symptoms at baseline but significantly lower in CBT group than control by week 7 (p < 0.001) and week 12 (p < 0.01). Significantly greater decrease in delusional conviction in CT group than control (p < 0.0001) *9-month results*: Significantly shorter time to recovery in CBT group compared to control. Time to recovery reduced 25% to 50% in CT compared to control, depending on definition used

Study	Description	Intervention	N	Patients	Intervention details	Results
London–East Anglia Study, 1997 [15, 78]	First large-scale controlled trial of cognitive therapy for schizophrenia	Cognitive behavioural therapy (CBT) Standard care	28 32	Patients with schizophrenia, schizoaffective disorder or delusional disorder, and distressing, medication resistant psychotic symptoms	Analysis of triggers, coping and context of symptoms, improving coping strategies, challenging delusions and dysfunctional schemas, management of social disability, relapse prevention	*9-month results:* Significantly greater decrease in total BPRS scores in CBT group compared with control ($p < 0.009$). Most change in suspiciousness, unusual thought content and hallucinations. 25% improvement in total BPRS in CBT group. 50% CBT, 31% control group classified as responders. Trend for decreases in measures of delusional conviction, delusional distress and frequency of hallucinations to favour CBT group, but not significant. Response to CBT predicted by cognitive flexibility at baseline ($p < 0.005$). No differential improvement between groups on measures of function or depression

continues overleaf

TABLE 3.2 (continued)

Study	Importance	Conditions	N	Subjects	Components of cognitive intervention	Results
Tarrier et al, 1998 [16]	Methodologically strict evaluation of cognitive therapy for schizophrenia	Cognitive behavioural therapy (CBT)	33	Patients with schizophrenia, schizoaffective disorder or delusional disorder, with medication-resistant psychotic symptoms and on stable medication	Coping strategy enhancement, problem solving training, relapse prevention	*3-month results:* Significantly greater improvements in severity ($p < 0.006$) and number ($p < 0.009$) of positive symptoms in CBT group compared with control.
		Supportive counselling	26			Supportive counselling group showed non-significant improvement in severity and number of positive symptoms relative to control.
		Routing care	28			33.3% CBT versus 12.9% control conditions combined achieved 50% reduction in severity and number of psychotic symptoms

| Hogarty et al, 1997 [79, 80] | Evaluates an individualized programme developed to buffer the impact of stress and combat late relapse | Trial 1 (patients living with family): Personal therapy — 23, Family therapy — 24, Personal therapy/family therapy — 26, Supportive therapy — 24. Trial 2 (patients not living with family): Personal therapy — 29, Supportive therapy — 25 | Patients with schizophrenia or schizoaffective disorder | 30 to 45 minute sessions weekly for 2 years and less frequently in third year. Treatment was individualized focusing on the patient's individual response to stress, and affective changes prodromal to relapse. Divided into three stages progressing from control of prodromes, through stress management, criticism management, conflict resolution and attempts to improve social roles | *3-year results: Trial 1:* Personal therapy associated with significant overall effect in delaying adverse effects ($p < 0.06$), especially in the first year of treatment. Widespread significant improvements in social functioning *Trial 2:* Personal therapy associated with significantly more relapse than supportive therapy ($p < 0.02$). Circumscribed significant improvements in work functioning domain |

the experimental and control conditions but was statistically treated as a separate group.

Methodological Issues

Some methodological problems emerge in these studies. Firstly, there is difficulty in establishing an appropriate control group. In two of the six studies [15, 72], the cognitive intervention was examined against a standard care control, leaving the study open to suggestions that non-specific factors, such as the increased amount of therapist contact in the intervention group, were responsible for the positive results. Conversely, in the absence of a standard care condition, it might be argued that certain control interventions have impeded recovery from psychosis, perhaps through the provision of an over-stimulating environment [76, 77] (although in Drury et al's study "standard care" in chaotic inner-city wards was considered more stressful than their control condition).

Secondly, the study by Tarrier et al [16] is the only one of the six which explicitly states that symptom ratings were conducted by assessors who were blind to the subjects' experimental allocation, although in all studies these assessors were independent of the provision of treatment, and close attention was paid to ensuring the reliability of ratings.

Thirdly, there was difficulty in ensuring that subjects in both groups received similar medication regimes during the intervention. This was despite the fact that most studies explicitly limited subject selection to patients on stable medication [16, 75] or at least to those with treatment-resistant symptoms [15, 72]. In both the London–East Anglia Study [15, 78] and the study by Drury et al [76, 77], medication use was somewhat different in the CBT and the control groups. However, in the former study, the direction of the difference could be expected to mask any treatment effects of CBT relative to control, while in the latter, the significant findings were still preserved after adjusting for medication use.

The Effectiveness of Cognitive Behavioural Therapy on the Positive and Negative Symptoms of Schizophrenia

Despite the above methodological problems, the six studies reviewed are consistent in their findings that CBT for schizophrenia can result in a statistically significantly greater improvement in psychotic symptoms relative to control conditions.

Three early studies used a relatively limited range of CBT techniques and relatively short periods of intervention and showed modestly positive results. In the first controlled trial of CBT for schizophrenia, Tarrier et al [75] found that, immediately after a 5-week intervention, the change in a measure of total positive symptoms was significantly greater in their group treated with CSE than in the control group who had been instructed in problem solving. Examination of subscales, however, showed that it was only in the area of delusions, and not in those of hallucinations, depression or negative symptoms, that a significantly different improvement had taken place between the groups. Despite this, the results were clinically promising: immediately after the intervention, 60% of the CSE group versus 36% of the control group had achieved a 50% or greater reduction in total symptom severity score from baseline, and 42% of the CSE group remained similarly improved at 6-month follow-up.

Using a slightly broader intervention, that involved cognitive therapy to challenge delusions and dysfunctional assumptions as well as the enhancement of coping strategies, Garety et al [72] also demonstrated a rate of decrease in total BPRS scores that was significantly greater in the CBT group than in the waiting list control. A detailed examination of the dimensions of delusional belief showed that improvements in some measures of delusional conviction, preoccupation and distress were significantly different between the two groups over the study period. Importantly, as in Tarrier et al's [16] study, hallucinations appeared more difficult to modify. Improvement in a measure of hallucinatory experience did not significantly differ between the two groups over the study period.

Drury et al [76, 77] focused more explicitly on challenging delusions and dysfunctional beliefs than on identifying precipitants and coping mechanisms for psychotic symptoms. They too found that cognitive therapy was associated with a significantly greater rate of decline in positive symptoms relative to control in the immediate post-intervention period. By the seventh week after entry to the intervention, the cognitive therapy group showed significantly lower mean scores on a measure of positive symptoms of psychosis, and also had significantly shorter times to recovery than did the control group. In fact, depending on the definition of recovery used, the time was reduced by 25%–50%. The improvement was maintained: at 9 months after the intervention, the cognitive therapy group showed fewer positive symptoms than did the control.

Following these early studies, there have been three further randomized controlled trials of CBT for schizophrenia. Unlike the earlier studies, they have employed broader combinations of cognitive behavioural methods to result in treatment packages that have been examined with increasing methodological rigour.

The London–East Anglia Study [15, 78] built upon the early work of Garety et al [72], and employed a manual-based treatment strategy involving enhancement of coping strategies, challenging of delusional and dysfunctional beliefs, management of social disability, and relapse prevention over a treatment period of 9 months. Like other investigators, it found that there was a significantly greater improvement in BPRS scores in the CBT group over the 9 months of the intervention relative to a standard care control. The improvement was clinically significant for the CBT group: by 9-month follow-up their total BPRS score had improved by 25%, and 50% of the CBT group could be classified as treatment responders versus 31% in the control group. Unlike the previous studies, BPRS items concerning hallucinations were among the most changed in the CBT group compared with the control. The authors, however, failed to find any significant differential treatment effect on self-reported measures of delusional conviction, delusional distress and frequency of hallucinations. This raises the possibility that the positive results of the behaviour therapy may have been due to non-specific factors, such as therapist attention, rather than being mediated by changes in dysfunctional beliefs.

The methodologically strict study by Tarrier et al [16] explicitly addresses this issue by evaluating CBT against both a supportive counselling and a routine care condition. They found significantly greater improvements in the severity and number of positive symptoms (measured by the BPRS) in the CBT condition compared with the control condition over a 3-month follow-up period. The supportive therapy condition also resulted in greater improvement than the control, but this was not significant. This suggests that part, but not all, of the effects of CBT on positive symptoms of schizophrenia may be explained by non-specific factors. Again, the improvement in symptoms in the CBT group was clinically significant: receipt of CBT resulted in almost eight times greater odds of showing a reduction in psychotic symptoms of 50% or more compared with routine care. Importantly also, while the total number of days spent in hospital was only one for the CBT group and one for the supportive counselling group, it was 204 for those receiving routine care.

Finally, Hogarty et al [79, 80] evaluated a somewhat different cognitive behavioural intervention for schizophrenia: Personal Therapy. This was developed on the basis of the results of their previous studies explicitly to prevent psychotic relapse in the second year of treatment. It consisted of an individualized and graded approach to stress management, involving, in particular, the identification and management of affect dysregulation preceding a psychotic relapse. The programme was divided into three steps, titrated to individual performance so that not all participants completed all sections. It progressed from a focus on therapeutic engagement and psychoeducation, through stress management, selected social skills training, relaxation training, and conflict and criticism management.

The investigators found that, for patients living with their families, Personal Therapy resulted in circumscribed but positive effects. There was a significant overall effect of Personal Therapy in delaying adverse effects, including psychotic or affective relapse or treatment-related termination, relative to supportive therapy. This effect was most pronounced in the first year after treatment. The effect in delaying psychotic or affective relapse alone was not significant, but the authors attribute this to the large number of treatment-related terminations in the supportive therapy group, leaving only the hardy individuals to act as a control group. Importantly, however, for patients living with their families, the authors found that participation in Personal Therapy actually increased the risk of relapse relative to the supportive therapy condition. In their discussion they suggest that the experience of Personal Therapy may have been too stressful for this group of patients, some of whom were in unstable social or accommodation situations.

Thus, in summary, there is consistent evidence from five studies [15, 16, 72, 75, 76] that CBT for schizophrenia can reduce positive psychotic symptoms to a greater extent than that which can be achieved with standard care or non-specific counselling alone. The effect appears clinically significant, with proportions of recipients in the range of 50% [15] to 60% [75] achieving good treatment responses and reductions of 25–40% in time to recovery from an acute episode of psychosis [77]. Those studies which have examined changes in measures of hallucinations and delusions separately have generally found more promising results for delusions, but conclusions must be tentative due to limited data.

There is suggestive evidence [16, 75–77] that some, if not all, of these positive effects are due to the specific effects of CBT on dysfunctional beliefs. However, it has not always been possible to demonstrate changes in the detailed dimensions of the symptoms of psychosis despite positive overall changes in psychotic symptomatology [15, 72, 78]. Garety et al [15], however, report that patients who had a "chink" of insight — who were willing to consider that they may be wrong — were most likely to respond to CBT, supporting the notion that part of the therapeutic action comes from a direct impact on delusional thinking.

Finally, data with respect to prolongation of relapse are mixed, and definite conclusions cannot be drawn, as they are based on the evaluation of a single, specific intervention [79].

Currently there is insufficient evidence to recommend a particular method of CBT for schizophrenia. Those interventions reviewed above have moved towards employing a variety of techniques as a therapeutic package. Similarly, there is insufficient evidence to determine which subgroups of patients with schizophrenia do and do not benefit from treatment, although at present Personal Therapy could not be recommended to people not living with their families [79, 80]. In each of these studies a considerable number of patients initially referred for entry into the trial were excluded due to factors such as non-compliance with medication, refusal to participate or persecutory ideation which interfered with engagement, suggesting that this treatment will not be suitable for all patients. Similarly, Kuipers *et al* [78] report that response to CBT in their study was associated with greater cognitive flexibility concerning delusions at baseline. This suggests that the sufferer may need some small degree of insight into the fact that he or she might be mistaken to benefit from cognitive therapy for delusions.

The Effectiveness of Cognitive Behavioural Therapy on Broader Outcome Measures

Despite the success of CBT in reducing positive psychotic symptoms, three of the four studies which examined its effects on measures of social functioning [72, 75, 78] did not find any significant therapeutic advantage relative to standard care or non-specific counselling controls. The exception to this was the study of Personal Therapy [80], which found a positive main effect attributable to receipt of Personal Therapy on a composite measure of social functioning after 18 months of intervention. For patients who lived with their families, there were widespread main effects of Personal Therapy on measures of global functioning, leisure activities and self-care. For those who did not live with their families, however, significant main effects were limited to measures of work-related activities. It is possible that these positive findings are due to the unusual length of the intervention (3 years), a focus which was broader than the management of medication-resistant symptoms of psychosis, and the use of a broad range of therapeutic techniques, including psychoeducation, social skills training, and stress and conflict management.

Finally, it appears that the management of depression associated with schizophrenia is not amenable to the cognitive behavioural interventions reviewed above, since only one [72] of the three studies [72, 75, 78] that examined changes in depression found a significant treatment effect attributable to the cognitive behavioural intervention.

Depression and Suicidal Thinking

The failure of the CBT interventions on psychotic symptoms to make any significant impact on associated depression is surprising, given that these symptoms are so distressing to patients. It is surprising still because some theories argue that depression is an "intrinsic" part of the psychotic process, so that one might expect a reduction in depression concomitant with psychotic symptoms. There has been, however, a revival of interest in the phenomenon of depression in schizophrenia. Recent studies suggest that depression is more closely tied not to the psychotic process itself but to patients' beliefs about psychosis and beliefs about themselves as sufferers from psychosis.

Depression in the context of a schizophrenic illness has been studied since Bleuler described certain "basic moods" of schizophrenia [81] and has its own place in the *International Classification of Diseases*, 10th revision (*Post-schizophrenic Depression*). Depression is a common clinical problem among people with schizophrenia and may be somewhat resistant to antidepressant medication [82]. It is understood to precede suicide, particularly if associated with hopelessness [83]. Depression in schizophrenia has not been studied within either the cognitive or psychosocial frameworks which have been so productive in unipolar depression [13, 84]. This is possibly due to a nosological confusion that surrounds it [85]. Various hypotheses have been proposed that explain depression in schizophrenia as a response to neuroleptics [86], as intrinsic to the schizophrenic process itself [82, 87], or as a result of "phenomenological overlap" with negative symptoms [88]. The "intrinsic" theory suggests that depression is an essential aspect of the schizophrenic process and as such should be discernible at one or more stages during the course of an acute psychotic episode [89, 90]. However, studies have reported a lack of a significant temporal relationship between the emergence of depression and the span of a psychotic episode [91]. "Pharmacogenic" theories suggest that depression observed in psychosis may be simply a drug-induced akinesic dysphoria that is well maintained by antiparkinsonian medication [92]. The suggestion is therefore that medication side effects may play a contributory factor in the high prevalence rates reported in some studies. However, a 10-year follow-up study by Berrios and Bulbena [93] refutes the claim that neuroleptic drugs are a causal factor in the onset of depression in psychosis. In addition, Leff [89], among others, provides results which suggest that patients' depressive symptoms *decrease* as acute psychotic pathology is combated by the administration of neuroleptic drugs.

The lack of a clear-cut theory may be due to the poor consensus for diagnosing schizophrenia and/or a failure to eliminate cases of schizoaffective disorder [94]. Munro [95] highlights "grey areas" where errors occur in the differentiation between affective disorders and schizophrenia. Although this argument may provide an answer to the considerable variation in incidence rates for depression in psychosis, it is highly unlikely that every study has employed consistently poor diagnostic classification.

A further possibility suggests that depression following a psychotic illness may be a reaction to the changes associated with the psychosis itself. Barnes *et al* [88] observed that subjective experiences of deficits in chronic schizophrenia, such as thinking, feeling and perception, were associated with vulnerability to depression. Birchwood *et al* [96] show that depression following acute psychosis may be viewed as a psychological response (demoralization) to an apparently uncontrollable life event (the psychosis) and all its attendant disabilities. Siris's [97] review of nearly 30 studies investigating secondary depression in schizophrenia suggest a rate of depression varying from 7% to 65%, with a modal rate of about 25%.

Leff [89] proposes three types of clinical course for secondary depression in schizophrenia: (a) depressive symptoms at the acute stage that are ameliorated as psychotic pathology recedes, and do not re-emerge after discharge; (b) depressive symptoms that emerge at the point of discharge following the remission of the acute psychosis; (c) depressive symptoms that emerge independently of the acute psychosis and at a point several months after discharge.

The consistent features found in recent studies to accompany depression in schizophrenia are suicidal ideation, attempt or completion [83, 98]. The latter of these studies concluded that depressed mood and the psychological aspects of depression (hopelessness, guilt and low self-esteem), not the vegetative symptoms, were important risk factors linked to later suicidal behaviour.

Recent research on the role of life events in triggering unipolar depression in community samples of women [84] provides a framework to help understand the link between a putative life event ("psychosis") and depression. This work has pointed clearly to the *appraisal* of the life event as being of primary importance particularly where the event involves loss (e.g. of status or cherished ideal) or threat and is further appraised as humiliating or entrapping (i.e. from which there is no escape). Whereas cognitive theory [13] argues that the lowering of self-regard has early developmental origins, recent ideas based on social ranking and power from ethology [99, 100] argue that certain situations are likely to be depressogenic, including: a direct attack on the individual's self-esteem linked to acceptance of a forced subordinate role ("loss"); events which undermine the person's rank, attractiveness or status ("humiliation"); and entrapment in a punishing situation or a disbelief in the ability of the individual to reaffirm an identity or sense of belonging ("entrapment" or defeat).

We have argued that placing the individual at the centre of our thinking locates psychosis as a major life event whose appraisal may involve all of the above elements. The onset of psychosis can limit activity in the interpersonal and achievement domains, thus leading to loss of valued roles or goals; the social stereotypes of mental illness may be viewed as a direct attack on the individual's attractiveness and rank [96, 101], and finally, individuals may feel a sense of entrapment in their symptoms (e.g. voices [73]) or in a relapsing psychotic illness [96], such that the achievement of desired roles or goals are constrained, and the individual feels entrapped. Two studies have found strong evidence for this model [96, 102].

The lack of impact of CBT on depression may be due to a failure to focus on patients' critical beliefs. We argue that it is the person's *appraisal* of psychosis which is vital to understand the meaning of depression in psychosis, and it is these beliefs or appraisals which need to be focused upon in CBT [17].

SOCIAL SKILLS TRAINING FOR SCHIZOPHRENIA

The poor social adjustment achieved by many people with schizophrenia [103] and the low correlation between adjustment and symptoms [104] have provided a rationale for efforts aimed at directly improving these patients' social functioning. Research has also highlighted the importance of premorbid social competence as a predictor of outcome in schizophrenia [104], suggesting that its remediation may also be accompanied by improved prognosis. Furthermore, the stress-vulnerability model of schizophrenia implies that the acquisition of adequate skills for dealing with the social environment will reduce its stressfulness and, thus, decrease the risk of psychotic relapse.

Social skills have been defined in a variety of ways, with reference to the internal states of patients, the topography of their behaviours, their goals and the effects of their interactions on others [105]. A representative definition states that they are those skills which allow the individual to "promote problem solving, engage others in successful affiliative and instrumental relationships, mobilize supportive networks and engage in work" [106]. They have been shown to predict social functioning independent of the severity of psychotic symptoms [107]. Social skills are composed of multiple verbal and non-verbal component skills, including both observable behaviours and skills in the social perception and cognitive domains [108]. Social skills training involves the systematic teaching of these component skills and the facilitation of their smooth integration [108].

Common content areas targeted for intervention include holding conversations, friendship making, conflict resolution, leisure and recreational activities, medication management and dealing with substance-abuse-related situations. Methods of social skills training are based largely on social learning principles, and interventions are generally specified in detail in treatment manuals. They use structured educational methods, such as behavioural rehearsal, modelling, role playing and positive social reinforcement, to teach skills in the presence of disruptive symptoms and cognitive deficits. They also aim to maximize generalization of skills to the real-life setting, by the use of homework exercises and *in vivo* training, and generally involve repeated practice until criteria for progress to the next treatment stage are met.

Numerous investigations of social skills training programmes among the patients with chronic psychiatric illness have been conducted since the 1970s. There have also been a number of reviews [105, 109, 110] and two meta-analyses [111, 112]. Early reviewers concluded that there was consistent evidence that social skills training is effective in increasing participants' feeling of ability, comfort and assertiveness in social situations, and in changing the topographical elements of social skills. However, this latter effect generally only occurred when the assessment situation was very similar to the training setting. Often the generalization of changes in social behaviour to natural settings was not assessed. Available evidence suggested that social skills training could improve symptoms and reduce rates of relapse in patients with serious mental illness, but the treatment effect appeared to be weak and based on few studies [105, 111, 112]. From the small number of studies of overall psychosocial functioning among these patients, it did not appear that social skills training had any effect on this variable [112]. Furthermore, the paucity of studies in an outpatient setting was noted [111].

These early studies, however, were hampered by poor methodology. Most importantly, many concerned "chronic psychiatric patients", and used poorly specified mixtures of patients. This limits the extent to which research findings can be summarized into a coherent whole. For example, in the widely cited meta-analysis by Benton and Schroeder [112], only 41% of the studies reviewed restricted their sample population to patients with schizophrenia only, and many of these studies were unpublished. Similarly, even in studies restricted to patients with schizophrenia, the method by which this diagnosis was reached was rarely standardized or even specified.

Since the mid-1980s, however, there have been a number of randomized controlled trials of social skills training in well-specified samples restricted to patients with schizophrenia. This chapter will review these studies, which are presented in Table 3.3.

Methodological Issues

These studies represent a considerable methodological improvement on those previously conducted in the field, through their use of standardized methods of diagnosis to screen subjects for entry to the study. Furthermore, by their choice of control groups, they attempt to evaluate the specific therapeutic effects of social skills training over and above the non-specific effects of therapist and group contact. However, generally they are not as methodologically rigorous as those evaluating other psychotherapies for schizophrenia. For example, not all ratings were performed by assessors who were blind to subject treatment condition [12, 113] and only two studies [11, 113] specifically mentioned the comparability of medication use in the two groups or examined treatment effects independent of medication compliance.

The study by Bellack et al [10] has particular methodological problems which are worthy of comment. The investigators began their analysis by a series of t-tests contrasting social skills training and standard day hospital care with respect to change scores derived from a series of outcome measures.

TABLE 3.3 Randomized controlled studies of social skills training

Study	Importance	Conditions	N	Subjects	Components of social skills intervention	Results
Bellack et al, 1984 [10]	Pioneering study	Day hospital treatment plus social skills training	44	Patients with schizophrenia attending a day hospital	3 hours per week for 12 weeks. Training involved conversation skills, assertiveness, social perception and special topics such as job interview skills and dating according to needs of patients	No differential treatment effect on skills, symptoms or psychosocial function at immediate follow up. Significant differential treatment effect on some symptoms favouring social skills condition at 6-month follow up. (Attrition rate 65% control; 50% social skills group). No significant difference in rates of hospitalization between conditions at 12-month follow up
		Day hospital treatment only	20			
Liberman et al, 1986 [12]	Early well-designed study	Social skills training	14	Patients with schizophrenia, with two or more prior hospitalizations and stable symptoms	10 hours per week for 9 weeks. Sessions involved training in "receiving skills", "processing skills" and "sending skills". Instrumental, friendship and dating situations covered	*Skills:* Significantly superior performance on behavioural tests in social skills group up to 9 months after intervention. No consistent pattern of superiority in self-report instruments
		Holistic health treatment	14			

continues overleaf

TABLE 3.3 (continued)

Study	Importance	Conditions	N	Subjects	Components of social skills intervention	Results
						Symptoms: Fewer relapses over 2 years in social skills group than control (not significant) *Psychosocial functioning*: Improvements in relatives' ratings of patients' social adjustment significantly favouring social skills
Hogarty et al, 1986, 1991 [11, 45]	Compares family intervention and social skills training against standard individual care	Family treatment and medication	22	Patients with schizophrenia or schizoaffective disorder living in a high EE household	Weekly to fortnightly sessions for 2 years. Flexible training in social behaviours and social perception skills, initially focusing on social skills in dealing with family, progressing to social and vocational interpersonal relationships	*Symptoms*: Significant main effect of social skills training in reducing relapse at 12-month follow-up, not preserved at 2 years *Psychosocial functioning*: Significant main effect of social skills training on some measures of social adjustment at 12-month follow-up but little effect at 2 years
		Social skills training and medication	23			
		Family treatment, social skills treatment and medication	23			
		Medication only	35			

Study	Aim	Interventions	N	Patients	Intervention details	Results
Dobson et al, 1995 [113]	Investigates effects of social skills training on both positive and negative symptoms	Social skills training / Social milieu treatment	15 / 13	Patients with schizophrenia who were not experiencing high levels of psychotic symptoms	4 hours per week for 9 weeks. Sessions covered basic communication skills, assertiveness training, individual communication and assertive goal setting	*Symptoms:* No significant differential effect on total or positive PANSS. Significantly lower negative PANSS in social skills group at 9 weeks follow-up but not at 3 months
Hayes et al, 1995 [114]	Evaluates programme with emphasis on facilitating generalization of skills	Social skills training / Discussion groups	63 total	Patients with schizophrenia, not significantly troubled by psychotic symptoms but with significant residual functional impairment	45 hours over 18 weeks and then nine booster sessions during 6-month follow-up period. Sessions emphasized interpersonal skills, social problem solving, symptom self-management, positive time use	*Skills:* Significantly greater improvement on one of two behavioural measures in social skills group at immediate follow-up, preserved at 6 months *Symptoms:* No differential improvement in BPRS or SANS. No differential effect on relapse rate *Psychosocial functioning:* No differential improvement in measures of general functioning or quality of life between groups. Little differential change in use of time

continues overleaf

TABLE 3.3 *(continued)*

Study	Importance	Conditions	N	Subjects	Components of social skills intervention	Results
Marder *et al*, 1996 [115]	Part of a larger study investigating skills-based psychosocial treatment and low dose medication	Social skills training Supportive group therapy	43 37	Male patients with schizophrenia and at least two previous psychotic episodes or 2 years of ongoing symptoms	Three hours per week for 6 months, then 90 minutes per week for further 18 months. Training modules covered medication self-management, symptom self-management, social problems solving and successful living skills	*Symptoms:* No significant difference in relapse rates between conditions at 1 or 2 years *Psychosocial adjustment:* Significant effects on social and leisure activities, personal well-being and total areas favouring social skills condition but only in subgroup given supplemental neuroleptics at first sign of relapse. Significant effect on total social adjustment scores seen only for patients with young age of illness onset

Study	Evaluates	Therapies compared	N	Population	Intervention	Outcomes
Liberman et al, 1998 [116]	Evaluates UCLA Social and Independent Living Skills Programme	Skills training Psychosocial occupational therapy	80 total	Male patients with "persisting and unremitting forms of schizophrenia"	12 hours per week for 6 months, followed by case management. Training modules covered basic conversation, recreation for leisure, medication management, and symptom management	*Skills*: Significantly greater improvement in self-report measure of total independent living skills averaged over 2-year period favouring skills training condition. *Symptoms*: Significantly greater decrease in distress favouring life skill training condition over 2 years. No significant difference in change in BPRS scores. *Psychosocial functioning*: No significant differences in changes in self-esteem, social activities or quality of life between groups over 2 years

They report that these tests "were almost uniformly nonsignificant, reflecting a consistent lack of differences in the degree of improvement" [10]. They then proceeded to examine pre- and post-test change for each variable within the two intervention conditions separately, and concluded that, since there were a large number of significant improvements in variables in the social skills group but fewer in the day hospital group, the effects of social skills training were discernible over and above those of the core treatment programme. The validity of this second statistical analysis may be questioned, since the repeated use of a univariate statistical analysis on measures likely to co-vary probably inflated the type one error rate. The larger sample size in the social skills group also gave the t-tests in this group greater power, possibly explaining the slightly larger number of significant score changes reported in this group over time. Furthermore, although they did find some significant between-group differences in change scores when calculated from baseline to 6-month follow-up, the attrition rate was over 50%, and the internal validity of these findings is suspect.

The Effectiveness of Social Skills Training in Improving Life Skills

Of the four studies that examined changes in the performance of specific social skills [10, 12, 114, 116], all except that of Bellack *et al* [10] reported pre- to post-test changes that were convincingly significantly greater in the social skills group than in the control condition, on at least some of the measures tested. Superior performance was most consistently, but not uniformly, demonstrated in behaviour tests such as role plays [12, 114]. The results concerning generalization of social skills to the real-life setting were inconsistent. Studies which reported results of a generalization test involving observed conversation with a stranger [12, 114] showed that social skills training had a significantly superior treatment effect to the control conditions. However, self-reported improvement in social skills in the real-life setting varied. Bellack *et al* [10] reported no differential improvement in self-reported assertiveness between their two experimental conditions. Similarly, Liberman *et al* [12] showed significant differential improvements in only some self-report measures of social skills. Both of these studies involved relatively brief periods of intervention, however. In a later study of a much more comprehensive intervention, Liberman *et al* [116] showed significantly greater improvements in a self-report measure of total indepen-dent living skills averaged over the 2-year period of follow-up, favouring those subjects treated in the social skills condition. They point out that the skills taught in the training programme were not isomorphic with those measured in the assessment instrument, suggesting some generalization of both stimulus and response. The authors attribute this to the fact that the treatment programme not only involved 6 months of intensive social skills training, but also assigned subjects to case managers who were charged with ensuring that they put their skills into practice over the ensuing 18 months.

Clearly, the above findings are limited by the self-report nature of some of the data. However, the research suggests that there is consistent evidence that people with schizophrenia can be taught a variety of social skills and that these can generalize, at least to situations in which the behaviours called upon are similar to those taught in the training situation. There is suggestive evidence that wider generalization can be obtained, provided the training programme is of sufficient duration and continuing efforts are made to encourage the participants to put their skills into practice.

The Effectiveness of Social Skills Training in Reducing Symptoms of Psychosis and Rates of Psychotic Relapse

All of the studies in Table 3.3 examined this question. With respect to reduction of relapse, the results are disappointing. The brief intervention by Bellack et al [10] showed no significant difference between experimental conditions in rates of psychotic relapse over the 12 months following the intervention (both conditions had relapse rates of approximately 50%). Similarly, in the 2 years following Liberman et al's [12] brief intervention, although the members of the control group were hospitalized twice as often as were members of the social skills group, this difference failed to make statistical significance (possibly due to the small sample size). The longer social skills interventions by Hayes et al [114] and Marder et al [115] also failed to significantly reduce relapse rates over periods of 6 months to 2 years.

However, the most detailed and informative exploration of the relationship between social skills training and psychotic relapse comes from the well-designed study by Hogarty et al [11, 45]. In this study, patients receiving both social skills training and family therapy had significantly lower rates of psychotic relapse at 1- and 2-year follow-up assessments than did patients receiving antipsychotic medication only. The effects of the two interventions were found to be additive, not interactive. A significant main effect of social skills training in reducing psychotic relapse was found at the end of the first year of follow-up, both in the entire sample and in patients who completed sufficient treatment sessions to be considered "treatment takers". The mechanism of this effect is unclear, however, as, when the subset of patients who faithfully complied with their antipsychotic medication was examined alone, the main effect of social skills training was no longer significant in the full sample and could be considered only marginally significant in the "treatment takers" (p < 0.09). In any case, the significant effect of social skills training in forestalling relapse appeared temporary, as at the 2-year follow-up the significant main effect of social skills training was no longer evident.

Thus, there is only very modest evidence that social skills training is effective in forestalling relapse. It may offer some benefit in combination with family therapy, but its effect appears to be temporary and may occur indirectly through increased compliance with medication.

Four of the studies in Table 3.3 also examined the effects of social skills training on the level of psychotic symptoms independent of rates of relapse.

The brief intervention by Bellack *et al* [10] showed no convincing benefits of social skills training in reducing a variety of psychiatric symptoms compared with the control condition, given the methodological limitations of their study. Two other brief interventions did show some significant benefits of the social skills condition in decreasing symptomatology, however: Liberman *et al* [12] demonstrated improvements in BPRS and Present State Examination ratings over the 2 years following the intervention, significantly favouring the social skills group over the control. Similarly, while Dobson *et al* [113] found that total and positive scores on the Positive and Negative Symptom Scale (PANSS) were not significantly different between their social skills and social milieu groups immediately following the intervention, negative PANSS scores were significantly lower in the social skills group. This effect, however, was no longer evident at the 3-month follow-up.

The intensive social skills training programmes were ineffective in causing reductions in schizophrenic symptomatology over that which could be obtained with the control interventions, despite patients' successful acquisition of social skills. Both the studies by Hayes *et al* [114] and Liberman *et al* [116] found no differential improvement in BPRS between the social skills and control conditions over follow-up periods ranging from 6 months to 2 years. However, there was a significantly greater improvement in a measure of distress in the social skills group compared with control following the intervention by Liberman *et al* [116].

Thus, currently the evidence is contradictory. Most favours the proposition that social skills training does not result in large or sustained decreases in core psychotic symptoms, but may result in changes in minor psychiatric symptomatology or possibly short-lived changes in negative symptoms. Clarification of these results must await better designed studies investigating subgroups of patients and controlling for such factors as medication use between groups.

The Effectiveness of Social Skills Training on Patient Psychosocial Functioning

All studies in Table 3.3 examined the impact of the social skills training programmes on broad measures of patient psychosocial functioning.

For example, Hogarty et al [11, 45], in the most methodologically sound of the studies, examined a broad range of indicators of psychosocial functioning in patients who had not relapsed over the 1 to 2 years of their study. In the first year, they found a significant main effect of social skills training on some of these measures, but by the 2-year follow-up, little of the effect remained, despite many of the subjects continuing to have weekly training sessions. This was consistent with their findings of the time-limited nature of social skills training in postponing relapse.

Liberman et al [116] also, despite a long training programme and evidence of generalization of social skills acquisition to the real-life setting, could not demonstrate that this impacted on patients' self-esteem, self-reported social activities or quality of life over the 2-year intervention period. Hayes et al [114] too failed to demonstrate any differential effect of their treatment conditions on quality of life or psychosocial functioning as measured by the Global Assessment Scale, despite their 6-month training programme.

The brief intervention of Bellack et al [10] found no significant advantage of social skills training over the control condition in improving psychosocial functioning, while Liberman et al [12], in contrast, did find that relatives' assessments of patients' social adjustment were significantly more improved after the intervention in the social skills group relative to control. This was validated to a certain extent by health worker ratings.

Interestingly, Marder et al [115] did find significant main effects of social skills training on a measure of total social adjustment and personal well-being, following a long training programme of 2-year duration. On measures of social and leisure activities, external family role and overall adjustment, there was a significant interaction between the two factors of the study (psychological therapy and drug condition). This indicated that significant benefits of social skills training were only seen in patients able to be stabilized on low dose medication who had shown themselves vulnerable to relapse but who were actively treated with neuroleptic medication at the first sign of exacerbation of symptoms. This suggests that social skills training may not demonstrate its effect on psychosocial functioning in patients who are either very well and unlikely to relapse, or treated with suboptimal medication. Interestingly also, when treatment effects on overall social adjustment were analysed by age of illness onset, it was found that the significant beneficial effects of the social skills condition were only present in patients whose illness had had its onset before the age of 24.

Thus, the best evidence that social skills training exerts an effect on overall psychosocial functioning was obtained in two programmes of 2 years' duration. At the best these advantages seem modest, but their importance in subgroups of patients may be obscured by analyses using total samples.

The Effectiveness of Social Skills Training in Subgroups of Patients with Schizophrenia

Little work has been conducted on the effectiveness of social skills training in subgroups of patients with schizophrenia apart from that of Marder et al [115]. Kopelowicz et al [117], in a small pilot study of social skills training in three patients with the deficit syndrome of schizophrenia and three with non-deficit negative symptoms, found a significant difference in the acquisition of behavioural skills favouring the non-deficit syndrome group. There is also evidence that cognitive deficits interfere with the acquisition of social skills in patients with schizophrenia [118, 119]. This has prompted the development of treatment strategies such as Integrated Psychological Therapy (ITP) [120], which consists of hierarchically organized subprogrammes ranging from those targeting basic cognitive skills to training in social skills and complex interpersonal problem solving. Most evidence exists for the effectiveness of ITP on elementary cognitive processes, but overall social adjustment has been found to improve significantly after ITP in an inpatient setting [121].

INDIVIDUAL PSYCHOEDUCATION FOR SCHIZOPHRENIA

Psychoeducation refers to the provision of information about psychosis and skills of self-management. It has generally been targeted either at neuroleptic medication compliance and/or improving understanding and insight into psychotic illness itself.

A randomized controlled trial by Eckman et al [122] randomly assigned 41 DSM-III-R patients to a modularized psychoeducation programme or to supportive psychotherapy. Two modules were taught including symptom self-management (identification of early signs of relapse, coping with persistent symptoms, avoiding street drugs) and medication management (information about medication, knowing correct doses, identifying side effects, negotiating medication with professionals). Outcomes were evaluated in terms of "skills performance in a series of role-played tests". No data on medication compliance were available, but BPRS measures of mental state were available. Fewer experimental subjects dropped out (5/20 vs. 9/21) and, in those that remained, skills acquisition was greater in the experimental group and retained over 12 months. No improvements in BPRS symptoms were seen in the psychoeducation group. Smith *et al* [123] report a similar study of a group psychoeducation approach comparing patients with and without positive symptoms. They demonstrated an improvement in retention of information but no improvement in insight or attitude to medication.

Patients with symptoms were also less likely to acquire "information about symptoms", which the authors felt was a result of patients' resistance to information which is dissonant with their current beliefs. Goldman and Quinn [124] report a study of psychoeducation about schizophrenia and its treatment. One group completed a 3-week programme while another randomly assigned control group continued to receive routine ward activities. Again, while an improvement in knowledge was demonstrated, no impact on symptoms was apparent. These early studies demonstrate that patients can acquire information and skills, but they still beg the question as to whether such information and skills internalize such that these are seen as relevant to the individual and his or her own situation. This requires an improved focus on outcome measures with greater clinical validity (see also Hornung *et al* [125]).

Some recent well-controlled studies have departed from this approach and have developed an individualized form of therapy with an explicit focus on medication compliance.

This approach known as "compliance therapy" has been developed in the UK by Kemp *et al* [126]. Compliance therapy uses the motivational interviewing approach pioneered in the drug and alcohol field. The first phase involves reviewing the history of illness and the patient's conceptualization of his/her own problem. The next phase focuses on symptoms and the side effects experienced by the individual. The benefits and drawbacks of drug treatment are considered, and the patient's ambivalence explored, with the therapy highlighting discrepancies between the patient's actions and beliefs, so as to create a form of "cognitive dissonance" which is resolved through a change in behaviour towards greater compliance. The last phase is concerned with the stigma of drug treatment and is tackled by considering that drugs are seen as a freely chosen strategy of the patient to enhance his/her quality of life. The intervention uses metaphors such as a "protective layer" and "insurance policy" in an attempt to distance the patient from otherwise more stigmatizing implications.

In Kemp *et al*'s randomized controlled trial [127], patients were drawn from an acute psychiatric ward ($n = 47$), and 25 were randomly assigned to compliance therapy with the remainder receiving non-specific counselling. Compliance was measured by the patient and by an objective method involving information derived from relatives, community psychiatric nurses, pharmacies, etc. Insight and attitudes towards medication were also measured. Results showed not only a major improvement in compliance in up to 40% of those receiving the therapy (10% for controls), but also in insight and attitude to medication, which persisted over 6 months' follow-up. No difference in psychiatric symptoms was apparent at 6 months. An 18-month follow-up has been reported [127], which showed that these effects were retained but, crucially, survival in the community prior to readmission/relapse was significantly longer in the compliance therapy group, with 50% of the latter surviving within an 18-month follow-up versus 30% for controls. These effects were also shown in a subsequent paper to be cost-effective when costs of admissions were balanced against the treatment costs [128]. There was a high readmission rate overall but the clinical reality of this sample was ensured by the use of minimal selection criteria. Around one third of the sample refused to enter the study or dropped out (the analysis used was "intention to treat"), which is broadly comparable with studies of CBT in general [75, 76). The group differences in insight/attitude to drugs averaged approximately 15.6% in the measures used.

This compliance therapy approach points to a clear benefit in short-term risk of relapse, but not in psychotic symptoms, which was linked to the receipt of compliance therapy. Many of the psychoeducational interventions have assumed that patients have, as it were, a deficit in knowledge or skills assumed to be responsible for poor compliance. Kemp *et al*'s trial, on the other hand, focused on patients' existing beliefs (i.e. fears or concerns about medication) and used these in a positive and individualized way to promote compliance.

SUMMARY

In this paper we have reviewed the evidence for the effectiveness of the four most commonly used psychotherapies for schizophrenia in order to guide clinicians in their appropriate application. This evidence can be summarized as follows.

Consistent Evidence

Family Interventions

- Family education alone does not reduce rates of psychotic relapse, but provides a non-threatening medium for engagement, increases knowledge, and results in short-term reduction in carer distress and increase in optimism.
- Printed or video materials and *in vivo* educational sessions are equally effective in increasing knowledge.
- Comprehensive psychoeducational and skills-based family interventions postpone psychotic relapse and rehospitalization if of sufficient duration

(generally at least 9 months). Most benefits occur during the most intensive phases of intervention.
- The beneficial effects of family intervention in forestalling relapse are most evident in patients from high EE homes.
- Family interventions can be implemented in non-Western settings with few resources.
- There is no evidence for the effectiveness of family interventions not involving a psychoeducational skills-based model.

Cognitive Behavioural Therapy

- Cognitive behavioural therapy for schizophrenia can reduce psychotic symptoms and/or distress associated with them to a greater extent than that which can be achieved with standard care or non-specific counselling alone.
- Despite this, it has little effect on social functioning or depressed mood.

Social Skills Training

- People with schizophrenia can be taught a wide variety of social skills which generalize to a certain extent to the real-life situation.
- The effect of social skills training in forestalling relapse is modest and temporary.
- The effects of social skills training on psychosocial functioning and quality of life are modest and found in programmes of long duration.

Individual Psychoeducation

- People with schizophrenia can learn about their illness and treatment, but this is generally not accompanied by changes in psychotic symptoms.

Incomplete Evidence

Family Interventions

- The duration of the beneficial effects of family intervention in postponing relapse beyond 2 years is based on few data and needs further investigation.
- There is suggestive evidence that family interventions reduce carer distress and burden, based on one study which requires extension.
- There is suggestive evidence that patients from low EE households may benefit from family interventions, but this requires more research.

Cognitive Behavioural Therapy

- Delusions may be easier to modify than hallucinations with cognitive interventions.
- There is suggestive evidence that some, if not all, of the positive effects of cognitive interventions on symptoms of schizophrenia are due to the specific effects on dysfunctional beliefs.
- It is likely that a "chink of insight" is helpful for the success of cognitive therapy for delusions.

Social Skills Training

- The extent to which social skills training affects the symptoms of schizophrenia is uncertain. Most evidence suggests that it does not result in large or sustained decreases in core psychotic symptoms but may result in changes in minor psychiatric symptomatology or possibly short-lived changes in negative symptoms.

Individual Psychoeducation

- Currently an individualized approach to psychoeducation (Compliance Therapy), focusing on patients' existing beliefs, appears most promising in increasing knowledge about illness and postponing relapse. Further work focusing on the relevance of psychoeducational material to the individual and his or her own situation needs to be conducted.

Areas Still Open to Research

Family Interventions

- While there is suggestive evidence that family interventions improve patients' psychosocial functioning, whether this is independent of their effect on relapse is unknown.
- The effects of family interventions among families from minority ethnic groups or among patients experiencing first-episode psychosis are relatively unknown.

Cognitive Behavioural Therapy

- There is insufficient evidence to recommend a particular method of cognitive therapy other than interventions which have employed a wide variety of techniques as a therapeutic package.

- There is insufficient evidence to determine which subgroups of patients with schizophrenia do and do not benefit from cognitive therapy.
- Depression and suicidal thinking do not respond to treatment focused on psychotic symptoms: CBT interventions need to be developed focusing on patients' appraisal of their psychosis and self-evaluative beliefs.

Social Skills Training

- The mechanisms by which social skills training exerts its positive mild positive effects on relapse and symptoms is not clear.
- The subgroup of patients who might benefit most from social skills training is unclear.

REFERENCES

1. Fromm-Reichmann F. (1948) Notes on the development of treatment of schizophrenics by psychoanalytic psychotherapy. *Psychiatry*, **11**: 263–273.
2. Mueser K., Berenbaum H. (1990) Psychodynamic treatment of schizophrenia. Is there a future? (Editorial). *Psychol. Med.*, **20**: 253–262.
3. McGlashan T.H. (1994) What has become of the psychotherapy of schizophrenia? *Acta Psychiatr. Scand.*, **90** (Suppl. 384): 147–152.
4. Leff J.P., Wing J.K. (1971) Trial of maintenance therapy in schizophrenia. *Br. Med. J.*, **111**: 599–604.
5. Johnson J.A.W. (1976) The duration of maintenance therapy in chronic schizophrenia. *Acta Psychiatr. Scand.*, **53**: 298–301.
6. Liberman R.P., Foy D.W. (1983) Psychiatric rehabilitation for chronic mental patients. *Psychiatr. Ann.*, **113**: 539–545.
7. Mueser K.T., Bellack A.S., Douglas M.S., Morrison R.L. (1991) Prevalence and stability of social skills deficits in schizophrenia. *Schizophr. Res.*, **5**: 167–176.
8. Brown G.W., Birley J., Wing J. (1972) Influence of family life on the course of schizophrenia: a replication. *Br. J. Psychiatry*, **121**: 241–258.
9. Vaughn C.E., Leff J.P. (1976) The influence of family and social factors on the course of psychiatric illness: a comparison of schizophrenic and depressed neurotic patients. *Br. J. Psychiatry*, **129**: 125–137.
10. Bellack A.S., Turner S.M., Hersen M., Luber R.F. (1984) An examination of the efficacy of social skills training for chronic schizophrenic patients. *Hosp. Comm. Psychiatry*, **35**: 1023–1028.
11. Hogarty G.E., Anderson C.M., Reiss D.J., Kornblith S.J., Greenwald D.P., Jabna C.D., Medonia M.J. (1986) Family psychoeducation, social skills training and maintenance chemotherapy in the aftercare treatment of schizophrenia. I. One-year effects of a controlled study on relapse and expressed emotion. *Arch. Gen. Psychiatry*, **43**: 633–642.
12. Liberman R.P., Mueser K.T., Wallace C.J. (1986) Social skills training for schizophrenic individuals at risk of relapse. *Am. J. Psychiatry*, **143**: 523–526.
13. Beck A.T., Rush A., Shaw B., Emery G. (1979) *Cognitive Therapy of Depression*. Guilford, New York.

14. Beck A.T. (1952) Successful out-patient psychotherapy of a chronic schizophrenic with a delusion based on borrowed guilt. *Psychiatry*, **25**: 305–312.

15. Garety P., Fowler D., Kuipers E., Freeman D., Dunn G., Bebbington P., Hadley C., Jones S. (1997) London–East Anglia randomized controlled trial of cognitive-behavioural therapy for psychosis. II: Predictors of outcome. *Br. J. Psychiatry*, **171**: 420–426.

16. Tarrier N., Yusupoff L., Kinney C., McCarthy E., Gledhill A., Haddock G., Morris J. (1998) Randomized controlled trial of intensive cognitive behavioural therapy for patients with chronic schizophrenia. *Br. Med. J.*, **317**: 303–307.

17. Birchwood M., Iqbal Z. (1998) Depression and suicidal thinking in psychosis: a cognitive approach. In *Outcome and Innovation in Psychological Management of Schizophrenia* (Eds T. Wykes, N. Tarrier, S. Lewis), pp. 81–100. Wiley, Chichester.

18. Zubin J., Spring B. (1977) Vulnerability — A new view of schizophrenia. *J. Abnorm. Psychol.*, **86**: 103–126.

19. Nuechterlein K.H., Subotnik K.L. (1998) The cognitive origins of schizophrenia and prospects for intervention. In *Outcome and Innovation in Psychological Management of Schizophrenia* (Eds T. Wykes, N. Tarrier, S. Lewis), pp. 18–41. Wiley, Chichester.

20. Birchwood M., Jackson C. (2000) *Schizophrenia*. Psychology Press, London.

21. Heinrichs D.W., Hanlon T.E., Carpenter W.T. (1984) The Quality of Life Scale: an instrument for rating the schizophrenic deficit syndrome. *Schizophr. Bull.*, **10**: 388–398.

22. Chadwick P.D.J., Birchwood M. (1995) The omnipotence of voices. II: The beliefs about voices questionnaire. *Br. J. Psychol.*, **165**: 773–776.

23. Smith J., Birchwood M. (1990) Relatives and patients as partners in the management of schizophrenia: the development of a service model. *Br. J. Psychiatry*, **156**: 654–660.

24. McGill C.W., Falloon I.R.H., Boyd J.L., Wood-Silverio C. (1983) Family educational intervention in the treatment of schizophrenia. *Hosp. Comm. Psychiatry*, **34**: 934–938.

25. Berkowitz R., Eberlein-Fries R., Kuipers E., Leff J. (1984) Educating relatives about schizophrenia. *Schizophr. Bull.*, **10**: 419–428.

26. Smith J.V., Birchwood M.J. (1987) Specific and non-specific effects of educational intervention with families living with a schizophrenic relative. *Br. J. Psychiatry*, **150**: 645–652.

27. Cozolino L.J., Goldstein M.J., Nuechterlein K.H., West K.L., Snyder K.S. (1988) The impact of education about schizophrenia on relatives varying in expressed emotion. *Schizophr. Bull.*, **14**: 675–687.

28. Abramowitz I.A., Coursey R.D. (1989) Impact of an educational support group on family participants who take care of their schizophrenic relatives. *J. Consult. Clin. Psychol.*, **57**: 232–236.

29. Pakenham K.I., Dadds M.R. (1987) Family care and schizophrenia: the effects of a supportive educational program on relatives' personal and social adjustment. *Aust. N. Zeal. J. Psychiatry*, **21**: 580–590.

30. Posner C.M., Wilson K.G., Kral M.S., Lander S., McIlwraith R.D. (1992) Family psychoeducational support groups in schizophrenia. *Am. J. Orthopsychiatry*, **62**: 206–218.

31. Solomon P., Draine J., Mannion E., Meisel M. (1996) Impact of brief family psychoeducation on self-efficacy. *Schizophr. Bull.*, **22**: 41–49.

32. Birchwood M., Smith J., Cochrane R. (1992) Specific and non-specific effects of educational interventions for families living with schizophrenia: a comparison of three methods. *Br. J. Psychiatry*, **160**: 806–814.
33. Tarrier N., Barrowclough C., Vaughn C., Bamrah J.S., Porceddu K., Watts S., Freeman H. (1988) The community management of schizophrenia: a controlled trial of a behavioural intervention with families to reduce relapse. *Br. J. Psychiatry*, **153**: 532–542.
34. Lam D.H. (1991) Psychological family intervention is schizophrenia: a review of empirical studies. *Psychol. Med.*, **21**: 423–441.
35. Goldstein M.J., Rodnick E.H., Evans J.R., May R.P.A., Steinberg M.R. (1978) Drug and family therapy in the aftercare of acute schizophrenics. *Arch. Gen. Psychiatry*, **35**: 1169–1177.
36. Glick I.D., Clarkin J.F., Spencer J.H., Haas G.L., Lewis A.B., Peyser J., De-Mane N., Good-Ellis M., Harris E., Lestelle V. (1985) A controlled evaluation of inpatient family intervention. I. Preliminary results of the six month follow-up. *Arch. Gen. Psychiatry*, **42**: 883–886.
37. Haas G.L., Glick I.D., Clarkin J.F., Spencer J.H., Lewis A.B., Peyser J., De-Mane N., Good-Ellis M., Harris E., Lestelle V. (1988) Inpatient family intervention: a randomized clinical trial. II. Results at hospital discharge. *Arch. Gen. Psychiatry*, **45**: 217–224.
38. Vaughan K., Doyle M., McConachy N., Blaszcynski A., Fox A., Tarrier N. (1992) The Sydney intervention trial: a controlled trial of relatives' counselling to reduce schizophrenic relapse. *Soc. Psychiatry Psychiatr. Epidemiol.* **27**: 16–21.
39. Leff J., Kuipers E., Berkowitz R., Eberlein-Vries R., Sturgeon D. (1982) A controlled trial of social intervention in the families of schizophrenic patients. *Br. J. Psychiatry*, **141**: 121–134.
40. Leff J., Kuipers E., Berkowitz R., Sturgeon D. (1985) A controlled trial of social intervention in the families of schizophrenic patients: two year follow-up. *Br. J. Psychiatry*, **146**: 594–600.
41. Falloon I.R.H. (1982) Family management in the prevention of exacerbations of schizophrenia. *N. Engl. J. Med.*, **306**: 1437–1440.
42. Falloon I.R.H. (1985) Family management in the prevention of morbidity of schizophrenia: clinical outcome of a two-year longitudinal study. *Arch. Gen. Psychiatry*, **42**: 887–896.
43. Falloon I.R.H., Pederson J. (1985) Family management in the prevention of morbidity of schizophrenia: the adjustment of the family unit. *Br. J. Psychiatry*, **147**: 156–163.
44. Falloon I.R.H. (1987) Family management in the prevention of morbidity of schizophrenia: social outcome of a two-year longitudinal study. *Psychol. Med.*, **17**: 59–66.
45. Hogarty G.E., Anderson C., Reiss D., Kornblith S., Greenwald D., Ulrich R., Carter M. (1991) Family psychoeducation, social skills training and maintenance chemotherapy in the aftercare treatment of schizophrenia. II. Two-year effects of a controlled study on relapse and adjustment. *Arch. Gen. Psychiatry*, **48**: 340–347.
46. Linszen D., Dingemans P., Van der Does J.W., Nugter A., Scholte P., Lenior R., Goldstein M.J. (1996) Treatment, expressed emotion and relapse in recent onset schizophrenic disorders. *Psychol. Med.*, **26**: 333–342.
47. Tarrier N., Barrowclough C., Vaughn D., Bamrah J.S., Porceddu K., Watts S., Freeman H. (1989) Community management of schizophrenia: a two-year follow-up of a behavioural intervention with families. *Br. J. Psychiatry*, **154**: 625–628.

48. Barrowclough C., Tarrier N. (1990) Social functioning in schizophrenic patients. I. The effects of expressed emotion and family intervention. *Soc. Psychiatry Psychiatr. Epidemiol.*, **25**: 125–129.
49. Leff J., Berkowitz R., Shavit N., Strachan A., Glass I., Vaughn C. (1989) A trial of family therapy versus a relatives' group for schizophrenia. *Br. J. Psychiatry*, **154**: 58–66.
50. Leff J., Berkowitz R., Shavit N., Strachan A., Glass I., Vaughn C. (1990) A trial of family therapy versus a relatives' group for schizophrenia: two year follow up. *Br. J. Psychiatry*, **157**: 571–577.
51. Zastowny T.R., Lehman A.F., Cole R.E., Kane C. (1992) Family management of schizophrenia: a comparison of behavioural and supportive family treatment. *Psychiatr. Quarterly*, **63**: 159–186.
52. Randolph E.T. (1994) Behavioural family management in schizophrenia: outcome of a clinic-based intervention. *Br. J. Psychiatry*, **164**: 501–506.
53. McFarlane W.R., Lukens E., Link B., Dushay R., Deakins S.A., Newmark M., Dunne E.J., Horen B., Toran J. (1995) Multiple-family groups and psychoeducation in the treatment of schizophrenia. *Arch. Gen. Psychiatry*, **52**: 679–687.
54. McFarlane W.R., Dushay R.A., Stastny P., Deakins S.M., Link B. (1996) A comparison of two levels of family-aided assertive community treatment. *Psychiatr. Serv.*, **47**: 744–750.
55. Schooler N.R., Keith S.J., Severe J.B., Matthews S.M., Bellack A.S., Glick I.D., Hargreaves W.A., Kane J.M., Ninan P.T., Frances A. *et al* (1997) Relapse and rehospitalisation during maintenance treatment of schizophrenia: the effects of dose reduction and family treatment. *Arch. Gen. Psychiatry*, **54**: 453–463.
56. Xiong W., Phillips M.R., Hu X., Wang R., Dai Q., Kleinman J., Kleinman A. (1994) Family-based intervention for schizophrenic patients in China: a randomized controlled trial. *Br. J. Psychiatry*, **165**: 239–247.
57. Xiang M., Ran M., Li S. (1994) A controlled evaluation of psychoeducational family intervention in a rural Chinese community. *Br. J. Psychiatry*, **165**: 544–548.
58. Zhang M., Wang M., Li J., Phillips M.R. (1994) Randomised-control trial of family intervention for 78 first-episode male schizophrenic patients: an 18-month study in Suzhou, Jiangsu. *Br. J. Psychiatry*, **165** (Suppl. 24): 96–102.
59. Telles C., Karnon M., Mintz J., Paz G., Arias M., Tucker D., Lopez S. (1995) Immigrant families coping with schizophrenia: behavioural family intervention vs. case management with a low-income Spanish-speaking population. *Br. J. Psychiatry*, **167**: 473–479.
60. Kottgen C., Sonnichsen I., Mollenhauer K., Jurth R. (1984) Group therapy with the families of schizophrenic patients: results of the Hamburg Camberwell-Family-Interview Study III. *Int. J. Fam. Psychiatry*, **5**: 83–94.
61. Levene J.E., Newman F., Jefferies J.J. (1989) Focal family therapy outcome study I: Patient and family functioning. *Can. J. Psychiatry*, **34**: 641–647.
62. De Giacomo P., Pierri G., Santoni R., Buosante M., Vadruccio F., Zavioanni L. (1997) Schizophrenia: a study comparing a family therapy group following a paradoxical model plus psychodrugs and a group treated by the conventional clinical approach. *Acta Psychiatr. Scand.*, **95**: 183–188.
63. Mari J.J., Streiner D. (1998) Family intervention for schizophrenia. In *Schizophrenia Module of the Cochrane Database of Systematic Reviews* (Eds C.E. Adams, L. Duggan, K. Wahlbeck, P. White). The Cochrane Collaboration, Oxford.
64. Tarrier N., Barrowclough C., Porceddu K., Fitzpatrick E. (1994) The Salford Family Intervention Project: relapse rates of schizophrenia at five and eight years. *Br. J. Psychiatry*, **165**: 829–832.

65. Fadden G. (1998) Family intervention in psychosis. *J. Ment. Hlth*, **7**: 115–122.
66. Mazillier J.S., Birchwood M. (1981) Behavioural treatment of cognitive disorders. In *Future Perspective in Behaviour Therapy* (Eds L. Michelson, M. Hersen, S.M. Turner), pp. 38–91. Plenum Press, New York.
67. Falloon I.R.H., Talbot R. (1981) Persistent auditory hallucinations: coping mechanisms and implications for management. *Psychol. Med.*, **11**: 329–339.
68. Tarrier N. (1987) An investigation of residual positive symptoms in discharged schizophrenic patients. *Br. J. Clin. Psychol.*, **26**: 141–143.
69. Chadwick D., Birchwood M. (1994) The omnipotence of voices. A cognitive approach to auditory hallucinations. *Br. J. Psychiatry*, **164**: 190–201.
70. Chadwick P.D., Birchwood M., Trower P. (1996) *Cognitive Therapy for Delusions, Voices and Paranoia*. Wiley, Chichester.
71. Brett-Jones J., Garety P., Hemsley D.R. (1987) Measuring delusional experiences: a method and its application. *Br. J. Clin. Psychol.*, **26**: 257–265.
72. Garety P.A., Kuipers L., Fowler D., Chamberlain F., Dunn G. (1994) Cognitive behavioural therapy for drug resistant psychosis. *Br. J. Med. Psychol.*, **67**: 259–271.
73. Birchwood M., Chadwick P.D. (1997) The omnipotence of voices. III: Testing the validity of the cognitive model. *Psychol. Med.*, **27**: 1345–1353.
74. Bentall R.P., Kinderman P. (1998) Psychological processes and delusional beliefs: Implications for the treatment of paranoid states. In *Outcome and Innovation in Psychological Treatment of Schizophrenia* (Eds T. Wykes, N. Tarrier, S. Lewis), pp. 119–144. Wiley, Chichester.
75. Tarrier N., Beckett R., Harwood S., Baker A., Yusupoff L., Ugarteburu I. (1993) A trial of two cognitive-behavioural methods of treating drug-resistant residual psychotic symptoms in schizophrenic patients: I. Outcome. *Br. J. Psychiatry*, **162**: 524–532.
76. Drury V., Birchwood M., Cochrane R., MacMillan F. (1996) Cognitive therapy and recovery from acute psychosis: a controlled trial. I. Impact on psychotic symptoms. *Br. J. Psychiatry*, **169**: 593–601.
77. Drury V., Birchwood M., Cochrane R., MacMillan F. (1996) Cognitive therapy and recovery from acute psychosis: a controlled trial. II. Impact on recovery time. *Br. J. Psychiatry*, **169**: 602–607.
78. Kuipers E., Garety P., Fowler D., Dunn G., Bebbington P., Freeman D., Hadley C. (1997) London–East Anglia randomized controlled trial of cognitive-behavioural therapy for psychosis. I: Effects of the treatment phase. *Br. J. Psychiatry*, **171**: 319–327.
79. Hogarty G.E., Kornblith S.J., Greenwald D., DiBarry A.L., Cooley S., Ulrich R.F., Carter M., Flesher S. (1997) Three-year trials of Personal Therapy among schizophrenic patients living with or independent of family. I: Description of study and effects on relapse rates. *Am. J. Psychiatry*, **154**: 1504–1513.
80. Hogarty G.E., Greenwald D., Ulrich R.F., Kornblith S.J., DiBarry A.L., Cooley S., Carter M., Flesher S. (1997) Three-year trials of Personal Therapy among schizophrenic patients living with or independent of family. II: Effects of adjustment of patients. *Am. J. Psychiatry*, **154**: 1514–1524.
81. Bleuler E. (1911) *Dementia Praecox and the Group of Schizophrenias* (Transl. J. Zinkin). International Universities Press, New York.
82. Siris S.G. (1991) Diagnosis of secondary depression in schizophrenia: implications for DSM-IV. *Schizophr. Bull.*, **15**: 179–188.
83. Drake T., Cotton T. (1986) Suicide among schizophrenics: a comparison of attempted and completed suicides. *Br. J. Psychiatry*, **149**: 784–787.

84. Brown G.W., Harris T.D., Hepworth C. (1995) Loss, humiliation and entrapment among women developing depression: a patient and non-patient comparison. *Psychol. Med.*, **25**: 7–21.

85. DeLisi L.E. (1990) *Depression in Schizophrenia*. American Psychiatric Press, Washington, DC.

86. Harrow M. (1995) Vulnerability to delusions over time in schizophrenia and affective disorders. *Schizophr. Bull.*, **21**: 95–109.

87. Johnson D. (1981) Studies of depressive symptoms in schizophrenia. *Br. J. Psychiatry*, **139**: 89–101.

88. Barnes T.R., Curson D.A., Liddle P.F., Patel M. (1989) The nature and prevalence of depression in chronic schizophrenic in-patients. *Br. J. Psychiatry*, **154**: 486–491.

89. Leff J. (1990) Depressive symptoms in the course of schizophrenia. In *Depression and Schizophrenia* (Ed. L.E. DeLisi), pp. 1–25. American Psychiatric Press, Washington, DC.

90. Hirsch S.R., Jolley A.G. (1989) The dysphoric syndrome in schizophrenia and its implications for relapse. *Br. J. Psychiatry*, **5** (Suppl.): 46–50.

91. Green M.F., Neuchterlein K.H., Ventrua J., Mintz J. (1990) The temporal relationship between depressive and psychotic symptoms in recent-onset schizophrenia. *Am. J. Psychiatry*, **147**: 179–182.

92. Van Putten T., May P. (1978) "Akinetic depression" in schizophrenia. *Arch. Gen. Psychiatry*, **35**: 1101–1107.

93. Berrios G.E., Bulbena A. (1987) Post-psychotic depression: the Fulbourn cohort. *Acta Psychiatr. Scand.*, **76**: 89–93.

94. Pope H.G. (1983) Distinguishing bipolar disorder from schizophrenia in clinical practice: guidelines and case reports. *Hosp. Comm. Psychiatry*, **34**: 322–328.

95. Munro A. (1987) Neither lions nor tigers: disorders which lie between schizophrenia and affective disorders. *Can. J. Psychiatry*, **32**: 296–297.

96. Birchwood M., Mason R., MacMillan F., Healey J. (1993) Depression, demoralisation and control over psychotic illness: a comparison of depressed and non-depressed patients with a chronic psychosis. *Psychol. Med.*, **23**: 387–395.

97. Siris S.G. (1995) Depression and schizophrenia. In *Schizophrenia* (Eds S.R. Hirsch, D.R. Weinberger), pp. 184–221. Blackwell, Oxford.

98. Addington D., Addington J. (1992) Attempted suicide and depression in schizophrenia. *Acta Psychiatr. Scand.*, **85**: 288–291.

99. Gilbert P. (1993) *Depression: The Evolution of Powerlessness*. Erlbaum, Hove.

100. Price J., Sloman L., Gardner R., Gilbert P., Rohde P. (1994) The social competition hypothesis of depression. *Br. J. Psychiatry*, **164**: 309–315.

101. Estroff S.E. (1989) Self identity and subjective experience of schizophrenia: in search of the subject. *Schizophr. Bull.*, **15**: 189–196.

102. Rooke O., Birchwood M. (1998) Loss, humiliation and entrapment as appraisals of schizophrenic illness: a prospective study of depressed and non-depressed patients. *Br. J. Psychol.*, **37**: 259–268.

103. Sylph J.A., Ross H.E., Kedward H.B. (1977) Social disability in chronic psychiatric patients. *Am. J. Psychiatry*, **134**: 1391–1394.

104. Strauss J.S., Carpenter W.T. (1974) The prediction of outcome in schizophrenia: II. The relationship between predictor and outcome variables. *Arch. Gen. Psychiatry*, **31**: 39–42.

105. Wallace C.J., Nelson C.J., Liberman R.P., Aitchison R.A., Lukoff D., Elder J.P., Ferris C. (1980) A review and critique of social skills training with schizophrenic patients. *Schizophr. Bull.*, **6**: 42–63.

106. Anthony W.A., Liberman R.P. (1986) The practice of rehabilitation: historical, conceptual and research base. *Schizophr. Bull.*, **12**: 542–559.
107. Halford W.K., Hayes R.L. (1995) Social skills in schizophrenia: assessing the relationship between social skills, psychopathology and community functioning. *Soc. Psychiatry Psychiatr. Epidemiol.*, **30**: 14–19.
108. Mueser K.T., Drake R.E., Bond G.R. (1997) Recent advances in psychiatric rehabilitation for patients with severe mental illness. *Harvard Rev. Psychiatry*, **5**: 123–137.
109. Brady J.P. (1984) Social skills training for psychiatric patients. I: Concepts, methods and clinical results. *Occup. Ther. Ment. Hlth*, **4**: 51–68.
110. Brady J.P. (1984) Social skills training for psychiatric patients. II: Clinical outcome studies. *Am. J. Psychiatry*, **141**: 491–498.
111. Dilk N.M., Bond G.R. (1996) Meta-analytic evaluation of skills training research for persons with severe mental illness. *J. Consult. Clin. Psychol.*, **64**: 1337–1346.
112. Benton M.K., Schroeder H.E. (1990) Social skills training with schizophrenics: a meta-analytic evaluation. *J. Consult. Clin. Psychol.*, **58**: 741–747.
113. Dobson D.J.G., McDougall G., Busheikin J., Aldous J. (1995) Effects of social skills training and social milieu treatment on symptoms of schizophrenia. *Psychiatr. Serv.*, **46**: 376–380.
114. Hayes R.L., Halford W.K., Varghese F.T. (1995) Social skills training with chronic schizophrenic patients: effects on negative symptoms and community functioning. *Behav. Ther.*, **26**: 433–449.
115. Marder S.R., Wirshing W.C., Mintz J., McKenzie J., Johnston K., Eckman T.A., Lebell M., Zimmerman K., Liberman R.P. (1996) Two-year outcome of social skills training and group psychotherapy for outpatients with schizophrenia. *Am. J. Psychiatry*, **153**: 1585–1591.
116. Liberman R.P., Wallace C.J, Blackwell G., Lopelowicz A., Vaccaro J.V., Mintz J. (1998) Skills training versus psychosocial occupational therapy for persons with persistent schizophrenia. *Am. J. Psychiatry*, **155**: 1087–1091.
117. Kopelowicz A., Liberman R.P., Mintz J., Zarate R. (1997) Comparison of efficacy of social skills training for deficit and nondeficit negative symptoms in schizophrenia. *Am. J. Psychiatry*, **154**: 424–425.
118. Mueser K.T., Bellack A.S., Douglas M.S., Wade J.H. (1991) Prediction of social skill acquisition in schizophrenic and major affective disorder patients for memory and symptomatology. *Psychiatry Res.*, **37**: 281–296.
119. Kern R.S., Green M., Satz P. (1992) Neuropsychological predictors of skills training for chronic psychiatric patients. *Psychiatry Res.*, **42**: 223–230.
120. Brenner H.D., Rodel V., Kienzle N., Hodel B. (1991) *Treatment and Rehabilitation of Schizophrenic Patients: An Integrated Psychological Therapy Program.* Huber, Toronto.
121. Brenner H.D., Hodel B., Roder V., Corrigan P. (1992) Treatment of cognitive dysfunctions and behavioural deficits in schizophrenia. *Schizophr. Bull.*, **18**: 21–25.
122. Eckman T.A., Wirshing W.C., Marder S.R., Liberman R.P., Jonston-Cronk K., Zimmerman K., Mintz J. (1992) Technique for training schizophrenic patients in illness self-management: a controlled trial. *Am. J. Psychiatry*, **149**: 1549–1555.
123. Smith J., Birchwood M., Hadrell A. (1992) Informing people with schizophrenia about their illness: a comparison of symptomatic and non-symptomatic patients. *J. Ment. Hlth*, **1**: 13–21.
124. Goldman C.R., Quinn F.L. Effects of a patient education program in the treatment of schizophrenia. *Hosp. Comm. Psychiatry*, **39**: 282–286.

125. Hornung W.P., Klingberg S., Feldman R., Schonauer K., Schulze Monking H. (1998) Collaboration with drug treatment by schizophrenic patients with and without psychoeducational training: results of a 1-year follow-up. *Acta Psychiatr. Scand.*, **97**: 213–219.

126. Kemp R., Hayward P., Applewhaite G., Everitt B., David A. (1996) Compliance therapy in psychotic patients: randomised controlled trial. *Br. Med. J.*, **312**: 345–349.

127. Kemp R., Kirov G., Everitt B., Hayward P., David A. (1998) Randomised controlled trial of compliance therapy: 18-month follow-up. *Br. J. Psychiatry*, **172**: 413–419.

128. Healey A., Knapp M., Astin J., Beecham J., Kemp R., Kirov G., David A. (1998) Cost-effectiveness evaluation of compliance therapy for people with psychosis. *Br. J. Psychiatry*, **172**: 420–424.

Commentaries

3.1
Relevant Methods, Goals, Time-dimensions and Emotional Influences in the Psychotherapy of Schizophrenia

Luc Ciompi[1]

The overview presented by Birchwood and Spencer marks important progress in current knowledge on psychotherapy of schizophrenia. It confirms the effectiveness of psychoeducational and skills-based family interventions, of cognitive behavioural therapy, of social skills training, and of individual psychoeducation. It also separates areas of robust knowledge from areas of still insufficient evidence concerning, for example, the effects of family interventions in low expressed emotions (EE) households, or the effectiveness of the studied methods beyond 2 years. Finally, it identifies important questions for future research, among them differential effects on different subgroups, and correlations between psychosocial functioning and relapse rates.

Certain problems may, however, deserve some additional reflection, among them the focused field of psychotherapy itself, the question of relevant dependent variables, the influence of time, and the possible key role of emotional factors in schizophrenia and its psychotherapeutic implications.

The range of psychotherapy is reduced in the overview to the four methods which are best explored by empirical research. While certainly justified from a methodological standpoint, this procedure has also possible disadvantages: it perhaps prematurely excludes other methods, such as systemic and psychodynamic approaches, which are statistically less well explored, but appear as efficient in a number of cases according to clinical experience. Therapy-relevant insights into relations of psychotic symptoms with biographic and sociodynamic factors, too, might thus get lost, as well as valuable information from different well-studied psychotherapy-based approaches in the community, such as the "need-adapted treatment" in Finland [1], the "Soteria" projects in the USA and Switzerland [2–4], and

[1]La Cour, Cita 6, CH-1092 Belmont-sur-Lausanne, Switzerland

comprehensive rehabilitation programmes which also include social skills training and psychoeducation [5].

Concerning the problem of dependent variables, the question arises whether a certain hierarchy among the adopted criteria of success (mainly positive and negative psychotic symptoms, relapse rates, social and occupational functioning, family burden) should not be established. Statistical correlations between psychopathology and social functioning are rather loose. As certain schizophrenics function quite well in the community in spite of severe symptoms such as hidden hallucinations and/or delusions, improving social autonomy and survival in the community may be a more relevant general goal of psychotherapy than psychopathologic and/or cognitive improvement. Variables such as housing situation and working situation, which are probably the most valid indicators for social autonomy, could therefore be considered as supraordinated dependent variables towards which all therapeutic efforts should converge. Under this perspective, too, psychotherapy and rehabilitation are broadly overlapping.

For obvious methodological reasons, most of the reviewed studies have a time horizon of 2 years or less. As the usual duration of schizophrenic disturbances is, however, much longer, and ongoing psychotherapeutic and/or sociotherapeutic support is usually needed according to clinical experience, future research should extend beyond that limit.

Long-term research has, on the other hand, revealed a remarkable potential for unforeseen changes and improvements in the long run [6]. There is growing evidence that the evolution of schizophrenia follows complex nonlinear dynamics [7, 8]. Under this perspective, the level of emotional tension appears as a crucial control parameter capable of provoking sudden bifurcations from normal to psychotic functioning in vulnerable individuals.

Other converging evidence, including clinical observation, the reported importance of Expressed Emotions, of personal trust and therapist attention, and innovative concepts on the emotional bases of thinking supported by recent neurobiological findings [9] speaks for a considerably greater pathogenetic and therapeutic impact of emotional factors in schizophrenia than hitherto believed. Schizophrenia may even be understood as an "affective psychosis" of, however, another type than depression and mania [10]. This assumption is also supported by the fact that systematically reducing emotional tensions by combined psychotherapeutic–milieutherapeutic methods, such as those employed in the mentioned Soteria houses, had in two controlled studies similar 2-year effects on acute psychotic symptomatology, relapse rates, and social functioning as standard hospital treatments with 3–5 times higher total doses of neuroleptics [2–4]. Additional psychotherapeutic, preventive and theoretical implications of a higher emphasis on emotions are discussed in other contributions [9, 10].

REFERENCES

1. Alanen Y.O. (1997) *Schizophrenia. Its Origins and Need-adapted Treatment*. Karnac, London.
2. Mosher L.R., Menn A.Z. (1978) Community residential treatment for schizophrenia: two-year follow-up data. *Hosp. Comm. Psychiatry*, **29**: 715–723.
3. Ciompi L. (1997) The Soteria-Concept. Theoretical bases and practical 13-year experience with a milieu–therapeutic approach of acute schizophrenia. *Psychiatr. Neurol. J.*, **99**: 634–650.
4. Ciompi L., Kupper Z., Aebi E., Dauwalder H.P., Hubschmid T., Trütsch K., Rutishauser C. (1993) The pilot-project "Soteria Berne" for the treatment of acute schizophrenics. II. Results of a comparative prospective study over two years. *Nervenarzt*, **64**: 440–450.
5. Hoffmann H., Kupper Z. (1997) Relationship between social competence, psychopathology and work performance and their predictive value for vocational rehabilitation of schizophrenic outpatients. *Schizophr. Res.*, **23**: 69–79.
6. Ciompi L. (1988) Learning from outcome studies. Toward a comprehensive biological–psychological understanding of schizophrenia. *Schizophr. Res.*, **1**: 373–384.
7. Globus G.G., Arpaia J.P. (1994) Psychiatry and the new dynamics. *Biol. Psychiatry*, **35**: 352–364.
8. Ciompi L. (1997) Non-linear dynamics of complex systems. The chaos–theoretical approach to schizophrenia. In *Toward a Comprehensive Therapy of Schizophrenia* (Eds H.-D. Brenner, W. Böker, R. Genner), pp. 18–31. Hogrefe & Huber, Seattle.
9. Ciompi L. (1997) The concept of affect logic. An integrative psycho-sociobiological approach to understanding and treatment of schizophrenia. *Psychiatry*, **60**: 158–170.
10. Ciompi L. (1998) Is schizophrenia an affective disease? The hypothesis of affect-logic and its implications for psychopathology. In *Emotions in Psychopathology: Theory and Research* (Eds W.F. Flack, J.D. Laird), pp. 283–297. Oxford University Press, New York.

3.2
Family and Individual Cognitive–Behavioural Interventions
Nicholas Tarrier[1]

The review of indications and planning of psychotherapies for schizophrenia provided by Birchwood and Spencer is thorough and comprehensive. Some further comments may be helpful to add to the literature review carried out by these authors.

There is good evidence to support the efficacy of family intervention in reducing relapse in schizophrenia. However, the published studies involve

[1] *Department of Clinical Psychology, University of Manchester, Withington Hospital, West Didsbury, Manchester M20 8LR, UK*

research teams evaluating a novel treatment, which may represent high levels of skill and motivation that may be absent or difficult to sustain within a standard clinical setting. This is clearly an important issue in effecting the dissemination and availability of innovative non-drug treatments. In Manchester, we have considerable experience in developing and evaluating psychosocial and psychological treatments and it is an issue that has concerned us. A randomized controlled trial was conducted to test the effectiveness of a family intervention delivered within a routine service setting [1]. Patients and their carers were recruited through screening of a geographical sample and randomized either to a needs-based psychosocial intervention service including family support (treatment group) or to family support alone (control group). Patients and carers in the treatment group were offered specific psychosocial interventions, the focus and content of which were determined by a systematic assessment of carer need for psychosocial intervention. This was determined by use of a specially designed assessment instrument, the Cardinal Needs Schedule (RCNS) [2]. Ten intervention sessions were regarded as the minimum "dose" to produce a treatment effect. Of the control group, 46% relapsed compared to 24% of the treatment group, with fewer days in relapse being experienced by the treatment group. Survival analysis demonstrated that there was a significantly better outcome in survival time to relapse in the treatment group. There were also significant benefits of treatment in terms of global outcome of patients and a decrease in identified needs of their carers.

There is little evidence available regarding the durability of treatment effects of cognitive–behaviour therapy. Perhaps this is unsurprising given the recent origins of these treatments. Follow-up of 97% of chronic schizophrenic patients who had participated in the Manchester trial comparing cognitive–behaviour therapy, supportive counselling and routine care [3] found that, 12 months after the end of treatment, significant advantages for cognitive–behaviour therapy over routine care were sustained in both positive and negative symptoms [4]. Initial analysis of 2-year follow-up data suggests that there is a significant disadvantage for patients who receive only routine care. Thus, evidence is beginning to accumulate to suggest that treatment benefits are durable over time.

We have examined whether different symptoms may respond differentially to cognitive–behaviour therapy [5]. There were indications that while both delusions and hallucinations showed improvements, delusions responded better to non-drug treatments. There was no evidence that patients suffering from paranoid delusions were more difficult to treat than those suffering from other types of delusions. Thought disorder also showed an improvement with treatment as did negative symptoms. Improvements in depression were associated with improvements in positive symptoms.

If there is strong evidence for the efficacy and effectiveness of non-drug treatments for schizophrenia, how can these treatments be made widely available? In Manchester and London, training courses that train mental health professionals in family and cognitive–behavioural interventions have been developed, which have provided a model for a large number of satellite courses within the UK [6]. Despite evidence that mental health staff can acquire specific therapy skills [7] and that the use of these therapies by staff can have clinical benefits for their patients [6], the success of such training courses in making these therapies widely available has been disappointing. Although it has been assumed that staff training is the key to dissemination, it is probable that organizational and management aspects of mental health services are as important. Given the potential benefits of the widespread availability of these non-drug treatments, the ways in which the workforce can obtain these skills and the organizational factors, which would facilitate their implementation, deserve closer attention.

REFERENCES

1. Barrowclough C., Tarrier N., Lewis S., Sellwood W., Mainwaring J., Quinn J., Hamlin C. (1999) Randomised controlled effectiveness trial of a needs-based psychosocial intervention service for carers of people with schizophrenia. *Br. J. Psychiatry*, **174**: 505–511.
2. Barrowclough C., Marshall M., Lockwood A., Quinn J., Sellwood W. (1998) Assessing relatives' needs for psychosocial interventions in schizophrenia: A relatives' version of the Cardinal Needs Schedule (RCNS). *Psychol. Med.*, **28**: 531–542.
3. Tarrier N., Yusupoff L., Kinney C., McCarthy E., Gledhill A., Haddock G., Morris J. (1998) A randomised controlled trial of intensive cognitive behaviour therapy for chronic schizophrenia. *Br. Med. J.*, **317**: 303–307.
4. Tarrier N., Wittkowski A., Kinney C., McCarthy E., Morris J., Humphreys L. (1999) Durability of the effects of cognitive–behavioural therapy in the treatment of chronic schizophrenia: 12-month follow-up. *Br. J. Psychiatry*, **174**: 500–504.
5. Tarrier N., Kinney C., McCarthy E., Wittkowski A., Yusupoff L., Gledhill A., Morris J. The cognitive–behavioural treatment of persistent symptoms in chronic schizophrenia: are some types of psychotic symptoms more responsive to CBT? Unpublished manuscript.
6. Lancashire S., Haddock G., Tarrier N., Baguley I., Butterworth A., Brooker C. (1997) Effects of training in psychosocial interventions for community psychiatric nurses in England. *Psychiatr. Serv.*, **48**: 39–41.
7. Devane S., Haddock G., Lancashire S., Baguley I., Butterworth A., Tarrier N., James A., Molyneux P. (1998) The clinical skills of community psychiatric nurses working with patients who have severe and enduring mental health problems: an empirical analysis. *J. Adv. Nursing*, **27**: 253–260.

3.3
It is no Longer Surprising that Cognitive–Behavioural Therapy Reduces Distressing Psychotic Symptoms

Philippa A. Garety[1]

Recently, I presented the results of the London–East Anglia study of cognitive–behavioural therapy (CBT) for medication-resistant psychosis to an audience of British psychiatrists [1, 2]. This study is one of the six included in Birchwood and Spencer's review of CBT. The first comment from the floor intrigued me. The questioner acknowledged that the results showed good evidence that CBT is effective to reduce distressing positive symptoms, but expressed surprise that the results did not show a corresponding significant improvement in depression. These two points are consistent with the conclusions drawn by Birchwood and Spencer. What intrigued me was the questioner's lack of surprise or doubt about the results concerning positive symptoms. In a few years, and with rather few studies (only six rather disparate controlled trials), there has been a major change in the understanding most British psychiatrists have of psychosis and of the relevance of psychological therapies to its treatment. Now, it is recognized widely that distressing psychotic symptoms, particularly delusions and hallucinations, previously thought to be inaccessible and intractable, are amenable to cognitive approaches. This proposition, which used to be unthinkable, is no longer surprising.

The conclusion that CBT is effective for positive symptoms seems to be robust. Indeed, the findings of the recently published London–East Anglia follow-up study, to which Birchwood and Spencer were not able to refer, add further encouragement [3]. It was found that the improvement in positive symptoms was sustained or even augmented 9 months after treatment had terminated, so that, whereas at the end of the treatment phase 50% of patients showed significant clinical improvements, at 18 months follow-up, 65% showed reliable and significant clinical benefits. Specific measures of delusions and hallucinations, not significantly different from controls at the end of treatment, also showed significant reductions. Furthermore, an economic evaluation found a preliminary indication that the costs of CBT were offset by reductions in service use, particularly inpatient days, in the CBT group.

Therefore, in addition to psychotic symptom reductions, the London–East Anglia study noted a preliminary finding that CBT may reduce rehospitalization. A review of CBT for schizophrenia [4], which draws on most of the studies discussed by Birchwood and Spencer, but which also includes a study on "compliance therapy" as a variant of CBT [5], reports a meta-analysis.

---

[1]*Department of Psychology, St Thomas' Hospital, London SE1 7EK, UK*

This found that CBT groups were significantly less likely to deteriorate or relapse and that the differences in comparison with standard care were considerable, suggesting that CBT may reduce the risk of relapse by 54% (number needed to treat 6, confidence interval 3–30). It is therefore possible, but by no means established, that, like family therapy, CBT may have an impact on relapse and rehospitalization.

However, even if the findings of future studies are consistent with regard to CBT leading to psychotic symptom reduction and support the suggestion of relapse reduction, there are a number of important further questions. First, why are there no changes in depression? Birchwood and Spencer suggest that to be effective with depression the focus needs to shift to the appraisal of the psychosis and self-evaluative beliefs. It may also be that a CBT intervention may need to be of longer duration than the typical 6 to 9 months if it is to deal effectively with distressing positive symptoms, relapse reduction strategies *and* depressogenic beliefs. Secondly, do the two different CBT approaches clearly described by Birchwood and Spencer differ in effectiveness, in general or in specific outcomes? The distinctive results of personal therapy in terms of social functioning may indicate this [6]. Thirdly, do outcomes differ as a function of therapy duration, as is the case for family interventions? Current studies describe therapy which varies from 10 weeks' to 3 years' duration. These are but three of the possible research questions. The results of new studies will doubtless continue to surprise, but seem likely to offer support for a well-grounded claim that CBT for schizophrenia is, for some people and for some outcomes, a valuable intervention.

REFERENCES

1. Kuipers E., Garety P., Fowler D., Dunn G., Bebbington P., Freeman D., Hadley C. (1997) London–East Anglia randomised controlled trial of cognitive–behavioural therapy for psychosis. I: Effects of the treatment phase. *Br. J. Psychiatry*, **171**: 319–327.
2. Garety P., Fowler D., Kuipers E., Freeman D., Dunn G., Bebbington P., Hadley C., Jones S. (1997) London–East Anglia randomised controlled trial of cognitive–behavioural therapy for psychosis. II: Predictors of outcome. *Br. J. Psychiatry*, **171**: 420–426.
3. Kuipers E., Fowler D., Garety P., Chisolm D., Freeman D., Dunn G., Bebbington P., Hadley C. (1998) London–East Anglia randomised controlled trial of cognitive-behavioural therapy for psychosis III: Follow-up and economic evaluation at 18 months. *Br. J. Psychiatry*, **173**: 61–68.
4. Jones C., Cormac I., Mota J., Campbell C. (1998) Cognitive behaviour therapy for schizophrenia (Cochrane review). *The Cochrane Library*. Update Software, Oxford.
5. Kemp R., Kirov G., Everitt B., Hayward P., David A. (1998) Randomised controlled trial of compliance therapy. 18-month follow-up. *Br. J. Psychiatry*, **172**: 413–419.
6. Hogarty G.E., Greenwald D., Ulrich R., Kornblith S.J., DiBarry A.L., Cooley S., Carter M., Flesher S. (1997) Three-year trials of personal therapy among schizophrenic patients living with or independently of family, II: Effects on adjustment of patients. *Am. J. Psychiatry*, **154**: 1514–1524.

3.4
Serious Questions Remain Concerning Efficacy, Effectiveness and Scope of Family Interventions in Schizophrenia

George Szmukler[1]

Birchwood and Spencer offer a most valuable review of the place of psychological treatments in schizophrenia. Clinicians and service planners will find it a boon. I restrict my comments to family interventions since I am most familiar with these. There are three issues I wish to raise.

The first is: are family interventions making less difference today? When looking at family intervention studies over the 15 years or so of their history, I observe that the gap in efficacy between the family treatment and control treatments so evident in earlier studies has all but disappeared in the most recent studies. Three of the latest [1–3], each large and carefully designed, show few differences between the "formal" family treatment condition and controls, and certainly not in relapse or rehospitalization rates. These studies also cover between them a broad range of patients with schizophrenia — recent onset cases [1], the especially difficult [2], and a broad spectrum but favouring the less persistently ill [3]. Their generalizability is thus presumably greater than the earlier studies treating smaller groups of high expressed emotion (EE) families. To these studies can be added another negative study [4]. Again quite large, it failed to show differences in relapse between regular relatives' groups (without patients, and therefore perhaps of questionable efficacy) and standard treatment only. Relapse rates were high.

What is the explanation? Interpretation is complicated by the move from treating high EE families only (although this has the advantage of helping clinicians who no longer have to worry about how they might detect high EE in routine practice). The control groups in recent studies have been better specified, and in each case received a high level of care including elements of family involvement. "Standard" treatment has over the years become better and thus differences are harder to show. This is supported by lower relapse rates in these studies than among controls in the early studies. One is then left with the questions: is there a "ceiling effect" for family interventions, and what interventions are adequate to achieve it? Perhaps "intensive" family treatments are unnecessary.

A second issue is: effectiveness, cost effectiveness and the service provider's perspective. Even if family interventions show "efficacy" under experimental conditions, are they "effective" under routine clinical conditions? We do not know since there have not been any "effectiveness" studies. What about cost effectiveness? A useful measure of treatment effects is the "number-needed-to-treat" (NNT). The figure given by Mari and Streiner [5] is 6; that is,

---

[1]Bethlem and Maudsley NHS Trust, Maudsley Hospital, Denmark Hill, London SE5 8AZ, UK

six families need to be treated to prevent one relapse or rehospitalization over 9–12 months. I have made some calculations for my own service in South London. We know that in a service sector for a population of around 45 000 we have around 250 patients with a psychosis, 80% being non-affective [6]. Of the 200 patients with schizophrenia or related disorders, 55% have a carer with whom they are in regular contact. Of these 110 families about 50% (55) are likely to accept a family intervention [7]. With an NNT of 6 for rehospitalization over 1 year, family treatment will prevent nine admissions. Admissions average 20 days and cost £200 per day; the service will thus save £36 000 per year. But to treat 55 families will require 2.75 therapists (at 20 families per therapist, fortnightly sessions). At £25 000 per therapist, this will cost £68 750. Thus costs will exceed savings by about £30 000. If the NNT holds for multiple family groups, the position is better; 1.5 therapists will result in the service breaking even. The review indicates there is no evidence that intensive family interventions result in better coping with fewer relapses after the cessation of treatment. Support for families will thus need to be maintained. The above analysis, though crude and taking no account of other values associated with providing intensive family interventions, gives an indication of the scale of the problem for a cash-strapped service. If, as suggested by recent studies, a lesser quantum still of family input achieves similar results, substantial savings may occur. I hope future research will address these questions.

The third issue is: what about other members of the family? It is disappointing that family interventions continue to neglect outcomes for other family members. Families are a cornerstone of community care and their new status as "carers" may require new obligations from services. As the authors point out, the evidence on family interventions reducing carer distress or improving family functioning is meagre. A further randomized controlled trial (RCT) showing a modest gain in carer outcomes from a family intervention is omitted in Birchwood and Spencer's review [7]. There are difficulties in measuring such outcomes, but there are now some promising instruments [8]. I find the term family "burden" unacceptable: it is pejorative, conceptually unsatisfactory as a basis for measurement, and fails to capture important dimensions of caregiving by focusing purely on the negative. A neutral term such as "caregiving" is less constraining and more appropriate.

REFERENCES

1. Linszen D., Dingemans P., Van der Does J.W., Nugter A., Scholte P., Lenior R., Goldstein M.J. (1996) Treatment, expressed emotion and relapse in recent onset schizophrenic disorders. *Psychol. Med.*, **26**: 333–342.
2. MacFarlane W.R., Dushay R.A., Stastny P., Deakins S.M., Link B. (1996) A comparison of two levels of family-aided assertive community treatment. *Psychiatr. Serv.*, **47**: 744–750.

3. Schooler N.R., Keith S.J., Severe J.B., Matthews S.M., Bellack A.S., Glick I.D., Hargreaves W.A., Kane J.M., Ninan P.T., Frances A. *et al* (1997) Relapse and rehospitalization during maintenance treatment of schizophrenia: the effects of dose reduction and family treatment. *Arch. Gen. Psychiatry*, **54**: 453–463.
4. Buchkremer G., Schulze Monking H., Holle R., Hornung W.P. (1995) The impact of therapeutic relatives' groups on the course of illness of schizophrenic patients. *Eur. Psychiatry*, **10**: 17–27.
5. Mari J.J., Streiner D. (1996) Family intervention for schizophrenia. Cochrane Database of Systematic Reviews, Cochrane Collaboration, Oxford.
6. Thornicroft G., Strathdee G., Phelan M., Holloway F., Wykes T., Dunn G., Mc-Crone P., Leese M., Johnson S., Szmukler G. (1998) Rationale and design. PRiSM Psychosis Study 1. *Br. J. Psychiatry*, **173**: 363–370.
7. Szmukler G.I., Herrman H., Colusa S., Benson A., Bloch S. (1996) A controlled trial of a counselling intervention for caregivers of relatives with schizophrenia. *Soc. Psychiatry Psychiatr. Epidemiol.*, **31**: 149–155.
8. Szmukler G.I., Burgess P., Herrman H., Benson A., Colusa S., Bloch S. (1996) Caring for relatives with serious mental illness: the development of the Experience of Caregiving Inventory. *Soc. Psychiatry Psychiat. Epidemiol.*, **31**: 37–48.

3.5
The Interaction of Psychotherapy and Drugs in the Management of Schizophrenia: A Neglected Field

Heinz Katschnig[1]

Summarizing the evidence about the efficacy of psychotherapeutic measures in schizophrenia is a much more difficult task than reviewing the evidence of the efficacy of drugs. Not only does there exist a much broader diversity of psychotherapeutic interventions than of neuroleptic drugs (although on the basis of some superficial characteristics psychotherapeutic interventions might be grouped into a few types), but it is much more difficult to keep fidelity of the intervention over time and across study sites than it is for drug treatment. What makes generalization so difficult in this field is the mostly neglected possible interaction between drugs and psychotherapy.

While research protocols addressing the issue of the efficacy of new *drugs* explicitly exclude patients who are currently undergoing psychotherapy of any form (and at most allow "psychosocial support"), most studies testing the efficacy of *psychotherapeutic treatment* techniques in schizophrenia explicitly allow or even encourage the simultaneous use of neuroleptic drugs. There are good reasons to do so, since the efficacy of neuroleptic treatment, both for treating acute episodes of schizophrenia and preventing relapse, is beyond doubt, and not using neuroleptics could be an ethical problem. In fact, today,

[1]*Department of Psychiatry, University of Vienna, Waehringer Guertel 18–20, A-1090 Vienna, Austria*

most scholars and advocates of psychotherapeutic treatment techniques (in a broad sense) favour the concomitant use of drug treatments. In clinical practice usually "treatment packages" are applied which include drugs.

However, while drugs are allowed in most clinical studies which aim at testing the efficacy of psychotherapies, the use of these drugs is rarely controlled for. Issues such as whether drugs are taken at all, which drugs are taken and in which dosages, are often not considered — and this creates a problem of interpretation of the results. Thus, although it is suggested by common sense to combine drug and psychosocial treatments, and although the combination is practically used in clinical routine in many places, very little systematic knowledge exists about the efficacy of the combination. In our own review of randomized long-term studies explicitly combining drug treatment and psychosocial measures (and fulfilling minimal methodological standards), only five of fifteen identified trials controlled for drug treatment or introduced drug treatment as a separate treatment variable; all other studies allowed "routine drug treatment" [1].

One might assume that randomization renders this problem irrelevant, but interaction between drugs and psychotherapy might develop over the course of the trial and this might influence the drop-out rate and the study results. Such interactions might occur only after a lengthy period of treatment: in their classical combination study, Goldberg et al [2] could show that the effect on relapse prevention of combining chlorpromazine with "major role therapy" became only apparent after 1 year of treatment.

Interaction issues are probably especially relevant if the atypical antipsychotics are used. We know from clinical experience that one consequence of using these new drugs is that patients are getting more interested than before in taking part in psychosocial programmes, in other words: the new antipsychotic drugs increase compliance with such programmes. Why this is so, is not quite clear — it might be the lack of extrapyramidal side effects (with a possible change in self-perception in the sense of becoming more attractive to other people), the efficacy of the new drugs for negative symptoms and the possible antidepressant effect of some of the new agents.

The net result is that patients are more and more actively asking us for "psychotherapeutic" help and we have to respond to this request — and this might even lead us to develop new types of psychotherapies. It is our experience that, if we offer such programmes, they should not just be of the disease-centred psychoeducational type, but give more prominence to positive quality of life aspects. For 1 year we have been running such a programme in Vienna. It is called "Knowing — Enjoying — How to live better" and — besides the usual psychoeducational topics (centred around the issue of how to understand schizophrenia and its treatment) — typical topics are "How to make friends", "How to create a pleasant surrounding" and "Where to go to feel well".

Systematic studies controlling for both psychotherapy and drug treatment are necessary, because their combination could also be harmful (e.g. drugs might prevent a patient from profiting from psychotherapy because of their impairment of learning processes). Falloon and Liberman [3] have pointed out the possible outcomes of such combinations, including "no additional effect" of one of these treatments if added to the other, additive effects, multiplicative effects, but also the possibility that one treatment might reduce the effect of the other.

But such combination studies are easier suggested than carried out, especially if one considers the necessity to have study periods of many months or even years and to get sufficiently large numbers of patients for the many subgroups required for such studies. Also, patients who will participate in such studies and do not drop-out before the end constitute a highly selected group. The same applies to the researchers, who are usually well trained because research funds are available. Before such studies become available, we have at least to be modest in generalizing about the efficacy or non-efficacy of psychotherapeutic interventions in schizophrenia.

REFERENCES

1. Katschnig H., Windhaber J. (1998) Die Kombination einer Neuroleptika-Langzeit-medikation mit psychosozialen Maßnahmen. In *Neuropsychopharmaka. Ein Thera-pie-Handbuch*, *vol. 4. Neuroleptika* (Eds P. Riederer, G. Laux, W. Pöldinger), pp. 249–272. Springer, Wien.
2. Goldberg S.C., Schooler N.R., Hogarty G.E., Roper M. (1977) Prediction of relapse in schizophrenic outpatients treated by drug and sociotherapy. *Arch. Gen. Psychiatry*, **34**: 171–184.
3. Falloon I.R.H., Liberman R.P. (1983) Interactions between drug and psychosocial therapy in schizophrenia. *Schizophr. Bull.*, **9**: 543–554.

3.6
How Effective are Psychotherapies for Schizophrenia?
Michael G. Madianos[1]

The heterogeneity of the clinical forms of schizophrenia has had implications in the treatment modalities [1]. Drug treatment has proved not to affect sufficiently patients suffering from specific symptoms. On the other hand,

[1]*Laboratory of Psychopathology and Social Psychiatry Unit, 123 Papadiamatopoulou Str., Athens 115–28, Greece*

therapies based on interpersonal communication in the form of insight psychotherapy have largely failed to find support to their efficacy [2].

In the years since 1970, a number of individual, group and family psychotherapies focusing on the "restoration" of social and cognitive deficits of schizophrenia have been developed. The current body of literature on this subject provides evidence that these types of psychotherapies are consistently effective.

It appears that patients suffering from schizophrenia, despite all the serious psychopathologic background and the variety of impairments in information processing, are capable of actively participating in therapy, and successfully respond to the various therapeutic stimuli. However, this positive agreement on the effectiveness of cognitive–behavioural therapy, social skills training and individual or family psychoeducation, as shown is several studies, raises several questions.

First of all, to what extent is the improvement of symptoms and social functioning of the patient by the application of these models of psychotherapy independent from some good prognostic features of the illness and the patient?

Among several good prognostic features of illness are prominent affective symptoms [3]. In Birchwood and Spencer's review of literature, the majority of the randomized trials of cognitive therapy and family interventions also included patients with schizoaffective disorder [3]. Additionally, one study included only first-episode patients, a second only patients with stable or low levels of symptoms, and another married, non-chronic patients. Only three studies out of a total of 32 focused on patients with persisting or unremitting forms of schizophrenia or poor response to medication. A limited number of patients had a range of negative symptoms. The approach of treating patients with negative symptoms is rather multidimensional, requiring a long-term community-based aftercare programme with a variety of therapeutic activities [4]. Since, among psychotherapeutic variables, there are several which have been considered as being influenced by the good prognostic features of the illness and the patients' characteristics, future researchers should eliminate any risk of critique of their methodologically "sound" results.

Second, how long are the benefits gained from these psychotherapies maintained? Is the follow-up time span sufficient to provide robust results?

In Birchwood and Spencer's review of literature, the follow-up study period ranged from 9 to 24 months. Only one study provided 5-year relapse rates. Several randomized controlled studies on social skills training suggest that the extent over time to which this training affects psychotic symptoms is uncertain. In addition, in the area of family interventions, the follow-up period in preventing relapses and readmissions, in the majority of studies, rarely exceeded the 24 months.

It seems that the factor of time is a very important element in the practice and research of the new psychotherapeutic approaches in schizophrenia. On the other hand, the "suitability" of the patients to psychotherapy is a significant factor. This issue generates the following question: to what extent do cognitive–behavioural therapies engage patients who perhaps do not benefit from therapy? Is there sufficient evidence for a particular psychotherapeutic model with patients with a dual diagnosis [5]? Are there any psychotherapeutic approaches for patients and families with low sociocultural background? The issue of individualized approach to psychoeducation dealing with pre-existing stereotypes and beliefs has only recently been taken into consideration by the therapists [6].

A final question is related to efficacy of psychotherapy when the patient is in the early stage of the illness. Research carried out up to now has focused on patients with a long-term duration of the illness [7]. Further studies are needed to explore this area.

In sum, it becomes evident that there is a consensus that the four most commonly used psychotherapies have beneficial effects for the patient and the family. Nevertheless, some issues still remain unresolved. Research in this area should incorporate the following key elements: individualization, socioculturally responsive realistic expectations, implementation at a monitoring system of care level, and convergence between psychotherapeutic models and the identification of which patients will optimally benefit from psychotherapy.

REFERENCES

1. Tsuang M.T., Lyons M.J., Faraone S.V. (1990) Heterogeneity of schizophrenia: conceptual models and analytic strategies. *Br. J. Psychiatry*, **156**: 17–26.
2. Mueser K., Berenbaum H. (1990) Psychodynamic treatment of schizophrenia. Is there a future? (Editorial). *Psychol. Med.*, **20**: 253–262.
3. Angst J. (1986) The course of schizoaffective disorders. In *Schizoaffective Psychoses* (Eds A. Marneros, M.T. Tsuang), pp. 63–93. Springer Verlag, Berlin.
4. Madianos M., Economou M. (1988) Negative symptoms in schizophrenia: The effect of long-term community-based psychiatric intervention. *Int. J. Ment. Hlth.*, **17**: 22–35
5. Mueser K.J., Bellak A.S., Blanchard J.J. (1992) Comorbidity of schizophrenia and substance abuse: implications for treatment. *J. Consult. Clin. Psychol.*, **60**: 845–856.
6. Telles C., Karnon M., Mintz J., Paz G., Arias M., Tucker D., Lopez S. (1995) Immigrant families coping with schizophrenia: behavioural family intervention versus case management with a low-income Spanish-speaking population. *Br. J. Psychiatry*, **167**: 473–479.
7. Haddock G., Morrison A.P., Hopkins R., Lewis S., Tarrier N. (1998) Individual cognitive-behavioural interventions in early psychosis. *Br. J. Psychiatry*, **172** (Suppl. 33): 101–106.

3.7
Need for an Integrated and Need-adapted Approach in Treating Schizophrenia

Ville Lehtinen[1]

The extensive review by Birchwood and Spencer is a noteworthy document because it shows clearly that psychosocial measures are effective in ameliorating symptoms, reducing risk of relapse and improving functioning in schizophrenia. This is an important message, because many still believe that the only effective means to treat this severe mental disorder is neuroleptics. The review focuses exclusively on those therapies for which the evidence of efficacy is based on randomized controlled trials (RCTs). This may, perhaps, give a too limited picture of the meaning and possibilities of psychosocial measures in the comprehensive treatment of schizophrenia. Therefore, in this comment, I will focus on two different topics. First, I will consider the question of evidence, and secondly, I will describe the development of the so-called Finnish model for treating schizophrenia.

The stress–vulnerability model of the aetiology of schizophrenia is widely accepted. In individual cases there are usually several predisposing and precipitating factors contributing to the disorder. Furthermore, these factors vary from one patient to the other. The treatment implication here is that the intervention must always be individually tailored and a standard treatment regimen is seldom the optimal. It also means that, in most of the cases, a single treatment mode is not enough but one must combine several different treatment measures, including drugs, family involvement and psychotherapies, to receive the best possible outcome [1]. Furthermore, the treatment of schizophrenic psychoses is usually a long-term (perhaps a lifelong) process in which the intervention should be adapted to the individual needs of the patient and his/her family and social network.

How to achieve clinically relevant evidence in a condition with an often chronic course and with needs varying over time? The paradigm of evidence-based medicine, relying on research data from RCTs only, has been extended rapidly from somatic medicine to psychiatry during recent years [2]. The idea is in itself adequate: it is important to know that the treatment we provide to our patients is effective and does not harm. There is no doubt, either, that RCTs can in many cases give the best evidence. The question is how to apply these principles in all situations, and whether it is always even possible or relevant. I belong to those who think that RCTs are not the only way to obtain the necessary evidence, and in some cases their use may not be appropriate [3]. Treatment of schizophrenia partly seems to belong here.

[1] The National Research and Development Centre for Welfare and Health, STAKES, Mental Health R&D Group, PO Box 220, FIN-00531, Helsinki, Finland

Traditionally, double-blind RCTs have been used in testing the efficacy of drugs, and in this situation they are clearly the most adequate. Also in other cases, where the treatment in question can be reduced to a circumscribed and well-defined action (e.g. the cognitive–behavioural therapy with 10 sessions in a major depressive episode), the RCT is a feasible design to test the efficacy. The problem is, however, that the treatment of schizophrenia in everyday practice cannot be pressed into a circumscribed and well-defined package.

An alternative approach to assess psychotherapeutically orientated treatment of patients with schizophrenic psychoses can be brought, for example, from the more than 30-year action research, conducted in the Department of Psychiatry of the University of Turku, Finland by Prof Yrjö O. Alanen and his co-workers [4]. The result of this research is the so-called Finnish Integrated Model for Early Treatment of Schizophrenia and Related Psychoses [3]. The overall goal of this model has been to develop a treatment for new schizophrenic patients that is predominantly psychotherapeutic, family centred and comprehensive, with a psychodynamic and systemic basic orientation. One of the central premises of the model has been the fact that schizophrenia is a very heterogeneous entity. This also leads to a diversity of therapeutic challenges. They should be met flexibly and individually in each case, on the basis of both an individual and interactional interpretation of the situation, and of the consequent definition of the therapeutic needs. This need-specific or need-adapted treatment approach has been described intensively elsewhere [4, 6].

A different approach has also been chosen in assessing the efficacy of this model. It has been done by several follow-up studies of incidence cohorts of consecutive first-time patients in the schizophrenia group from 1960s up to 1990s in the catchment area of Turku [5]. Because of the priority of the development goals, RCTs were not applied in these prospective follow-up studies. It was felt that the main principle of the model, adaptation of the treatment to the patients' and their network's needs, made use of randomized patient groups impractical. Instead, the strategy chosen allowed comparison of the outcomes in different stages of the development of the model. These comparisons show a continuously increasing improvement of the outcome. For example, in the cohorts from the 1980s and 1990s no psychotic symptoms were present at the 5-year follow-up after admission in more that 60% of the patients. This figure is in clear contrast with the corresponding figure from the 1970s (about 40%), and it is also satisfactory when compared to other first-episode follow-up studies.

My main conclusion is that we should not forget the manyfold needs of the schizophrenic patients in seeking for the most effective treatment. Most importantly, psychosocial measures should always be included in the comprehensive treatment regimen of these patients.

REFERENCES

1. Fenton W.S., McGlashan T.H. (1997) We can talk: individual psychotherapy for schizophrenia. *Am. J. Psychiatry*, **154**: 1493–1495.
2. Chalmers I. (1998) Unbiased, relevant, and reliable assessment in health care. *Br. Med. J.*, **317**: 1167–1168.
3. Kerridge I., Lowe M., Henry D. (1998) Ethics and evidence based medicine. *Br. Med. J.*, **316**: 1151–1153.
4. Alanen Y.O. (1997) *Schizophrenia. Its Origins and Need-adapted Treatment*. Karnac Books, London.
5. Alanen Y.O., Lehtinen V., Lehtinen K., Aaltonen J., Räkköläinen V. (1999) The Finnish model for early treatment of schizophrenia and related psychoses. Submitted for publication.
6. Alanen Y.O., Räkköläinen V., Laakso J., Rasimus R., Kaljonen A. (1986) *Towards the Need-specific Treatment of Schizophrenia*. Springer, Berlin.

3.8

To Integrate the Psychotherapy of Schizophrenia into the Activities of the Multidisciplinary Team, and to Base it on the Principles of Evolutionary Biology

John Price[1]

In their comprehensive and scholarly review of the application of psychotherapy to schizophrenia, Birchwood and Spencer have revealed two outstanding achievements of recent years. First, they show that psychotherapeutic techniques are able to modify the course of a schizophrenic illness, albeit to a moderate extent; and, secondly, they provide detailed evidence that these improvements have been confirmed in well-conducted, randomized controlled trials. In view of the nature of schizophrenia, and of the extreme difficulty in mounting a controlled trial of any psychiatric treatment, these results are a tribute to the ingenuity and perseverance of a generation of clinicians and researchers.

In the brief space allocated to me, I should like to make only two points. The first is that the psychotherapy of schizophrenia should be integrated into the activities of the multidisciplinary team, rather than carried out in a separate psychotherapy department. Much important psychotherapy is carried out in the daily work of psychiatrists, community nurses, social workers, occupational therapists, art therapists and others who regularly come into contact with patients. It is virtually impossible to evaluate the effect of this "everyday psychotherapy", let alone subject it to randomized

[1]*Odintune Place, Plumpton, East Sussex, BN7 3AN, UK*

trials; but common sense would suggest that it is responsible for the fact that most schizophrenic patients live reasonable lives and do not end up in prison, or sleeping rough, or committing suicide. If it is possible to have a clinical psychologist in the multidisciplinary team, so much the better, for he or she can act as a catalyst to orientate the team to new approaches; but even lacking such a specialist, the team can profit from some of the literature now available [1].

A current trend in psychotherapy is for integration, both the integration of different theoretical models [2], and the integration of different disciplines within the therapeutic team [3]. In the case of schizophrenia, even more than in other conditions, it is important to avoid the splitting that may be introduced when the main management of the patient is by a multidisciplinary team, but the patient is sent off for "psychotherapy" to a specialized department. All mental health professionals dealing with schizophrenic patients should feel comfortable with family interventions and with cognitive behavioural therapy, and most importantly, they should all regard themselves as psychotherapists.

My second point is that in planning the psychotherapy of schizophrenia, we should be prepared to go back to the drawing board and rethink psychotherapy from basic premises; there is no reason why techniques developed for the treatment of depression, anxiety and personality disorders should be applicable to schizophrenia. We should start by trying to conceptualize the biological function of the schizophrenic diathesis [4, 5].

One can discern in schizophrenia and the schizotypal personality a "dispersal phenotype"; that is, an evolved strategy which in the past has served to disperse the organism around the full range of its potential habitat. In the schizophrenic process, we can discern a vector influencing the individual to leave the natal group (into which he or she has been born and indoctrinated) and to disperse into uncharted terrain. Both attractive and repulsive forces promote this vector. On the one hand, the patient is drawn to some destination which is often conceptualized as a "promised land", and goes there under the influence of Messianic delusion, hopefully with a following of disciples to take care of the more practical aspects of life and performing much the same function as psychiatric nurses. On the other hand, the patient is driven from the natal area by paranoid delusions of persecution, often accompanied by hostile voices. The end result is a new community, with a new world view, incompatible with the natal group. Unfortunately, the process often goes astray, and the patients end up, not in a promised land, but in a shop doorway or a psychiatric ward. Or there may be a more benign outcome, and they may remain in the natal group as shamans, mystics and holy men [6].

In dealing with the schizophrenic patient, we encounter within a social group phenomena which are characteristic of relations between groups: languages do not coincide, and arguments are made from different premises. For this reason, too, it is important that psychotherapy should be the responsibility of the team rather than an individual, both for the sake of the patient, so that the team can decide how, and how much, the patient can be encouraged to rejoin the main stream of society, and for the sake of the therapist, so that professional identity can be firmly based in team membership. We are on the threshold of a psychotherapy which is firmly rooted in the principles of evolutionary biology: a truly biological psychotherapy [7].

REFERENCES

1. Kingdon D.G., Turkington D. (1995) *Cognitive–Behavioral Therapy of Schizophrenia*. Psychology Press, London.
2. Albeniz A., Holmes J. (1996) Psychotherapy integration: its implications for psychiatry. *Br. J. Psychiatry*, **169**: 563–570.
3. Knobloch F., Knobloch J. (1979) *Integrated Psychotherapy*. Aronson, New York.
4. Stevens A., Price J. (1996) *Evolutionary Psychiatry: A New Beginning*. Routledge, London.
5. Price J.S., Stevens A. (1998) The human male socialisation strategy set: cooperation, defection, individualism, and schizotypy. *Evol. Human Behav.*, **19**: 58–70.
6. Jackson M. (1997) Benign schizotypy? The case of spiritual experience. In *Schizotypy: Relations to Illness and Health* (Ed. G. Claridge), pp. 227–250. Oxford University Press, Oxford.
7. Stevens A. (1998) *An Intelligent Person's Guide to Psychotherapy*. Duckworth, London.

3.9
Psychotherapy for Schizophrenia: An Important Addition to Medication Alone?
Jan Scott[1]

Many researchers and clinicians regard the recent introduction of atypical antipsychotics as the most important advance in the treatment of schizophrenia. However, atypical antipsychotics are not appropriate or effective for all people with schizophrenia and, crucially, rates of medication

[1]*Department of Psychological Medicine, University of Glasgow, Gartnavel Royal Hospital, Glasgow G12 0XH, UK*

non-adherence with these drugs remain high (up to 70%). It is, therefore, timely to explore the evidence for and acceptability of psychological interventions. Clinicians want to know which psychotherapy to select, while researchers wish to answer outstanding questions about such interventions.

Effective psychological interventions for schizophrenia appear to share a number of characteristics with the brief therapies that are of proven effectiveness in other mental disorders [1]. Knowledge of these factors is important. It helps clinicians make reasoned judgements about which therapy to select, and offers criteria against which to assess any new psychosocial approaches that are advocated. The shared features of effective short-term therapies are: (a) therapy is based on a coherent theoretical model and is highly structured; (b) interventions are selected on the basis of the case conceptualization; (c) the model provides a clear rationale for the interventions employed; (d) psychological interventions are introduced in a logical sequence; (e) therapy promotes the development and the independent use of new skills; (f) change is attributed to the individual rather than the therapist's skilfulness; (g) therapy is collaborative and enhances the individual's sense of self-efficacy.

Birchwood and Spencer suggest that there is robust research evidence endorsing the use of behavioural family therapy (BFT) or cognitive behavioural therapy (CBT) in schizophrenia. These approaches clearly fulfil the criteria for an effective psychotherapy. The evidence supporting the use of social skills training (SST) is equivocal. Also, the data presented indicate that educational approaches, with the exception of compliance therapy, are the least effective interventions.

Choosing which evidence-based psychological approach to employ may be influenced by cultural and social factors. The need to change the patterns of interaction between the patient and his or her family or to reduce levels of expressed emotion may increase the likelihood of choosing family therapy. Alternatively, patient preference may mean that individual therapy is more appropriate. Importantly, the lack of an available and fully trained therapist may rule out the use of a particular approach. It is critical that the therapist offering the identified intervention has both the knowledge and the *skill level* required to deal with the complexity of the case referred. About 30% of the variance in patient outcome is attributable to therapist expertise and fidelity to the treatment model [2].

Finally, clinicians must review whether the patients they are assessing are comparable with those included in research studies. Patients who are homeless, physically unwell, have a "dual diagnosis", or those at the extremes of the age range, are rarely included. As such, clinicians will have to rely on their own judgement when deciding which patients from "difficult to treat" subpopulations should be offered psychotherapy.

Birchwood and Spencer's review allows gaps in our current knowledge to be highlighted:

1. Given the duration of follow-up in the studies described, we can only conclude that effective psychological interventions reduce time to recovery or increase time to relapse. We cannot unequivocally state that relapses are prevented.
2. We cannot state which particular model of CBT should be used for which particular patient. Differential predictors of treatment response need to be identified.
3. It is unclear whether BFT or CBT have specific or non-specific benefits. A recent study of CBT versus befriending [3] found that at the end of the acute treatment phase both groups of patients had improved. However, at 2-year follow-up, significant differences in outcome emerged which all favoured the CBT group.
4. The mechanisms of action of psychotherapy in schizophrenia need exploring. It is unclear whether specific psychotherapies improve outcome by enhancing medication adherence, reducing symptom levels or changing how the individual copes with symptoms.
5. Given the importance of reducing the rate of suicide in people with schizophrenia it is important to modify further the psychotherapies employed to ensure that depression and suicidal ideation are targeted.
6. We need to explore the adverse effects as well as the benefits of different psychotherapy models.

Considerable funds have been invested in seeking newer, more effective treatments of schizophrenia. New medications are important, but research suggests that psychotherapy for schizophrenia is a clinically effective and cost-effective alternative [3]. Guidelines for the use of such therapies, including criteria for allocating patients to briefer interventions (such as compliance therapy), as well as more sophisticated approaches, urgently need to be identified. If psychotherapy is to become a treatment option in schizophrenia, there will need to be a dramatic expansion in the training available for mental health professionals.

REFERENCES

1. Scott J. (1995) Psychological treatments for depression: an update. *Br. J. Psychiatry*, **167**: 289–292.
2. Roth A., Fonagy P. (1996) *What Works for Whom?* Guilford Press, London.
3. Sensky T., Turkington D., Kingdon D., Scott J., Siddle R., O'Carroll M., Barnes T. A randomized controlled trial of cognitive-behavioural therapy for persistent symptoms in schizophrenia resistant to medication. Submitted for publication.

3.10
The Effectiveness of Cognitive–Behavioural Therapy in Schizophrenia

Pier Maria Furlan[1]

Birchwood and Spencer's paper provides a useful overview of the main research contributions on the psychotherapy of schizophrenia, from family interventions to individual ones. However, it needs to be pointed out that the authors restrict psychotherapy to behavioural, cognitive and assertive techniques. They select the most methodologically correct studies, revealing at the same time the many methodological uncertainties. This leads to a first consideration: how difficult it is to apply the strict criteria of "hard" sciences to the "human sciences", not because of carelessness by researchers, but because of the methodological difficulty of encapsulating humans and their evolving events in variable free experimental conditions. This is evident in those techniques based on guidelines aiming at simplifying and standard-izing interventions whose efficacy, as regards the patient's symptomatology (or quality of life) or family distress, is more or less recognized, but whose therapeutic factors are still far from being identified in detail.

It is not surprising that when an empirical technique tries to construct a theoretical framework, it rediscovers existing paradigms discarded along with the global theories they were associated with. An example is provided by the defensive role of delusions, which has always been maintained by psychoanalysis and is now attributed to all of the main streams of cognitive therapy. The prognostic importance attributed to insight also re-emerges in a number of studies, as a resurrection of this psychological function.

All the different research areas reviewed by Birchwood and Spencer include at least one paper which contradicts the results of the others, being carried out with a similarly high degree of accuracy. Thus the reader is likely to conclude that each area, whether it concerns family, individual or social interventions, requires further research. What might lie behind these contradictions could be the conception of schizophrenia as a situation standing on its own, as an illness existing "per se". Yet, perhaps no psychiatric illness should be analysed without bearing in mind the context of the environment in which it occurs. The selective comparison of positive and negative findings in psychotherapy research results could suggest further studies aimed at better understanding of the nature–nurture interaction of "schizophrenias". For instance, the efficacy of individual approaches in the area of delusions, but their limited success as regards hallucination, depression or negative symptoms, could enable us to revise the hierarchy of symptoms and perhaps several aetiologic and pathogenetic theories. Likewise, in studies on the effectiveness of medication versus placebo, there

---

[1]University Department of Mental Health, San Luigi Gonzaga Hospital, ASL Collegno, University of Turin, 10043 Orbassano (Turin), Italy

is a consistent percentage of patients who get better despite the lack or reduction of treatment. The identification of specific rather than non-specific therapeutic factors remains an open question also in cognitive–behavioural therapy (CBT), as correctly pointed out by Birchwood and Spencer.

Certainly, remembering how strict the psychoanalytical setting used to be towards possible interference by patients' families, it is worth noticing the emphasis laid today on a supportive family milieu, whether or not under therapy.

While the importance of psychological treatment in schizophrenias clearly emerges, it is also evident that we are still far from a satisfactory answer to the question of which treatment for which patient, because no treatment can be suitable for all patients.

Birchwood and Spencer's paper includes very useful tables comparing and summarizing the main studies. Some reservations arise, however, about the low number of papers quoted by the authors to justify their exclusion of psychoanalytical techniques (just two) in comparison with the high number used to support CBT.

The importance of family therapy is evident in several research lines. Social skills training does not reduce significantly the rates of psychotic relapses. On the contrary, studies carried out on psychotic patients who had been exposed both to social skills training and to family therapy showed significantly lower relapse rates at the 1- and 2-year follow-up compared to patients receiving antipsychotic medication only. The effects of the two interventions were found to be summative, not interactive.

This research evidence of the importance of family therapy should lead to a reconsideration of the organization and the allocation of resources in mental health departments. For instance, in Italy, family therapies are often not available and 60–70% of the budget covers residential costs. This is especially true now that decision makers are strengthening rehabilitation programmes in many mental health services.

Thanks to meta-analysis of research on depression and schizophrenia, some other considerations could be made. Diagnostic criteria for the definition of psychoses are still uncertain. Is depression a primary or a secondary symptom of schizophrenia? Does depression improve along with schizophrenic symptoms? Can social skills training actually improve the quality of life?

A correlation probably exists between improvement on the one hand, and length and complexity of interventions on the other, which deserves some reflection, especially in those countries where psychiatry is closely controlled by financial companies. Resources for mental disability are being curtailed more and more and decision makers consider the possibility of financing only those therapies and interventions which are evidence based.

The shortage of studies demonstrating a positive effect of CBT on social functioning (the only exception was a study in which interventions on patients living with their families were complex and articulated), may demonstrate that schizophrenias need a holistic and multidimensional approach, as close as possible to the natural milieu of the patient, as the Italian psychiatric reform emphasizes.

3.11
Family: A System which Cannot be Neglected

János Füredi[1] and Janice Abarbanel[2]

Many years ago, the discovery of penicillin proved a great success without any controlled, randomized, or double-blind study. At that time it was enough to notice the full recovery of some patients from pneumonia. Most probably we will see the same when the right drug is found to solve the mystery of carcinoma. However, the situation is completely different today. For many disorders there is no unique remedy and, to achieve a relative improvement, we have to combine different methods.

Three large groups of interventions are at our disposal in psychiatry: biological–psychopharmacological, social and psychotherapeutic. In neuropharmacology, the rivalry is so intense that better and better research methods have to be developed to verify the effectiveness of the different drugs. This competition produces more and more scientific data to judge the efficacy of developed drugs. On the contrary, in the field of social and psychotherapeutic treatments, the variables are so numerous that truly satisfactory answers are missing from the so-called "evidence based" studies. Here it is difficult, if not impossible, to isolate one factor when there are many factors involved. The clinical experiences are still decisive in all practitioners' everyday routine.

The following comments will address our work with families. Chronic illness is interpersonal, social and cultural, not merely the story of only one patient's experiences. When a severe illness enters the family, like an unwelcome intruder, there is a disruption of the pre-existing homeostasis of the family system (roles, boundaries, expectations, wishes and hopes). The genetic road and the psychosocial road of the patient's family development both play a role. One cannot neglect the family system. If we neglect this agent, families will work against us with their prejudices, denials, stigma, ambivalence, mistreatments, etc. Family therapy intervention helps

[1]Department of Psychiatry Imre Haynal University of Health Sciences, Nyéki út 10, 1021 Budapest, Hungary
[2]Private practice, Budapest, Hungary

to integrate the illness into the family's changing identity. Psychotherapy can help the family grieve — mourn the loss of pre-illness expectations by sharing feelings about helplessness, anger, disbelief and fate. It is not unusual for a family to become isolated when a chronic illness appears in one of its members, and the accompanying shame can contribute to the development of a family "secret" in an effort to be "normal" to the outside world. Without the family intervention, the family is unable to express its fears and ends up with less capacity to adapt to the demands of the illness.

From studies in sociology, we know that life circumstances and the family's composition are important factors for the young individual [1]. Our observations during the political changes in Hungary at the end of 1980s have shown great evidence of the complexity of these factors [2]. When schizophrenia occurs, parents do not understand what has happened. They worry that they have done something wrong. According to research in Norway, relatives' guilt proneness may be a determinant of their criticism, hostility and emotional overinvolvement [3]. All these features are part of expressed emotion (EE), which is today the most investigated factor (besides biological research) of the course of schizophrenia. A recent study [4] shows the relationship of EE to affective style (AS) and communication deviance (CD), and another [5] calls attention to the most important component of the critical comments. Our own research (together with Z. Danics) calls attention to the expressed expectation (ExEx), of which we found three elements: unreality, intensity and confusion.

Evidence is still needed to determine which combinations of interventions are best. For clinicians, it goes without saying today that schizophrenics and their families need intervention throughout the course of the disease. Solomon et al, in their randomly assigned and controlled study, found that increasing family members' contact with community resources on behalf of their ill relative may increase the benefit of the intervention to the family as well as to the ill relatives [6].

Many data support our work with families [7, 8]. There is enough evidence now that major psychiatric illnesses are general stressors for families, concluding that family interventions should always be considered. The role of the family in the course of chronic illness is a crucial one which, with skilled intervention, can be turned to an extremely helpful resource.

REFERENCES

1. Füredi J., Kapusi G., Novák J. (1989) Macrosocial conflicts and the family: a Hungarian case study. *Fam. Syst. Med.*, **7**: 30–41.
2. Füredi J., Barcy M., Kapusi G., Novák J. (1993) Family therapy in a transitory society. *Psychiatry — Interpers. Biol. Proc.*, **56**: 328–336.

3. Bentsen H., Notland T.H., Munkvold O.G., Boye B., Ulstein I., Bjorge H., Uren G., Lersbryggen A.B., Oskarsson K.H., Berg-Larsen R. *et al* (1998) Guilt proneness and expressed emotion in relatives of patients with schizophrenia and related psychoses. *Br. J. Med. Psychol.*, **71**: 125–138.
4. Nugter M.A., Dingemans P.M., Linszen D.H., Van der Does A.J., Gersons B.P. (1997) The relationship between expressed emotion, affective style and communication deviance in recent-onset schizophrenia. *Acta Psychiatr. Scand.*, **96**: 445–451.
5. Shimodera S., Inoue S., Tanaka S. (1998) Critical comments made to schizophrenic patients by their families in Japan. *Compr. Psychiatry*, **39**: 85–90.
6. Solomon P., Draine J., Mannion E., Meisel M. (1998) Increased contact with community mental health resources as potential benefit of family education. *Psychiatr. Serv.*, **49**: 333–339.
7. Stricker K., Schulze Mönking H., Buchkremer G. (1997) Family interaction and the course of psychiatric illness. Results of a multivariate prospective study. *Psychopathology*, **30**: 282–290.
8. Friedmann M.S., McDermut W.H., Solomon D.A., Ryan C.E., Keitner G.I., Miller I.W. (1997) Family functioning and mental illness: a comparison of psychiatric and nonclinical families. *Fam. Process*, **36**: 357–367.

3.12
Psychological Interventions for Schizophrenia in Developing Countries
R. Srinivasa Murthy[1]

The inclusion of psychological interventions in the treatment of schizophrenia has been constantly part of the caring process in developing countries in general and India in particular. This has occurred mainly because of the extremely limited institutional facilities and specialized manpower in the country. As a result, there has been very little rivalry between the professionals and the families. It can be said rightly that there is no antipsychiatry movement in countries of Asia or Africa [1].

Most of the patients with schizophrenia live with their families and they get married and work in the community [2]. In India, the involvement of family members in the therapy has been a reality in psychiatry from the early 1950s. In some centres, like Vellore, it is a routine since 1959 to admit all patients with a family member. Currently most of the psychiatric centres utilize this approach as part of their psychiatric care in different settings.

There has been a greater effort towards providing active support to families subsequent to the beginning of the community mental health movement and due to the evidence of the important role of families in the course and

[1]*National Institute of Mental Health, Department of Psychiatry and Neuroscience, Post Bag 2700, Bangalore 56002-9, India*

outcome of schizophrenia. The current range of activities in India in the area of support to families include:

1. Active involvement of the significant family members as soon as the illness is identified and in all stages of treatment.
2. Admission of family members along with the patient for inpatient care.
3. Development of educational materials for family members.
4. Formation of self-help groups of carers.

However, possibly because of the widely accepted practice of working with families, to date no large-scale systematic efforts have been made to evaluate the role of family involvement both in terms of its level of effectiveness and the limitations of its value [3]. This is an area which has to be taken up on a priority basis by professionals.

Another aspect which is special to developing countries is the lack of any organized social welfare support to the ill individuals and their families. Consequently, most of the professional care occurs with a largely medical orientation [4]. There is an urgent need for creating professional roles for non-medical mental health professionals, namely, clinical psychologists, psychiatric social workers, psychiatric nurses, to take up the psychological interventions like family intervention, cognitive behavioural psychotherapy, social skills training and psychoeducation.

There is also a need for the complex and differing patterns of family structure and functioning to be reflected in the interventions. It is fortunate for the professionals working in developing countries to have this focus on psychotherapies for schizophrenia, which are easier to integrate in these countries because of the existing system of community care as the primary method of care for persons with schizophrenia.

The development of systematic efforts in Western countries will give a significant support to the organization of the psychological interventions in developing countries.

REFERENCES

1. Srinivasa Murthy R. (1996) Economics of mental health in developing countries. In *International Review of Psychiatry*, vol. 2 (Eds F. Lieh Mak, C.C. Nadelson), pp. 43–62. American Psychiatric Press, Washington, D.C.
2. Sharma V., Srinivasa Murthy R., Kumar K., Agarwal M., Wilkinson G. (1998) Comparison of people with schizophrenia from Liverpool, England and Sakalawara — Bangalore, India. *Int. J. Psychiatry*, **44**: 225–330.
3. Pai S., Kapur R.L. (1983) Evaluation of home care treatment for schizophrenic patients. *Acta Psychiatr. Scand.*, **67**: 80–88.
4. Government of India (1982) National Mental Health Programme for India. New Delhi.

4

Prevention of Disability and Stigma Related to Schizophrenia: A Review

Robert Cancro and Arthur T. Meyerson

Department of Psychiatry, New York University Medical Center,
New York, USA

INTRODUCTION

While the focus of this chapter is on schizophrenia, it is useful to understand that many of the issues concerning both stigma and rehabilitation are equally pertinent to most mental disorders. Schizophrenia in many ways is the most dramatic and destructive of these and hence receives special attention. All mental disorders by definition affect thinking, feeling and behaviour in varying degrees and admixtures. It follows then that all manifestations of mental illness have the capacity to impact on the patient's adaptation. Serious mental illness is persistent and/or recurrent. It is rare to see a full recovery with no risk of future relapse. Schizophrenia, in particular, is characterized by chronicity and in the thinking of many people, these patients never achieve a full restitution of mental functioning. This is a critical conceptual issue. The treatment of schizophrenia has to be understood as essentially life-long following the onset of an episode. It is worse than arbitrary to separate conceptually so-called acute management from so-called long-term management. It is best to think of *correct* management throughout the course of a life-long disorder in the same way as one would conceptualize the life-long management of diabetes.

The thesis of this chapter is that the prevention of disability in a chronic and persistent mental disorder such as schizophrenia involves the totality of management from the onset of the first manifestations of illness until death or full recovery, whichever occurs first. For didactic purposes, one can speak of acute and longer-term management. For practical purposes, the treatment of the individual patient must be continuous and integrated,

Schizophrenia, Second Edition. Edited by Mario Maj and Norman Sartorius.
© 2002 John Wiley & Sons Ltd.

because we have no cure. When this review speaks of rehabilitation it is referring to the longer-term treatment of the patient in an effort to reduce disability. Rehabilitation is ongoing treatment of the symptoms of this illness and their consequences. It is necessary because at the present time schizophrenia is a chronic illness. The prevention of disability involves the utilization of a variety of techniques ranging from diminution of pathological symptoms to decreasing vulnerability factors. It involves pharmacology and environmental regulation. It also involves the proper organization of health care services including meeting the psychosocial needs of the patient. The utilization of a full range of methodologies, including medical, psychosocial, legislative and political, constitutes the appropriate care and treatment of schizophrenia. It is only in this fashion that we can diminish and strive to eliminate disability.

HISTORY OF TREATMENT

Historically, Gheel in Belgium was providing family-based care of chronic mental patients as early as the fourteenth century. Under the influence of Pinel of France and Duke of Great Britain, the era of moral treatment began in Europe and subsequently spread to the United States. By the 1700s patients were seen as the victims of noxious environmental factors and if they were treated with respect and dignity, that is, moral treatment, they might recover. In the United States during the 1800s, the movement towards removing patients from jails and poorhouses resulted in the creation of hospitals under state jurisdiction that treated these individuals. By the turn of the century, mental hospitals had grown to be large and ineffective in most parts of the developed world, although they served as asylums to some extent.

A brief review of the post-moral era efforts to treat the schizophrenic disorders may be revealing. The therapeutic response of society and of the healing community to a particular disorder tells a great deal about the attitudes held by that society and those professionals concerning the disorder. Mental illness has evoked hostile responses for many centuries. This hostility is not restricted to society at large. One of the founders of the American Psychiatric Association, Benjamin Rush, devised the tranquillizing chair in which the patient was strapped and forced to remain immobile. This enforced immobility was intended to slow the heart rate and thereby decrease the blood supply to the head. The failure of this device was followed by the development of the gyrator, which spun the patient about on a board and increased the blood supply to the head. More revealingly, Rush wrote that the induction of terror was necessary in the treatment of madness. Other methods of inducing terror included immersion in water to instil the fear of death. A governor of Bethlehem Hospital would order patients to be thrown from great heights into water because the shock would be therapeutic.

It is easy enough to attribute these treatments to the physiologic ignorance of the time, although one must question why other medical diseases were not so treated. But if we look at the period of medical treatment of mental disorders since World War I, we find that the "scientific era" has been selective in which disorders received scientific, that is, data-based care. During World War I, for example, psychiatrists began to treat post-traumatic stress disorders although they were then called shell-shock. This short-term crisis intervention was quite effective in returning troops to combat. Subsequent to World War I, there began the development of psychiatric units in general hospitals as well as the opening of clinics associated with medical schools and hospitals. Nevertheless, much of the care was hospital based and custodial in nature and pseudoscientific in its approach. The focal infection theory of schizophrenia was popular at that time and involved removing tonsils, appendices and teeth. Older psychiatrists can remember how the search for these occult infections filled the chronic facilities with edentulous patients who had to remain on soft diets. The irrigation of sinuses and, in particular, intestines was also a popular treatment without a sound basis.

By the 1930s, the use of aseptic meningitis through the introduction of inactivated horse serum into the subarachnoid space was a commonly practised treatment. The surgeons were not to be outdone. They not only performed vasectomies and hemithyroidectomies, but were glad to remove other tissues that were perfectly normal. If one continues to review the history and looks at the use of intravenous gold salts, fever therapy, insulin, metrazol, lobotomies, renal dialysis and other unscientific treatments, it is very difficult not to draw the conclusion that these patients mobilize considerable ambivalence in the healer [1]. This is not an effort to condemn, but rather to recognize the nature of the response to mental illness. Mental illness is unique in its ability to alter the fundamental characteristics that define the human being and, hence, to mobilize the greatest anxiety in the observer. This insight may help us to understand the degree and intensity of the stigma associated with these disorders.

A combination of forces coalesced in the 1960s to move the emphasis of care from the hospital to the outpatient clinic. A major emphasis of treatment became the prevention of hospitalization or, if prevention was not possible, to reduce the length of stay dramatically. This philosophical change in the conception of treatment meant that social and vocational skills which were of little practical importance in an institution, were of major importance if the patient was to survive in the community. Behaviour that could be ignored in a long-term hospital was unacceptable outside and could lead to rehospitalization. In addition to reducing functional disabilities, it was necessary to reduce the social handicaps of schizophrenia. In this way the paradigmatic shift from living in an asylum to living in the community necessitated the learning and unlearning of various behaviours that would make living outside of an institution possible. Control of agitation, delusions and hallucinations was no longer sufficient. In some ways, the control of negative symptoms is of even greater importance for community adaptation.

COURSE OF SCHIZOPHRENIA

The *Diagnostic and Statistical Manual of Mental Disorders*, fourth edition (DSM-IV) [2] and the *International Classification of Diseases*, tenth revision (ICD-10) [3] provide essentially identical descriptions of the course and clinical features of schizophrenia. Even a cursory review of these nosologic efforts, reveals that this group of disorders tends to be persistent and often life-long. It logically follows that treatment must be continuous and not intermittent. The treatment will vary over time as a function of the pathologic manifestations present at that time. Unfortunately, few if any patients diagnosed with modern criteria reach a prolonged stage of full remission. This is a consequence of the inclusion of social and vocational disability as defining aspects of diagnosis. Utilizing DSM-III criteria, a number of long-term follow-up studies [4] indicated that positive symptoms appeared to lessen after a decade or more, in a significant number of patients, and that some of these patients sufficiently improved in social and vocational function to survive independently in the community.

In addition to the classical signs and symptoms of this group of disorders, several associated features are of great significance. These include a shorter life expectancy than the general population in developed countries, partially explained by the high suicide risk [5]; a typical lack of insight which may contribute to non-compliance; and a high comorbidity with substance abuse. Although the public perception of schizophrenia includes a markedly increased risk of violence, there is conflicting scientific evidence for this notion which is a significant source of the stigma associated with this illness.

TERMINOLOGY

It appears that the vulnerability in a schizophrenic disorder tends to be enduring. It seems to be present before the psychotic decompensation and can emerge during periods of reasonable symptom remission. The goal of long-term treatment is to move the patient from a poorer outcome to the best possible outcome. This requires not only treatment of acute symptoms, but the organization of protective components in the environment of that individual, including support services. Prior to reviewing preventive and rehabilitative strategies, it is best to define several terms that are central to the process of reducing disability. These terms are: impairment, disability and handicap. While they are not interchangeable terms, they are frequently misused as synonyms.

Impairment

Impairment can be thought of as the most readily observable and objectively demonstrable phenomenon. It is usually defined as a loss of mental or physical function. Thus, one individual with a single or multiple impairments may be disabled or handicapped, while another with similar impairments may be neither disabled nor handicapped. An example is a person engaged in the work of loading trucks, who as a consequence of osteoarthritis suffers an impairment of joint mobility, with a consequent loss of the capacity to lift heavy objects, and thus becomes vocationally disabled. An attorney or psychiatrist suffering the exact same illness and impairment, might not be disabled in any fashion. In the psychiatric sphere, using schizophrenia as an example, the classical positive and negative symptoms which affect cognition, appropriate affect and social skills are often defined as prototypical impairments. Some definitions of impairment in psychiatry, such as the one used by the Community Support Program of the National Institute of Mental Health (NIMH) [6] utilize the concept of an impaired role function for purposes of specifying those who are severely disabled. To meet that definition a patient must have at least two of the following difficulties on an intermittent or continuous basis for a minimum of 2 years: (a) unemployment, employed in a sheltered setting, or markedly limited work skills and a poor work history; (b) the need for public financial support and the inability to access such support without help; (c) severe limitation in the ability to establish and/or maintain a social support system; (d) need for assistance with basic survival skills; (e) inappropriate social behaviour calling for mental health or judicial intervention.

Disability

Definitions of disability vary widely depending on context. Different entitlement programmes in the United States use different definitions as do different rehabilitation programmes. All definitions, however, seem to share common principles. Disabled persons suffer from an illness, disease or disorder. They suffer signs and symptoms of that disorder which are impairments. As a consequence of those impairments they suffer a loss of ability or competence in a significant life function such as employment, finances, recreation, social role, socially acceptable behaviour and/or basic survival skills. Techniques utilized to diminish impairments and disabilities include neuroleptic drugs, social skills training, family education and therapy, supportive psychotherapy and cognitive therapy.

Handicap

In the United States, the term handicap is defined by the Rehabilitation Services Administration, which uses the statutory requirements of the Rehabilitation Act of 1973, reauthorized in 1993, as a "disability which requires multiple services over an extended period of time". Since this definition is for severe handicap, less stringent definitions usually require a disability based on an illness-caused impairment which requires either personal intervention (e.g. medical treatment, case management, rehabilitation, etc.), and/or environmental intervention (e.g. wheel chair accessibility, job accommodations, supported employment, etc.) for the handicapped person to achieve adequate functional capacity. It is best conceptualized as a limitation in the fulfilment of normal roles such as student, worker, spouse, etc. A range of activities, including family support, housing options, case management, psychosocial clubs, vocational rehabilitation and employment, all can be utilized to minimize handicap. The overcoming of handicap is essential to the overcoming of stigma.

Primary Prevention

Prevention in medical illness has traditionally been separated into primary, secondary and tertiary activities. Primary prevention is meant to reduce the incidence of the disease by preventing the development of new cases. This is done through the elimination of aetiologic factors, increasing host resistance, the reduction of risk factors, and blocking modes of disease transmission. Infectious diseases represent the classic example of the effectiveness of primary prevention where, for example, vaccines have essentially eliminated certain disorders. The aetiologic factors in mental illnesses such as schizophrenia are not known with sufficient certainty to make primary prevention possible as it was with conditions such as pellagra, tertiary syphilis and myxoedema madness. The aetiologies and pathogeneses in the schizophrenic disorders are extraordinarily complex. The complexity is increased by the limitation of our diagnostic methods, which are based exclusively on phenomenology.

Secondary Prevention

Early identification and prompt treatment of illness is the definition of secondary prevention. The goal is to reduce the total number of existing cases by more rapid effective intervention which shortens the duration of illness.

Tertiary Prevention

Tertiary prevention involves the reduction in the prevalence of residual defects or disabilities that are consequences of the illness. It may not be possible to eliminate fully the sequelae of the illness, but the goal of tertiary prevention is for individuals to reach their highest level of functioning. In the case of schizophrenia, the disabilities associated with the illness tend to be chronic and have major consequences both socially and economically. In that sense tertiary prevention is rehabilitation — as it has been traditionally understood — and is an integral part of the management of a life-long disease. It is not appropriate to delay the initiation of rehabilitative techniques until acute treatment is complete, because it is not always clear whether the symptoms being treated are merely part of the acute process or will continue after acute treatment. Anhedonia, for example, may be an exclusive component of the acute illness or may persist as a residual symptom.

REHABILITATION

Psychiatric rehabilitation is a continuous treatment of indefinite duration for a disorder which tends to be life-long in its manifestations. Rehabilitation emphasizes the maximization of the patient's strengths, including those of family and friends, and the minimization of the support necessary from health professionals. Before rehabilitation can be initiated, basics such as food and shelter must be available. The goal remains maximization of the quality of life and the maximization of the normality of that life.

A spectrum of services is necessary for tertiary prevention. These include acute inpatient facilities, emergency services, partial hospitalization, outpatient programmes, supervised graduated living arrangements, peer and family support organizations, case management services, and a variety of fiscal support mechanisms. The components of the rehabilitative system must be integrated so that the full range of necessary services is available and utilized. The rehabilitation of the chronic patient requires the assignment of a high priority to this activity. Rehabilitation requires the selection and training of staff members who are comfortable with chronic patients whose improvements are slow and often minimal. It is essential to implement methods of increasing staff satisfaction so that there is less turnover and burn-out in professional personnel. Medical students and specialists are not trained in the techniques of rehabilitation, that is, long-term care. The general goal of medical treatment is cure and little training emphasis is placed on the deficits that do not respond. Rehabilitation programmes, as all other medical interventions, must be evaluated for efficacy and cost-effectiveness.

Given that persons diagnosed with schizophrenia typically suffer from a variety of impairments in mental function, leading to disability and handicaps in the areas of social, vocational, educational, recreational, housing and survival skills, the goals of tertiary prevention for patients with this illness are to minimize the impact of the impairments, maximize the patients' coping skills and reduce the vulnerability to stress-induced exacerbation. To the degree that one is successful in accomplishing these goals, patients will have maximum tenure in the community and the fullest possible quality of life and freedom of choice.

The foundation of rehabilitation in schizophrenic patients is based on a therapeutic alliance between the patient and the caregiver, as it is in any treatment. This must involve mutual respect and trust. Rehabilitation is labour intensive and also requires a deep degree of commitment on the part of the care giver. There must be a working therapeutic alliance between the recipient of rehabilitation and the care giver. Rehabilitation cannot proceed until the goals and life roles are identified by the patient. It is also essential that the patients be assessed to determine whether they have the skills necessary to achieve those goals. This is all part of a functional assessment as opposed to a symptom assessment. The specific techniques, in addition to pharmacology, case management and therapy, which are mobilized to achieve these goals, are generally termed psychiatric rehabilitation.

Anthony and Liberman [7] postulate a vulnerability, stress, coping and competence model of disabling mental illness. This model is designed to account for the relationships between signs and symptoms, impairments, underlying biological vulnerability and consequent disability. These are seen to be modified by the patient's coping skills, adaptive abilities, and social and family supports. Protection against the impact of biological vulnerability to stress is thought to be provided by antipsychotic medication, psychosocial approaches and rehabilitation techniques. When these therapies are fully utilized, by reducing the impact of the biological vulnerability, decompensation is minimized and adaptive function is enhanced.

Developed Countries

While attempts were made to treat some schizophrenic patients in the community before the advent of modern psychopharmacology, these generally involved the development of non-hospital-based therapeutic communities or retreats. The major philosophical principle employed was a type of normalization within a protective environment. Despite these sporadic attempts at developing models of non-hospital care, most Western countries and some others had thousands (600 000 in the United States) hospitalized over long periods. With the advent of the effective pharmacology of schizophrenia, most developed countries found themselves in the position to discharge many patients into the community. However, two drawbacks emerged which gave this process of deinstitutionalization a negative connotation. First, the communities were ill prepared to cope with people who still retained some positive and negative symptoms and who required outpatient services to treat them. Second, even where funds were made available to provide adequate follow-up of medication and psychotherapeutic support, the patients often simply lacked the social skills to cope with community life. Disabilities in social skills, vocational skills, activities of daily living and survival skills were unaddressed, and patients frequently suffered exacerbations because they simply could not cope with the demands of community life. Even for those few who remained well enough to survive in the community, the quality of life was often tragically inadequate. Thus, the need to modify and strengthen patients' coping skills and to modify the environment to meet their needs came to the fore.

There is no single ideal, prototypical model or programme which defines the rehabilitation approach in the developed countries. There is agreement as to the usefulness of several models that have widespread application, including the clubhouse model, the high expectancy model, and others which will be described [8, 9]. Anthony *et al* [10] state that the goal of psychiatric rehabilitation is to:

> assume that the person with a psychiatric disability possesses those phys-
> ical, emotional and intellectual skills needed to live, learn and work in his
> or her particular environment. The major interventions by which this goal is
> accomplished involve either developing in patients the particular skills that
> they need to function in their environment, and/or developing the environ-
> mental resources needed to support or strengthen the person's present level of
> functioning.

In 1987, Rutman [9] developed a definition of psychosocial rehabilitation for the NIMH:

> Psychosocial rehabilitation refers to a spectrum of programs for persons with
> long-term mental illness. The programs are designed to strengthen individuals'
> abilities and skills necessary to meet their needs for housing, employment,
> socialization, and personal growth. The goal of psychosocial rehabilitation is to
> improve the quality of life of psychiatrically disabled individuals by assisting
> them to assume as much responsibility over their lives and to function as
> actively and independently in society as possible.
>
> Major psychosocial rehabilitation services, which are offered on a continuum,
> include socialization, recreational, vocational, residential, training in the skill
> of daily community living, and case management. In addition to psychoso-
> cial rehabilitation facilities may also provide assessment and goal planning,
> activities, educational programs, advocacy training and family support. The
> individual may need to use these programs on a short term basis or indef-
> initely. The programs are (ideally) offered in the context of a supportive,
> non-stigmatizing environment in the community, and in a manner that empha-
> sizes the "personhood" rather than the "patienthood" of the individual,

maximizes the individual's feeling of responsibility and self-worth, and encourages ownership in the rehabilitation process. The services are coordinated with those offered by other mental health and human service agencies.

There are a number of signs, symptoms and maladaptive behaviour patterns which are characteristic of many patients with schizophrenia and are thought to be responsive to rehabilitation approaches. In addition, the illness carries a considerable stigma in the minds of many in both developed and developing countries and as a consequence barriers to community adjustment may be erected which require environmental intervention. Examples of signs and symptoms as well as some typical maladaptive behaviours of the disorder which cause disability are listed in Table 4.1 alongside the frequently associated disability.

Since the goals of rehabilitation are functional in nature one might incorrectly assume that rehabilitation approaches do not address the signs and symptoms of the illness. This is a result of the false distinction between treatment and rehabilitation, which fails to understand that every treatment which is not curative is ameliorative and rehabilitative. While medication and psychotherapeutic interventions may be effective enough to allow a patient to live in the community and begin participation in a rehabilitation effort, the patient usually has some residual degree of one or more of the signs or symptoms listed in Table 4.1. As an example, patients with inappropriate affect could participate in a rehabilitation programme having already achieved the optimal response to the earlier interventions. Psychosocial rehabilitation would then attempt to help the patients modify their expression of affect to a socially-acceptable and vocationally-adaptive level. As will be described in the section on rehabilitation techniques, a combination of behavioural approaches (positive reinforcement of adaptive behavioural changes), educational style feedback, and guided practice can augment traditional approaches to modification of these symptoms

TABLE 4.1 Signs, symptoms or behaviours and related disability in schizophrenia

Sign, symptom, or behaviour	Related disability
Loosening of associations	Social, vocational and ADL*
Delusional thinking	Social, vocational and ADL*
Social withdrawal (autistic behaviour)	Social, vocational and ADL*
Flat affect	Social
Inappropriate affect	Social and vocational
Bizarre behaviour	Social and vocational
Disorganized behaviour	Social, vocational and ADL*

*ADL indicates activities of daily living, including hygiene, grooming, nutrition, etc.

and consequently lessen associated disabilities. Other techniques have been developed to focus specifically on typical disabling behaviours and disabilities rather than signs and symptoms. These latter techniques (including supportive housing, vocational rehabilitation, supportive employment and supportive education) involve attempts to modify the environment as well as the patient's specific, maladaptive signs, symptoms, and behaviours as they bear on specific functional capacities such as work or school. Vocational rehabilitation typically focuses on work-related functions such as coming on time, persistence and concentration on the work task, and relating to co-workers, supervisors and customers. Unemployment is a major factor in reducing quality of life for schizophrenic patients. Reduction in the barriers to employment for psychiatric patients is an important social handicap to be overcome. The techniques which will be discussed below may attempt to modify a patient's behaviour, but may also attempt to modify the tolerance and specific requirements of the potential worksite to enable the patient to succeed.

Specific Rehabilitation Approaches

Pharmacotherapy

The importance of good pharmacotherapy in the long-term management of patients cannot be overemphasized. The goal of pharmacologic treatment is not just to reduce positive and negative symptoms, but also to reduce the level of vulnerability to future acute episodes. Patients who are less vulnerable to the stresses of living will be better able to access various support services, which will assist their coping skills in a variety of functional areas. It was demonstrated by the University of Pittsburgh team [11] that the use of psychotropic agents in combination with family psychoeducation and patient social skills training achieved the best reduction in relapse rates. Patients treated with neuroleptics alone had a 38% relapse rate during the first year following discharge. Those treated with neuroleptics and a combination of family psychoeducation and patient social skills training had a 0% relapse rate. The difference was even more striking at the 2-year point, when their respective rates were 62% versus 25%. Finally, those who received the combined psychosocial and pharmacologic approach were more likely to be employed or in school versus those who did not receive such a combination of care.

An essential element of rehabilitation is the continuous monitoring of the patient and the patient's adjustment. This requires a close working relationship with the patient. The rehabilitation team must be sensitive to the patient's complaints about drug side effects. There is a tendency among professionals to minimize the importance of these side effects when talking to the patients and this can contribute to non-compliance. The very recognition on the part of the professional that the drug is producing undesirable side effects is a demonstration of respect for the patient. Even if efforts to reduce the side effects fail, the fact that the effort was made shows regard for the patient's wishes and needs. It is also true today that the newer antipsychotic agents have a less noxious side effect profile for many patients. In particular, the newer compounds do not interfere with the sexual life of the patient to the same degree as the older compounds. The principles of good pharmacologic management have been described elsewhere in this volume and need not be repeated. The principle that must be articulated in this context is that good pharmacologic management is an essential feature of psychiatric rehabilitation.

Assessment is an integral part of the long-term management of patients. It is impossible even to tell whether the psychopharmacology being utilized is appropriate unless the patient is being assessed over time. Similarly, the effectiveness of various psychosocial interventions, which are intended to enhance the patient's functioning, cannot be determined unless the level of functioning is monitored on a regular basis. Comprehensive evaluation and appropriate treatment planning require a full integration of both biologic and psychosocial factors. The patient must be involved in the assessment process actively and other important individuals in the patient's life, such as family or friends, must be involved as well.

Models and Settings

Over the past 30 or 40 years, the field has undergone a gradual shifting and sorting process of many different and disparate approaches. Five basic paradigms have emerged, due to a combination of support in the published literature and/or popularity among patients, families and professionals. Each of the five has a specific philosophical orientation and specific programme elements. They include the clubhouse, the consumer guided [9], the high expectancy, the intensive case management, and the Boston University [6] model of psychiatric rehabilitation.

Clubhouses. Clubhouses provide a supportive environment with a full continuum of available services. The expectation is that the patient will feel as if among family. Thus, persons are considered members as distinguished from patient or client. Members choose the intensity of contact including the frequency of their attendance. Rutman [9] summarized the essential programme components as follows:

> an accepting climate that establishes an unwavering sense of welcome; help
> in developing job related skills that can lead to placement in regular jobs in

business and industry, either through one or more transitional employment placements or in regular competitive employment; provision for those who need housing with an appropriate, normalized place to live, and a milieu which stimulates active and meaningful participation on the part of all members in all phases of the program, from performing housekeeping chores, assisting in the cafeteria or at the reception desk, to maintaining the agency's fiscal and clinical records.

These programmes achieve a community of cooperation and family feeling with members and staff sharing and interchanging roles. When a member cannot attend a transitional employment position, a staff member or other patient may fill in for a period. Fountain House is the most prominent example in the United States. It was founded in 1948 in New York City. It grew out of the patient self-help movement and therefore emphasized the role of the patient in its operation. Discharged patients from nearby state hospitals began the programme with the credo "mutual support was the norm and rejoining ordinary society as workers and friends was the goal" [12]. While there are staff members who offer assistance, the focus is on self-help. There are a variety of activities provided in this model, which include problem-solving groups, vocational services and welfare assistance. The patients provide work to the clubhouse including maintenance, kitchen and clerical. The patients are referred to as members and are seen as a part of a community. It is their responsibility to work in the maintenance of the clubhouse. This is seen as part of the recovery process. Fountain House contracts for jobs in the community and guarantees the employer that the job will be done — if not by the member then by the staff person who accompanies the member to the job.

Outcome studies have not been adequately controlled. One study which was uncontrolled showed that after 18 months 16% of the members were in full-time independent employment, with an additional 45% either in vocational programmes or attending school. In a 2-year follow-up study which was not randomized, the clubhouse members experienced fewer rehospitalizations and fewer days in hospital than did a comparison group.

In the decades since the inception of Fountain House, many European and Asian countries have seen the development of similar programmes modelled on the original. The basic ideology of Fountain House has been successfully established at Fountain House in Pakistan. Twenty years of experience has shown that despite the difference in cultural settings the fundamental model is applicable, that is, reduction of the patient's isolation from society.

Consumer run or sponsored programmes. These programmes have often been the outgrowth of patients and families who were dissatisfied with professionally organized services. In some cases they are part of independent living programmes which serve other disabled populations. The NIMH has funded programmes and studies of the outcomes of consumer case management, consumer run clubhouses, and other consumer run models including businesses. The guiding credo is the belief that those with a disabling condition will best understand and be sensitive to the needs of similarly affected individuals. George Fairweather established a lodge in San Francisco in the 1960s as a setting for a group of chronic patients discharged from a state hospital. Small patient groups were formed while still in the hospital in which training in daily living skills was emphasized. They were encouraged to function as a semi-autonomous group. The intent was to foster mutual responsibility and interdependent skills. Research on this experiment indicated that there was reduced recidivism and an increased rate of full-time employment. This model has not been replicated because of the difficulty of creating and educating groups of patients prior to their discharge from the hospital. Hospital discharges are performed still on an individual rather than a group basis.

There are day programmes, businesses, drop-in centres, community support activities and group vocational activities which are operated on this principle. Specialized neighbourhood social clubs have been developed by Project Return with professional staff who then turn them over to consumers [9].

The high expectancy model. This approach has modular elements or components which are often time-limited and highly structured. Patients move through these training elements at a pace which often offers little flexibility. Patients and staff set the individual's goals in terms of skills to be achieved, at the beginning of the programme, and these goals may be modified as the patient proceeds. The ultimate goals and process are similar to educational modules, or courses, in that patients are expected to graduate to working, independent housing and social lives [9, 13, 14]. This model has been most highly developed at the University of California, Los Angeles (UCLA). It starts with a demonstration of the skills followed by guided role play, including active coaching with critical feedback. This is then supplemented by homework assignments to facilitate the transfer of these skills into a community setting. Indeed, thorough training in real-life settings is strongly encouraged. Considerable reinforcement is required to maintain these skills once they have been acquired. Patients are also taught verbal and non-verbal skills which are essential to social interactions. Things such as eye contact, intonation, physical distance and appropriate level of curiosity are taught.

Vigilance and short-term memory are important to the individual's learning of psychosocial skills. Efforts at cognitive remediation are now an integral part of the rehabilitation of schizophrenics. Behavioural training can improve components of cognition such as reaction time, span of apprehension and vigilance. Positive reinforcement is utilized, usually in the form of tokens that can be redeemed for money, cigarettes, etc. There is no doubt that these techniques can improve functioning as measured by neuropsychologic tests, but there is only meagre evidence as yet to link these test improvements to clinical improvement.

Liberman *et al*'s [13] studies support the efficacy of such an approach. It is useful in decrease of symptoms, reduction of relapse and the avoidance of rehospitalization. Yet, it is important to note that some patients experience such expectations as stressors and withdraw or occasionally decompensate. Rehabilitation workers should be flexible and tolerant of slow and unsteady progress and, where necessary, modification of the original plan.

A hypothetical example may help to illustrate the model. A patient who has had difficulty with social and vocational adaptation because of inappropriate social behaviours might undergo the following sequence. A social skills training programme with focus on job-related social skills might be the first module, with emphasis on conversation, proper attire, punctuality, relationships with co-workers, customers and supervisors. Upon completion of the module, the patient may enter a sheltered workshop (not acceptable in some models, such as the consumer-run programmes who view this as demeaning work) or a transitional employment position. Additional modules are available related to job seeking for persons on the threshold of competitive employment and focus on the job search activities, preparation of a resumé, job interviews, etc. Housing goals may follow a similar graded progression from halfway house with *in vivo* training in cleanliness, meal preparation, etc., followed by a shared apartment with staff involvement, leading to independent living. Some modules are thought to be generally useful such as Liberman's [13] involving symptom control and medication management. Here patients are educated to observe and note their own changing clinical picture, use medication accordingly, speak to the psychiatrist about side effects and clinical changes, etc. Some programmes are entirely built around these modules while others [8, 9] use selected elements.

The intensive or case management model. While case management suffers from a variety of definitions and variability in implementation, it has as a general goal a reduction in social handicaps through improving the patient's access to existing services and resources. The patients receiving intensive clinical case management, which is also known as assertive community treatment (ACT), were studied in Madison, Wisconsin (15). Patients receiving intensive clinical case management versus standard treatment had lower rates of hospitalization, higher levels of functioning and greater life satisfaction. Other studies suggest that the intervention is not necessarily cost-effective. It is essential that the patients be sorted in such a fashion as to identify which subgroups will benefit from case management and which will not. This is an undone piece of research.

As a consequence of the fluctuating course, and the wide variations in programmatic needs of these patients, they must have access to the appropriate level and intensity of care, as their clinical and social state changes and their needs are consequently altered. Since many, if not most schizophrenic patients lack the capacity to negotiate the wide range of clinical programmes and life supports that they require, case management is almost always required. Some family members or other social contacts may be able to carry out this role to some degree but, generally, professional case managers are the glue which holds the long-term management together. Case management functions can include helping the patient identify and access appropriate life supports and treatment options. Public financial assistance, housing, disability payments, general health care, etc., may require the intervention of the case manager if a schizophrenic patient lacks the will, logical thinking, reality testing, or organization independently to obtain these vital supports. Psychiatric case managers also can do supportive counselling, crisis intervention, home visits, outreach and *in situ* rehabilitation. As a component of the rehabilitation process, they may do psychoeducation of patients, family members or other appropriate persons. Depending on the patient's clinical needs, the minimal function of the case manager is to help the patient access the appropriate clinical programming. The five functions which are usually considered the essential elements of case management are: assessing, planning, linking, monitoring and advocacy [16].

Case management is seen as helping patients obtain the necessary supports, resources and skills to improve functioning, deal with environmental barriers and achieve personal goals. Goals usually are focused on specific skill attainment for working, living or socializing [17, 18]. Robinson and Toff-Bergman [17] assert that "rehabilitation-oriented case management is a process of assisting clients to become successful and satisfied in the social environment of their choice with the least amount of professional help". Case management in the United States has moved from being a service broker to that of a provider and advocate.

The initial focus of this approach is functional assessment consisting of identifying the patients' current levels of function, strengths, skill deficits, abilities, and resources in relation to their chosen environment [18]. Case managers then help with "support in dealing with crises, coping with bureaucratic confusion, and acquiring personal and social skills" [19]. The case manager works with patients until they can take responsibility for their own care and coordinate their own needed resources aided by a natural support network. Several other models of case management such as the assertive community team originally developed in Wisconsin, USA [15, 20] use elements of skills training *in situ* but the emphasis is balanced with the acquisition of other rehabilitation programming.

Good case management may appear to be fiscally counterproductive because it may move homeless mentally ill from the inner city streets into treatment settings. Nevertheless, by any rational standard, removing the mentally ill from the street to treatment in the community makes excellent sense and can lead to patients becoming tax producers rather than tax consumers.

The Boston University rehabilitation model. Anthony *et al* [21, 22] have used a three-phase model of psychiatric rehabilitation consisting of diagnostic, planning and intervention phases. With the aid of a rehabilitation specialist, the patient defines overall goals in a selected area, potentially including housing, social life, self-care, work and/or education. Usually the achievement of a specific goal is expected or planned for in a framework of 6 months to 1 year. The patients must assume a major role in defining the goals of rehabilitation. Questions such as where they want to live, do they want to work, what problems do they see as impeding their happiness, etc., can only be determined by the patients themselves. The next step is a functional assessment during which a list of the patient's strengths, assets, weaknesses and deficits is made relevant to the specific goal to be achieved. In other words, what skills does the patient have to achieve the goal, and what additional skills or changed skills will be necessary? A third aspect of assessment is of the patient's environment and support networks. Are these helpful and supportive to the achievement of the goal? Does the person need part-time work rather than full-time work? Does the person have sufficient social contacts to find a date?

Once the diagnostic assessment is done, priorities for skill development are decided upon by the worker and patient who also identify needs for environment and resource modifications. These then become the basis for the initial rehabilitation plan. Written plans for interventions are made and signed by the patient. Skill development and resource development are used in this model. Direct teaching of skills is done when the functional assessment demonstrates that the patient lacks the required skill. A step-by-step process of using the skill in the chosen environment and modifying the environment when necessary is then undertaken.

Specific Rehabilitation Techniques

While the general principles of psychosocial rehabilitation, and their expression in the prototypical programmes, have been discussed, there are several specific techniques which have developed that will be described individually. These include social skills training, vocational rehabilitation and the place and train models, supportive education, and family psychoeducation. Each of these can stand alone in a programme format or be a component of a more comprehensive rehabilitation programme such as described above in the section on models.

The nature of the schizophrenic illness results in the patient having an impairment in interpersonal skills. These skills are critical for community adaptation and hence their acquisition will be described in more detail. Social skills training has as its goal the patient's development of specific interpersonal skills by the use of methods that promote maintenance and generalization of the new or relearned competencies. In order to live in the community persons must have interpersonal, self-care and coping skills. Social skills training is a method of enabling the patient to acquire those skills necessary to remain in the community. This most often can be provided in a specialized setting. Motivation is obviously important. If an individual understands the importance of interpersonal skills in obtaining a job or in getting a date, that person will be much more motivated to acquire the necessary skills. When a patient assumes significant responsibility in determining the goals of the programme, there is marked enhancement in the patient's motivation and willingness to follow the treatment regimen. Largely derived from social learning theory, the training is done with specific educational procedures. Group social experiences offer an opportunity to practise interpersonal skills and get consensual feedback with validation or constructive criticism. The typical format is a training group led by a worker, but involves dances, outings and homework assignments to help generalize the learned or relearned skills.

Specific behavioural techniques are utilized by the rehabilitation workers in the group and sometimes individual context, such as role playing, feedback about communication style and perceptions, modelling, didactic instruction, problem solving and attention focusing. A complex piece of interpersonal behaviour, for example, asking someone for a date or a job, is broken down into discrete elements which are then trained by employing the various techniques. Liberman [14] states that these techniques are designed to "promote the acquisition, generalization, and maintenance of skills required in interpersonal situations". The problem-solving approach used by Liberman's group and others derives from the observation that disabled persons with schizophrenia appear to have problems in cognitive problem-solving abilities which produce failing performances in social situations [23]. In Liberman's basic social skills training model, the rehabilitation worker acts out and models the appropriate use of the target skill. The patient then role plays the skill and gets direct, corrective feedback from the worker (and/or members of the group when this is done in group format). Videotaping is frequently used and useful in dealing with the three dimensions of social communication and interaction which are conceptualized as receiving (accurate perception from others), processing (producing and selecting response options), and sending (involving verbal and non-verbal skills to send an appropriate and effective social message). Other models are directed at skills other than communication, including medication management, dealing with physicians, independent living and grooming skills [13].

Social skills training has been extensively researched. According to Liberman [14], it is most effective as part of a comprehensive rehabilitation approach. Bellack and Mueser [24] reviewed psychosocial treatments for persons with schizophrenia and concluded that this approach is the most researched and promising one in the alleviation of disability for this population. Case studies, small group studies and clinical trials have shown efficacy in teaching a range of behaviours, including conversational skills, heterosocial skills, assertiveness and medication management. Bellack and Mueser [24] found that newly learned skills have been maintained for 6–12 months following intervention in follow-up studies. Other research support for the generalization and efficacy of skills training comes from studies, reviews and meta-analysis [25–29]. To ensure generalizability of acquired skills from the programme context to real-life environments, homework assignments are made with demonstrated efficacy [30, 31]. Family members, co-workers, and peers may become allies in providing feedback and cues in real situations, although this requires some education and training for them. Anderson *et al* [32] indicated that social skills training may be particularly effective when done together with family psychoeducation. In an extensive review of the research in this area, Lehman *et al* [33] concluded that, while evidence for positive impact on relapse and rehospitalization is inconclusive, the effects on social function appear generally positive. No conclusive process research has been done to determine the best frequency and duration of training sessions [24].

Social skills training is usually a needed dimension of rehabilitation prior to vocational function. Vocational rehabilitation is targeted to work-related skills including punctuality, habits of work (concentration, perseverance, pace, etc.), and relationships with bosses, co-workers and customers. The goal is to improve the individual's functional capacity for work through training and/or environmental support and manipulation, so that competitive employment is achieved and maintained [34]. Lehman *et al* [35] found that having no work contributed to poor quality of life as rated by persons with psychiatric disability. Patients with schizophrenia and other major psychiatrically-disabling conditions have been reported to have employment rates as low as 20–30% on discharge from a psychiatric admission to a hospital, and less than 20% of those who find work can retain it a year or two later [6]. Bond and McDonel [36] found that less than 20% of psychiatrically-disabled persons find work in the competitive market. Many who are employed are working at menial jobs, often below what their premorbid educational or vocational levels would suggest was appropriate.

A traditional train-and-place model assesses and trains patients in general work habits such as punctuality. They are then trained to do a particular kind of work, such as clerical or maintenance, and placed at a regular job site. The advantages are obvious, in that any attitudinal and behavioural factors that contribute to unemployability can be corrected before the patient goes into the job market. Disadvantages include limitations as to the range of work training available. The train-and-place model does not allow for adequate transition from the rehabilitation centre to the real world. Finally, patients find the delays in being able to have an income frustrating and this contributes to a high drop-out rate.

Bond and Dincin [37] found that many patients prefer to be rapidly placed in a job in the competitive marketplace rather than undergo prevocational and vocational training as a prerequisite. This preference has led to the development of the place-and-train model of supported employment. The place-and-train model involves evaluation of the patient's vocational preferences and the identification of a job setting willing to accept psychiatric patients as employees. The patient is then placed at the job site and trained on site to do a specific job for which the patient is being paid. This is also referred to as supported employment, in that the patient works with a job coach. The obvious disadvantages of this programme are that it is labour intensive, costly and requires employers who are willing to make a commitment to the employment of disabled individuals. Work can have many benefits for the psychiatrically disabled besides the financial rewards of a paycheck. These include self-esteem, productive use of time, increased social contacts, decreased empty time, and consequently the patients who work report a better quality of life [38]. Anthony et al [38] suggest a paradigm of choose, obtain and keep a job. Patients are involved in the assessment of their ability to accomplish the tasks and their need for rehabilitation interventions. This assessment then leads to the appropriate choice of specific vocational rehabilitation models and techniques.

A variety of vocational rehabilitation programmatic approaches is located in settings throughout the mental health system in the USA and elsewhere. Among the approaches which will be discussed are sheltered work settings, transitional employment, job enclaves, job clubs, mobile work crews, consumer-run businesses and supported employment. Any of these can be hospital based, community based, or tied to a case management programme, such as the assertive community team approach, with the addition of a vocational specialist to the team.

Sheltered work settings were among the earliest vocationally-oriented programmes and began in psychiatric hospitals. In some instances the programme was in the community but some hospitalized patients would attend as well as those attending outpatient programmes. This approach appears to have achieved some increase in patient self-esteem, with hope for reduced symptomatology, but little vocational adaptation to competitive employment was accomplished [34]. Unskilled work is utilized to train patients in personal and social skills that are work related. The setting is segregated, often in a mental health agency, and patients are paid less than the minimum legal wage in many instances. Many patients are seen as in a final placement but some expectation exists that this will be a transitional phase on the way to competitive employment for others. In some agencies, prevocational work crews doing housekeeping, meal preparation, or clerical chores are used to develop work-related skills. These are often unpaid, with the objective of helping the patient to develop relevant attitudes and behaviours and to experience success in a work-like situation. According to Bond [39], these programmes do not focus on specific job skills which are relevant to the competitive workplace.

Transitional employment (TE) is the placement of a patient in a job on a time-restricted basis (usually no more than 6 months). This allows for the on-site learning of relevant skills which are both general and job-specific, like punctuality, concentration, productivity, appropriate social behaviours, and whatever is required for the specific job which is one that exists in the real world market. This approach is typical of the train-and-place approach. Cooperative employers are willing to reserve a job for patients. Placements may be of individuals or of small work groups. Restaurant work, manual labour and clerical work are the typical placements [34]. Patients are paid prevailing wages but may work part time or may share a job, almost always at an entry level position regardless of employment history. The goal is for the patient to be provided with a successful work experience [40]. Some patients may have a number of placements which provide a broader array of opportunities for choice of jobs when they enter the competitive marketplace [41]. Staff may occasionally fill in for patients who are too ill or otherwise cannot fulfil the position for a time. This may keep the job available to the programme where otherwise an employer might discontinue hiring the mentally ill, even in a transitional placement. Limitations of TE include the focus on entry-level jobs, frequent failure to move to competitive employment and possible dependency on staff [34].

Job clubs have been touched on earlier in this chapter. A group approach is used to train patients to employ various strategies in job seeking. These include contacting relatives and friends about jobs, writing resumés and job applications, reading want ads, and job-related interviewing. Liberman [14] utilized group practice, lectures, homework, role playing and other group techniques to develop skills necessary to achieve employment. The club provides real infrastructure such as word processing equipment, classified sections of newspapers, telephones, etc. The rehabilitation workers develop a job-seeking plan for each patient and provide feedback. Peer support is also utilized. Job clubs have proven effective in job acquisition [14] but not in job retention [36]. Some patients find the pressure of the job club to be distressing [34]. Liberman [14] reported that two-thirds of participants were in a job at 6-month follow-up, although not necessarily in the same job they obtained initially.

Job enclaves and mobile work crews are forms of transitional and occasionally permanent employment. Contracts are obtained by an agency or group of patients for work which may be done in an enclave if appropriate, such as large mailings, or may require moving a crew of patients such as is required for commercial cleaning operations in office buildings. Some small businesses have been developed by patients with staff help, attached to mental health agencies. Restaurants, bulk mailing houses and cookie factories are examples. These can be used for TE or permanent employment [41].

Consumer run businesses may be started by patients in groups with or without staff assistance. Examples are restaurants, film laboratories and studios. In the USA, some consumer groups offer their own vocational counselling and rehabilitation "with minimal or no support from mental health professionals" [41].

The approach of supported employment derives from rehabilitation of the developmentally disabled and is defined by US Federal Law (P.L. 99–506) as:

> competitive work in integrated settings (a) for individuals with severe handicaps for whom competitive employment has not traditionally occurred, or (b) for individuals for whom competitive employment has been interrupted or intermittent as a result of a severe disability and who, because of their handicap, need ongoing support services to perform work. Supported employment is further defined by the refinement of its components (i.e. competitive work, integrated settings, severe handicaps, and ongoing support services) [42].

Support services may be continuing or periodic and work must be for at least 20 hours per week and may occur on or off the work site depending on individual need. Support services include transportation, personal care, counselling to the patient and family, but significantly to supervisors and co-workers as well. Strengths of this approach include job-related training that happens after the patient is placed and may be job-specific and bypasses the concerns about the schizophrenic's ability to generalize skills learned in one setting to another. Support includes assessment of the match between the person and the job prior to its selection, and may include specific job requirements such as co-worker's attitudes, travel requirements, etc. The patient earns competitive wages in this approach, and co-workers and supervisors may experience positive changes in prior prejudicial attitudes. Some drawbacks or potential drawbacks exist, including high dependency on staff, consequent staff burn-out, and high cost [39].

The rehabilitation worker in supported employment is called a job coach and he/she visits the worksite for support, counselling, and advocacy for some time after the job has begun. The coach learns the job and in turn trains the patient in the necessary skills. Clearly, this provides highly relevant information about a patient's adaptive capacities, as well as needed environmental foci including stigma. Job coaches relate to employers and co-workers to provide information about mental illness, rights such as those provided under the Americans with Disability Act, and deal with negative attitudes. The coach may gradually leave the worksite as the patient succeeds and may return when necessary.

Supportive education derives from the recognition that some disabled psychiatric patients may require additional, formal, post-secondary education in order to achieve their educational and vocational ambitions [42]. The goal is the integration of this population into colleges and universities [43]. This concept is relatively new, although educational interventions for the mentally ill were described as early as the 1970s [44]. Schizophrenia has a typical age of onset in the late teens and early twenties, the peak years of higher education. Thus, many educational careers are interrupted. The absence of education and the appropriate credentials make vocational choices markedly restricted. This is believed to account, in some measure, for the underemployment or unemployment of many patients with a schizophrenic illness. Patients are often intimidated at the prospect of re-entering school, and anticipate stigma, rejection, social isolation, difficulty concentrating and thinking. They are concerned about the stresses of exams, classroom performance and social demands. Cooper, in 1993 [45], described patients' fears, including the absence of anyone at the school who will be available to counsel and support them. On the other hand, college officials, faculty, and students may fear mentally ill persons as dangerous, inappropriate and disruptive. Administrators may be unable to distinguish disciplinary issues from signs and symptoms of a mental disorder like schizophrenia [46, 47]. The goal is a successful completion of the educational programme and development of a career plan, as well as development of a system of other students who provide peer support [48]. Hopefully, the patients come to accept a new identity as students. Techniques utilized by the rehabilitation worker include on-site behaviour modification, skills training, study habits, role playing, crisis therapy for school-related stress, and where possible modification of negative attitudes and unhelpful behaviours of administrators, faculty and fellow students. Supported education generally uses one or more of three basic structures: the self-contained classroom with a special curriculum for a group of disabled patients; on-site support with the patient in the regular college classroom and the worker providing services on campus; and a mobile supported education model with regular off-site psychiatric rehabilitation services, usually a group, with the availability of on-site supports [42, 48]. Some hospitals and some community-based comprehensive rehabilitation programmes have developed relationships with colleges in their areas to develop a continuum of educational services from intra-agency classes, to supported education, to independent enrolment. Academic activities are integrated into the full psychiatric treatment plan in these programmes and the belief is that education and treatment go hand in hand in the patient's adaptation [49, 50].

Families are usually intensely interested in information about mental disorders. Family psychoeducation involves more than a transmission of information about mental disorders and ways to obtain professional services. Families must be assisted in how to communicate with the ill relative and to use these skills in a way to improve the quality of the relationship. Estimates of the percentage of families of seriously mentally ill persons who must participate in their care have varied between 30 and 60% in the United States [51–54]. Moving patients from the hospital to the community has put emotional and financial burdens on family members [55, 56]. Once families were viewed by the field as potential causative agents in schizophrenia. As biological and stress diathesis models have come to the fore, families have become allies in advocacy and treatment with mental health professionals. Because modification of the environment is a focus of traditional rehabilitation, psychoeducation of families is legitimately viewed as a rehabilitation strategy.

This has received support from the classic studies of expressed emotion (EE) in families. These identified that families rated as highly critical, hostile or emotionally overinvolved with their schizophrenic family member, had much higher rates of patient relapse [57–59]. Patients who live with families rated high on EE do receive some protection from neuroleptics and reduced contact with family [58]. When families are educated about schizophrenia, its course and treatment, and the need to modify high expressed emotion related behaviours, some studies indicate a reduced rehospitalization and relapse rate from approximately 50–75% over 2 years to 11% over 2 years for patients living with families with high EE [32]. Families are seen as a group with the patient or in the conjoint family model with several families in attendance. After direct observation of family function to rate communication and expectations, interventions used include behavioural analysis of family members, education about the illness and its treatment, training in communication skills, and training in problem-solving skills. Some models actually enlist family members as part of the formal rehabilitation process providing job counselling, friendship skills, feedback, etc.

While this approach has been widely accepted, some families still express concern about feeling blamed for the patient's illness, and this must be addressed directly. Families can serve as an early detection system for recognition of the onset of symptoms before they have achieved a dangerous level. Family psychoeducation skills training can be conducted in multiple family groups, which is more cost-effective. It also is a means of strengthening interfamilial networks. Dealing with other families who are sharing the burden of a mentally ill member not only reduces stress and isolation, but reduces the sense of stigma experienced by that family.

Shelter

All humans require shelter. The specific form of that shelter varies as a function of culture and economic development. In some cultures the extended family provides shelter, whereas in others it is more the role of the nuclear family. In many of the most economically-evolved societies, independent living can become a role function. Clearly, it is necessary to identify the role of shelter in a particular setting, rather than to attempt to develop guidelines that will be of only limited generalizability.

In recognizing the need for forms of shelter which maximize the quality of the patient's life, it is important to understand that in the name of offering shelter we can create highly artificial environments for the patients. These artificial environments may label the patient as a subhuman individual and thereby contribute to a significant degree of stigma. The more a housing environment differs from the norm of a particular culture, the greater the effort must be to make that a transient environment. The planning of housing must take into account the need to reduce stigma. Placing former mental patients in slum housing in dangerous neighbourhoods only stigmatizes the patients as not deserving of appropriate and decent housing. It devalues the patient and says to the public only mentally-ill people need to reside under these conditions. A major failure of community mental health programmes in the United States has been the placement of patients in substandard housing environments. The more normal the housing arrangement, the less the associated stigma for the patient.

Patients require different levels of housing support at different phases of their illness. There are some individuals who can live in a normal setting with little or no assistance other than fiscal. There are individuals who require a community residence in which a variety of social and medical services including supervision are readily available. In other words, there are housing arrangements which simply consist of subsidized housing to housing arrangements which involve significant service provision along with the housing. The traditional halfway house follows this latter model. It provides 24-hour supervision, including a planned programme of patient activities. It is seen as a transient form of housing, and it is expected that the patient will ultimately be able to move into a less restrictive setting. In a sense, this type of housing is viewed as a transition between a hospital and full community living. Unfortunately, there are patients for whom this kind of housing is not a transient need, but rather is required for the long term.

Not every patient can move from a halfway house to more normal living circumstances.

There is a very strong need for research on every aspect of residential placement. The need includes identification of means by which patients are matched to housing alternatives, duration of each alternative, means of identifying when the patient is ready to move to a less restrictive environment, and the cost-effectiveness of such programmes.

Psychological Well-being

A critical element in all psychiatric rehabilitation is the psychological status of the patient. Traditionally, rehabilitation has focused on employment and shelter. In recent years, particularly under the influence of the UCLA group, there has been considerable emphasis on the acquisition of interpersonal skills. Nevertheless, it is clear that being able to hold a conversation, be employed, and to maintain an apartment, which are essential elements of life, are far from the totality. The only valid measure of the patient's satisfaction with his/her life is the patient's self-image. If a patient realistically feels proud of himself/herself, then the rehabilitation effort is going in a good direction. There are many factors that contribute to a sense of well-being, including being employed, having an apartment, having friends, etc. Yet, one can have all of these and still find life to have little existential meaning. The psychological rehabilitation of patients must receive greater attention. This is not a call for individual psychotherapy for all patients, but rather the need to recognize that all people, including patients, have to feel useful to and needed by other people in order to maintain their dignity. It is the task of the rehabilitation team to identify and assist the patient to engage in activities that will enhance self-confidence and a sense of personal worth. Obviously, this task will be very much influenced by cultural variables. That which is sustaining in one culture may very well be of little value in another.

Developing Countries

The goals and principles of psychiatric rehabilitation do not vary as a function of economic development. Economically developing countries will define normal life differently from countries which have developed further economically. Cultural factors will contribute significantly to the definition of what constitutes a normal life. Adult roles differ among different countries as a function of both culture and economic development. Nevertheless, every group has its own definition of what are appropriate roles for an adult in that particular social setting. While the society defines the roles, it remains the task of rehabilitation to help psychiatric patients fulfil those roles as fully as is possible.

Shinfuku [60] warned about the tendency in some of the rapidly developing Asian economies to create long-term psychiatric beds as a way of dealing with the problem of the mentally disabled. His warning is more explicitly stated by Deva [61], who fears that the rapidly developing countries are turning to the warehousing of patients rather than towards proper treatment. Deva warns that this practice is more of value to families who wish to be relieved of the burden of their mentally-ill relative rather than focusing on the needs of the patient. It may be premature to raise an alarm. However, the danger in a rapidly expanding economy is that all other values can be swept aside by the opportunity to become rich.

When it is understood that rehabilitation is merely an aspect of the treatment of the schizophrenic, it becomes clear that economic development does not change theoretical understanding, but merely may limit application of established techniques. Developing countries often have a less complex social order which makes fewer demands on the schizophrenic. This fact probably explains the better prognosis of the schizophrenic in the developing world. Schizophrenics can adapt to a simpler life more easily. Furthermore, many developing countries benefit from the existence of extended families. The schizophrenics can move among several family members over time, thereby reducing the burden on any given family member.

STIGMA

The term stigma refers to a mark or sign that denotes a shameful quality in the individual so marked. As such, stigma serves as a means of social control. As with all forms of social control, the use of stigma can be either constructive or destructive. Every society will define certain behaviours as unacceptable. In associating stigma with those behaviours, they make them less likely to occur. Social opprobrium is a very effective means of social control. The psychologic dynamic of stigma is the branding of a person as "the other". Otherness in virtually every society is seen negatively. There are many languages in which the term for stranger and enemy are synonymous. Difference is something that is not readily accepted by humans. Tolerance of difference is an acquired socially-conditioned trait that is not easily achieved.

Virtually every serious medical illness has been associated with stigma at sometime in its history. Illnesses that involve personal responsibility, such as sexually transmitted diseases, were as likely to be associated with stigma as diseases such as cancer which bore no such responsibility. There are certain general features of medical disorders that lead to stigma. The disorder must be dangerous to the person's life, appearance or productivity. Diseases, such as the plague, which were rapidly life threatening were very much associated with stigma. Deforming disorders such as leprosy were associated with stigma. Disorders that rendered the persons unable to care for themselves, such as mental retardation, were associated with stigma. It is important to understand that stigma is not a problem only of mental illnesses, but rather a consequence of fear induced in the person not so afflicted.

The mental illnesses, however, do have a unique disadvantage that contributes to stigma. More so than most medical illnesses, the mental disorders alter the most fundamentally human characteristics of the person. The person's way of thinking, expressing feelings, understanding social cues, etc., are significantly changed. It is this alteration of the basically human characteristics of the individual that incites so much fear and even animosity in many of the observers of the mentally ill. It is in some ways easier to observe persons losing muscle mass than it is to observe persons losing their ability to communicate. The more severe the capacity to behave in a way that is similar to other people, the more likely the person is to be treated with hostility and to be stigmatized. There are cultural differences in the societal response to human difference. Some cultures are more tolerant of deviation from the norm. Historically, there were cultures that even valued madness and saw these individuals as closer to the Gods. Nevertheless, the preponderant response to people with mental illnesses has been negative.

When one gets beyond the individual case, one finds that the mental illnesses represent a threat to much of the public. They are not diseases that, for example, can be avoided by a proper diet. They cannot be avoided by economic development. In fact, they cannot be avoided. Mental illness can strike anyone at anytime. No family is immune. This egalitarian feature of mental illness does not make it more attractive, but rather more frightening. The limited effectiveness of treatment also contributes to public fear and therefore stigma. As medical treatments of a disease improve, the public fear is reduced as is the stigma.

Mental illness in the public's mind has long been associated with irrational and unpredictable violence. Research studies concerning this purported relationship have not been consistent. As schizophrenia, in the developed world, has begun to show considerable comorbidity with abuse of drugs, the risk for violence has increased. The reduction of violence in this population will assist greatly in reducing stigma. The media portrayal of mentally ill people as violent and dangerous contributes to the problem. This is not a recommendation for censorship, but rather for responsible media behaviour. The media must temper sensationalism in the search for higher ratings.

There is no single answer to the reduction and control of stigma. There are many approaches and they must go on simultaneously. A better understanding of the aetiopathogenic factors that contribute to mental illness will help. Blaming society only increases public hostility and stigma. Interestingly, the identification of a breast cancer gene for certain types of breast cancer has helped to reduce stigma. It is as if society can say it is the fault of the gene and not of society. Science can be of assistance in reducing stigma by increasing the understanding of the nature of schizophrenia.

Improved treatments will help enormously. The stigma on recurrent depression has diminished sharply as treatments have improved dramatically. A good prognosis is an excellent counterweight to stigma, as is a rapid response to treatment. There is a fundamental difference between spending a year in a hospital waiting for the depression to run its course and waiting several weeks for the antidepressant to take effect.

The family movement has had an extraordinary effect in reducing stigma. Openness has contributed to the reduction. Treating mental illness in the family as a secret, makes the illness appear shameful and deserving of stigma. When people speak openly of the illness of family members without shame, there is an automatic reduction in stigma through this process of self-demonstration that stigma is not warranted. Families have worked to educate the public as well as themselves. They have mobilized the public against the illness, rather than against the patient who has suffered from the illness. Family groups have played a very important role in influencing the media so that the mentally ill are not routinely portrayed as dangerous individuals.

Finally, the fact that so many patients are living successfully in the community is having a very powerful effect on stigma. Studies have shown that 20–40 years after the onset of schizophrenia, from one half to two-thirds of the patients can function reasonably adequately in their community. This finding supports the importance of psychiatric rehabilitation as a means of improving the spontaneous improvement rates. Living and working with people who are in the process of overcoming their mental disabilities is an excellent antidote to the problem of stigma.

SUMMARY

This paper has reviewed the definition of schizophrenia, its various courses, a history of its past treatment, and its current treatment. The purpose of this review was to establish clearly that schizophrenia represents a chronic and persistent disorder which is essentially life-long. The recognition of the life-long nature of the disease requires acceptance that treatment is also going to be life-long. The distinction that has traditionally been made between acute and long-term treatment can be useful, but is quite arbitrary. This distinction has frequently led psychiatrists to see the management of an acute decompensation as medical, and the management of the longer-term features of the illness as the domain of other non-medical disciplines. The very use of terms such as residual symptoms can suggest that medicine has done all that is possible and now it is up to "rehabilitation" specialists to help the patient to adapt to his/her limitations. While there is some truth in this formulation, it frequently leads to a separation of services and a lack of continuity for the patient suffering from a life-long illness. It also leads to a hierarchy in treatment values, with the management of the acute decompensation being seen as more skilled and important than the management of the long-term features of the illness.

In the absence of a rapid cure, most medical disorders have long-term consequences. This is true for diabetes, hypertension, cardiovascular disease, etc. The fact that a diabetic must follow a particular diet is best conceptualized as an integral part of the management of the illness and not as a rehabilitative technique. Obviously, the intent of dietary management is to prevent negative consequences that would otherwise occur. The recognition that what is called rehabilitation is an integral part of the active treatment of schizophrenia, but at different phases of the disorder, is essential to the thesis of this chapter. What is special about schizophrenia is that it leads to disabilities in the area of cognition, interpersonal skills, vocational skills and employability. These disabilities lead to a variety of social and vocational handicaps. The disabilities and handicaps are integral to the disease and must be treated as actively as an acute decompensation.

With the introduction of neuroleptics in the 1950s, the management of schizophrenia changed dramatically. Many patients who previously faced hospitalizations of many years were now able to be discharged to the community. One unexpected consequence of this was that the disabilities that did not prevent a person from remaining in hospital, could prevent a person from remaining in the community. Behaviours which were acceptable on a chronic hospital ward were not acceptable in the real world outside of the hospital. This led to an increasing awareness of the importance of ongoing treatment of the total picture. It was not enough to control agitation and violence, but it was now essential to control the gamut of symptoms associated with this disorder. The recent introduction of the newer antipsychotics offers considerable promise. The side effect profile of these compounds is much more comfortable for the patients. The diminished extrapyramidal manifestations may also reduce the risk of the complication of tardive dyskinesia. Furthermore, these compounds appear to have a beneficial effect on the negative symptoms of the disorder. Compliance with medication is in part a function of how comfortable the patient is with side effects of the drug. Any movement towards reducing side effects and increasing patient comfort will contribute towards compliance.

The non-pharmacologic treatments are as essential in the continuing treat-ment of schizophrenia as is the neuroleptic treatment. As indicated earlier, many of the manifestations of schizophrenia appear in the area of cognition, interpersonal skills, vocational skills and employability. Disabilities in these areas diminish the capacity of the patient to fulfil culturally-determined adult roles in a given society. Functional restoration is the goal of all medical treatment. If some symptoms are controlled, but the patient remains disabled, it is inappropriate to call that a successful outcome. The non-pharmacologic treatments have been demonstrated to be very useful in the acquisition and/or relearning of social skills. These social skills are vital not only for interpersonal relationships, but for vocational training as well. It has also been demonstrated that a significant percentage of patients can be vocationally trained and become tax producers rather than tax consumers. Research has shown improvements in cognition on psychological tests in patients receiving cognitive training, but it is yet to be demonstrated that this makes a difference in the real life of the individual. It is important to note in this context that the failure to demonstrate does not mean the absence of an effect. Finally, the entire area of self-esteem is critical, not only for role functioning, but for an adaptive life. The proper use of non-pharmacologic interventions can contribute to the patient's sense of well-being, which is an integral part of the goal of treatment.

Much of the research on psychosocial interventions in schizophrenia does not approach the methodologic rigour of the psychopharmacologic studies. This chapter required, as a minimum for a study to be included, that it should have a pre/post design utilizing a comparison of quality of life issues such as community survival or patient welfare. There are several areas of rehabilitation which have been subjected to more rigorous designs including control groups, random assignment and outcome including standardized measures of recidivism, community longevity, productive work, as well as quality of life measures. In the arena of case management, the work of Stein and Test [15] has had widespread acceptance as scientifically valid and replicated in a variety of settings. In the area of job club and related prevocational and vocational modules, the work of the UCLA group, under the direction of Robert Liberman, has been exemplary in its design and use of clear, measurable outcome variables [14, 30], as well as the work of Bond and his group [36, 40]. In the area of family psychoeducation, several groups, most notably the original describers of high EE, Vaughn, Brown, Birley, and Leff [57–59], and later on, the work of the group at the University of Pittsburgh [32] have been widely replicated, well designed, and demonstrated major efficacious effects in recidivism, community tenure, and quality of patient and family life.

While pre- and post-designs have been useful in pointing the way to such techniques as supported education and supported employment, the attempts at controlled studies have revealed work outcomes which affect small percentages of patients so treated. However, given the morbidity of these patients' depleted lives, the small percentage of successful patients who return to work, or work for the first time, or complete an educational programme, can surely justify the interventions in humanistic terms. The process may include later attempts for today's treatment failures, which may prove successful in a different phase of the disease process. In addition, as we learn to use modern neurochemical, neuropsychological, genetic and imaging techniques to subtype schizophrenia and other disabling illnesses, we can be more specific as to which patients may respond to which interventions. We are at the threshold of realizing those possibilities.

The problem of stigma is not unique to schizophrenia, nor is it even unique to the mental illnesses. Whether it is bubonic plague, leprosy, AIDS, etc., there are many medical illnesses that have been the recipient of stigma. These illnesses tend to be life threatening, or disfiguring, or role incapacitating. Obviously, the need to reduce stigma is essential to reduce the handicap faced by schizophrenic patients. Public education is important. Family education is equally important. When families stop being embarrassed about their schizophrenic child, it makes an enormous difference to the attitude of the public. The improved integration of the schizophrenic patients into real community life will also reduce stigma. Ultimately, as our treatments improve and as disability is reduced, then the reduction of stigma will automatically follow.

Consistent Evidence

Psychopharmacologic interventions, utilizing traditional neuroleptics, can reduce and to some degree control positive symptoms, thereby decreasing disability. The more recently developed, so-called atypical, antipsychotics also have an impact on negative symptoms, thereby leading to less disability. The more comfortable side-effect profile of these drugs contributes to better compliance. Continuous psychopharmacologic management throughout the course of the illness is essential.

Bizarre behaviours that are "acceptable" in a hospital setting are not socially acceptable in the community. The combination of psychopharmacology, family psychoeducation and social skills training gives the best reduction of exacerbations and rehospitalizations, thereby reducing both disability and stigma. Social skills training can yield an improvement in the patient's level of social skills and can improve the patient's employability and social acceptability. Families with high EE can be assisted to reduce this level, thereby reducing disability in the patient.

All of the psychosocial techniques reviewed in this paper have been shown to reduce rehospitalization. Psychosocial and vocational training improves community adaptation for only a relatively small percentage of the patient cohort.

Many illnesses, not only mental, suffer from stigma. Cultures differ in their tolerance of deviation. The family movement has reduced stigma appreciably. Slum housing for the mentally ill contributes to stigma. Stigma is a product of fear, ignorance and prejudice.

Incomplete Evidence

Social skills training when administered alone has an unclear impact on relapse. The evidence of job retention beyond 6 months is uncertain. Male schizophrenics may have a tendency towards greater disability. Schizophrenics in developed countries appear to suffer greater disability. Structural brain changes appear to be associated with greater disability. The value of cognitive remediation in real-life situations is not clear.

Areas Still Open to Research

The need for reduction of the aetiopathogenic heterogeneity in the population is essential. It is necessary: (i) to identify subtypes of schizophrenia which are more responsive to specific neuroleptic agents; (ii) to develop new neuroleptic agents which will be more effective for particular subtypes; (iii) to identify the specific non-pharmacologic interventions for specific subtypes; (iv) to develop new non-pharmacologic interventions and to identify the subtypes for which they are the optimal treatments; (v) to develop cost–benefit analyses for particular interventions in particular cases, such as the frequency and duration of a particular psychosocial intervention.

REFERENCES

1. Cancro R. (1979) The healer & madness. *J. Nat. Assoc. Priv. Psych. Hosp.*, **10**: 5–15.
2. American Psychiatric Association (1994) *Diagnostic and Statistical Manual of Mental Disorders*, 4th edn. American Psychiatric Association, Washington, DC.
3. World Health Organization (1992) *The ICD-10 Classification of Mental and Behavioural Disorders. Clinical Descriptions and Diagnostic Guidelines.* World Health Organization, Geneva.
4. McGlashan T.H. (1988) A selective review of recent North American long-term follow up studies of schizophrenia. *Schizophr. Bull.*, **14**: 515–542.
5. Roy A. (1982) Suicide in chronic schizophrenia. *Br. J. Psychiatry*, **141**: 171–177.
6. Anthony W.A., Cohen M.R., Farkas M. (1990) *Psychiatric Rehabilitation.* Boston Center for Psychiatric Rehabilitation, Boston.
7. Anthony W., Liberman R.P. (1986) The practice of psychiatric rehabilitation. *Schizophr. Bull.*, **12**: 542–558.
8. Dincin J. (1975) Psychiatric rehabilitation. *Schizophr. Bull.*, **13**: 131–147.
9. Rutman I.D. (1987) The psychosocial rehabilitation movement in the United States. In *Psychiatric Disability* (Eds A.T. Meyerson, T. Fine), pp. 131–147. American Psychiatric Press, Washington, DC.
10. Anthony W.A., Cohen M.R., Cohen B.F. (1983) Philosophy, treatment, process, and principle of the psychiatric rehabilitation approach. In *Deinstitutionalization* (Ed. L.L. Bachrach), pp. 67–79. Jossey-Bass, San Francisco.

11. Hogarty G., Anderson C., Reiss D., Kornblith S.J., Greenwald D.P., Ulrich R.E., Carter M. (1991) Family psychoeducation, social skills training, and maintenance chemotherapy in aftercare of schizophrenia: II. Two year effects of a controlled study of relapse and adjustment. *Arch. Gen. Psychiatry*, **481**: 340–347.
12. Propst R. (1992) Introduction. *Psychosoc. Rehab. J.*, **161**: 3.
13. Liberman R.P., Jacobs H.E., Blackwell G.A. (1987) Overcoming psychiatric disability through skills training. In *Psychiatric Disability* (Eds A.T. Meyerson, T. Fine), pp. 221–249. American Psychiatric Press, Washington, DC.
14. Liberman R.P. (1988) Social skills training. In *Psychiatric Rehabilitation for Chronic Patients* (Ed. R.P. Liberman), pp. 147–198. American Psychiatric Press, Washington, DC.
15. Stein L.I., Test M.A. (1980) Alternatives to mental hospital treatment conceptual model 1: Treatment program and clinical evaluation. *Arch. Gen. Psychiatry*, **37**: 392–397.
16. Hargreaves W., Shaw R., Shadoan R., Walker E., Surber R., Gaynor J. (1984) Measuring case management activity. *J. Nerv. Ment. Dis.*, **172**: 296–300.
17. Robinson G.K., Toff-Bergman G. (1990) *Choices in Case Management: Current Knowledge and Practice for Mental Health Programs*. Mental Health Policy Resource Center, Washington, DC.
18. Hodge M., Draine J. (1993) Development of support through case management services. In *Psychiatric Rehabilitation in Practice* (Eds R.W. Flexer, P. Solomon), pp. 155–169. Andover, Boston.
19. Goering P., Wasylenki D., Farkas M., Lancee W.J., Ballantyne R. (1988) What difference does case management make? *Hosp. Comm. Psychiatr.*, **39**: 272–276.
20. Test M. (1992) Training in community living. In *Handbook of Psychiatric Rehabilitation* (Ed. R.P. Liberman), pp. 153–170. Macmillan, New York.
21. Anthony W.A. (1982) Explaining psychiatric rehabilitation by an analogy to physical rehabilitation. *Psychosocial Rehab. J.*, **6**: 61–65.
22. Anthony W.A., Cohen M.R. (1987) Training and technical assistance in psychiatric rehabilitation. In *Psychiatric Disability* (Eds A.T. Meyerson, T. Fine), pp. 251–269. American Psychiatric Press, Washington, DC.
23. Platt J.J., Spivak G. (1972) Problem solving thinking of psychiatric patients. *J. Consult. Clin. Psychol.*, **28**: 3–5.
24. Bellack A., Mueser K. (1993) Psychosocial treatment for schizophrenia. *Schizophr. Bull.*, **19**: 317–326.
25. Wallace C.J., Nelson C., Liberman B.P., Aitchison R.A., Lukoff D., Elder J.P., Ferris C. (1980) A review and critique of social skills training with chronic schizophrenics. *Schizophr. Bull.*, **6**: 42–63.
26. Bellack A., Hersen M., Turner V. (1976) Generalization effects of social skills training in chronic schizophrenics: an experimental analysis. *Behav. Res. Ther.*, **14**: 391–398.
27. Goldsmith J.C., McFall R.M. (1975) Development and evolution of an interpersonal skill training program for psychiatric inpatients. *J. Abnorm. Psychol.*, **84**: 51–58.
28. Corrigan P. (1991) Social skills training in adult psychiatric populations: A meta-analysis. *J. Behav. Ther. Exp. Psychiatry*, **22**: 203–210.
29. Halford W., Hayes R. (1991) Psychosocial rehabilitation of chronic schizophrenic patients: recent findings on social skills training and family psychoeducation. *Clin. Psychol. Rev.*, **11**: 23–44.

30. Liberman R.P., Reueger D.B. (1984) Drug–psychosocial treatment interactions: comprehensive rehabilitation for chronic schizophrenics. *Psychosoc. Rehab. J.*, **3**: 3–15.
31. Finch B., Wallace C.J. (1977) Successful interpersonal skills training with schizophrenic inpatients. *J. Consult. Clin. Psychol.*, **45**: 885–890.
32. Anderson C.M., Hogarty G.E., Reiss D.J. (1980) Family treatment of adult schizophrenic patients: a psycho-educational approach. *Schizophr. Bull.*, **6**: 490–505.
33. Lehman A., Dixon L., LeVine J. (1994) *Literature Review: Schizophrenia Patient Outcomes Research Team.* Center for Mental Health Services Research. University of Maryland, Baltimore, MD.
34. Simmons T.J., Selleck V., Steele R., Sepetauc F. (1993) Supports and rehabilitation for employment. In *Psychiatric Rehabilitation in Practice* (Eds R. Flexer, P. Solomon), pp. 119–135. Andover, Boston.
35. Lehman A.F., Ward N.C., Linn L.S. (1983) Chronic mental patients: the quality of life issue. *Am. J. Psychiatry*, **133**: 796–823.
36. Bond G., McDonel E. (1991) Vocational rehabilitation outcomes for persons with psychiatric disabilities. *J. Voc. Rehab.*, **1**: 9–20.
37. Bond G., Dincin J. (1986) Accelerating entry into transitional employment in a psychosocial agency. *Rehab. Psychol.*, **32**: 143–155.
38. Anthony W.A., Howell J., Danley K. (1984) Vocational rehabilitation of the psychiatrically disabled. In *Chronically Mentally Ill: Research & Services* (Ed. M. Mirabi), pp. 215–237. Spectrum, New York.
39. Bond G. (1987) Supported work as a modification of the transitional employment model for clients with psychiatric disabilities. *Psychosoc. Rehab. J.*, **11**: 55–73.
40. Bond G., Boyer S. (1988) Rehabilitation programs and outcomes. In *Vocational Rehabilitation of Persons with Prolonged Psychiatric Disorders* (Eds J. Ciardiello, M. Bell), pp. 231–263. Hopkins, Baltimore, MD.
41. National Institute on Disability and Rehabilitation Research (1992) *Consensus Statement*, vol. 3.
42. Unger K. (1993) Introduction. *Psychosoc. Rehab. J.*, **17**: 11–23.
43. Unger K., Anthony W., Sciarappa K., Rogers E.S. (1991) A supported education program for young adults with long term mental illness. *Hosp. Comm. Psychiatry*, **42**: 838–843.
44. Lamb H.R. (1976) An educational model for teaching living skills to long-term patients. *Hosp. Comm. Psychiatry*, **12**: 875–877.
45. Cooper L. (1993) Serving adults with psychiatric disabilities on campus: a mobile support approach. *Psychosoc. Rehab. J.*, **17**: 25–38.
46. Unger K. (1990) Supported education for young adults with psychiatric disabilities. *Comm. Supp. Network News*, **6**: 1–11.
47. Cook J.A., Solomon M.L. (1993) The community scholar program: an outcome study of supported education for students with severe mental illness. *Psychosoc. Rehab. J.*, **17**: 83–97.
48. Moxley D., Mowbray C., Brown S.K. (1993) Supported Education. In *Psychiatric Rehabilitation in Practice* (Eds R.W. Flexer, P. Solomon), pp. 137–153. Andover, Boston.
49. Hoffman F.L., Mastrianni X. (1992) The hospitalization of the college student: a model program for psychiatric treatment. *Am. J. Orthopsychiatry*, **62**: 297–302.
50. Hoffman F.L., Mastrianni X. (1993) The role of supported education in the inpatient treatment of young adults: a two site comparison. *Psychosoc. Rehab. J.*, **17**: 109–119.

51. Goldman H.H., Gatozzi A.A. (1981) Defining and counting the chronically mentally ill. *Hosp. Comm. Psychiatry*, **52**: 21–27.
52. Carpentier N., Lesage A., Goulet I., Lalonde P., Renaud M. (1992) Burden of care of families not living with young schizophrenic relative. *Hosp. Comm. Psychiatry*, **43**: 38–43.
53. Minkoff K. (1978) A map of chronic mental patients. In *The Chronic Mental Patient* (Ed. J.A. Talbott), pp. 11–37. American Psychiatric Press, Washington, DC.
54. Lamb H.R., Goertzel V. (1977) The long-term patient in the era of community treatment. *Arch. Gen. Psychiatry*, **29**: 803–809.
55. Hartfield A. (1978) Psychosocial costs of schizophrenia to the family. *Social Work*, **23**: 355–359.
56. Thompson E., Doll W. (1982) The burden of families coping with the mentally ill: an invisible crisis. *Fam. Rel.*, **31**: 379–388.
57. Brown G.W., Birley J.L.T., Wing J.K. (1972) Influence of family life on the course of schizophrenic disorders: a replication. *Br. J. Psychiatry*, **121**: 241–258.
58. Vaughn C., Leff J. (1976) The influence of family and social factors on the course of psychiatric illness. *Br. J. Psychiatry*, **129**: 125–137.
59. Vaughn C., Snyder K., Jones S., Freeman W.B., Falloon I.R. (1984) Family factors in schizophrenic relapse. *Arch. Gen. Psychiatry*, **41**: 1169–1177.
60. Shinfuku N. (1998) Mental health services in Asia: international perspectives and challenge for the coming years. *Psychiatry Clin. Neurosci.*, **52**: 269–274.
61. Deva M.P. (1998) Is rehabilitation losing out to warehousing in developing countries? *Bull. WAPR*, **10**: 1.

Commentaries

4.1

What Works for the Rehabilitation of Schizophrenia? A Brief Review of the Evidence

Kim T. Mueser[1]

Cancro and Meyerson provide a comprehensive overview of schizophrenia, including the nature of the illness, the extent of social disability, stigma and rehabilitation. The overriding theme of their review is that schizophrenia is a lifelong disorder that requires a long-term commitment to rehabilitation in order to optimize outcomes. Psychosocial rehabilitation focuses on helping patients to enhance their capacity for interpersonal relationships, to work, to live as independently as possible in the community, and to improve the quality of their lives. Ultimately, the most important way of reducing the stigma of schizophrenia is to improve the social impairment that characterizes this illness.

Cancro and Meyerson provide a broad overview of different rehabilitation approaches for patients with schizophrenia. In addition to understanding the range of available options, clinicians need to be informed about the empirical evidence supporting different methods of psychosocial rehabilitation. This information can serve as a guide to clinicians in selecting front-line interventions in their work with patients. Researchers also need to know which rehabilitation strategies have been demonstrated to be effective at improving specific domains of functioning in order to determine appropriate priorities for research.

To facilitate clinicians and researchers in understanding the effectiveness of psychosocial rehabilitation for schizophrenia, Table 1 provides a brief summary of those strategies which have received the most empirical support. Effective strategies include family intervention, supported employment, social skills training, assertive community treatment, integrated treatment for comorbid substance abuse, and cognitive therapy for psychosis. Each of these rehabilitation strategies has received support from at least three controlled studies.

[1]NH-Dartmouth Psychiatric Research Center, Main Building, 105 Pleasant Street, Concord, NH 03301, USA.

TABLE 1 Empirically supported psychosocial rehabilitation strategies for schizophrenia

Rehabilitation model	Brief description	Areas of improvement	Who benefits?	Supporting references
Family psychoeducation	Long-term family work aimed at educating relatives about illness, reducing family stress, improved monitoring of illness, and helping all members achieve goals	Lower relapse rates and family burden	Patients in regular contact with their relatives	1
Supported employment	Employment specialists help patients find competitive jobs rapidly in their areas of interest, and provide ongoing job support as needed	Higher rates of competitive employment	Unemployed patients	2
Social skills training	Systematic teaching of interpersonal skills using principles of social learning (e.g. modelling, role playing, etc.)	Improved quality of social relationships	Patients with poor social functioning	3
Assertive community treatment	Case management with low staff: patient ratios (1:10), using shared caseloads among clinicians, with services provided to patients in their natural environments, and 24-hour coverage	Fewer hospitalizations, more stable housing, lower symptoms, better quality of life	Patients with a history of high service utilization	4
Integrated dual diagnosis treatment	Mental health and substance abuse treatment provided by the same clinicians, concurrently, with the clinicians taking responsibility for integrating treatment	Decreased substance abuse	Patients with substance abuse or dependence	5
Cognitive therapy for psychosis	Individual or group therapy aimed at helping patients evaluate the evidence supporting delusional thoughts and developing alternative explanations	Decreased severity of psychosis, fewer relapses	Patients with hallucinations and delusions	6, 7

Over the past two decades tremendous advances have been made in the psychosocial rehabilitation of schizophrenia. Despite these advances, significant social disability continues to be a problem, and many patients do not receive state-of-the-art rehabilitation. There is a need to improve our systems of care, and to increase patients' access to empirically supported rehabilitation methods. The advances made in recent years towards developing and evaluating effective rehabilitation models, combined with an increased focus on community-based approaches for working with patients with schizophrenia, bodes well for the future. Professionals, families and patients have good reasons for being optimistic concerning the progress towards the ultimate goal of helping patients with schizophrenia assume responsibility for themselves and reclaim their lives.

REFERENCES

1. Mueser K.T., Glynn S.M. (1998) Family intervention for schizophrenia. In *Best Practice: Developing and Promoting Empirically Supported Interventions* (Eds K.S. Dobson, K.D. Craig), pp. 157–186. Sage, Newbury Park, California.
2. Bond G.R., Drake R.E., Mueser K.T., Becker D.R. (1997) An update on supported employment for people with severe mental illness. *Psychiatr. Serv.*, **48**: 335–346.
3. Dilk M.N., Bond G.R. (1996) Meta-analytic evaluation of skills training research for persons with severe mental illness. *J. Consult. Clin. Psychol.*, **64**: 1337–1346.
4. Mueser K.T., Bond G.R., Drake R.E., Resick S.G. (1998) Models of community care for severe mental illness: a review of research on case management. *Schizophr. Bull.*, **24**: 37–74.
5. Drake R.E., Mercer-McFadden C., Mueser K.T., McHugo G.J., Bond G.R. (1998) A review of integrated mental health and substance abuse treatment for patients with dual disorders. *Schizophr. Bull.*, **24**: 589–608.
6. Drury V., Birchwood M., Cochrane R., MacMillan F. (1996) Cognitive therapy and recovery from acute psychosis: a controlled trial: I. Impact on psychotic symptoms. *Br. J. Psychiatry*, **169**: 593–601.
7. Kuipers E., Garety P., Fowler D., Dunn G., Bebbington P., Freeman D., Hadley C. (1997) London–East Anglia randomised controlled trial of cognitive–behavioural therapy for psychosis: I. Effects of the treatment phase. *Br. J. Psychiatry*, **171**: 319–327.

4.2
The Stigma of Mental Illness: Some Empirical Findings
Jo C. Phelan[1]

Cancro and Meyerson remind us that people with schizophrenia are people, not merely a collection of psychiatric symptoms, and that adequate treatment

[1]*Division of Sociomedical Sciences, Joseph L. Mailman School of Public Health, Columbia University, 600 W. 168th St, New York, NY 10032, USA*

of schizophrenia must focus not only on symptom management but also on helping the ill person, as far as possible, to live a happy, socially connected and fulfilling life. As the authors note, one important impediment to this goal is stigma. In this commentary I review empirical evidence that underscores the authors' concerns about the problem of stigma, and unfortunately, in some cases, amplifies those concerns.

As noted by the authors, people with schizophrenia are often viewed with fear and animosity. A recent indication of this is provided by the 1996 General Social Survey's Mental Health Module, a nationally representative survey of nearly 1500 Americans. Responding to a vignette describing an individual displaying symptoms of schizophrenia but no indications of violence, over 60% of respondents thought the person was likely to commit violence; nearly half thought the person should be legally forced to receive psychiatric treatment; and respondents were significantly less willing to interact with the person than with someone without psychiatric symptoms [1, 2].

On an optimistic note, Cancro and Meyerson mention several factors they believe are working to significantly reduce stigma. These include increasingly effective treatments, increased openness about mental illness generated by the family movement, and increased knowledge of biological aetiological factors. On each point, evidence suggests that optimism must be tempered.

Psychotropic medications have been enormously effective in helping persons with schizophrenia and other disorders behave more normally and function better. However, a recent study of men dually diagnosed with major mental disorder and substance abuse cautions that reductions in stigma cannot be expected to follow automatically from symptom reduction. After a year in treatment, the men's substance use and psychiatric symptoms had declined significantly from baseline levels. However, perceptions of devaluation and discrimination, experiences of stigma, and coping strategies of secrecy and withdrawal did not decline [3].

The family movement, exemplified by groups like the National Alliance for the Mentally Ill, has strongly championed the idea that mental illness is an illness like any other and not a cause for shame or secrecy. Nevertheless, a comparison of two studies published 20 years apart shows that family members of psychiatric patients were twice as likely to report concealing the illness in 1981 as in 1961 [4, 5] and a currently ongoing study of families of persons treated for psychosis indicates that half the family members concealed the hospitalization from others to at least some degree [6].

Knowledge about biological contributors to schizophrenia is growing rapidly. While it is often argued that biological understandings of mental disorder are destigmatizing, the limited available evidence paints a more complicated picture. When mental disorder is understood in biological terms, the ill person is perceived as less blameworthy and amoral, but the illness is perceived as more serious, less likely to change, and more psychotic. Biological attributions also result in greater disruption of social interactions and the delivery of more intense shocks in "learning" experiments [7, 8].

Finally, to the extent that the stigma-reducing forces referred to above are operative, we should observe reductions in stigma over time. Again, however, available evidence does not indicate such change. Examining results from comparable surveys conducted in 1950 and 1996, Phelan *et al* found that the proportion of respondents describing people with psychosis as being violent increased by nearly $2\frac{1}{2}$ times over this period [9].

While the tone of this commentary may seem pessimistic, I do not mean to suggest that the problem of stigma is totally intractable. Rather, my purpose has been to underscore the seriousness and stubbornness of the problem, to point out that assumptions about what will reduce stigma or what has reduced stigma must be empirically tested, to suggest that stigma-reducing efforts must be intelligently and strategically planned, and to strongly underscore Cancro and Meyerson's point that stigma must be addressed if people with schizophrenia are to live successfully and happily in the community at large.

REFERENCES

1. Link B.G., Phelan J.C., Bresnahan M., Stueve A., Pescosolido B. (1999) Public conceptions of mental illness: Labels, causes, dangerousness, and social distance. *Am. J. Public Hlth*, **89**: 1328–1333.
2. Pescosolido B., Monahan J., Link B.G., Stueve A., Kikuzawa S. (1999) The public's view of the competence, dangerousness, and need for legal coercion of persons with mental health problems. *Am. J. Public Hlth*, **89**: 1339–1345.
3. Link B.G., Rahav M., Phelan J.C., Nuttbrock L. (1997) On stigma and its consequences: evidence from a longitudinal study of men with dual diagnoses of mental illness and substance abuse. *J. Hlth Soc. Behav.*, **38**: 177–190.
4. Freeman H.E., Simmons O.G. (1961) Feelings of stigma among relatives of former mental patients. *Social Problems*, **8**: 312–321.
5. Thompson E.H., Doll W. (1982) The burden of families coping with the mentally ill: a hidden crisis. *Family Relations*, **31**: 379–388.
6. Phelan J.C., Bromet E.B., Link B.G. (1998) Psychiatric illness and family stigma. *Schizophr. Bull.*, **24**: 115–126.
7. Mehta S.I., Farina A. (1997) Is being "sick" really better? Effect of the disease view of mental disorder on stigma. *J. Soc. Clin. Psychol.*, **16**: 405–419.
8. Furnham A., Rees J. (1988) Lay theories of schizophrenia. *Int. J. Soc. Psychiatry*, **34**: 212–220.
9. Phelan J.C., Link B.G., Stueve A., Pescosolido B. (1997) Public conceptions of mental illness in 1950 and today: Findings from the 1996 General Social Survey Module on Mental Health. Presented at the Annual Meeting of the American Sociological Association, Toronto, August.

4.3
Reducing the Stigma Associated with Schizophrenia
Richard Warner[1]

Media hyperbole and biased reporting tend to perpetuate negative attitudes toward schizophrenia. Entertainment and news media in Britain, America and elsewhere often portray the mentally ill as dangerous and evil, at best figures of fun.

Modern communication technology, however, also offers the possibility of reducing stigma. Since the unsuccessful anti-stigma campaigns of the postwar period, public education methods and techniques for health promotion have improved dramatically. "Social marketing" campaigns have been used successfully to advance a variety of causes including AIDS prevention, family planning, smoking cessation and reducing infant mortality. Effectiveness is increased by "audience segmentation" — partitioning a mass audience into sub-audiences that are relatively homogeneous and devising promotional strategies and messages that are more relevant and acceptable to those target groups [1].

In developing such campaigns, it is important to conduct a needs assessment, using focus groups, telephone surveys or opinion leaders, to gather information about cultural beliefs, misapprehensions, and frequently used media. Objectives, audiences, messages and media are selected, materials are pre-tested and revised. An action plan is implemented and, with continuous monitoring of impact, constantly refined [1].

Entertainment media, such as popular songs and soap operas, are especially useful for socially taboo topics such as mental illness. Soap operas have been successful in advancing social messages in several countries. A TV soap opera in China called "Ordinary People", which promotes smaller family size and AIDS education, began broadcasting in 1995 and will, in due course, reach 16% of the world's population. A radio soap opera encouraging AIDS awareness and family planning gained a wide audience in Tanzania and was effective in changing attitudes and sexual behaviour. Similarly, a TV programme centred on a character named Maria and aired in Mexico for 40 years has promoted, among other things, adult education [1].

Advocacy groups can lobby the entertainment media to include positive characters in existing programming. In the USA, a group calling itself the "Soap Summit" analyses the content of soap operas (looking at such topics as teenage sexual behaviour), lobbies script-writers to change the content of their programmes to create positive social messages, and measures the impact of their lobbying on soap-opera content. In Britain, a character with schizophrenia was recently introduced into the country's

---

[1]Mental Health Center, Boulder County, 1333 Iris Avenue, Boulder, Colorado 80304-2296, USA

most widely watched programme, *EastEnders*. The National Schizophrenia Fellowship reports that this storyline has attracted unprecedented attention and done more to reduce stigma than any number of worthy media appeals. The programme has humanized the illness and exploded the myths that schizophrenia means someone has a split personality and/or that it is likely to make someone violent.

The movie *Shine* is an example of the successful use of an entertainment medium to heighten awareness and communicate information about mental illness. It conveyed several stigma-breaking messages: (a) people recover from schizophrenia; (b) they can work even if they have symptoms; (c) work helps them recover; (d) people's responses towards someone with schizophrenia can influence the course of the illness; (e) people with schizophrenia can be included in the community (*Shine* can be criticized, however, for failing to communicate the message); (f) poor parenting does not cause schizophrenia.

Building on the advances in communication technology, the World Psychiatric Association has initiated a worldwide campaign to combat the stigma of schizophrenia. The 3-year programme will field-test materials in different settings and prepare them in multiple translations. The first pilot of the campaign was launched in Calgary, Alberta, in 1997. The local action committee, made up of consumers, mental health professionals, health policy makers, researchers and representatives of the press and the clergy, selected the following target groups: (a) health care professionals, including emergency-room personnel, medical students and health care policy makers; (b) teenagers in grades 9 and 11; (c) community change agents such as businesspeople, the clergy and journalists; (d) the general public.

For each target group, messages and media were selected. In the case of teenagers the messages were: (a) no one is to blame for schizophrenia; (b) people recover from schizophrenia; (c) people with schizophrenia are *people* with schizophrenia.

The media being used are: (a) speakers' bureaux of consumers, family members and professionals, organized by the local chapter of the Schizophrenia Fellowship, to address high school classes; (b) an attractively designed teaching guide on schizophrenia for high school health teachers; (c) an internet web page (www.openthedoors.com) with information on schizophrenia (developed by a World Psychiatric Association expert panel) with access doors for different users: teenagers, health professionals, consumers and family members; (d) a competition for high school students to produce anti-stigma materials; (e) posters in the high schools; (f) radio and bus advertising.

From this example, it is clear that a stigma-reducing campaign need not be expensive. Many interventions are low cost; more expensive media, such as radio and bus advertising, can be used if funding is available. The 2-year budget for the Calgary project, including a limited media campaign directed at the general public, is under $150 000. It is not expensive to introduce education about schizophrenia into the high school curriculum and thus reduce the massive ignorance about this condition throughout an entire generation.

Those who are interested in launching a similar campaign locally should contact Prof. Norman Sartorius, World Psychiatric Association Programme to Reduce Stigma Because of Schizophrenia, Hôpitaux Universitaires de Genève, Département de Psychiatrie, 16–18, Boulevard de St Georges, 1205 Geneva, Switzerland.

REFERENCE

1. Rogers E.M. (1995) *Diffusion of Innovations*, 4th edn. Free Press, New York.

4.4
The Influence of Stigma on Preventive Efforts in Psychotic Disorders
Patrick McGorry[1]

Stigma has been with us since the beginning of civilization. Erving Goffman characterized it as "spoiled identity", an evocative term which captures its impact on the individual, yet fails to convey its social origins. The latter derive from ignorance and fear, as well as the disempowerment which accompanies any devalued status. Non-medical forms of stigma deriving from power imbalances and shame have been seen in slavery, women, racial groupings characterized as "inferior", and in Vietnam veterans. In fact, inferior or shamed status is both a cause and effect of stigma. Medical examples have more to do with ignorance and fear, with inferior status and marginalization representing consequences. Cancro and Meyerson refer to the case of leprosy, which has been well studied by sociologists; however, another recent dramatic example has been the HIV-AIDS epidemic. The relatively successful destigmatizing responses which have occurred here may contain some lessons for us. Furthermore, they show that even though "a good prognosis is an excellent counterweight to stigma, as is a rapid response to treatment", this is only part of the story.

Stigma can be viewed as a powerful risk factor influencing the course of psychiatric disorders. In this commentary, I will examine the multiple ways that stigma undermines preventive endeavours in the identification and treatment of potentially serious mental illness, specifically psychosis. Early case identification, initial management and the recovery process will

[1]*Department of Psychiatry, University of Melbourne, Locked Bag 10 Parkville, Victoria 3052, Australia*

be considered as discrete stages in which stigma operates in somewhat different ways to delay treatment and compromise recovery.

Firstly, there are a number of preventive "stepping stones" involved in early case identification and the initiation of effective treatment. This is the current frontier for preventive efforts, since primary prevention is not yet feasible, and reducing delays in treatment offers substantial hope as a preventive strategy [1]. The first stepping stone is when there is a change in the person, usually initially subtle and subjective, who is at risk for the development of the fully fledged disorder. Stigma commonly operates here by stimulating fear and denial of the change if mental illness is perceived as a possibility, because the person holds the uniformly negative stereotype of "mental" patients and also of psychiatric treatments and professionals [2]. The next step of seeking help is also inhibited in most people because of the above fears and the desire to avoid stigma, particularly since there is a lack of confidence in mental health professionals and their treatments. General practitioners and counsellors, however, are much more likely to be consulted [2]. The third stepping stone is recognition by the doctor or counsellor, and the capacity and propensity to do so is likely to be influenced not only by skill and knowledge levels, but also by the attitudes and prejudices of the clinician. Despite training, these are often disturbingly similar to those in the general community, and strongly reflect stigma.

The fourth hurdle, potentially a large one, is referral to a mental health service or psychiatrist. Here stigma again operates in the mind of the doctor through his or her attitudes to psychiatrists and mental health services. These are variable and depend on several factors, especially prior experience and the quality of particular professional relationships. Nevertheless, those who work with stigmatized groups of people inevitably become stigmatized themselves, and this effect can inhibit the referral process, especially the referral threshold. It may also undermine the referee's confidence in the specialist treatment system, reinforcing any reluctance to accept such referral.

Once the patient reaches the specialist mental health system, he or she is affected by stigma in several ways. Firstly, the quality of facilities and the professional skills of the staff are affected by the long-standing neglect of this area of health care by society. This is reinforced if the services are separated geographically from other health care facilities. These factors derive in part from stigma and powerfully reinforce it. Secondly, the attitudes of the clinicians to the patients as well as to themselves will have been influenced by stigma. Even mental health professionals may carry at least residual or diluted prejudices regarding the patients which will influence their approach. It remains difficult for many to see people with psychosis as more like themselves than otherwise, as Sullivan urged many years ago. Sadly too, some will have accepted their own devalued status within the health care system, preventing them from applying their skills with full confidence.

During recovery from the first episode, stigma is a key influence to be tackled and neutralized in any prevention-orientated service. Here it operates through enhancing the corrosive pessimism which emanates from the Kraepelinian belief system, and which still influences the therapeutic attitudes of many psychiatrists. Stigma also undermines recovery in two other ways. Firstly, through its effects on the pre-illness attitudes of the recovering person, it makes it extremely difficult to accept the role of the mental patient and consequently treatment. This internalized operation of stigma stimulates an understandable defence against "spoiled identity". Meanwhile the person tries to retain faith in cherished "possible selves", which have been put at risk. This is intensified if early psychosis patients are treated side by side with the older and most disabled subgroup, because a stark and unacceptable future then confronts the young person struggling with these issues. Secondly, the stigma-laden external recovery environment is poisoned for the recovering psychotic person in the same way as it was for the returning Vietnam veteran. This effect lasts for the duration of the illness and further corrodes the quality of life of the person and the family.

If more effective preventive strategies are to succeed, stigma will need to be effectively countered, and we will need to learn from those who have achieved this in other areas. Some of the potential benefits can be clearly seen from the above analysis.

REFERENCES

1. McGorry P.D., Singh B.S. (1995) Schizophrenia: risk and possibility. In *Handbook of Studies on Preventive Psychiatry* (Eds B. Raphael, G.D. Burrows), pp. 491–514. Elsevier, Amsterdam.
2. Jorm A.F., Korten A.E., Jacomb P.A., Christensen H., Rodgers B., Pollit P. (1997) "Mental health literacy": a survey of the public's ability to recognise mental disorders and their beliefs about the effectiveness of treatment. *Med. J. Aust.*, **166**: 182–186.

4.5
Disability, Stigma and Discrimination: A View from Outside the USA

Heinz Häfner[1]

This commentary aims to complement Cancro and Meyerson's excellent review, by focusing on five issues concerning stigma and disability related to schizophrenia.

[1] *Schizophrenia Research Unit, Central Institute of Mental Health, PO Box 12 21 20, D-68072 Mannheim, Germany*

Stigma involves loss of prestige, social contacts and self-esteem and has an unfavourable effect on the social course of schizophrenia. Those stigmatized lose resources and power in society. Stigma results in discrimination at various levels: (a) individual (loss of partner, social isolation, etc.); (b) work (obstacles to finding work or returning to work, etc.); (c) family (loss of prestige, tense family atmosphere, etc.); (d) housing (landlords refuse rental, disabled schizophrenics cluster in city areas with high rates of unemployment, crime and homelessness); (e) legal (disadvantages in social security, health care and civil rights and liberties).

The WPA has launched a worldwide educational programme to reduce stigma and discrimination because of schizophrenia [1]. The aim is to promote knowledge of the disorder and its treatment, understanding for the patients and their families, and motivation to help and act. This is planned to be accomplished through educational programmes designed for schools, health care personnel and the public, an objective reporting in the media, and the support of political leaders and legislators. Patients' accounts of suffered discrimination and disadvantage have proved particularly effective. Cooperation with family and user organizations aims at empowering the mentally ill in the public domain and with politicians for a sustained fight against stigma and discrimination.

The few studies on the cultural variance of stigma and discrimination and their impact on the social course of schizophrenia show a high variation. Some cultures are more tolerant than others of bizarre thoughts and behaviour. This may either make the life of the chronically ill easier or cause them to be ignored. The finding of a better illness course in developing countries in the World Health Organization (WHO) studies contrasts with reports of total neglect and exclusion of schizophrenics. Therefore, the need for fighting stigma and discrimination is great in many developing countries.

Schizophrenia is responsible for a considerable amount of disability in the world and causes high costs [2]; it constitutes a major public health problem in developed countries, too. Contributing to the reduction of disability is the rehabilitation of long-stay psychiatric patients, as discussed in detail by Cancro and Meyerson. A series of model programmes, for example Fountain House, offer rehabilitation at various levels: relapse prevention, cognitive and social skills training, reintegration into work or alternative work settings, sheltered accommodation, family education, etc. From the public health aspect, however, the question is to what extent these needs are met. Before all needs for prevention and rehabilitation can be met in a community, there must be an easily accessible comprehensive community mental health service available for the population. Such services are well developed in the Scandinavian countries, Great Britain and Canada, but underdeveloped in the USA.

Services planning and evaluation requires epidemiological studies into the met and unmet need. The Team for the Assessment of Psychiatric Services (TAPS) study [3] showed that the majority of long-stay patients, 5 years after discharge from two public mental hospitals in London, were living in non-restrictive community settings and were able to lead a freer and socially more rewarding life. More than 80% rated their current arrangement as more satisfactory than a hospital stay. One year after discharge, negative symptoms and social disability were already significantly reduced and remained so.

Despite the impressive reduction in disability and improvement in quality of life, however, deinstitutionalization also causes problems. With a growing number of patients discharged the costs of community care increase [4], finally exceeding the costs of long-term inpatient treatment. At the same time, the number of severely disturbed patients in the community increases, which involves problems, such as sexual offences, violence and crime.

According to a nationwide analysis based on the Danish case register [5], the rate of psychiatric bed occupancy decreased from 2.36/1000 to 0.97/1000 (59%) between 1977 and 1997. The readmission rate for schizophrenics in the first year after discharge increased from 30% to 45%, clearly above the results of good therapy studies (about 20%). Involuntary admissions increased by 52%, involuntary treatment by about 300%. From 1988 to 1997, the proportion of schizophrenics under legal supervision because of crimes (80% involved bodily harm or death) increased. The standard mortality rate of schizophrenics because of suicide increased by 2.1%, while suicides in the population decreased. There obviously are vulnerable schizophrenics not sufficiently protected against suicide, violence and social deprivation by the current system of care. This raises the question whether it would be necessary to preserve part of the mental hospitals for the supervised care of these patients. The alternative would be more intensive supervision in the community. England is currently planning to render multiprofessional community mental health teams better equipped for this task and to intensify the supervision of high-risk patients. A supervision register is aimed at keeping the number of drop-outs low. Prevention of disability and asociality focuses on the main risk factors: drop-out from treatment, unfavourable social situation, comorbidity with substance and alcohol abuse. The comparison of the effectiveness and costs of these alternative strategies is topical in European health care research.

Treatment of schizophrenia is currently preceded by 1 year of psychotic symptoms and 5 years of prodromal phase on average. Schizophrenia starts primarily with negative symptoms and functional impairment [6]. Social disability appears on average 2 to 4 years before the climax of the first episode. The social consequences emerge in this early illness phase and on average persist in further illness without change, while individual illness courses vary greatly. Medium-term social course is significantly predicted by the level of social development at the climax of the first episode, whereas type of illness onset, symptoms, age and sex exert an indirect effect via social status at the end of the early illness phase [6]. Rehabilitation currently begins only after the disorder has produced most of its consequences. Early recognition of this risk and early intervention before disability emerges are therefore urgently needed. To this end programmes have been undertaken in Melbourne, Birmingham, Amsterdam, Cologne and Stavanger and successfully evaluated in Melbourne [7]. Besides the rehabilitation strategies discussed by Cancro and Meyerson, early cognitive and educational interventions are important to promote insight into the symptoms, coping with the illness and stress, and to prevent job loss or drop-out from education or vocational training. When the first attenuated positive symptoms emerge, preventive action can be supplemented by antipsychotic therapy.

REFERENCES

1. Sartorius N. (1998) Stigma: what can psychiatrists do about it? *Lancet*, **352**: 1958–1959.
2. Murray C.J.L., Lopez A.D. (1996) *The Global Burden of Disease*. Published on behalf of the World Health Organization and the World Bank by Harvard School of Public Health.
3. Leff J., Trieman N., Gooch C. (1996) Team for the Assessment of Psychiatric Services (TAPS) project. 33: prospective follow-up study of long-stay patients discharged from two psychiatric hospitals. *Am. J. Psychiatry*, **153**: 1318–1324.
4. Häfner H., an der Heiden W. (1996) Background and goals of evaluative research in community psychiatry. In *Mental Health Services Evaluation* (Eds H.C. Knudsen, S. Thornicroft), pp. 19–36. Cambridge University Press, Cambridge.
5. Munk-Jørgensen P. (1999) Has deinstitutionalization gone too far? *Eur. Arch. Psychiatry Clin. Neurosci.*, **249**: 136–143.
6. Häfner H., Löffler W., Maurer K., Hambrecht M., an der Heiden W. (1999) Depression, negative symptoms, social stagnation and social decline in the early course of schizophrenia. *Acta Psychiat. Scand.*, **100**: 105–118.
7. Yung A.R., Phillips L.J., McGorry P.D., McFarlane C.A., Francey S., Harrigan S. Patton G.C., Jackson H.J. (1998) Prediction of psychosis. A step towards indicated prevention of schizophrenia. *Br. J. Psychiatry*, **172** (Suppl. 33): 14–20.

4.6
The Toxic Effects of Stigma
Harold M. Visotsky[1]

Throughout the practice of medicine, the prevention and limitation of disability has been a primary element in the rehabilitative process following

---

[1]*Northwestern Medical School, 303 E. Superior Street, Chicago IL 60611, USA*

the acute phase of an illness. Medical history is replete with the limitation of recovery or rehabilitation due to ignorance, fear, prejudice or regional or cultural myths. These reactions to illnesses have limited the functional recoveries and the quality of life outcomes for certain categories of illness. Stigma has acted as a powerful toxic agent, thwarting the healing of the human spirit and the wounds of disorders. Such illnesses as leprosy (now Hansen's disease), cancer, the venereal diseases, and more recently human immunodeficiency virus (HIV) have been prime targets of stigma.

In our history, no disorder has been a greater target for stigma than the mental disorders. Over the centuries, fear and ignorance reduced the mental patients to outcasts, objects of derision, rejection and abandonment. The search for cures frequently resulted in particularly punitive and cruel attempts to drive the illness from the brains and bodies of such poor unfortunates. Stigma, in essence, limits the therapeutic efforts of science and its practitioners and contributes significantly to the chronicity of the disorder. Over the years false theories of genetics led to the term eugenics coined by Francis Galton, a British mathematician. He believed that only the most ethnically fit must be encouraged to survive. Many of the geneticists of the 1920s and 1930s as well as many academics felt that retarded persons and the mentally ill should be actively prevented from reproducing [1]. This was incorporated in public policy in the United States and abroad. These unfounded theories affected immigration laws and even led to widespread sterilization practices in mental hospitals. As recently as 1995 and 1996, China proposed eugenics law which was withdrawn after international publicity and outrage (the World Psychiatric Association cancelled a scheduled World Congress to be held in Beijing in protest).

There are many disorders which are impacted by the current state of our scientific knowledge and the limitations of treatment discoveries and advances. In psychiatry, psychotic illnesses such as schizophrenia frequently represent the limitation of our field to produce a full recovery and a return to a previous functional state. Chronicity is a feature which takes over after the acute phases of the illness and subsequent relapses. It is an element of the illness which requires a comprehensive array of treatment interventions over the extended lifetime of the illness. The array is not limited to the medical psychiatric interventions of therapy and psychoactive agents, but it must include the social rehabilitative efforts of community-sited education, social services for housing and supportive life services, interventions with families (when present and available), community agencies, courts and police. Every facet of our society must be utilized to improve the status and function of the individual afflicted by this disorder. Such rehabilitative efforts represent the true and valiant goals for the limitation and/or prevention of disability.

More and more psychiatry, in concert with behavioural specialities and professions, is creating treatment protocols and systematic approaches to the prevention of disabilities arising out of emotional and mental disorder. These professionals and community agents have made alliances with advocacy groups, made up of families of patients and former patients, to advance knowledge about mental disorders, and advocate for community-based services. Increased media time and exposure has improved the critical need for education.

The significant development of family and patient advocates has produced a powerful antidote to the problems arising from stigma. By speaking out in public forums, by approaching public decision-makers and by sharing their experiences with their communities, they have reduced the stigma by appreciable measures. In a very private society such as Japan, the development of a family-based advocate organization (the Zinkaren) has produced a significant reduction in the stigma which produced hidden populations of mentally and aged persons.

REFERENCE

1. Barker D. (1989) The biology of stupidity: genetics, eugenics and mental deficiency in the inter-war years. *Br. J. Hist. Sci.*, **22**: 347–375.

4.7

The Conceptualization of Long-term, Disabling Psychiatric Disorders

Pedro Ruiz[1]

The review by Cancro and Meyerson has stimulated me to reflect on the central theme of long-term, disabling psychiatric disorders. At the core of this theme, we find schizophrenia and the concept of stigma. Unfortunately, schizophrenia is perceived not only by the public at large but also by most members of the psychiatric profession as a chronic psychiatric disorder. As such, the treatment approaches most often offered to patients who suffer from schizophrenia tend to be primarily directed to the symptoms and the sequelae of this disorder, and much less so to the acute phases of the illness in an integrated and thorough manner. Relapses, within the context of this illness, tend to be perceived by most mental health professionals as a manifestation of the chronicity of the disorder rather than as an expression of an acute phase of a long-term, disabling mental illness. As a result of this perception, patients suffering from schizophrenia tend to be denied the

[1]*Department of Psychiatry and Behavioral Sciences, University of Texas Medical School at Houston, 1300 Moursund Street, Houston, TX 77030, USA*

opportunity to receive intensive care during the acute phases of the illness and, instead, are offered less comprehensive and insufficient services.

In many ways, this approach to care is quite discriminating when compared with other disorders that are more ingrained in the medical model. For instance, arthritic and diabetic conditions, although long-term, disabling diseases, tend to be treated intensively every time that is required. Needless to say, the priority and attention accorded to the investigation of chronic and disabling medical conditions, such as multiple sclerosis, muscular distrophies, Parkinson disease, etc., are rarely accorded to long-term, disabling psychiatric illnesses. It is stigma that makes schizophrenia, but not diabetes or arthritis, medically and publicly unacceptable. Stigma represents a "mark of shame", a "discredit", a "stain". We must understand, however, that stigma is not an integral part of the suffering schizophrenic patient but an integral part of ourselves. We/society are the ones who are afraid, who feel guilty, who feel ashamed, who worry about rejection. We/society are the ones who do not understand the feelings, the ways of thinking and the behaviour of schizophrenic patients and, thus, reject them because they are different to us/society. The mere possibility of us/society thinking that we can also be vulnerable and become like them, makes us afraid and frightened of them.

This situation is not unique to mental illnesses. People tend to be afraid of other people who are different from them, because of the colour of their skin, their language, their religion, or their culture. Discrimination, religious persecution and even racism are all rooted in the same phenomenon. At times, certain values and customs become the norm of a group. When this group becomes the majority, it evolves into the norms of a given society; that is, it becomes the culture of the majority group.

Since the origin of medicine and society, stigma has always prevailed. In the past, it happened with the plague, leprosy, mental retardation, epilepsy, and with many other illnesses that stimulated fear and guilt in us/society. Today, it is still happening with severe mental disorders, of which schizophrenia is the best example. It will certainly happen again in the future with other medical conditions that will not depict our/society's concept of beauty and/or "normality".

We, as clinicians, educators, researchers, scientists, physicians, psychiatrists and human beings, must reconceptualize the understanding of long-term, disabling conditions, particularly mental illnesses. Psychiatrists and other mental health professionals must be at the vanguard of this reconceptualization. We must advocate on behalf of the mentally ill; particularly, the mentally ill who suffers from long-term, disabling disorders like schizophrenia [1]. We must advocate for the application of the biopsychosocial model in the treatment of these patients, and also for the integration of the mind and body in the reconceptualization of mental illnesses [2, 3].

It is obviously clear that isolated state hospitals are not the answer to the treatment needs of the severely mentally ill patients. However, it is even more evident that the streets of the urban metropolis and/or the prison system are not the answer either. We/society must advocate for the humane treatment of the severely mentally ill patient in general hospitals and ambulatory medical clinics, since these patients are as medically ill as any other patients treated in these types of facilities. We/society must advocate for the allocation of adequate resources for research and treatment of mental conditions as they are also medical illnesses. The long-term, disabling mentally ill patient deserves to be offered a biopsychosocial approach as part of his/her treatment, with emphasis on rehabilitation and all aspects of prevention, as outlined in Cancro and Meyerson's review on prevention of disability and stigma.

REFERENCES

1. Grunebaum H., Friedman H. (1988) Building collaborative relationships with families of the mentally ill. *Hosp. Comm. Psychiatry*, **39**: 1183–1187.
2. Engel G.L. (1980) The clinical application of the biopsychosocial model. *Am. J. Psychiatry*, **137**: 535–544.
3. Goodman A. (1991) Organic unit theory: the mind–body problem revisited. *Am. J. Psychiatry*, **148**: 553–563.

4.8

Utility of Multiaxial Assessment in the Rehabilitative Work with Chronically Disturbed Patients

Marianne C. Kastrup[1]

Issues concerning both stigma and rehabilitation are pertinent to most mental disorders, as pointed out by Cancro and Meyerson, and all manifestations of mental illness have the capacity to have an impact on the patient's adaptation. Furthermore, we know that the prevention of disability in a chronic and persistent mental disorder involves the totality of management. This implies that a variety of techniques have to be utilized in the individual patient related to the manifestations of psychopathological phenomena as well as vulnerability and resilience factors. In that context, it is important to recognize that the rehabilitative intervention has to take place within the triangle consisting of the patient, the immediate environment/family and the society at large including its institutions and services.

[1] *Rehabilitation and Research Center for Torture Victims, Borgergade 13, 1300 Copenhagen K, Denmark*

Cancro and Meyerson conclude that functional restoration is the goal of all medical treatment and point to the fact that in order to consider an outcome as successful we have to take into consideration the social skills, the area of self-esteem, and the fulfilment of role functioning. Traditionally, psychiatrists, as other medical doctors, have had a tendency to focus on a reduction in pathological symptomatology as the core concern of any intervention. When dealing with disorders of a more chronic nature other goals may, however, become more pertinent and with a shift towards rehabilitative activities, the focus may shift. But, as Cancro and Meyerson point out, there is a false distinction between treatment and rehabilitation, failing to recognize that treatment which is not curative is ameliorative and rehabilitative.

In the rehabilitative process it is important continuously to monitor and assess the patient's condition. And the authors emphasize that a comprehensive evaluation as well as regular assessments of a patient's functional level are needed in order to determine the impact and effectiveness of a given intervention.

Hitherto, such medical assessments have usually been unidimensional, with the focus on symptom profiles and phenomenology, and with an eye to the fulfilment of diagnostic criteria. With the introduction of multiaxial classifications, a more comprehensive, multidimensional approach to assessment has materialized.

Multiaxial classification facilitates an understanding of the complexity of psychiatric conditions, recognizing that it is difficult to capture complexity of psychiatric conditions with a single diagnostic category. A multiaxial approach provides a more comprehensive picture, a better basis for planning treatment and enabling an improvement of outcome prediction [1, 2]. Furthermore, a systematic evaluation with attention paid to the total situation, including level of functioning, may ensure that the latter is not overlooked, which could be the case if focus were restricted to assessing a single presenting problem [3].

Presently, both the DSM-IV [3] and the ICD-10 [4] have developed multiaxial classifications, and both classifications comprise an axis on adaptive functioning of use in determining the level of functioning either globally or subdivided into independent areas. In the DSM-IV, the assessment is done using the GAF (Global Assessment of Functioning) Scale, with respect to psychological, social and occupational level of functioning, rated on a scale from 1 to 100. In the World Health Organization (WHO) classification, rating takes place on four independent axes: namely, personal care and survival; functioning with family; occupational functioning, that is, performance in expected role as remunerated worker or homemaker; and broader social behaviour, that is, functioning in other social roles and activities and interaction with other individuals and the community at large.

In the International Guidelines for Diagnostic Assessment that are presently being finalized by the Section on Classification, Diagnostic Assessment and Nomenclature of the World Psychiatric Association (WPA), the level of adaptive functioning or participation in society is suggested to be a domain of assessment with clinical relevance. The proposed axis comprises a rating of all impairment in adaptive functioning or participation in society, which may be a result of mental disorders, physical disorders or both [1].

Exercising such an approach and rating the level of social and adaptive functioning at different points in time may be a useful tool in the rehabilitative work with the chronically disturbed patients. Broadening the focus to cover all the major aspects of the total clinical condition is a further reflection of the complexity in evaluating health conditions.

In their very comprehensive review, Cancro and Meyerson emphasize that "if some symptoms are controlled, but the patient remains disabled, it is inappropriate to call that a successful outcome". Using a multidimensional approach would refrain from drawing such conclusions, and research on the feasibility and utility of multiaxial assessment in the rehabilitative work worldwide should be enhanced.

REFERENCES

1. Kastrup M., Skodol A., Mezzich J.E., Berganza C. (1999) Multiaxial formula-tion. In: *International Guidelines for Diagnostic Assessment* (Eds J.E. Mezzich, C. Berganza, M. Jorge, M. Kastrup, S. Murthy, A. Okasha, A. Skodol, M. von Cranach, M. Zaudig, N. Sartorius), in preparation.
2. Mezzich J.E. (1999) Architecture of clinical information and prediction of service utilisation and costs. *Schizophr. Bull.*, **17**: 469–474.
3. American Psychiatric Association (1994) *Diagnostic and Statistical Manual of Mental Disorders*, 4th edn. American Psychiatric Association, Washington, DC.
4. World Health Organization (1997) *The Multiaxial Presentation of ICD-10 for Use in Adult Psychiatry*. Cambridge University Press, London.

4.9
"Clanning" for Recovery
Ulf Malm[1]

The individual patient who successfully manages handicaps in life and living is the best envoy to combat and prevent the disability caused by stigma in the community. But, in the present situation and because of the illness-related

[1]*Department of Clinical Neuroscience, Section of Psychiatry, Sahlgrenska University Hospital, Kron-husgatan 2F, S-411 13 Gothenburg, Sweden*

impairments of the patient, there have to be joint ventures. Since many, if not most schizophrenic patients lack the capacity to negotiate the wide range of clinical programmes and life supports that they require, professional case management is almost always required.

On the road to recovery and integration into the community the patient cannot be alone, but needs the help of people — professionals as well as significant others. From the review by Cancro and Meyerson I have elected three topics of clear relevance to these needs: the absence of a supportive environmental social structure; the lack of communication skills in the patient; and communities that are ill-prepared to cope with people who still retain some positive and negative symptoms.

As emphasized by Cancro and Meyerson, five "basic paradigms" have emerged over the past 30–40 years. Professional case managers are the glue that holds the long-term management together in each of the five models.

For meeting the needs of the patient, specific programmes should offer the context of supportive, non-stigmatizing environments in the community, in a manner that emphasizes "personhood", rather than "patienthood", gradually maximizes the individual's feeling of responsibility and self-worth, and encourages ownership in the rehabilitation process. In the light of clinical experience and outcome data from a 5-year research project on the implementation of an assertive community outreach strategy, ".Integrated Care" [1], I will discuss some topics important for coping with stigma and social integration.

The resource group should be looked upon as a local social network "clan" for the individual patient. The patient can then "play in his or her own recovery team" coached by the psychiatrist and the clinical case manager. In a supportive and informed micro-cosmos, the patient can be prepared for integration into the community together with the people he or she knows and trusts.

The patient and the clinical case manager screen all kinds of potential resource persons from the patient's social network. The case manager meets individually with the nominated significant other people, such as family members, social-services staff, friends, to introduce and teach about the strategy. Together the case manager and the patient then initiate a first resource-group meeting. A proposal for a personal growth plan is the main agenda for a series of decisions on how to achieve the patient's main personal goal. Three prioritized short-term goals for the next 3–6 months of the rehabilitation process are set, as are how to evaluate the patient's adjustment and his or her intermediate as well as final outcome, ending up with a distribution of tasks to the members in the resource group — akin to setting up a theatre play. The written growth plan for the patient contains general techniques for problem solving and training in effective personal communication. Furthermore, there is information on specific methods for optimal medication for treating impairments, handling handicaps, providing around-the-clock support, promoting the fulfilment of social roles, cognitive psychotherapy against persisting psychotic symptoms, etc., as well as who is in charge of what. The outreach interventions may take place at home, in wards or wherever may be the best location.

The personal growth plan draft with its decisions is finalized by patient and case manager together and then distributed to all interested parties by the patient, in the first instance the resource-group members. The resource group, including the case manager, meet regularly for follow-up, monitored by continuous outcome assessments. Usually these meetings should take place every third month the first year, then every 6–12 months for long-term management. The non-professional participants of the resource group are encouraged to have regular meetings of their own according to the same concept, and should learn to use the case manager and psychiatrist more and more as consultants. The resource group acts as a kind of "one-stop-station" for acute and long-term management, continuous and integrated combination of medication and psychosocial treatment methods. Social and family support are also met by the resource groups, as are the patient's need of shelter and cover in crisis situations. In the case of unexpected events, extraordinary meetings may be called.

Group therapies can provide supportive and socializing experiences, and prepare for the performing of normal social roles in the community. In the 2-year randomized controlled trial (RCT) outcome study by Malm [2], communication-orientated group therapy was shown to be useful in promoting entries and re-entries into the community.

To have a job and employment is important for most people, as it is for persons with schizophrenia. Work gives opportunities to socialize, communicate and return to normal social roles, which also can help to reduce stigma. Two "clanning" strategies — consumer-run cooperatives and transitional employment — offer especially promising possibilities. Successful examples can be found in Vadstena, Sweden (carpeting), Athens (handicraft), Birmingham and San Francisco (restaurants).

Evidence-based managed psychiatry confirms clinical experience and common sense concerning the usefulness of combining the continuous personal efforts of informal carers and professionals, as well as of medication and psychosocial treatments. Now we have to combat healthy people's prejudiced attitudes to provide an environment in the community that is designed to help people who may be odd, but not mad.

REFERENCES

1. Falloon I.R.A. and the OTP Collaborators (1999) Optimal treatment for psychosis in an international multisite demonstration project. *Psychiat. Serv.*, **50**: 615–618.

2. Malm U. (1990) Group therapy. In *Handbook of Schizophrenia*, vol. 4 (Eds M.I. Hertz, S.J. Keith, J.P. Docharty), pp. 191–211. Elsevier, Amsterdam.

4.10
Stigma and Schizophrenia: The Greek Experience
Marina Economou[1]

It has long been realized that mental illness and especially schizophrenia is associated with a significant amount of stigma all over the world, but this stigma has many variations across cultures.

In Greece there are many folk beliefs, stereotyped ideas and scornful expressions about schizophrenia generated by strong religious and cultural values. These notions are mostly empirically noticeable in some aspects of interpersonal relationships in everyday life, the mass media and the civil laws [1, 2].

Despite the Greek origin of the words "stigma" and "schizophrenia", stigma attached to this severe mental illness has not been adequately studied in Greek society. Up to 1980, there were very few studies on people's perception of mental illness, mainly among relatives of the mentally ill [3, 4]. In the general population, two studies [5, 6] were conducted in 1964 and 1977, which showed some changes in public attitudes and beliefs about the various causes of mental illness. The majority of the respondents in the 1964 study believed that the main cause of mental illness was "poverty" and "bad socioeconomic conditions", whereas the 1977 study revealed that "everyday life stress" was the main cause and only older individuals expressed the view that mental illness is inherited. In the second study, in terms of seeking help, it was found that only young respondents raised and living in Athens would seek help from a psychiatrist in the case of a major psychological problem, while the rest of the population preferred other traditional means of seeking help such as priest, folk healers, relatives, etc.

In 1980, attitudes towards mental illness were measured in a probability sample of 1574 adults, but only involving residents of two boroughs in the greater Athens area where a community mental health service was to be established [7]. The younger and more educated respondents expressed humanism and tolerance towards deviant behaviour, while the older respondents with a low level of education expressed rejection and considerable fear of the mentally ill.

In 1994, 14 years after the development of the community mental health centre in the area, a replication study was carried out to explore the possible

[1]*Community Mental Health Center, 14 Delou Street, 161 21 Kessariani, Athens, Greece*

differences in public attitudes towards mental illness [8]. This study showed more positive attitudes towards the social integration of the mentally ill, more tolerance of deviant behaviour, less authoritarianism on issues concerning the civil rights of mental patients, better knowledge about the aetiology of mental illness and views supporting a humane approach to the treatment methods in psychiatry. These positive changes in public attitudes could be attributed partly to the social changes taking place in Greece generally, but mainly to the implementation of local community mental health intervention programmes.

On the other hand, results from another study measuring public attitudes to mental illness as opposed to physical illness, conducted in 1996 on a representative sample of 1000 adults from four parts of Greece, revealed negative attitudes towards a person with a history of severe mental illness, especially in the areas of employment and housing [9, 10]. More specifically, 23% of the respondents would never rent an apartment to mentally ill patients, in comparison with 2% for a person suffering from a chronic physical disease; 42.5% would not employ mentally ill persons, in comparison with 4–9% for those with chronic physical disease; and 36% would not live in an area with community services for mentally ill patients. This study, which is the only representative one from all over Greece, demonstrated that discrimination and stigma against the mentally ill still prevail in Greece.

It is obvious that people diagnosed with a "mental illness" inhabit a different space in public perception from those diagnosed with "physical illness" such as cancer or heart disease. Such negative perceptions not only create barriers for the mentally ill patients who wish to reintegrate into the community, but also seriously affect the families who, feeling stigmatized, conceal the mental illness, do not share their experiences outside the family circle and are reluctant to join self-help groups.

It can therefore be suggested that the stigma is one of the reasons why the family movement has been slow to gain ground in Greece. Although there is an organization, the Panhellenic Families Association for Mental Health, established in 1993, which has spread to several parts of the country, Greek families, fearful of local "gossip", hesitate to participate in its activities.

Moreover, it is widely known [9, 11] that the most efficient way of informing the public and changing people's attitudes is the mass media. It is important to know that practical approaches for fighting stigma exist. These approaches include examining the factors associated with variations in stigma within the specific sociocultural conditions, providing psycho-education for patients and families, developing good relations with the media and work with them to destigmatize mental illness, encouraging families to speak openly about the illness and promoting public awareness campaigns.

REFERENCES

1. Blum R., Blum E. (1965) *Health and Healing in Rural Greece*. Stanford University Press, Stanford.
2. Blum R., Blum E. (1970) *The Dangerous Hour*. Chatto and Windus, London.
3. Alevisatos G., Lyketsos G. (1964) A preliminary report of research into the families of hospitalized mentally ill patients. *Int. J. Soc. Psychiatry*, 10: 37–44.
4. Safilios-Rothschild C. (1969) Deviance and mental illness in the Greek family. *Family Process*, 8: 100–107.
5. Vassiliou G., Vassiliou V. (1968) Attitudes of the Athenian public towards mental illness. *Int. J. Ment. Hlth. Newsletter*, 7: 1–8.
6. Georgas T., Janakis M., Geratsidou O. (1978) Attitudes towards mental health in Athens and provinces. *Arch. Hygiene*, 1 (Suppl.): 114–119 (in Greek).
7. Madianos M., Madianou D., Vlachonikolis J., Stefanis C. (1987) Attitudes towards mental illness in the Athens area: implications for community mental health intervention. *Acta Psychiatr. Scand.*, 75: 158–165.
8. Madianos M., Economou M., Hatjiandreou M., Papageorgiou A., Rogakou E. (1999) Changes in public attitudes towards mental illness in the Athens area (1979/1980–1994). *Acta Psychiatr. Scand.*, 99: 73–78.
9. Parashos J. (1998) *Athenian's Views on Mental and Physical Illness*. Lundbeck Hellas, Athens (in Greek).
10. Theodotou R., Paraschos I. (1998) Public attitudes: Comparison between mental patients and patients suffering from chronic physical illness. Presented at the Panhellenic Congress of Psychiatry. Lemnos, Greece, 29 April–3 May.
11. Mayer A., Barry D.D. (1992) Working with the media to destigmatize mental illness. *Hosp. Comm. Psychiatry*, 43: 77–78.

4.11
Disability and Stigma Prevention: The Russian Experience

Vassily S. Yastrebov[1]

Cancro and Meyerson's review deals with one of the main problems of modern psychiatry. I would like to focus on the social and economic aspects of this problem.

In our professional practice, we are used to hearing that the problem of treatment of schizophrenia and of disability due to this illness are an exclusive domain of psychiatry and psychiatrists. In connection with this, demonstrating that schizophrenia is not only a clinical, but also a serious social problem, becomes an important task for psychiatrists.

I believe that this evidence can be constructed on the basis of a clear definition of the real dimensions of the problem. These dimensions include: (a) the high prevalence of schizophrenia; (b) the severity of the disease,

[1]*Mental Health Support Systems Research Centre, Russian Academy of Medical Sciences, 2 Zagorodnoje Shosse, 113152 Moscow, Russia*

which often leads to profound disability; (c) the serious economic and social consequences of the disease at the microsocial level; (d) the significant burden at the family level, which is expressed primarily by the decrease of the quality of life of patients and their relatives. The strategies to attract the attention of governmental bodies to the necessity of preventive measures should be designed proceeding from the above-mentioned dimensions.

Clearing up what is the influence of economic, social and political changes on the indices of disability is of a certain interest. The most illustrative discussion of this question can be made using a concrete example from the history of Russian psychiatry. By the end of the 1980s, in Russia, a well-developed network of psychiatric settings had been created. The availability of this system of psychiatric and rehabilitative services gave an opportunity to every patient in need of specialized medical care to get it in every region. As the result of the activity of these services it became possible in the 1970s and 1980s to involve up to 86% of disabled schizophrenic and other psychiatric patients in different forms of labour of social utility [1].

The socioeconomic crisis of the early 1990s in Russia led to the severe reduction of funds available for psychiatric service financing, and correspondingly to the reduction of the volume of care rendered, and in some regions to the closing of rehabilitation facilities. The negative consequences of this situation became obvious by 1996, when the number of disabled because of mental disorders increased by 16.1% in comparison with 1991.

Concerning the problem of stigma attached to schizophrenic patients, it is necessary to stress that the dimensions of this problem are also numerous. Actually, because of the complexity and multiform character of the problem, any society, independently from its level of development, will be unable to solve it satisfactorily in the visible future. Success in the solution of this problem depends on the level of economic development of the nation, cultural and religious traditions of the society, the level of its civilization and also the social and political situations.

The situation of stigma attached to schizophrenic patients in Russia can provide an illustrative demonstration of this statement. In the former Soviet republics, discussion of the problem of stigma was begun too late. In the late 1980s, due to the "glasnost", an opportunity of open discussion of actual questions of psychiatry became available. At the same time, a very strong anti-psychiatric campaign started, which contributed to shape a negative public opinion of psychiatrists and psychiatry as a whole [2]. An overwhelming part of the population, which had never got any information on psychiatry and its therapeutic opportunities from mass media, believed that "schizophrenics", as well as any other mentally ill, were extremely dangerous, unpredictable persons, and that it was necessary to avoid any contacts with them. Research which was carried out in that period by our group demonstrated that about 68% of the population believed that mentally ill persons do not have the right to drive a car, about 80% believed that they should not work in law bodies, and 84% that they should not work with children.

The development of such a negative image of the mentally ill in public consciousness can be explained not only by the exclusion of psychiatric subjects from public discussion, which had been taking place in the USSR during the previous 70 years, but also by the absence of legislative documents defending the rights of the mentally ill during all that period of time. It is understandable that in these conditions a long-term, thorough work is necessary in order to raise the level of awareness of population, revive the humanitarian traditions of tolerance towards the mentally ill, and broaden public initiatives for their support and defence, as well as to take advantage of the most recent experiences of foreign specialists in fighting the stigma attached to schizophrenic patients.

REFERENCES

1. Livshitz A.E., Arzamastzev Y.N. (1975) New forms of working capacity rehabilitation and employment of mental patients of a large industrial area. *J. Neuropathol. Psychiatr. Korsakov*, **5**: 752–756.
2. Rukavishnikov V.O., Rukavishnikova T.P., Bilzho A.G. (1990) Problems of the community mental health and psychiatric services according to the Soviet press. *J. Neuropathol. Psychiatr. Korsakov*, **11**: 110–114.

4.12

Are Western Models of Psychiatric Rehabilitation Feasible and Appropriate for Developing Countries?

Michael R. Phillips[1]

Cancro and Meyerson's review describes models for the treatment and rehabilitation of schizophrenic patients that are utilized in the United States, many of which are also employed in other economically developed countries. In most cases the rehabilitative interventions have proven useful, so the important question is why these models are not being promulgated more widely. Some research is still needed to refine the models and to tailor them to the changing needs of patients and families, but the focus of the research

[1]*Research Center of Clinical Epidemiology, Beijing Hui Long Guan Hospital, Beijing 100096, China*

effort in developed countries must now be on the socioeconomic factors that are limiting the widespread application of these models, *not* on the development of more models. Once we understand the factors that facilitate or obstruct the development and long-term survival of comprehensive and integrated rehabilitation services, we will be better able to intervene in ways that will improve the chances for promulgating the use of such services.

The review correctly emphasizes the need to include the provision of acute treatment as an integral part of the overall effort to prevent disability. But more than half of the individuals with schizophrenia in the world do not have access to (or do not utilize) basic psychiatric services, so their rehabilitation and the prevention of disability remain a remote goal. Estimates computed from *Global Health Statistics* [1] — collected as part of the Global Burden of Disease Study cooperatively conducted by the World Bank, the WHO and Harvard University — indicate that in 1990 23% of the 9.7 million individuals with schizophrenia in developed countries and 67% of the 17.2 million individuals with schizophrenia in developing countries received no treatment whatsoever. Clearly, the emphasis for the prevention of disability in individuals with schizophrenia in developing countries needs to be on the provision and utilization of basic treatments: making antipsychotic medications available, training primary care providers how to administer medications, and educating the public to utilize the available services. Every attempt should be made to incorporate ongoing rehabilitative measures as part of these basic interventions, but economic and personnel constraints in developing countries, particularly in rural areas, will make most of the rehabilitative measures described in the review infeasible for the foreseeable future.

Inpatient industrial work therapy and sheltered workshops have been employed in urban areas of several developing countries, and experimental models of clubhouses, half-way houses, and family psychoeducational approaches have been initiated in a few developing countries. However, this does not demonstrate the feasibility and appropriateness of Western rehabilitative methods for developing countries. The theory and practice of psychiatric rehabilitation described in the review is based on the characteristics of the mental health system in the West (largely the United States) and on the social and cultural values of Western society. In developing countries the prevalent beliefs about the causes and appropriate management of mental illnesses, the evolution and characteristics of the mental health system, and the overall sociocultural environment are fundamentally different [2]: (a) developing countries have not experienced the massive institutionalization and subsequent deinstitutionalization of the mentally ill seen in the West over the last several decades, so there has been no incentive to develop extensive community mental health services and inter-mediate care facilities; (b) the lack of mental health providers — particularly psychologists, social workers and occupational therapists — severely limits the types of rehabilitative services that can be provided in developing countries; (c) in many developing countries the majority of the popula-tion work as rural farm labourers (usually in family groups) in widely dispersed communities, so community-based rehabilitative measures that require congregating groups of patients and that train them to adapt to urban work conditions are both infeasible and inappropriate; (d) the Western focus on individual responsibility and individual rights implicit in many of the rehabilitative approaches conflicts with the collectivist values (still dominant in most developing countries) that emphasize the interdependence of family members and the responsibility of the society to control and supervise the mentally ill.

Increased urbanization, the globalization of Western values, and the rapid (often traumatic) conversion to a market economy are directly affecting the treatment and rehabilitation of schizophrenic patients in developing countries. For example, in China the economic reforms have been asso-ciated with a dramatic increase in the relative cost of inpatient care, an increasingly competitive job market that is less receptive to persons with disabilities, decreased social welfare provision from the state, and a decreased willingness on the part of families to provide lifelong support to disabled family members [3]. These changes are increasing professional and public awareness of the importance of rehabilitation for the mentally ill (primarily in urban areas) and may increase the feasibility of some of the Western approaches, particularly family psychoeducational approaches. But the type of psychiatric rehabilitative services available in developing countries is *not* a simple reflection of the level of economic development; it is also influenced by the history of mental health service development, by the imperatives driving the current provision of services, and by beliefs about mental illnesses prevalent in the community. The theory and estab-lished techniques of psychiatric rehabilitation will need to be extended to accommodate sociocultural differences between Western and non-Western countries.

REFERENCES

1. Murray C.J.L., Lopez A.D. (1996) *Global Health Statistics*. Harvard University Press, Cambridge.
2. Phillips M.R., Pearson V. (1994) Future opportunities and challenges for the devel-opment of psychiatric rehabilitation in China. *Br. J. Psychiatry*, **165** (Suppl. 24): 128–142.
3. Phillips M.R. (1998) The transformation of China's mental health services. *China Journal*, **39**: 1–36.

4.13
Is Schizophrenia a Chronic Illness? The Experience of Developing Countries

R. Srinivasa Murthy[1]

Schizophrenia is a major public health problem in both developed and developing countries. The wide variety of issues relating to the understanding of disability and stigma in different countries is providing a rich arena to understand the biological, psychological and social contributions to the illness. Of the many differences across countries and cultures, the most important is the issue of relatively better outcome of schizophrenia in developing countries [1]. It has been shown consistently that chronicity is not an essential part of the illness. For example, in the 10-year follow-up study of schizophrenia from Madras, it was found that 16% of patients had not suffered any relapse after the first remission, 38% had had one episode, and 34.5% had had two to five episodes, and that the average number of relapses in the cohort was about two. In addition, duration of illness at intake was strongly related to the likelihood of having a poor outcome, with those whose illness had preceded intake by 8–12 months or 19–24 months having twice the odds of having a poor course. This increased to 16 times with those with an illness duration of 13–18 months [2].

It is this and related observations which make it important not to consider schizophrenia as a chronic illness. The debate about chronicity is of great relevance to developing countries, as the currently available mental health resources, in terms of professionals and hospital beds, do not even cover 5% of the ill population [3]. In view of this, the approach adopted has been to integrate mental health with primary care. However, it becomes difficult, for non-specialist professionals, to deal with an illness which is looked at as a lifelong disorder. It is more likely that they would accept the care and responsibility for schizophrenia if it were presented as a treatable condition. One wonders whether we are overemphasizing that "we have no cure". Would it not be more appropriate to emphasize the value of early recognition, proper treatment and rehabilitation rather than the inevitability of chronicity? Studies done in India have also shown that disability is a function of treatment status. In addition, in clinical practice, even patients who have been ill for many years with significant negative symptoms have responded to the first-level antipsychotics, such as chlorpromazine, very dramatically. It is in this context that psychiatrists in developing countries could take a public health perspective, emphasizing the impact of treatment on both short-term and long-term outcome of the disorder. This approach can help fighting stigma, because any group with a lifelong disabling disorder

[1]*National Institute of Mental Health, Department of Psychiatry and Neuroscience, Post Bag 2900, Bangalore 56002-9, India*

is more likely to be stigmatized. There is need for rethinking about the chronicity of schizophrenia from the above viewpoints.

The alternative role of care to meet the needs of people with long-standing illness, in terms of day-care centres, half-way homes, hostels, is in the early stages of development. Professionals recognize that these needs will be there until universal coverage of mental health services becomes a reality. A very important point that is becoming an issue is the breakdown of the traditional families. Along with urbanization and modernization, both the supportive traditional societies and community tolerance are coming under strain. A rapidly expanding economy which can wipe out all of the values if it becomes a reality would have a tremendous impact on the care of schizophrenia. The developing countries also have a unique opportunity to develop welfare programmes that are user friendly and at the same time not stigmatizing. It has been often voiced by professionals from Europe and America that the availability of a wide variety of social welfare measures often contributes to the continuing ill status of individuals, and indirectly to the stigma attached to them. There is a need for professionals to combine imaginatively the needs of patients with all policy developments to support them.

REFERENCES

1. Kulhara P. (1994) Outcomes of schizophrenia: some transcultural observations with particular reference to developing countries. *Eur. Arch. Psychiatry Clin. Neurosci.*, **24**: 227–235.
2. Thara R., Henrietta M., Joseph A., Rajkumar S., Eaton W.W. (1994) Ten year course of schizophrenia: the Madras longitudinal study. *Acta Psychiatr. Scand.*, **90**: 329–336.
3. Srinivasa Murthy R. (1996) Economics of mental health in developing countries. In *International Review of Psychiatry*, vol. 2 (Eds F. Lieh Mak, C.C. Nadelson), pp. 43–62. American Psychiatric Press, Washington, DC.

4.14
Prevention of Disability and Stigma: Experience from a Developing Country

Muhammad Rashid Chaudhry[1]

The subject of schizophrenia has witnessed remarkable improvement in terms of its definition, diagnosis, treatment and management over the last 100 years. Apart from pharmacological advances, innovations in psychosocial treatments have also revolutionized the care of patients suffering

[1]Fountain House Foundation Trust, Fountain House, 37 Lower Mall, Lahore, Pakistan

from this illness. Cancro and Meyerson's paper describes the historical perspectives, especially the topics of prevention of disability and stigma, in a very comprehensive way. The work being done in this area is excellent.

During the past few decades, new horizons have been explored in the rehabilitation of the mentally ill. Technological innovations in the development of new drugs, modifications of treatment measures, use of psychosocial techniques for creating therapeutic milieux, developing vocational potentials and transitional employment placements have all given new hopes and promises and have opened up new vistas and pathways for treatment and rehabilitation of the mentally ill.

The interest of professionals in the mental health field has also been focused on the development of after-care facilities to assist discharged psychiatric patients to make a safe transition from hospital to community. One such type of facility is the halfway house. The rationale for the halfway house is based on the logical thinking that an environment intermediate between the hospital and the outside world would make up an important contribution to the rehabilitation of psychiatric patients [1]. The halfway houses are intended to provide the discharged mental patients, mostly schizophrenics, with a temporary home, with a peer group of other former patients to interact, socialize and share common experiences during the initial period of adjustment to non-hospital life.

Most of these innovations have taken place in developed countries [2]. The situation in developing countries, on the other hand, is also very promising. The spectrum of services for rehabilitation is taking a positive and forward step in many countries. The psychiatric scene in Pakistan has also witnessed such changes and in fact they have influenced the practice of psychiatry to a large extent. During the last 25 years, Fountain House, Lahore, based on the clubhouse model, has attained national as well as international recognition in the field of rehabilitation of schizophrenic patients [3]. Its functioning has created new awareness in the management of chronic mentally ill in this country and has also initiated a lot of collaborative work with many other countries. The experience of Fountain House, Lahore, a pioneering facility in psychiatric rehabilitation, has established its efficacy as a therapeutic community and has given a sense of direction to develop suitable programmes to achieve better management goals for chronic schizophrenics in the community. The self-awareness, that comes at Fountain House, of one's own contribution and capabilities is the beginning of the discovery that one is worth something and will be able to achieve reasonably full participation in the life of the community at large. It is intended to convey to the member (patient) that he is accepted and belongs to an auxiliary family structure that contains many of the same qualities of mutual concern, learning, discipline and expectation as might be found in a healthy family.

The experience of Fountain House, therefore, not only opens new avenues in the field of rehabilitation in developing countries, but also strongly recommends that all available resources should be utilized for the management of psychiatric patients. The modifications, which were made in the original concept of the Fountain House model and which were based on our own needs, also demonstrate that ideas originating from one country may have usefulness for other countries provided that they are adapted to the prevailing sociocultural needs. The reports about the usefulness of the agrotherapy programmes of Fountain House, which have also confirmed their effectiveness as a measure of rehabilitation, can be considered suitable for countries having agro-based economies [4].

It is hoped that community-based rehabilitation programmes for the schizophrenics will initiate, grow and thrive in developing countries and will also be fully incorporated with adaptations reflecting local conditions and circumstances in other countries. Institutions, like religion and the extended family system (joint family system), which are still preserved in many developing countries, are contributing to the successful rehabilitation of the chronic mentally ill [5].

It is true that the mental health professionals still have a long way to go in overcoming the problems in care of the mentally ill. Although progress in many spheres is being made in the treatment and management of chronic illnesses like schizophrenia, more work is still needed especially in the areas of prevention and stigma reduction. The situation in developing countries becomes even more important as lack of resources, fewer professionals and problems in attitudes of public towards mental illnesses still require a lot of work and input.

REFERENCES

1. Beard J.H., Malmud T.J., Rosmann E. (1978) Psychiatric rehabilitation and long term rehospitalization rates. *Schizophr. Bull.*, **4**: 622–635.
2. Chaudhry M.R., Beard J.H. (1979) Rehabilitation of schizophrenics — a collaborative study between Fountain House, New York and Fountain House, Lahore. *Int. J. Rehab. Res. Dev.*, **2** (Suppl. 2): 39–43.
3. Chaudhry M.R., Mirza L. (1983) Fountain House Lahore — a unique experiment in cross cultural collaboration. *Ind. J. Psychiatry*, **25**: 322–327.
4. Javed M.A., Chaudhry U.R., Sulaman T., Chaudhry M.R. (1993) Agrotherapy: new concepts of rehabilitation for chronic schizophrenics in Pakistan. *J. Pak. Med. Assoc.*, **43**: 251–253.
5. Chaudhry M.R., Javed M.A. (1998) Twenty years of experience of rehabilitation of chronic schizophrenics in a developing country like Pakistan. In *Social Psychiatry: A Global Perspective* (Eds V.K. Varma, P. Kulthara, C.M. Masserman, A. Malhotra, S.C. Malik), pp. 190–196. Macmillan, Delhi.

Schizophrenia Spectrum Disorders: A Review

Wolfgang Maier, Peter Falkai and Michael Wagner

Department of Psychiatry, University of Bonn, Germany

INTRODUCTION

Schizophrenia spectrum disorders are schizophrenia-like disorders which are not fulfilling the diagnostic criteria for schizophrenia but which are sharing symptoms, causes and risk factors with schizophrenia. The concept emerges from the recognition that the clinical syndrome of schizophrenia is too restrictive to tap the whole variation of symptoms and features induced by causes underlying schizophrenia.

The specific criterion for schizophrenia spectrum disorders is that they are aetiologically related to schizophrenia; particularly that they are driven by the same familial–genetic factors. Along this line, two types of syndromes were proposed as components of the schizophrenic spectrum: (a) personality features and disorders — sometimes the spectrum concept is restricted to personality traits; (b) psychotic symptoms and disorders, often with an episodic course, which are sharing clinical features with chronic schizophrenia without meeting the full diagnosis.

Personality Features and Personality Disorders

Soon after the familial aggregation of schizophrenia had been recognized, odd, eccentric, deviant and peculiar personality features and other behavioural traits not fitting into the diagnostic patterns of psychotic or affective disorders were observed to occur among the unaffected relatives of schizophrenics more often than expected by chance. Similar behavioural abnormalities were also observed in subjects who developed the full syndrome of schizophrenia subsequently [1]. In this

Schizophrenia, Second Edition. Edited by Mario Maj and Norman Sartorius.
© 2002 John Wiley & Sons Ltd.

context the concept of paranoid personality was introduced, and this personality type was characterized by unwarranted mistrust of others (suspiciousness). Simultaneously, Bleuler [2] observed milder behavioural deviations in untreated relatives of overt schizophrenics which were similar to schizophrenia by chronicity and by symptoms such as flat affect, ambivalence, bizarre thinking, poor contact and poor interpersonal relationships; positive symptoms were uncommon in this group of untreated relatives. He called this less severe variant of overt schizophrenia "latent schizophrenia" and considered the extended concept of schizophrenia as syndromes "with varying degrees and shading on the entire scale from pathological to normal". Latent schizophrenia was redetected by subsequent clinicians (e.g. as pseudoneurotic schizophrenia by Hoch and Polatin [3]) and included in the earlier versions of the ICD system; however, the nosological status of this concept remained controversial.

Following Kraepelin's observations of premorbid features of schizo-phrenia, Kretschmer [4] postulated schizophrenia to be one extreme of a continuum of social behaviour, with normal behaviour as the other extreme, and schizophrenia-like personality patterns (schizoid character) located in between; Kretschmer described schizoid character as unsociable, timid, nervous, socially indifferent and simultaneously hypersensitive, some-times eccentric. More severe and dysfunctional variants of this pattern were described as "personality disorder" (schizoid personality disorder). Schizoid personality became a widely accepted concept and was included — as person-ality disorder (PD) — in the DSM-I and -II (without well-defined diagnostic criteria).

Twin studies, particularly those by Kallmann [5], provided convincing evidence that schizophrenia is at least partly under genetic control. This result motivated the concept of the "schizophrenic genotype". Rado [6] coined the term "schizotype" for the range of phenotypes hypothetically expressed by the "schizophrenic genotype"; he assumed "anhedonia" (a reduced ability to experience pleasure and joy) to be the core phenotype. Meehl [7] also postulated that the boundaries of the phenotype transmitted in families are not as distinctly demarcated as expected from a clearly defined disease entity. Meehl considered the vulnerability to schizophrenia as the crucial phenotype which he called "schizotypy"; he defined schizotypy as an enduring personality condition, based on a genetically caused neurointe-grative deficit named "schizotaxia". The schizotypal personality may remain compensated, or may decompensate into schizophrenia, due to detrimental personal or environmental circumstances. Again, anhedonia was considered as the crucial symptom [7], but later on three other features were simultane-ously proposed [8]: cognitive slippage (a more or less pronounced loosening of associations); ambivalence (the co-occurrence of disparate experiences and feelings); and interpersonal aversiveness (a combination of social anxiety, suspiciousness, anticipated rejection by others and low self-esteem).

Meehl's conception that schizotaxia is the result of a single autosomal gene with low clinical penetrance has remained controversial and is untenable nowadays. However, the idea of a genetically determined underlying neurofunctional aberration (schizotaxia) common to schizotypal PD and schizophrenia is still prevailing, and possible neurobiological indicators which have been studied in spectrum disorder patients as well as in schizophrenic patients and their relatives are briefly reviewed below.

The first strict empirical approach to characterize schizotypal traits in unaffected relatives of schizophrenics emerged from the Danish Adoption Study (Extended Family Study) in chronic schizophrenia using the "adopted-away" strategy [9]. Given the twin studies-based evidence for genetic determination of schizophrenia, the only modest, insignificant excess of schizophrenia among biological parents of schizophrenics compared to controls came as a surprise. However, schizophrenia-like personality features (initially called "borderline schizophrenia") were not only substantially more common but occurred nearly exclusively among biological parents of schizophrenics compared to all control groups. Combining full manifestations and borderline cases of schizophrenia, the expected excess of affected biological relatives in comparison to controls was obtained. The "borderline cases" were too heterogeneous by psychopathological symptoms and signs to be sufficiently characterized by the pre-existing DSM-I and DSM-II categories of schizoid or paranoid PD. Instead, the psychopathological profile of the "borderline cases" showed a striking similarity with previously proposed clinical concepts of schizophrenia-like disorders in non-psychotic patients derived by Bleuler ("latent schizophrenia") and others [10]. Psychopathological analysis of these "borderline" conditions observed in the Danish Adoption Study delivered a list of eight diagnostic items characterizing "borderline schizophrenia" which was relabelled as "schizotypal PD" [11]. Schizotypal PD was first introduced in DSM-III and defined by diagnostic criteria based on these analyses. Thus, schizotypal PD is the first empirically derived diagnostic category.

There was some overlap with borderline PD (characterized by affective instability), which is aetiologically less strongly related to schizophrenia [12, 13]; this overlap was reduced in subsequent reanalyses. Although it was clear from the preexisting literature and empirically that the negative type symptoms/criteria of schizotypal PD were more common in and characteristic for the biological relatives of chronic schizophrenics, positive symptom-like criteria were retained in the definition of schizotypal PD; these symptoms turned out to be more common among patients with schizotypal PD in psychiatric treatment [14]. Minor changes of the diagnostic DSM-III criteria of schizotypal PD were undertaken in DSM-III-R [15] and DSM-IV [16], in order to reduce overlap with borderline PD (e.g. reference to "derealization, depersonalization" was discarded, and the criterion "odd behaviour" was introduced). Finally, the other leading diagnostic system (ICD) also adopted this concept as schizotypal disorder in the tenth edition [17].

Personality disorders may be considered as an extreme of a continuum of variation of a personality trait (dimension). Thus, "schizotype" as a PD motivated explicit dimensional approaches tracing schizotypal traits to a subclinical level [18]. A number of psychometric instruments have been developed to assess schizotypal personality features with self-report questionnaires, the primary tools of personality research. These scales are purportedly designed either to measure attenuated psychotic-like experiences, or to directly measure self-reported symptoms of schizotypal PD as delineated in diagnostic manuals. Both types of questionnaires are often used to identify in the population, for example in large groups of college students, subjects with high scores, and to further investigate these "schizotypal" groups with regard to neurobiological similarities with schizophrenic patients, prevalence of psychiatric disorders in relatives, and also with regard to long-term outcome. Subjects with high scores are thought to constitute a "psychometric high-risk" group, with an increased probability to later develop psychoses. Some evidence for the predictive validity of these scales has accrued [19, 20], in that subjects with high scores of social anhedonia or magical ideation were found to have more psychotic relatives than subjects with average scores, to have more psychotic symptoms and more often develop a psychosis several years later, but there seems to be no specificity with regard to schizophrenic psychosis. When several scales are given, factor analyses very consistently reveal at least a "positive schizotypy" factor representing unusual perceptual experiences (e.g. from the Perceptual Aberration/Magical Ideation Scale), and a "negative schizotypy" factor defined by social withdrawal and anhedonia (for a recent review of questionnaire measurement of schizotypy, see ref. [21]).

Psychotic Axis I Spectrum Disorders

Originally, the spectrum concept was limited to schizophrenia and related PD [10, 11]. Recently, the concept was extended to schizophrenia-related axis I disorders (e.g. ref. [22]). Some schizophrenia-like axis I disorders were included as spectrum disorders as the familial co-aggregation with schizophrenia is a consistent finding across most family and adoption studies. Unlike the schizophrenia spectrum PD, the diagnostic and clinical characterization of the axis I spectrum disorders occurred mostly independent of the genetic research on the boundaries of the phenotype transmitted in families of schizophrenics. These diagnostic concepts were derived on clinical grounds.

Three major candidates can be discussed as putative components of the schizophrenic spectrum because of sharing symptoms with overt chronic schizophrenia.

1. If schizophrenia is defined as a chronic disorder (as in DSM-III/-III-R/-IV) the non-chronic condition (duration 2 weeks to 6 months) is called schizophreniform disorder. By definition, a patient with schizophrenia was a patient with schizophreniform disorder before; therefore, schizophreniform disorder is automatically a component of the spectrum of schizophrenia ("good prognosis schizophrenia"). Furthermore, most widely used diagnostic criteria in research (e.g. Research Diagnostic Criteria, RDC [23]), as well as the most recent edition of ICD (ICD-10), are ignoring this difference by defining schizophrenia by a shorter minimal duration. Empirical studies are widely in agreement with this position by placing the schizophreniform group between the more chronic variant of schizophrenia (episode duration > 6 months) and affective disorder, but more closely to schizophrenia (e.g. regarding long-term course [24]). Therefore, this review ignores the difference between schizophrenia and schizophreniform disorder (as proposed in DSM-IV) and subsumes schizophreniform disorder to schizophrenia.

2. Schizoaffective disorders describe schizophrenic symptoms occurring consecutively or simultaneously with manic or depressive syndromes. In clinical settings both syndromes occur more frequently together in the same patients than expected by chance, challenging the validity of the nosological dissection between affective and schizophrenic disorders. This concept dates back to Kasanin [25] and has a controversial history with diagnostic ambiguities as a consequence. The most widely accepted diagnostic definitions during the last decades (e.g. RDC, DSM-III-R/-IV, ICD-10) reveal only limited overlap, and reliability for most definitions is relatively low. The crucial features is simultaneous presence of both psychotic, schizophrenia-like symptoms and full affective syndromes (depression, mania); the more schizophrenia-like subtype (as proposed by RDC and redefined for schizoaffective disorder in general in DSM-III-R/-IV) presents for a minimal time period with schizophrenia-like symptoms (delusions, hallucinations) only in absence of full-blown affective syndromes; the more affective-like syndrome (RDC) describes the reverse relationship. Despite these diagnostic inconsistencies, schizophrenia and schizoaffective disorders are co-aggregating in families independent of the diagnostic system used; strongest co-aggregation with chronic schizophrenia is observed for schizoaffective disorders sharing a maximum of features with schizophrenia (i.e. the schizophreniform and chronic subtype).

3. Other psychotic disorders are sometimes observed to co-aggregate with schizophrenia in families, but less strongly than schizoaffective disorder

or schizophrenia itself. Although there are some positive results, the whole body of evidence is not sufficient to consider these psychotic disorders as a component of the schizophrenic spectrum.

PHENOMENOLOGY AND DIAGNOSIS

Spectrum Personality Disorders

A broad variety of schizotypal traits, signs and symptoms characterizing unaffected relatives of schizophrenics and the premorbid states of schizophrenia were reported in classical clinical textbooks [1–4]. These traits, signs and symptoms can be assessed by two different methods:

1. Using semistructured clinical interview, for example the interview used in the Danish Adoption Study, including 17 possible schizotypal features, or the more recently developed SIS (Structured Interview for Schizotypy [26]) which defines 25 possible schizotypal signs and symptoms.
2. Self-rating by questionnaire; the most widely used scales were those developed by Chapman *et al* to assess physical and social anhedonia [27], perceptual aberrations [28], and magical ideation [29]; two other questionnaires, more closely oriented towards the criteria of schizotypal PD, are the Schizotypal Personality Questionnaire (SPQ) by Raine [30] and the Schizotypal Personality Scale (STA) by Claridge and Broks [31].

Assessment tools available for each of these approaches differ in the underlying phenomenological and clinical concept, comprehensiveness of content of symptoms and signs, and relative weight of various components of schizotypal traits. The possible schizotypal features cover social, emotional and cognitive functions. This most comprehensive set of schizotypal traits included in SIS comprises: poor rapport, aloofness/coldness, guardedness, odd behaviour, illusions, ideas of reference, magical thinking, depersonalization, suspiciousness, recurrent suicidal threats, inappropriate anger, affective instability, jealousy, impulsivity, chronic boredom, general lack of motivation, occupation functioning below expected, social isolation, social anxiety, hypersensitivity, anxiety, cognitive slippage, odd speech, hypervigilance and irritability. Not included in the SIS are two crucial features proposed by the classical papers: ambivalence [2] and anhedonia [6, 7, 27]. Multimethod–multitrait techniques are appropriate to explore the extent of similarity and discrepancy between the various approaches. Only one study explores this crucial methodological issue [32]. Only moderate consistency was observed.

The heterogeneous set of items is divided into multiple components, as demonstrated by factor analyses performed for various assessment instruments: using less comprehensive sets of signs and symptoms (than the SIS) in clinical settings, a two-factor model was proposed with a cognitive/perceptual- and a deficit-related factor [33], three-factor models with the factors cognitive/perceptual, paranoid and interpersonal [34], and alternatively with a disorganization instead of a paranoid factor [35]. In a general population sample using a self-assessment inventory, a two-factor model with positive and negative schizotypal signs, and a three-factor model with positive schizotypal traits, nonconformity and social schizotypal traits were obtained [36]. Gruzelier [37] proposed a four-factor model by using the questionnaire SPQ in the general population, with factors "activity", "withdrawal", "unreality" and "suspiciousness". As the schizotype concept emerges from deviations in unaffected relatives of schizophrenics, factor analyses in this population are particularly informative. Using the comprehensive 25 schizotypal items of the observer-rated SIS, Kendler et al [38] extracted seven factors: negative schizotypy, positive schizotypy, borderline symptoms, social dysfunction, avoidant symptoms, odd speech and suspicious behaviour. Among these factors "borderline symptoms" are not discriminative for relatives of schizophrenics, excluding this factor from the schizophrenic spectrum. Taken together, although most of these factor analyses were performed in a heterogeneous, broadly defined set of schizotypal and related items, the extracted factors are not in correspondence with the taxonomy of schizophrenia-related PD; thus, the empirical basis for separating schizotypal, schizoid and paranoid PD on the grounds of symptom patterns is not compelling.

Each of the three spectrum PDs is referring to overlapping subsets of schizotypal traits.

Schizotypal PD is the most heterogeneous category, covering social, emotional and cognitive function. Most diagnostic criteria were derived from the most common and discriminative schizotypal items found in relatives of schizophrenics. Most influential has been the reanalysis of the Extended Danish Adoption Study by Spitzer et al [11], who defined the basis for the schizotypal PD diagnosis in DSM-III. These criteria include ideas of reference and paranoid thinking, odd beliefs and magic thinking, unusual perceptions, odd thinking and speech, suspiciousness, constricted affect, lack of close friends, and excessive social anxiety. Schizotypal PD is referring to a heterogeneous set of behavioural abnormalities in biological relatives of schizophrenics, tapping social anxiety and constricted affective response, cognitive/perceptual distortions, suspiciousness and ideas of reference as well as odd speech. Another reanalysis of a more comprehensive sample derived from the same studies only partly confirmed Spitzer et al's results [12]. Particularly the high weight put on positive schizotypal criteria (e.g. ideas of reference, magical thinking, illusions, depersonalization, derealization) received critical comments [39]. On the other hand, it was argued that criteria for schizotypal PD in diagnostic manuals used by clinicians have primarily to deal with patients asking for treatment; therefore, it was argued that deviations in relatives of schizophrenics are not the only source to extract the most appropriate criteria [14]. Indeed, in clinical samples, transient psychosis, brief paranoid experiences, hallucinations and distinct delusions discriminated for schizotypal PD against other PDs [40].

A confirmatory factor analysis [41] explored the coherence of criteria defining schizotypal PD in non-psychotic outpatients. Best fit was obtained for three factors: cognitive–perceptual, interpersonal, and oddness factor. Raine *et al* [42] and Lenzenweger *et al* [43] also found support for a similar three-factor solution. These results propose that schizotypal PD does not present as an appropriate diagnostic entity in clinical settings; it might be useful to consider the three components separately as three dimensions. Future research might profit from this modified approach.

ICD-10 acknowledges the specific genetic relationship of schizotypal PD to schizophrenia. In contrast to DSM-IV, the ICD-10 relabels schizotypal PD as "schizotypal disorder" (F21) by shifting this category from the "PD section" (axis II) to the "schizophrenia and related psychoses" section (F2; axis I). In contrast to schizotypal PD, ICD-10 includes the other two spectrum PDs in the "PD section" (F6).

Schizoid PD is more homogeneous than schizotypal PD; it is characterized by social and environmental features as a low number of social contacts, friends and confidants, by a lack of interpersonal enjoyment and emotional aloofness/coldness; cognitive features are less characteristic. This characterization is most similar to the description of the schizoid character by Kretschmer [4]. Because of the similarities with residual and prodromal phases of schizophrenia, this PD is considered as a possible schizophrenia spectrum disease. Although ICD-10 and DSM-IV have most of the diagnostic criteria in common, ICD-10 in addition focuses on engagement in phantasies and introversion.

Paranoid PD is also substantially more homogeneous than schizotypal PD, and focuses on suspiciousness, mistrustfulness, distortions in cognition and perception, and reluctance to confide in others. Emotional factors are less relevant for the diagnosis of paranoid PD. Paranoid PD has an own history dating back to Kraepelin [44], who considered suspiciousness as the leading sign; Kretschmer [4] considered hypersensitivity to criticism as another crucial trait. Paranoid PD is considered as a possible schizophrenia spectrum disease because its leading symptom, suspiciousness, is a schizotypal trait clustering in biological relatives of schizophrenics. The diagnostic criteria in ICD-10 and DSM-IV are widely in agreement, with ICD-10 stressing more self-relatedness and excess of self-appreciation.

All three PDs cover overlapping personality traits; however, diagnostic criteria vary by complexity and scope between the disorders. These three PDs cluster together and are subsumed as bizarre and odd PDs (so-called cluster A-PDs). A diagnosis of each PD requires the presence of a minimum number out of a comprehensive list of criteria. Coexistence of these three PDs is not excluded by diagnostic manuals; comorbidity between these three PDs is very common in clinical samples (e.g. see ref. [45]): nearly half of the schizotypal PD patients are meeting criteria for each of the other two PD; comorbidity with schizotypal PD is particularly high for patients with schizoid PD (more than 50% in the majority of studies) [46]. One third of cases with paranoid PD also fulfil other cluster A-PD diagnoses [45], mainly schizotypal PD. As an exception, there is some disagreement concerning schizoid and paranoid PD in clinical samples: reports on large overlap [47] are contrasted by reports on small overlap (e.g. refs [48, 49]).

A great deal of overlap between schizotypal and borderline PD was observed in various samples by using DSM-III. After reducing similarity of diagnostic criteria between both disorders, the overlap was reduced to 20% [13]. Comorbidity between both diagnoses is particularly high in samples of hospitalized patients [40]. Some authors [13] consider the overlap as artificial and claim that it is due to the misconception of PDs as diagnostic categories instead of dimensions. In this perspective, the observed overlap is the consequence of the correlation of two dimensions: "borderline" and "schizotypal" personality traits. Schizoid PD, and to a less degree schizotypal PD, occur also more often than expected by chance in comorbidity with avoidant PD (excess social anxiety), because of overlap of diagnostic criteria. In addition, paranoid PD overlaps considerably with passive–aggressive PD [45].

Co-occurrence of these PDs and specific axis I disorders higher than expected by chance can also be observed (at least in treated samples): in samples of hospitalized patients the majority of cases with schizotypal PD are likely to suffer an episode of schizophrenia [50]; episodes of major depression are reported in 10–40% of the schizotypal cases [51]. Paranoid PD is often associated with major depression and paranoid disorder [52].

Schizophrenia-like Schizoaffective Disorder

Early diagnostic approaches to schizoaffective disorders focused exclusively on the simultaneous coexistence of full affective and schizophrenic syndromes (preferentially mood-incongruent delusions and hallucinations) excluding the diagnosis of either uncomplicated affective or schizophrenic disorders [53]. The RDC diagnoses of schizoaffective disorder received maximal acceptance; although more elaborated diagnostic systems are available in the meantime, the RDC diagnosis of schizophrenia/schizoaffective disorder is still common in genetic research. Most clinical papers on subtypes of schizoaffective disorders were dedicated to the validation of the unipolar depressive/bipolar subdivision [54, 55]; these papers do not specifically focus on the relationship to schizophrenia and are, therefore, not discussed in this context. The RDC were the first to shift emphasis on patterns of course, particularly in the "mainly schizophrenic" subtype; this subtype requires persistence of psychotic symptoms in absence of full affective syndromes for 2 weeks. The subdivision was particularly validated by family studies [56, 57]. In clinical samples of patients with broadly defined schizoaffective disorders (RDC), about a quarter is belonging to the mainly schizophrenic subtype in both the unipolar depressive as well as the manic subtype [58, 59].

Subsequently, DSM-III-R and DSM-IV restricted the diagnosis of schizoaffective disorder to modified versions of the RDC schizoaffective disorder subtype "mainly schizophrenic", which might be considered as a schizophrenia spectrum disorder. In contrast, the diagnostic definition of schizoaffective disorder by ICD-10 is substantially broader and covers also the mainly affective subtype.

One of the sources of diagnostic heterogeneity of schizoaffective disorders are differences in defining schizophrenia. The two currently most widely accepted diagnostic manuals, ICD-10 and DSM-IV, include subjects with schizophrenic symptoms who are simultaneously suffering from a depressive episode into the category of schizophrenia. DSM-III-R/-IV allocates priority to the relative duration of associated full affective syndromes (it should be short relative to the duration of psychotic symptoms); ICD-10 allocates priority to the time sequence of onset (psychotic syndromes should occur earlier).

Both manuals require coexistence of core symptoms of schizophrenia and of full episodes of affective disorders for the definition of schizoaffective disorders. According to DSM, schizophrenic symptoms have to persist in absence of mania or depression for at least 2 weeks, whereas ICD-10 includes all variants of coexistent schizophrenic and affective syndromes (if schizophrenic syndromes are *not* primary) into the schizoaffective disorder category.

Given these discrepancies between DSM-IV and ICD-10, schizoaffective disorders in DSM-IV might be diagnosed as schizophrenia by ICD-10 and vice versa. Therefore, it is difficult to tease apart schizophrenia and schizophrenia-like schizoaffective disorders in an unequivocal manner. Thus, differences between these two disorders might be difficult to recognize.

Family studies demonstrate that the affective subtype (RDC) of schizoaffective disorder is more closely allied with affective disorders in families [56, 57, 60]. Thus, the ICD-10 category of schizoaffective disorder is over-inclusive and less appropriate than the DSM-IV category to present as a schizophrenia spectrum disorder component.

EPIDEMIOLOGY AND COURSE

Spectrum Personality Disorders

Only a few well-designed studies report on the prevalence rate of spectrum PDs in the general population (Table 5.1). Four of these studies report prevalence rates in general population control groups of family studies [61–64]; the other study only applies self-rating techniques [65]. The prevalence rates vary considerably by setting and method. For example, the study by Zimmerman and Coryell reported higher rates by self-assessment by PDQ (Personality Disorders Questionnaire) compared to observer assessment by interview (SIPD — Structured Interview for Personality Disorders). Males are more often affected than females for all three cluster A-PDs. Overall, the lifetime prevalence rates of schizotypal PD are comparable or even higher than for schizophrenia; paranoid PD is more common and schizoid PD is less common.

Paranoid and schizoid PDs were the object of a small follow-up study [49]. The long-term course of schizotypal PD was systematically investigated in only a single follow-back study among former inpatients over one to three decades by McGlashan [50]. The status of schizotypal PD before first hospitalization was lower compared to other PDs and to schizophrenia in terms of social skills, social contact and adjustment. Overall, schizotypal PD was associated in this hospitalized sample with severe impairment and disability; schizotypal PD showed the worst long-term course compared to other PDs in terms of living situation at follow-up (dependent on others, not married, no children), psychopathology, social activity and employment during the follow-up period; in all these areas of functioning schizotypal PD did better than schizophrenia. Schizotypal PD occurring in comorbidity with borderline PD was surprisingly associated with a less severe course by all mentioned outcome criteria (exception: more alcohol abuse in the combined group). Systematic follow-up studies in more naturalistic samples (outpatients, general population samples) are not available.

Studies exploring the stability of odd PD diagnoses are also missing. However, in samples of inpatients, a major subgroup, perhaps the majority, experience at least one episode of schizophrenia [50]. Furthermore, some studies contribute to the relationship of schizotypal personality traits and schizophrenia in the early course of the disorder. Two possible relationships can be explored: (i) schizophrenia spectrum disorders, schizotypal traits and personality features (disorders) are precursors of schizophrenia; (ii) schizophrenia spectrum disorders and schizotypal traits are two alternative developments and share some of their precursors and causes.

TABLE 5.1 Prevalence of Specific Personality Disorders (PD) in Epidemiological Surveys

Type of PD	Authors	Country	Sample size	Classification system	Method of assessment	Prevalence (%)
Schizotypal	Baron et al, 1985 [61]	USA	374*	DSM-III	SIB; SADS-L	2.1
	Maier et al, 1992 [63]	Germany	447*	DSM-III-R	SCID	0.7
	Reich et al, 1989 [65]	USA	235	DSM-III	PDQ	5.1
	Zimmerman and Coryell, 1990 [62]	USA	697*	DSM-III	PDQ	5.6
					SIPD	3.0
	Kendler et al, 1993 [64]	Ireland	580	DSM-III-R	SIS	1.4
Schizoid	Baron et al, 1985 [61]	USA	374*	DSM-III	SIB; SADS-L	0
	Maier et al, 1992 [63]	Germany	447*	DSM-III-R	SCID	0.4
	Reich et al, 1989 [65]	USA	235	DSM-III	PDQ	0.8
	Zimmerman and Coryell, 1990 [62]	USA	697*	DSM-III	PDQ	0.9
					SIPD	0.7
Paranoid	Baron et al, 1985 [61]	USA	374*	DSM-III	SIB; SADS-L	2.7
	Maier et al, 1992 [63]	Germany	447*	DSM-III-R	SCID	1.8
	Reich et al, 1989 [65]	USA	235	DSM-III	PDQ	0.8
	Zimmerman and Coryell, 1990 [62]	USA	697*	DSM-III	PDQ	0.4
					SIPD	0.4
	Kendler et al, 1993 [64]	Ireland	580	DSM-III-R	SIS	0.4

*First-degree relatives of normal control probands.
SIB, Schedule for Interviewing Borderlines; SADS-L, Schedule for Affective Disorders and Schizophrenia-Lifetime; SCID, Structured Clinical Interview for DSM-III-R; PDQ, Personality Disorders Questionnaire; SIPD, Structured Interview for Personality Disorders; SIS, Structured Interview for Schizotypy.

Schizotypal Traits and Symptoms as Precursors of Schizophrenia

Evidence for a link between schizotypal traits and later development of schizophrenia comes from: (a) follow-back studies in schizophrenia; (b) follow-up studies in high-risk samples; and (c) birth cohort surveys in combination with case registers.

Only a minority of these studies used PD assessment tools, but most of them reported behavioural abnormalities preceding schizophrenia which might reflect premorbid personality traits. Particularly recent follow-back studies characterized later schizophrenics by depressive, negative and cognitive traits [66]. Follow-back studies also report higher rates of suspiciousness and unusual speech [67]. High-risk studies report poor affective control, social solitariness, irritability, maladaptive behaviour and cognitive disturbances to precede schizophrenia [68, 69]. Attentional deficits are the most common preceding characteristics of schizophrenia and schizotypal PD in the New York High-Risk Study [70], with anhedonia operating as a potentiating factor. These reports are backed up by prospective birth cohort studies linking large-scale assessments in children with case registers later in life: Crow *et al* [71] reported anxiety, depression, aversive behaviour, social withdrawal, cognitive underachievements (mainly verbal functions) and insufficient control of motor functions.

Prospective clinical studies in patients receiving the diagnosis of schizophrenia at a later stage found selected self-reported psychological deficiencies (basic symptoms) to be characteristic; syndromes of interpersonal sensitivity, of information processing, thought and perceptual aberrations were particularly predictive for schizophrenia [72–74]. Although these signs cannot unambiguously be considered as personality traits, these results point at schizotypal features as prerunners of schizophrenia. However, schizotypal or other spectrum PDs cannot be considered as obligatory precursors. A few follow-back studies were exploring the prevalence of PD premorbid to schizophrenia: in 44%, normal personality features were observed [75]. Unfortunately, no prospective study exploring the transition probability between schizotypal PD and other spectrum PDs to schizophrenia has been published up to now.

Are schizotypal traits in the premorbid personalities specific for schizophrenia or do they contribute also to the premorbid personalities of other disorders? Foerster *et al* [76] compared the same postulated premorbid features between patients with schizophrenia versus patients with affective psychosis. Poor educational achievement indicating reduced cognitive and attentional abilities discriminated both patient groups. Overall, the diagnostic specificity of pre-existing traits needs further study.

Evidence for Common Precursors for Schizophrenia and Spectrum PDs

Schizotypal personality and schizophrenia might be viewed as alternative developments emerging from the same pattern of vulnerability [77]. In the New York High-Risk Project [77], attentional deficit with subsequent inability to process interpersonal information are common preceding features of both schizophrenia and schizotypal PD; it is hypothesized that active avoidance of others leads to symptom control (i.e. schizotypal PD), whereas failed attempts to interact with others induces stress and provokes the symptoms of schizophrenia. Olin *et al* [78] compared childhood precursors (School Report Questionnaire) in the Copenhagen High-Risk Study between subjects presenting with schizophrenia and those with schizotypal PD: both groups were additionally more passive and unengaged and more socially anxious and withdrawn compared to low-risk controls; later schizophrenics were primarily characterized by hypersensitivity to criticism, whereas later schizotypal PD cases were characterized by disruptive and hyperexcitable behaviour (particularly males). In this study PDs other than schizotypal PD revealed no significant differences from low-risk normals on these childhood-behaviour dimensions. These conclusions are only partly in agreement with the New York High-Risk Project.

Schizophrenia-like Schizoaffective Disorder

Given the complexity of making a diagnosis of schizoaffective disorder, and of the schizophrenic subtype in particular, it is no surprise that the large-scale epidemiological surveys are not reporting prevalence rates of schizoaffective disorders. Control groups of family studies might be used as a substitute; it is apparent from those studies that the lifetime prevalence of schizoaffective disorder is in the range of schizophrenia (1% or less).

A substantial literature on the long-term course of schizoaffective disorders is available [55, 79]. Overall, schizoaffective disorders are located between schizophrenia and affective disorders by all indicators of course. Most of the follow-up studies in schizoaffective disorder are using a broad diagnostic concept which is preferentially subdivided by the unipolar/bipolar distinction. Unfortunately, only a minority of studies applies the schizophrenic subtype (RDC) separately or applies the more restrictive DSM-III-R/-IV definition.

The mainly schizophrenic subtype is characterized by a more severe course than the affective counterpart type [58, 59]. When using a broad diagnosis of schizoaffective disorder, the occurrence of schizophrenic symptoms at some stage of illness in absence of affective disorder and a family history of schizophrenia were key predictors of a worse outcome [80]. Whereas the occurrence of schizodepressive and schizophrenic episodes predicted worse outcome, the alternation between depressive and manic episodes was associated with relatively good outcome [80]. In another follow-up study (collaborative study), the patients with a schizophrenic subtype of schizoaffective disorder, particularly with a schizodepressive episode, had longer times to recovery from an acute episode, were more chronic, had more morbidity during follow-up (indicated by higher rehospitalization rates, more frequent suicidal behaviour, more affective symptoms and more psychosocial impairment) [58, 59]. Differences of follow-up indicators between the mainly schizophrenic and mainly affective subtype of patients with schizoaffective episodes were less pronounced. In contrast, subtyping by chronicity delivered more pronounced differences between subtypes in all indicators of course, with the chronic subtype demonstrating strong similarities with schizophrenia.

Only a few investigations studied the transition probabilities between schizoaffective disorders and schizophrenia [55] using a broad definition of schizoaffective disorders. Marneros *et al* [55] found that patients receiving the diagnosis of schizoaffective disorder later on partly started with an episode diagnosed as schizophrenia: 14% among unipolar depressive, 11% among bipolar schizoaffective disorders. During the whole course, 14% of cases finally diagnosed as unipolar depressive and 34% of those finally diagnosed as bipolar schizoaffective group experienced at least one episode diagnosed as schizophrenia. Despite this fluctuation, nearly 90% of patients with the diagnosis of schizophrenia in the first episode did not change the diagnosis in the long term; patients with the diagnosis of schizoaffective disorder (depressed type) in the first episode did not change their diagnosis across the whole long-term course [55]. The schizophrenic subtype was not analysed separately in this very carefully conducted follow-back study, but even higher proportions of schizoaffective patients with previous schizophrenic episodes can be expected in this more severe subgroup.

As a conclusion, there is some evidence that the schizophrenia-like subtype of broadly defined schizoaffective disorder (RDC) shares chronic course with schizophrenia; it is also likely that these episodes alternate with schizophrenic episodes in the same patients. The reported results support a nosological link between schizoaffective — defined by DSM-III-R/-IV or by RDC as mainly schizophrenic — and schizophrenic disorders and justify the inclusion into the schizophrenia spectrum.

FAMILIAL–GENETIC BASIS OF SPECTRUM CONCEPTS

Familiarity and Genetic Delineation of Spectrum Disorders

It is well documented that schizophrenia is familially mediated by a strong genetic component. There is also evidence that the other suggested spectrum disorders cluster in families if they are considered as distinct nosological entities. Several family studies demonstrated schizotypal PD and schizoaffective disorder (DSM-III-R/-IV) and schizoaffective disorder — mainly schizophrenic — (RDC), respectively, to cluster in families (Tables 5.2 and 5.3). One small family study [49] found schizoid traits to be more common among relatives of patients with schizoid PD; clustering of paranoid traits in paranoid PD families was less pronounced.

Very few studies explored if the familial aggregation of spectrum disorders is due partly to genetic factors. A small twin study is available for schizotypal PD [87], which reports an eight-fold higher monozygotic concordance rate, proposing a genetic component. Evidence also comes from adoption studies: a subgroup of index cases of the re-evaluated Danish Adoption Study was classified as schizotypal PD ($n = 41$); a substantially higher proportion of biological relatives of probands with this diagnosis were also classified as schizotypal PD (see Table 5.2) than of controls [22]. Thus, it can be concluded that schizotypal PD is partly under genetic control.

Three small twin studies including schizoaffective disorders were compiled by McCabe [88] with a four-fold higher concordance rate for monozygotic twins; as a limitation, this study used various older classification systems, and subdivision by the more schizophrenic type is not possible. In the re-evaluation of the Danish Adoption Study, a small subgroup ($n = 11$) of probands were diagnosed as schizoaffective disorder (DSM-III-R); although a substantial proportion of their biological first-degree relatives suffered from schizophrenia (9% vs. 1% among controls), not a single biological relative received the diagnosis of schizoaffective disorder (DSM-III-R). This result might be due to the slim sample size. However, the genetic basis of schizoaffective disorders becomes more evident if considered in the context of schizophrenia.

Familial Relationship of Axis I Spectrum Disorders and Schizophrenia

A familial relationship between schizophrenia and spectrum disorders can be evidenced by: (a) excess risk of a spectrum disorder in families of schizophrenics; (b) excess risk of schizophrenia in families of probands with a spectrum disorder; and (c) synergistic, interactive effects for schizophrenia as well as for spectrum diseases to relatives of families of a schizophrenic, given a second relative with a spectrum disorder.

TABLE 5.2 Lifetime prevalence rates (%) for schizophrenia-related disorders in families of probands with schizotypal personality disorder (PD).

Diagnosis in relatives	Relatives of probands with schizotypal PD vs. controls				
	Kendler et al, 1994 [22]	Kendler et al, 1993 [64, 81, 82]	Siever et al, 1990 [83]	Thaker et al, 1993 [84]*	Battaglia et al, 1995 [85]†
Schizophrenia	0 vs. 0.6	5.2 vs. 0.7	2.0 vs. 0	3.3 vs. 0	4.1 vs. 0
Schizoaffective disorder	2.4 vs. 0	3.9 vs. 0.7	0 vs. 0	5.6 vs. 1.4‡	2.0 vs. 0
Schizotypal PD	12.2 vs. 3.1	5.0 vs. 1.4	14.4 vs. 2.3	15.6 vs. 9.7	18.8 vs. 2.2

*Schizotypal PD and/or paranoid PD and/or schizoid PD.
†Control group: families of probands with non-schizotypal PD.
‡All functional psychoses with the exception of schizophrenia or schizophreniform disorder (DSM-III-R).

TABLE 5.3 Lifetime prevalence rates (%) for schizophrenia-related disorders in families of probands with schizophrenia spectrum diseases

Diagnosis in relatives	Relatives of probands with schizoaffective disorder (mainly schizophrenic) vs. schizoaffective disorder (mainly affective) and controls														
	Baron et al, 1982 [56] (RDC)			Kendler et al, 1986 [86]* (DSM-III)			Maj et al, 1991 [57] (DSM-III-R)			Maier et al, 1992 [60] (DSM-III-R)			Kendler et al, 1993 [81, 82] (DSM-III-R)		
	SA-S	SA-A	C	SA	PA	C	SA	PA	C	SA	PA	C	SA	PA	C
Schizophrenia/Schizophreniform disorder	4.1	0	—	5.6	4.3	0.2	8.7	3.8	0	3.8	2.0	0.5	4.4	2.5	0.7
Schizoaffective disorder (mainly schizophrenic)	0.7	0	—	2.7	0	0.1	—	—	—	2.4	1.1	0.2	3.9	5.7	0.7
Schizoaffective disorder (mainly affective)/Affective disorder with mood-incongruent psychotic features	0	3.2	—	—	—	—	—	—	—	2.3	2.5	0.5	3.0	3.1	2.7
Affective disorder	10.9	28.1	—	11.0	20.0	7.6	2.4	6.5	2.6	16.9	17.4	7.4	49.7	28.8	22.8

*Schizoaffective disorder (mainly affective) not reported: only psychotic affective disorder.
RDC, Research Diagnostic Criteria; SA, Schizoaffective; SA-S, Schizoaffective, mainly schizophrenic; SA-A, Schizoaffective, mainly affective; PA, Psychotic affective; C, Controls; —, No data available.

Spectrum Disorders in Families of Schizophrenics

A series of controlled family studies of schizophrenic probands, using structured clinical interviews for assessing the relatives, tried to replicate the Danish Adoption Study and explored the prevalence of the schizotypal PD among relatives [61, 89–96] (Tables 5.4 and 5.5). An excess of schizotypal PD in relatives of schizophrenics compared to controls is consistently observed in all controlled family studies. The effects are significant in all listed family studies with the exception of Coryell and Zimmerman [90]. Besides this strong qualitative result, the risk ratios are broadly varying. Limitations of sample sizes and different sensitivities of assessment instruments partly explain the variation of relative risk. Although the schizotypal PD criteria were mainly derived from the first subsample of the Danish Adoption Study, the relative risk in the extended sample using DSM-III-R criteria got attenuated with very low specificity. However, the Danish Adoption Study proposed in addition to demonstration of familial aggregation that this familial relationship is genetically mediated.

Paranoid and schizoid PDs were also investigated in some of the family studies (see Table 5.4). Consistently, paranoid and schizoid PDs were more common in relatives of schizophrenics compared to controls. On the other hand, paranoid and schizoid personalities were not more common among biological relatives of schizophrenics in the Danish Adoption Study, questioning a genetic relationship to schizophrenia [98]. These observations provide only limited evidence for an inclusion of these two PDs into the schizophrenia spectrum. Other family studies without controls from non-psychiatric populations support these results: for example, Onstad *et al* [92] found an excess of schizotypal PD and to a less degree also of paranoid PD in relatives of schizophrenics compared to relatives of depressed probands. Schizoid PD was equally distributed in this family study.

Although not consistently so, there is evidence for an excess of schizoaffective disorder among relatives of schizophrenics (either mainly schizophrenic subtype by RDC or by DSM-III-R/-IV definition); in favour for the hypothesis are the Danish Adoption Study, the high-risk studies and the majority of family studies, but not so the family study by Coryell and Zimmerman [90] (see Tables 5.4 and 5.5). Taking the limited sample size of the last study compared to the combined sample size of the other studies together, a familial link between schizoaffective disorder and schizophrenia can be concluded; the mainly affective schizoaffective disorder (RDC) and mood-incongruent psychotic affective disorder (DSM-III-R) are consistently less strongly related to schizophrenia but more strongly related to affective disorders (see Table 5.3); however (as a limitation), the two subtypes of schizoaffective disorder are overlapping in families and not breeding true.

TABLE 5.4 Aggregation of schizophrenia spectrum disorders (lifetime prevalence rates) among biological family members of schizophrenics

	Relatives of schizophrenics (index) (%)	Controls (%)
Danish Adoption Study		
• Kendler *et al*, 1994 [22]–DSM-III		
Schizophrenia	2.3	0.6
Schizoaffective disorder	1.1	0.0
Schizotypal personality disorder (PD)	4.5	3.1
All spectrum disorders	8.0	3.7
Family studies		
• Baron *et al*, 1985 [61]–DSM-III		
Schizophrenia	5.8	0.6
Atypical psychosis	0.5	0.0
Schizotypal PD, definite*	14.6	2.1
Schizoid PD, definite*	1.6	0.0
Paranoid PD, definite*	7.3	2.7
• Frangos *et al*, 1985 [89]–DSM-III		
Schizophrenia	3.3	0.6
Atypical psychosis	1.2	0.9
Schizotypal PD	0.9	0.3
Paranoid PD	1.4	0.1
Schizoid PD	2.1	0.9
• Coryell and Zimmerman, 1988 [90]–DSM-III		
Schizophrenia	1.4	0.0
Schizoaffective disorder	0.0	2.0
Schizotypal PD	2.8	2.5
Paranoid PD	1.4	0.6
• Kendler *et al*, 1993 [64, 81, 82]–DSM-III-R		
Schizophrenia	4.6	0.7
Schizoaffective disorder	2.3	0.7
Other psychoses	1.1	0.7
Schizotypal PD*	6.9	1.4
Paranoid PD*	1.4	0.4
• Maier *et al*, 1993, 1994 [95, 97]–RDC		
Schizophrenia	3.9	0.5
Schizoaffective disorder	2.2	0.7
Schizotypal PD	2.1	0.3
Schizoid PD	0.7	0.3
Paranoid PD	1.8	0.9

*Measured by an interview specifically designed for schizotypal personality traits (SIS).

TABLE 5.5 Lifetime risks for schizophrenia spectrum disorders (DSM-III-R) in children of a schizophrenic parent (high-risk studies)

	Copenhagen Study [93]		New York Study [96]	
	High risk (%)	Low risk (%)	High risk (%)	Low risk (%)
Schizophrenia including schizophreniform disorders	16.7	2.8	11.1	1.1
Schizoaffective disorder, schizophrenic type	0.5*	0.0*	1.9	1.1
Schizoaffective disorder, mainly affective/ psychotic affective			3.7	0.0
Other psychoses	3.6	0.9	5.6	0.0
Personality disorders				
schizotypal	18.8	5.0	4.5	0.0
schizoid	0.5	0.0	6.8	1.1
paranoid	2.6	0.0	6.8	1.1

*All schizoaffective disorders (including affective type).

Schizophrenia in Families of Probands with Spectrum Disorders

Evidence for aggregation of schizophrenia in families of spectrum disorder probands is less strong. Among spectrum PDs, informative studies are only available for schizotypal PD, but not so for paranoid and schizoid PD. All family studies with schizotypal PD index cases have a very limited sample size. In spite of this limitation, schizophrenia was more common among schizotypal PD relatives than among controls, with the single exception of the Danish Adoption Study (with only 41 relatives of schizotypal PD probands investigated) (see Table 5.2). The relative risk for schizophrenia in schizotypal PD families is overall lower than in families of schizophrenics. This result support the view that schizotypal PD is a less severe variant of schizophrenia. The increased prevalence of another spectrum disorder, schizoaffective disorder (DSM-III-R), among the biological relatives of schizophrenics also supports this view (see Table 5.2).

Most surprising is the relatively high prevalence of schizotypal PD in families of schizotypal PD patients, which exceeds the prevalence rate in relatives of schizophrenics. This is particularly the case for the Danish Adoption Study. In addition, the prevalence rates for schizotypal PD in relatives of probands in the other studies listed in Table 5.2 are higher than predicted from family studies in patients with schizophrenia (see Tables 5.4 and 5.5).

Similarly, in families of patients with schizoaffective disorder (DSM-III-R) or schizoaffective disorder, mainly schizophrenic (RDC), schizophrenia is more common than among control families (see Table 5.3). The relative risk for schizophrenia is overall higher among relatives of probands with schizoaffective disorder compared to relatives of probands with mood-incongruent disorder or with psychotic affective disorder.

Synergistic Effects

Only two studies explored the combined effects, on the other relatives, of schizophrenia in one and spectrum disorders in another relative of the same family. Baron *et al* [61] found that the diagnosis of schizotypal PD in a parent of a schizophrenic index case increases the risk for schizophrenia as well as for schizotypal PD in the sibling of the index case (compared to families without parental schizotypal PD) in a superadditive manner. Kendler *et al* [99], in the Roscommon Family Study, also found this synergistic effect: given two affected relatives (schizophrenia in the proband, schizotypal PD in one of the parents), the risk for schizophrenia, for schizotypal PD and for all spectrum disorders together increased substantially by a factor between two and five compared to families with only a schizophrenic index case. In this particular study, synergistic effects on other disorders (e.g. affective disorders) were not observed. However, this diagnostic specificity of synergistic effects on other family members is not in agreement with other studies [100].

In summary, there is currently no conclusive familial–genetic evidence on how restrictively the spectrum of schizophrenia should be defined. The Roscommon Family Study is proposing the broadest variant by including all psychotic disorders (including psychotic affective disorder), schizotypal PD and paranoid PD in the spectrum [99]. In contrast, the Danish Adoption Study is proposing the most restrictive concept, including only schizotypal PD and schizoaffective disorder (DSM-III-R) [22, 98]. There is consensus by familial–genetic studies that schizotypal PD as well as schizoaffective disorders (mainly schizophrenic) are related to schizophrenia. Evidence to date for including paranoid and schizoid PDs is not convincing in a familial–genetic perspective. Future twin and adoption studies should focus on the genetic relationship between these two PDs and schizophrenia. Concluding evidence also requires additional family studies starting with paranoid and schizoid PD probands to explore the risk for schizophrenia among the relatives.

Diagnostic Specificity of the Familial Relationship to Schizophrenia

The Relationship of Non-affective Psychotic Disorders to Schizophrenia

Symptomatic overlap between schizophrenia/schizoaffective disorders on the one hand, and delusional disorders on the other hand motivate the hypothesis of a familial–genetic link between these groups of disorders. Again, a familial link between schizophrenic and delusional disorders can be demonstrated by: (a) excess risk of delusional disorders in families of schizophrenics; and (b) excess risk of schizophrenia in families of patients with delusional disorders.

There is one study observing an excess risk of delusional disorders in families of schizophrenics of the Iowa family study [101]. This result is also supported by a previous analysis of a subsample of the Danish Adoption Study [102], whereas a more recent analysis in the extended sample came to the opposite conclusion [98]. A familial relationship to schizotypal PD was also excluded [103]. However, the familial relationship to paranoid PD is stronger. Two reports provided evidence for aggregation of paranoid PD or paranoid personality features (e.g. suspiciousness) in relatives of delusional patients [103, 104], proposing that schizotypal PD and paranoid PD are related to nosologically different axis I disorders.

The majority of studies were unable to report a substantial excess of schizophrenia among relatives of delusional disorder patients: three family studies [103, 105, 106] found no excess of schizophrenia nor of other spectrum disorders in families of delusional patients. Thus, there is no strong evidence to include delusional disorders in the schizophrenic spectrum.

Other non-affective psychotic disorders seem to be more closely related to schizophrenia than to delusional disorders [82]. However, this group seems to be heterogeneous in clinical and familial–genetic respect [107]. Thus, a familial–genetic link to schizophrenia can be postulated at most for a subgroup of non-affective disorders.

The Relationship of Spectrum Disorders to other Disorders

Schizophrenia spectrum disorders do not only occur in the familial context of schizophrenia; their risk might also be increased in families of probands with non-spectrum diagnoses.

Schizophrenia-related PDs. One high-risk study reports an excess of this disorder in children of affective disorder probands [108]. In another study, an increased risk for paranoid PD disorder in relatives of patients with unipolar depression was also reported, but the risk for schizotypal PD in relatives of depressed probands was not substantially increased [95]. A third family study found excess rates of schizophrenia-related PDs (schizotypal and paranoid PDs) also among relatives of borderline PD (not comorbid for schizotypal PD) comparable to relatives of schizophrenics by quantity; in contrast, the prevalence of chronic schizophrenia did not differ between both groups of relatives [109]; a more detailed analysis of this study concluded that schizotypal PD without comorbid affective PD traits (as borderline

PD) may more specifically describe the characteristics familially related to schizophrenia.

Schizophrenia-related axis I disorder. Schizoaffective disorders (DSM-III-R) or schizophrenic type-schizoaffective disorder (RDC) are slightly more common among relatives of affective disorder probands, particularly those with psychotic features, compared to controls (see Table 5.3). The New York High-Risk Study reports the maximal excess of schizophrenia-like schizoaffective disorder (RDC) among children of patients with affective disorders (6.8% vs. 0% in controls) [110]. Some studies found psychotic affective disorders (particularly mood-incongruent psychotic) to be related to schizoaffective disorder (DSM-III-R/-IV): the risk for schizophrenia in relatives of probands with psychotic affective disorder is slightly increased; the risk for psychotic affective disorder is increased in relatives of probands with schizoaffective disorder (DSM-III-R/-IV) (see Table 5.3). A clear exception of this constellation is the family study by Baron *et al* [56] using the RDC system. A series of family, high-risk and adoption studies [22, 90, 93] are not considering psychotic affective disorder separately. Therefore, there is no consensus to include these subtypes of affective disorder in the schizophrenia spectrum.

Schizotypal Traits with High Familial Specificity

Given that the familial relationship between schizophrenia and spectrum disorders is less specific than ideally expected, a symptom-specific approach might be instrumented for sharpening this relationship. This criteria-specific strategy was up to now only applied to the various versions of the diagnostic definitions of schizotypal personality. Those criteria are defining the strongest familial relationship to schizophrenia which are most discriminative between schizophrenics and controls. Oddness of behaviour as well as negative-like features of the schizotype are most discriminative in this respect.

Examples from more Recent Studies

- Gunderson *et al* [12] reanalysed the discriminative power of traits proposed for schizotypal personality (including the DSM-III criteria) for the borderline relatives in the Danish Adoption Study. Maximal discriminative power was found for social isolation, poor rapport, undue social anxiety, social dysfunction at work, odd appearance and suspiciousness, whereas magical thinking and illusions were substantially less discriminative. Psychotic-like symptoms which are included in all current and previous definitions of schizotypal PD were less useful; these symptoms were particularly not able to define the border between schizotypal and borderline PD. Furthermore, "somatization" was observed in the Danish Adoption Study as a characteristic of biological relatives of schizophrenics without being integrated in any assessment instrument.

- Kendler *et al* [38] found the strongest discrimination between relatives of schizophrenics and controls for a factor comprising odd speech and cognitive slippage, for social dysfunction and lack of motivation, and for the negative schizotype factor comprising poor rapport, oddness and aloofness. Borderline features (affective instability, impulsivity and boredom) did not differ between the two groups of relatives, and positive schizotypy (illusions, ideas of reference, magic thinking, suspiciousness and depersonalization) were only weak discriminators.

- Squires-Wheeler *et al* [108] and Maier *et al* [95] explored the discriminative power for relatives of schizophrenics versus controls in combination with the diagnostic specificity (by comparison between relatives of probands with depression versus controls). The first study found odd behaviour, odd speech, inappropriate affect and recurrent illusions to distinguish non-psychotic relatives of schizophrenics and controls. Although less pronounced, all of these differentiating traits were also more common in relatives of patients with affective disorders. In the second study, odd behaviour, odd speech and affective flattening were the only DSM-III-R criteria for schizotypal PD which were substantially more common among relatives of schizophrenics compared to controls and to relatives of depressed probands. Suspiciousness and undue social anxiety clustered strongly in relatives of schizophrenics but also in relatives of depressed probands.

- Lyons *et al* [111] compared schizotypal PD in relatives of patients with schizophrenia to the same disorder in relatives of patients with affective disorder. They found more inadequate rapport to characterize schizophrenia related to schizotypal PD; impulsive behaviour and comorbidity with histrionic PD were less common in this group.

- Thaker *et al* [112] administered the Chapman scales to familial schizophrenia spectrum personality-disordered subjects (SSPD), who were family members of schizophrenic patients, and to non-familial SSPD patients without a family history for schizophrenia. The non-familial SSPD subjects scored higher on "magical ideation", "perceptual aberration" and "impulsive nonconformity" than the familial SSPD and non-SSPD groups. "Physical anhedonia" was especially pronounced in the familial SSPD group, while "social anhedonia" was elevated in both groups of SSPD. Importantly, only in the non-familial group was it possible to predict statistically a spectrum disorder diagnosis from extreme scores in the Chapman scales. This implies that the self-reported schizotypal experiences of subjects with spectrum disorders according to DSM-III differ depending on whether or not they have a family member suffering from schizophrenia. Importantly, "positive" schizotypal traits, like those assessed with the Perceptual Aberration and Magical Ideation Scales, do not seem to be elevated in familial SSPD. This is very much in agreement with the study of Clementz et al [113], who found only "physical anhedonia", but not "perceptual aberration", to be elevated in a sample of 146 first-degree relatives of schizophrenic patients. Franke et al [114] replicated this result with a smaller sample of siblings of schizophrenic patients, and within the siblings also found evidence for a correlation of only this "negative" schizotypal trait with reduced performance on tests sensitive to frontal lobe dysfunction. Thus, most studies agree that negative schizotypal traits run in families of schizophrenics.

Consequently, focus on odd behaviour and negative schizotypy in the definition of schizotypal PD would increase the specificity of the relationship between schizophrenia and schizotypal PD. But the definition of schizotypal PD in the widespread diagnostic manuals is a compromise between characterization of non-psychotic relatives of schizophrenics and characterizing patients with schizophrenia-like personality patterns asking for treatment [14]. Thus, the currently available definition of schizotypal PD is suboptimal in a familial–genetic perspective and might include multiple nosologically different subgroups.

Spectrum Disorders and Traits: Less Severe Variants of Schizophrenia

Spectrum diseases are conceptualized as less severe variants of schizophrenia, with causes of spectrum disorders operating also as causes of schizophrenia; the number of risk factors contributing to spectrum disorders is smaller than it is assumed for schizophrenia. This concept can be hypothetically extended to include subclinical signs and symptoms occurring in the absence of a lifetime diagnosis of a psychiatric disorder more frequently among biological relatives of schizophrenia than among controls. These subclinical psychopathological, neuropsychological and neurophysiological features might be assumed to be also determined by familial risk factors which also influence schizophrenia; however, the number and weight of involved risk factors is lower.

The multiple threshold model combines contributing aetiological factors into a hypothetical vulnerability dimension, the liability to develop schizophrenia, which is graded by severity; the model assumes that all of the disorders assigned to the spectrum are influenced by the same liability which combines familial and genetic factors. The liability predisposing to a specific spectrum disorder is located between two disorder-specific thresholds. Beyond a hypothetical threshold schizophrenia will occur; submaximal values are associated with less severe variants of schizophrenia. Lower values are not associated with any impairment induced by aetiological factors contributing to schizophrenia. Given inconsistent evidence that paranoid PD and atypical psychoses belong to the spectrum, these conditions are not included in the model.

The model predicts that: (a) given the strong familial impact on the liability dimension, the risk for schizophrenia as well as for all assumed minor variants of schizophrenia are co-aggregating and clustering in families of schizophrenics; (b) the strongest familial aggregation of schizophrenia and of all of its minor variants occurs in the condition with maximal liability (i.e. in schizophrenic probands); (c) the risk for schizophrenia as well as for all assumed minor variants of schizophrenia is also increased in relatives of probands with all indicated minor variants (i.e. all spectrum disorders).

Points (a) and (b) are supported by the reviewed literature for schizotypal PD as well as for schizoaffective disorder. However, it is uncertain if (c) is true. Particularly, schizotypal PD is more common among relatives of patients with schizotypal PD than among relatives of schizophrenics in the majority of studies investigating both groups of relatives. In contrast to schizotypal PD, the patterns of familial aggregation of schizoaffective disorders are more in concordance with this model. Therefore, this model might be too simple. According to the majority of studies, a modification (e.g. including only subgroups of schizotypal PD) might be more appropriate. Furthermore, the majority of studies do not support the inclusion of paranoid PD and delusional disorder (because evidence for (c) is missing). A possible explanation for the discrepant results of family studies is that only subtypes of paranoid PD and delusional disorder belong to the spectrum.

However, there is one major study which behaves differently from the majority of comparable studies. Kendler *et al* [99] proposed a multiple threshold model including — besides schizophrenia, schizoaffective disorder and the combination of schizotypal/paranoid PD — also other non-affective psychoses and psychotic affective disorder. Although there remain inconsistencies, for example no excess of schizophrenia in families of non-affective psychotic disorder [106], this proposed model fitted the family data emerging from the Roscommon Study. It remains an unresolved issue why conclusions from other very carefully conducted studies, for example the re-evaluation of the Danish Adoption Study by the same author [22] with the maximal risk for schizotypal PD in biological relatives of schizotypal PD probands, but not in schizophrenic probands, are at variance with this multiple threshold model.

NEUROBIOLOGICAL CORRELATES

The inclusion of a brief overview of neurobiological findings in studies on schizotypal PD and schizotypy is motivated by three assumptions. First, as pointed out above, the spectrum concept is based on phenomenolog-ical similarities with schizophrenic psychoses and on familial aggregation of spectrum disorders in families of schizophrenic patients. Neurobiology is another level of description. Similar neuropsychological, neurophysio-logical, neuromorphological and neurochemical changes in schizophrenia and in schizophrenia spectrum disorders or in schizotypal subjects would strengthen the case of spectrum disorders to be aetiologically and nosolog-ically related to schizophrenia. Second, this approach might also be fruitful regarding the question of heterogeneity within the group of spectrum disor-ders. Finally, delineation of neurobiological changes in spectrum disorders is important for the development and refinement of treatment strategies, which will be discussed in the next section. Raine *et al* [115] provide more detailed information about empirical findings in schizotypy and schizotypal PD.

Neuropsychology

Executive Functioning

The Wisconsin Card Sorting Test (WCST) requires executive functioning and is widely used to assess frontal lobe integrity. Schizophrenic patients generally are impaired in the WCST. In one study [116], interesting because of the range of patient groups and neuropsychological measures, patients with schizotypal PD, patients with other PD, schizophrenic patients and normal controls were given a battery of neuropsychological tasks including the WCST, a test of verbal fluency and Trails B (all three measures are sensitive to frontal dysfunction). In addition, tests of more general intellectual functioning (vocabulary and block design subtests of the Wechsler Adult Intelligence Scale-Revised) were administered. The data revealed significant differences between schizotypal PD patients and patients with other PDs for the WCST and for Trails B, but not for general intellectual functioning, which suggests that prefrontal functions are particularly impaired in patients with schizotypal PD [116]. In a study which controlled for selection bias, by employing personality-disordered subjects from an epidemiological study (rather than schizotypal PD subjects identified by a schizophrenic relative), Tien *et al* [117] found schizotypal personality traits to be strongly correlated with perserverative responses on the WCST. Furthermore, Tien *et al* noted differences between schizotypal, paranoid and schizoid traits with regard to WCST performance, suggesting differences in frontal functioning within the group of spectrum disorders. There is at least one study where schizotypal PD patients did not differ from normal controls in the WCST [118].

Studies of the relatives of schizophrenic patients who may display schizo-typal psychopathology suggest that these individuals often perform worse than controls on measures of set alternation and verbal fluency as well as abstraction and verbal memory [119]. In a study employing frontal lobe tasks and self-ratings of schizotypal experiences, siblings of schizophrenics performed worse than healthy controls in the WCST, verbal fluency and Trail Making Tests (TMT) [114]. Furthermore, the score on the Physical Anhedonia Scale (but not the Perceptual Aberration Scale) was increased in the siblings of schizophrenics and correlated with the impairments in WCST and TMT. Volunteers selected by virtue of their schizotypal characteristics [120, 121] also have been shown to perform worse than controls in the WCST.

Miller *et al* [122] employed the Luria-Nebraska Neuropsychological Battery (which includes tests of executive functioning like Trails B and the Halstead Category Test) to compare the cognitive performance of schizoaffective and schizophrenic patients. No differences emerged between these groups.

Working Memory

Working memory, the ability to temporarily hold in mind and to operate on information, is impaired in schizophrenic patients [123, 124] and their relatives [125]. No studies employing schizotypal PD patients have been published so far, but students scoring high on the Perceptual Aberration Scale, thus showing some schizotypal symptoms, were less accurate in delayed spatial responding and also had more failures in maintaining response set during the WCST [126].

Sustained Attention

A popular test of attentional performance is the Continuous Performance Task (CPT), where subjects have to react when target stimuli appear in a rather lengthy series of stimuli presented at regular intervals. CPT performance is generally impaired in schizophrenic patients and their relatives [127, 128] (see ref. [129] for a review). Offspring of schizophrenic patients, schizotypal volunteers and schizotypal patients make more errors during the CPT [130]. A very informative study of Roitman *et al* [131] compared 30 subjects with schizotypal PD, 35 subjects with other PD (from the non-odd cluster), 36 subjects with schizophrenia, and 20 healthy controls without psychiatric disorder. Only schizotypal PD patients, but not patients with other PD, performed worse than the healthy group on two identical pair versions of the CPT, as did the schizophrenic group. In a large community sample, low CPT performance was associated with high scores on the Perceptual Aberration Scale and in the SPQ [132]. A similar association between CPT performance and positive schizotypal symptoms (assessed with clinical interview) was found in a group of first-degree relatives of schizophrenic patients [133].

No such association between CPT performance and self-reported perceptual aberration or physical anhedonia was found in another study with first-degree relatives [128].

Backward Masking

Backward masking (BM) is a procedure to assess "early" visual perception by masking a relevant stimulus display after a brief (e.g. 30–120 ms) interval. The BM performance of schizophrenic patients is often found to be impaired. A recent study of Green *et al* [134] found reduced BM performance in a group of unaffected siblings of schizophrenics, as compared to healthy controls, which shows that reduced BM performance is an enduring vulnerability indicator. Patients with schizotypal PD have also been found to be impaired with regard to BM [135]. A later study did not find BM performance differences between schizotypal PD patients and controls [136], but did find significant correlations of "negative" schizotypal PD features (like social deficit symptoms) with BM performance and critical stimulus duration (another measure of sensory processing). Schizoaffective patients were found to be even more impaired in the BM task than schizophrenic patients, while patients with a borderline PD performed like healthy controls [137].

Declarative Memory

Declarative memory is another domain of cognitive functioning where schizophrenic patients [138] and their first-degree relatives are often impaired [119]. There are few data on memory functioning in schizotypy and schizotypal PD. Voglmaier *et al* [139] found schizotypal PD patients to have a reduced performance in the California Verbal Learning Test, in addition to being impaired on the WCST. Cannon *et al* [140] studied siblings of schizophrenics with a comprehensive neuropsychological battery including verbal memory, and found the subgroup of siblings with a schizotypal PD to be more impaired than siblings without schizophrenia spectrum symptoms. A normal memory performance in schizotypal subjects identified by high scores on the Chapman's scales was found by La Porte *et al* [141]. Manschreck *et al* [142], in a carefully controlled study, compared context memory in schizoaffective, schizophrenic, depressive and healthy groups. Schizoaffective and schizophrenic patients both attained smaller improvements in performance with increasing context than the other groups. Beatty *et al* [143] found that schizophrenic patients did show accelerated forgetting on delayed recall of verbal material, which was not present in the schizoaffective group.

Thought Disorder and Cognitive Inhibition

Cognitive slippage is one of the characteristics of schizotypy according to Meehl [8]. Cognitive slippage denotes a mild form of formal thought disorder, corresponding to the loosening of associations already noted by Bleuler. Several methods have been proposed to measure changes in associative processes, which may underly formal thought disorder [144], but only a few have been applied to study this aspect of schizotypal thinking. Perhaps the method most closely reflecting the loosening of associations noted by clinicians is the Thought Disorder Index (TDI), derived by formal analysis of Rorschach protocols [145]. Siblings of schizophrenics show more thought disorder, measured with the TDI, than control subjects [146]. The same is true for subjects with high scores on the Perceptual Aberration Scale [147]. Edell [148] found an equally elevated TDI in subjects with schizotypal PD (DSM-III criteria) and in patients with a schizophrenic disorder, as compared to a non-psychiatric control group. Duchene et al [149] reported that students with above average scores in the Magical Ideation (MI) Scale produced more words with a low probability of occurrence in a verbal fluency task, while the total number of words uttered did not depend on the MI score; the authors interpreted this finding to indicate reduced inhibitory semantic network functioning, which may underly creativity as well as thought disorder. Several studies used the "negative priming" procedure to study semantic activation and inhibition processes in relation to schizotypal symptoms in non-clinical populations. Beech et al [150] found reduced negative priming in subjects scoring high on the Schizotypal Personality Scale (STA) [31] which reflects mostly positive schizotypal symptoms. Similar results were obtained by Peters et al [151] and by Moritz and Mass [152]. Reduced negative priming has also been found in schizophrenic patients [153], especially in those with present or past positive symptoms [154], but no data are yet available for subjects with spectrum disorders.

Neurophysiology

Smooth Pursuit Eye Movements

Dysfunction of the smooth pursuit eye movement (SPEM) system has been consistently reported in 50–85% of chronic schizophrenic patients [155, 156] and in relatives of schizophrenics [157]. Siever et al [158] employed a "biological high-risk approach" to study the psychopathological correlates of SPEM dysfunction in the population. Almost 300 college students were screened for their tracking accuracy electro-oculographically. Those with the least accurate tracking were restudied in the laboratory by both electro-oculographic and infrared tracking recorders. They also participated in an extensive series of clinical interviews and ratings. The low-accuracy or impaired trackers exhibited a significantly higher prevalence of DSM-III schizotypal PD and a higher prevalence of schizotypal characteristics than the high-accuracy trackers [158, 159]. Comparing schizophrenics, patients with schizotypal PD and control subjects, about 50% of the first two groups but only 25% of the controls show impaired eye tracking performance. In addition, there seems to be a relation between eye tracking impairment and more severe enduring symptoms across the spectrum of schizophrenic and schizophrenia-related disorders [160]. Impaired SPEM performance in subjects with schizotypal PD (according to DSM-III-R) was also reported by Lencz et al [161]. Impaired tracking is associated with deficit-like symptoms, but not with psychotic-like symptoms in schizotypal PD [162]. In another study, an additional group of other non-schizophrenia-related PDs was included. The results demonstrated that only patients with clinically defined schizotypal and not other non-schizophrenia-related PDs are biologically related to schizophrenia [130]. To understand the precise oculomotor mechanism underlying the abnormality of SPEM in schizophrenia spectrum disorders, the traditional smooth pursuit gain measure and the target velocity were obtained in first-degree relatives of probands with schizophrenia and in subjects recruited from the community. Relatives of patients with schizophrenia, particularly those with schizotypal PD, have specific deficits in predictive pursuit based on only extraretinal motion signals. Normal smooth pursuit gain in response to both retinal and extraretinal motion signals is likely due to compensation based on retinal motion information. The latter suggests normal retinal motion processing and smooth pursuit motor output [163]. Subjects with increased scores on either the Perceptual Aberration or the Physical Anhedonia self-report scales also have an impaired SPEM performance [164].

Antisaccade Errors

Another consistent finding in schizophrenic patients with regard to oculo-motor functioning is a disinhibition of reflexive saccades when the task calls for an "antisaccade" to a position opposite of a stimulus [165]. Relatives of schizophrenic patients also have an increased proportion of antisaccade errors [165–167]. Studies including subjects with schizotypal PD have not been published to date, but recently O'Driscoll et al [168] reported that subjects scoring high on the Perceptual Aberration Scale made more antisac-cade errors and also had reduced SPEM quality, as compared to controls. Interestingly, Ross et al [169] found the disinhibition of reflexive saccades during an antisaccade task to occur specifically in parents of schizophrenic patients who themselves had a positive family history for chronic psychosis, as compared to their spouses with a negative family history. Since the former are more likely to be carriers of susceptibility genes, this finding supports the assumption that saccadic disinhibition is a genetically based trait. Conceptually replicating this result with another procedure, Ross et al [170] found also a failure to suppress anticipatory saccades during SPEM in likely genetic carriers.

Neurological "Soft Signs"

Meehl [8] has argued that neurological "soft signs" (NSS) may also be indicators for the basic neurointegrative defect common to schizophrenia and schizotypal personality. Neurological soft signs, like dysdiadochokinesis, are more frequent in schizophrenic patients than in controls with other psychiatric disorders, although the latter groups often have also more neurological soft signs than healthy subjects [171]. NSS are more frequent in healthy relatives of schizophrenic patients [172], and several high-risk studies have found neuromotor abnormalities in children of schizophrenic patients. Barbara Fish has coined the term "pandysmaturation" to describe early developmental peculiarities in these high-risk groups, and has found pandysmaturation in childhood often to be associated with schizotypal disorder in adulthood [173, 174]. Neuromotor precursors of schizophrenia have also been described by Walker et al [175] using home movies of children who later became schizophrenic.

Evoked Potentials

A reduction of the amplitude of late evoked brain potentials (ERP), as well as a latency delay, while certainly not being pathognomonic, has often been reported in schizophrenia patients and their relatives [176, 177]. In the latter study, most relatives who were presumed obligate gene carriers showed a delayed auditory P300, suggesting that some ERP abnormalities may be genetically based. The results of high-risk studies with children of schizophrenics are inconsistent [178, 179]. Amplitude of P300 and N200 has also been reported to be reduced in volunteers scoring high on the Chapman Anhedonia Scales [180]. In two studies, a delayed P300 was noted in schizotypal PD patients [181, 182], but the delay was also found in individuals with borderline PD. In another study of clinically selected schizotypal patients, the P300 amplitude was intermediate between schizophrenics and normal controls, but, in contrast to the amplitude of P300 in schizophrenic patients compared with that in controls, the P300 amplitude in schizotypal patients did not significantly differ from that of adequate controls [162, 183]. Trestman et al [184] again found schizotypal PD patients to have a P300 amplitude in between that of schizophrenics and healthy subjects, and not significantly different from P300 amplitude in the latter group.

Pre-pulse Inhibition

Inhibition of the startle reflex by a weak pre-pulse (PPI) is a paradigm to investigate sensorimotor gating in humans and animals [185]. Because schizophrenic patients have reduced PPI, and all effective antipsychotic drugs normalize PPI in animal models, PPI is an attractive paradigm for pharmacological research. Schizotypal PD patients, whether treated with neuroleptic medication or not, were found to have reduced PPI [186]. However, subjects selected for hypothetical "psychosis proneness" by having extreme scores either on the Perceptual Aberration/Magical Ideation or on the Physical Anhedonia Scales, were not found to have reduced PPI, and did not differ from controls with regard to backward masking [187]. Subjects with high scores on these self-report measures of schizotypy had more psychotic and affective symptoms, but they did not have schizotypal PD. Less PPI has also been demonstrated with the auditory P50 component of the auditory evoked potential in biological relatives of schizophrenics [188, 189], but has not yet been studied in spectrum disorder.

Correlations Between Neurofunctional Deficits and Schizotypal Symptoms

While ample evidence suggests that schizotypal personality traits and neurofunctional dysfunctions similar to those found in schizophrenic patients are more frequent in relatives of schizophrenics, few data are available concerning the question of whether psychopathological and neuropsychological/neurophysiological deviations correlate in these samples. This is important with regard to the question of whether psychopathological and neurofunctional deviations, as far as they are genetically influenced, are expressions of the same or different genes conferring susceptibility for the disease. A recent report from the New York High-Risk Project [190], studying young adults with parents from different parental groups, found that negative (e.g. interpersonal) schizotypal personality traits were more frequent in children of schizophrenic parents compared with children of affectively disordered or healthy parents, and that these negative features correlated with verbal working memory and P300 decrement. Interestingly, positive (e.g. perceptual) schizotypal traits were more frequent in both groups with parental psychiatric disorders and did not correlate with working memory or P300 amplitude scores. This might imply that positive and negative schizotypal personality traits may be based on different pathophysiological processes. A similar conclusion was reached by Siever *et al* [183], who stated after a review of the literature:

> The study of patients with schizotypal personality disorder suggests that a dimension of deficit-like or "negative" symptoms of asociality and interpersonal impairment may be associated with neuropsychological and psychophysiological correlates of altered cortical, particularly frontal, function. On the other hand, the psychotic-like or "positive" symptoms seem to be more related to increases in dopaminergic activity that may be partially responsive to neuroleptic treatment.

Data from the same High-Risk Project also show that the correlation between psychopathological and neurocognitive deviations may show up over time in longitudinal analyses. Attentional impairment, assessed in childhood, was more frequent in children of schizophrenic parents, and was found to be related to physical anhedonia in adolescence [191]. Attentional impairment and physical anhedonia both were related to worse social outcome in young adulthood [70]. Thus, attentional dysfunction may be an early indicator of later negative schizotypal personality features, possibly because social interactions require information-processing skills, such as detection of subtle emotional cues regulating social exchange.

Neurotransmitters and Neuroendocrinology

Schizophrenia is a severe neuropsychiatric disorder and there is solid literature for a neurochemical basis. However, the disease is heterogeneous, and the findings often subtle, leading to non-replicable results. In addition, there are many confounding variables, like the treatment with neuroleptics, which are difficult to rule out. Therefore, it is promising to research schizophrenia spectrum disorders — especially using biochemical markers — as they show a considerable phenomenological overlap with schizophrenia but usually are not confounded by treatment variables.

Schizoid and Paranoid Personality Disorders

Performing a Medline literature research between 1966 and November 1998, using the term "schizoid personality disorder", 455 publications were listed. Of these, only four dealt with the topic of dopamine and related terms. One found that dyskinesia and dyskinetic-like movements are more common in subjects with schizophrenia spectrum personality (primarily schizotypal, less schizoid) than in normal subjects and are related to positive symptoms. Furthermore, a failure of normal behavioural sensitization mechanisms after dextroamphetamine challenge was seen in subjects with schizophrenia spectrum personality [192]. In two further publications, only a hypothetical relation was drawn between schizoid PD and dopamine, while reviewing posterior fossa lesions associated with neuropsychiatric symptoms [193] or examining the blink rate in childhood schizophrenia spectrum disorder [194]. Dealing with schizoid PD not like a disorder but rather like a personality trait, one study described an association between the dopamine D_2 receptor *Taq A1* allele and schizoid/avoidant behaviour. Additionally, a weaker association between the *480-bp VNTR 10/10* allele of the dopamine transporter *(DAT1)* gene and schizoid/avoidant behaviour was similarly found [195]. However, until now this finding seeks replication.

Searching the same period of time with Medline, no article was found dealing with paranoid PD.

Schizotypal Personality Disorder

The dopamine "hypothesis" of schizophrenia, which in its simplest form states that schizophrenia is associated with excessive dopaminergic function in the central nervous system, has persisted — despite relevant criticism — as the predominant neurochemical hypothesis of schizophrenia for three decades [196]. Therefore, it seems feasible to examine the dopaminergic system in schizophrenia spectrum disorders where one might hypothetically find similar but less severe changes as described in schizophrenia.

Homovanillic acid (HVA) is a product of the dopaminergic metabolism and often used as a peripheral indicator of dopamine function. Plasma HVA concentrations have been found to be significantly higher in schizotypal PD patients compared with normal controls and other PD comparison groups, but do not seem to be related to any of the usual confounding variables endemic to schizophrenia studies, such as neuroleptic treatment, etc. [197]. Plasma HVA concentrations are significantly positively correlated with the psychotic-like symptoms of schizotypal PD, but not with other deficit-related symptoms of schizotypal PD. Similarly, cerebrospinal fluid HVA concentrations have been found to be elevated in schizotypal PD patients compared with patients with other PD; they again correlate with psychotic-like schizotypal PD symptoms, but not deficit-like symptoms [198, 199]. In contrast, in the relatives of schizophrenic patients with schizotypal PD who are primarily characterized by negative or deficit-like symptoms, concentrations of plasma HVA were in fact lower than those observed in non-schizotypal relatives of schizophrenia patients or controls. The reductions in HVA correlated with the degree of deficit-like symptoms and with neuropsychological measures sensitive to frontal dysfunction [130].

Patients meeting criteria for borderline and schizotypal PDs demonstrated a worsening of psychotic-like symptoms and anxiety after an amphetamine infusion [200]. Patients with schizotypal PD receiving amphetamine demonstrated an improvement in neurocognitive performance, for example measured as an improvement of WCST performance [201], although there was no marked worsening of psychotic-like symptoms.

In conclusion, there is some evidence for an overactivity of the dopaminergic system in patients with schizotypal PD, which is correlated with positive symptoms. Very interesting is the preliminary result from amphetamine challenges, demonstrating improved cognitive functioning in schizotypal PD patients without affecting the other florid symptoms. It is interesting to note that there is some overlap between schizotypal PD and borderline PD.

Schizophrenia-like Schizoaffective Disorder

Specific morphological, physiological, neuropsychological or biochemical studies have rarely been undertaken in schizoaffective disorder. That lack is probably due to diagnostic inconsistencies and disagreements over the years and to the general assumption to characterize such issues first in the well-defined pure mood disorders and schizophrenia. Nevertheless, a number of biological studies of schizophrenia have included patients with schizoaffective disorder, where internal data analyses failed to distinguish them from the larger group of schizophrenic patients under study. The exceptions are some endocrine studies, like one where the 24-h plasma cortisol response to dexamethasone in 19 patients with coexisting depressive and psychotic features, and 12 non-depressed patients with only psychotic features were examined [202]. The rate and degree of abnormal dexamethasone suppression was greatest in patients who met RDC criteria for primary depressive disorder. Patients who met criteria for schizoaffective (mainly schizophrenic), depressed and other psychotic disorders did not differ from each other in their response to dexamethasone.

Neuroimaging

Neuroimaging studies have helped considerably to introduce the concept of schizophrenia as being a brain disorder. Meta-analytical studies of structural imaging [Computed Tomography (CT) and Magnetic Resonance Imaging (MRI)] have established the enlargement of the ventricular system [203] and the reduction of the hippocampal volume [204] as robust findings in schizophrenia. No correlation with disease duration and no tendency for progression of subcortical pathology in follow-up studies are arguments that these morphological changes are a consequence of disturbed brain development, rather than being based on an ongoing brain disease [205]. At the moment, the underlying causes for these changes are widely unclear. Therefore, in order to study the aetiopathogenetic factors, schizophrenia spectrum disorders are very promising, as there is a phenomenological overlap on one hand, and, furthermore, the confounding variable of treatment can easily be excluded.

Schizoid and Paranoid Personality Disorder

Reviewing the literature between 1966 and November 1998 in the way shown above, no article was found specifically researching these disorders with the means of brain imaging.

Schizotypal Personality Disorder

Initial studies of schizotypal patients from clinical populations have suggested increases in ventricle-to-brain ratio (VBR) in schizotypal patients compared with other PD patients and/or normal controls. Furthermore, an increase was found in lateral VBR (particularly the left lateral VBR) in the schizotypal patients compared with the patients with other PDs [183, 197]. In a subsequent, well-controlled CT scan study [206], the VBR was obtained in 36 male schizotypal PD patients, in 23 males with other PDs, in 133 male schizophrenic patients, and in 42 male normal volunteers. The mean body of the lateral VBR was significantly greater in the schizotypal PD patients than in the patients with other PDs. The VBR of the schizotypal PD patients did not differ significantly from either that of the normal volunteers or the schizophrenic patients but was intermediate between the two groups. To investigate possible genetic determinants of ventricular enlargement in schizophrenia, the VBRs were compared in schizophrenic patients with their own siblings, some with ($n = 69$) and some without ($n = 56$) other schizophrenia-related disorders (e.g. schizotypal PD), as well as with a group of unrelated normal controls ($n = 22$) [207]. The VBRs were significantly different across the groups, but the only significant pairwise group difference was between the schizophrenics and the family member group without schizophrenia-related disorders. In the within-sibship analyses, however, the VBRs of those with schizotypal PD and schizophrenia were similar, and both groups had significantly larger VBRs than their own siblings without schizophrenia-related disorders. In addition, siblings with a negative family history for schizophrenia-related disorders had larger VBRs than family-history-positive siblings.

MRI gives a more detailed view of the brain including the ventricular system. Comparing the MRI scans of patients with schizotypal PD, patients with chronic schizophrenia and normal volunteers, schizophrenics revealed a larger left anterior and temporal horn compared to the controls, while schizotypal PD patients demonstrated the same abnormalities in an attenuated form, lying between the two groups [208].

However, the most elegant way to examine the influence of genetic and environmental factors on brain morphological changes in schizophrenia is the high-risk strategy. In a very decisive study, the offspring of schizophrenic patients were evaluated as to whether they had neither, one or both parents in the schizophrenia spectrum (e.g. one schizophrenic and one schizotypal) and/or whether they had birth complications. Increases in the genetic risk for schizophrenia, as indicated by the number of parents with schizophrenia or schizophrenia spectrum disorders, were associated with increased VBR values, and with particular prominence of the cortical sulci in temporal and other cortical areas. In contrast, birth complications were more associated with increases in ventricular size. Offspring with schizotypal diagnoses, who had fewer perinatal complications than the chronic schizophrenic patients, demonstrated a ventricular size that did not differ from normal, while sulcal enlargement was common to both schizotypal and schizophrenic offspring [209–211]. These results demonstrate that genetic susceptibility and perinatal complications interact with each other, resulting in ventricular and sulcal enlargement. It is interesting to note that the common neuropathological basis of schizotypy and schizophrenia is the sulcal enlargement, which is mainly determined by genetic susceptibility, while ventricular enlargement is more pronounced in the more severe syndrome [212]. Recent MRI studies support the notion that children [213], siblings [214] and first-degree relatives of schizophrenic patients [215] demonstrate volumen reductions of certain brain regions which are in their extent comparable to patients suffering from schizophrenia.

Beside structural imaging, there are methods like magnetic resonance spectroscopy (MRS) or single photon emission computed tomography (SPECT) allowing a non-invasive measure of the biochemistry or regional blood flow of the human brain. There is some evidence from MRS studies for frontotemporal changes in schizophrenia. Therefore, children with symptoms of schizophrenia spectrum disorders and a comparison group took part in a proton-MRS study examining the left frontal lobe [216]. The mean ratio of N-acetylaspartatecreatine (NAA/Cre) was significantly lower in schizophrenia spectrum subjects, suggesting that the metabolic changes associated with adult schizophrenia are observed in children with some or all of the symptoms of schizophrenia. Furthermore, regional cerebral blood flow (rCBF) was measured by SPECT in patients with schizotypal PD and normal volunteers under the condition of the WCST and a control task. At least some schizotypal PD patients demonstrated abnormal patterns of prefrontal activation, perhaps as a compensation or dysfunction in other regions.

In summary, structural brain imaging studies of schizotypal PD patients demonstrate cortical and ventricular changes which are similar to schizophrenia, but in an attenuated extent. Mainly genetic factors seem to influence the cortical atrophy, while ventricular enlargement is more prominent in schizophrenia and additionally influenced by environmental factors like birth complications. First functional imaging studies describe fronto-temporal changes similar to schizophrenia, but the findings are preliminary and the whole field of neuroimaging is open for research.

Schizophrenia-like Schizoaffective Disorder

As already pointed out above, there are no studies in the literature specifically researching schizophrenia-like schizoaffective disorder with brain imaging. Usually, studies on schizophrenia include patients with schizoaffective disorder on purpose, and the internal analysis does not reveal any significant difference between schizophrenic and schizoaffective disorders.

TREATMENT OPTIONS

The treatment of schizophrenia rests on three columns: pharmacotherapy, psychotherapy and sociotherapy. The pharmacotherapy of acute schizophrenia is based on the use of neuroleptics, being effective mainly against positive symptoms [217]. Therefore, one would predict that patients with schizophrenia spectrum disorders will benefit from similar approaches. However, most people with schizotypal PD do not seek psychiatric treatment. Those who do seek treatment often suffer from associated symptoms, such as depression, dysthymic disorder, anxiety or substance-related disorders. Therefore, treatment regimens developed recently focus on subsyndromes such as psychotic-like features.

Schizoid Personality Disorder

The role of drug therapy in this disorder has not been investigated; however, medications may be required to treat concurrent depression or other disorders, and low-dose antipsychotics may be used occasionally to diminish the symptoms of anxiety. There are no controlled data on psychotherapeutic interventions either. As people with schizoid PD avoid relationships, they will only seek help if an acute stressor or the encouragement of a family member urges them to do so. Some of them profit from psychodynamic psychotherapy and some from psychoeducation, especially those having a poor grasp of social conventions.

Paranoid Personality Disorder

Case reports suggest that patients sometimes benefit, especially in the treatment of psychotic decompensation, from low doses of antipsychotic medication, but there are no controlled data available. There are no controlled studies of psychotherapy in the literature. Case reports suggest that cognitive therapy might be helpful. Group therapy may enable relatively healthy patients to improve their social skills. Family therapy may be indicated where the family dynamics are contributing to the patient's difficulties.

Schizotypal Personality Disorder

There are no controlled data in the literature of psychotherapy, but some controlled studies on the pharmacotherapy of schizotypal PD. The literature concerning the treatment with neuroleptics and anxiolytics is reviewed, as these seem to be the only effective principles in improving psychotic-like and anxiety symptoms.

In spite of the fact that the literature on the pharmacotherapy of personality-disordered subjects goes back at least three decades, there are only few clear-cut results in terms of clinical outcome [218]. Overall, most agents are non-specific in mechanism and non-specific in effect. This is due both to the non-selective nature of the drugs and to the heterogeneity of schizotypal PD. A review of the literature [218] suggests that symptom, or personality, dimensions are best correlated with central biological systems and treatment effects. One example is that serotonin re-uptake inhibitors are effective for treating impulsive–aggressive behaviour despite the heterogeneous nature of the personality-disordered sample. There are some general conclusions from the literature which are summarized here.

While neuroleptics have generally been useful in treating positive schizotypal symptoms in personality-disordered subjects, early studies found little efficacy for neuroleptic agents. Some years later, an open-label study of pimozide in DSM-II PD subjects suggested that this drug was associated with good to excellent global improvement in 69% of subjects, with the best results in subjects with paranoid or schizoid PD [219]. The first placebo-controlled study along these lines was published in 1986, followed by a study examining treatment response to thiothixene in a predominantly schizotypal PD outpatient population with pretreatment history of brief psychotic disturbances, reporting a clear therapeutic effect associated with the neuroleptic [220]. Further studies examining treatment response to haloperidol reported moderate efficacy by measures of psychoticism, paranoid ideation, hostility, depression and anxiety, for example ref. [221]. Studies examining atypical agents in schizotypal PD patients found, for example that clozapine treatment ranging from 2 to 9 months resulted in significant improvement in global functioning and in seven of eight "positive symptom" items and significant improvement in three of five "negative symptom" items of the Brief Psychiatric Rating Scale (BPRS) [222]. Studying amoxapine, five schizotypal PD subjects and five subjects with borderline PD were treated for at least 3 weeks, adding oxazepam as a sedative. Only the schizotypal PD subjects demonstrated any benefit in global psychopathology, in BPRS "schizophrenia-like" symptom score, or in the Hamilton Rating Scale for Depression score.

Although often used, anxiolytics have not been widely studied in subjects with schizotypal PD. Early reports suggested that they may offer some global benefit to personality-disordered subjects [223], which has to be proven in controlled studies.

Concerning the use of tricyclic agents, monoamine oxidase inhibitors, lithium, anticonvulsants and selective serotonin re-uptake inhibitors (SSRIs), there is a growing literature for the treatment of borderline PD, but not for schizotypal PD [218].

The effect of psychotherapy on schizotypal PD has not been studied in detail. First attempts have suggested that exploratory psychotherapeutic approaches might have the potential effect of facilitating decompensation, but more structured approaches like psychoeducation may be helpful [224]. Models for the psychoeducational treatment of schizophrenia, if extended to patients with schizotypal PD, suggest that patients and their family members should be encouraged to allow the patients to remove themselves from stressful situations, particularly situations that may require an activation of attention and information processing that is beyond the patient's capacities [225].

In conclusion, there is preliminary evidence that low doses of antipsychotic medication (1–2 mg per day of haloperidol equivalent) are effective in at least temporarily reducing or relieving the psychotic-like symptoms of schizotypal PD. In psychotherapy there is only clinical experience available and, therefore, controlled studies are needed to adapt the specific methods used in schizophrenia.

Schizophrenia-like Schizoaffective Disorder

There is a considerable overlap between the treatment regimes in schizoaffective disorders and schizophrenia as well as affective disorders. In spite of this, it is interesting to note that the evidence in the literature for the treatment of schizoaffective disorders is weak. One important column of treatment is the pharmacotherapy.

Acute treatment of schizomania. Antipsychotics and lithium are the psychopharmacological agents most often used in the treatment of schizoaffective mania. The efficacy of a monotherapy with neuroleptics is proven, while for using lithium on its own clear evidence is lacking [226]. Combining both strategies is often done in clinical practice, but the evidence for this approach is weak based on double-blind trials [227].

Acute treatment of schizodepression. There is some evidence for greater efficacy of neuroleptics over antidepressants in the treatment of acute schizodepression, but a combination of both agents is preferred in clinical practice. The superiority of such a combination compared with the monotherapy is not proven, but there are some studies pointing in this direction [228].

Long-term-treatment. The efficacy of lithium to prevent a relapse is well documented for schizoaffective disorders. Lithium is more effective in cases with prevailing affective symptoms [229], while in cases where psychotic symptoms prevail neuroleptics have to be added [230]. Studies demonstrating a superiority of neuroleptics over lithium should be taken cautiously because of the small number of cases and the short duration of treatment under examination [231]. In the case of a lithium non-response, carbamazepine can be used instead. The efficacy of valproate is not proven for the long-term treatment of schizoaffective disorders.

The *psychotherapeutical interventions* are based on building up a relationship of trust with the patient and helping him or her through the acute phases of the disease. If longer interactions are possible, psychoeducation is the first-line treatment to allow the patient to understand the basis of the disorder and the necessity of the treatment.

In summary, there is very little consolidated knowledge about the effective treatment of schizophrenia spectrum disorders. As a matter of fact, there is no single well-designed placebo-controlled treatment study with an appropriate number of patients in any of the three spectrum PDs. Instead, the similarity of psychopathology, neurobiology and aetiology between schizotypal PD and schizophrenia motivates similar treatment strategies. This procedure is validated by some small studies including patients with schizotypal PD. Using low-dose neuroleptics may be an effective way to improve or relieve psychotic-like symptoms in this disorder. This statement is partially true for schizophrenia-like schizoaffective disorders, where the literature is broader. Lithium and/or antipsychotics are useful in schizomania, while the combination of antidepressants and antipsychotics is the first-line treatment in schizodepression. Lithium is proven to be effective in long-term treatment. In the case of non-response, carbamazepine can be substituted for lithium. The field of treatment of schizophrenia spectrum disorders is wide open to research.

SUMMARY

Schizophrenia shares symptoms, precursors, causes and risk factors with other disorders. These disorders are combined in the schizophrenia spectrum. There is consensus that besides schizophrenia and schizophreniform disorder the following disorders belong to the spectrum: schizoaffective disorder (as defined by DSM-III-R/-IV or the mainly schizophrenic type as defined by

RDC), and schizotypal PD; limited evidence is available for further including paranoid and schizoid PD. There might also be a yet unspecified subgroup of atypical psychoses related to schizophrenia. Adoption studies demonstrate that the familial cosegregation of these spectrum disorders is at least in part genetically mediated; the specific nature of the involved genes is still obscure.

Consistent evidence has been compiled during nearly a century of research that not the productive signs of schizotype but more the negative signs (such as social and emotional behaviour and basic cognitive dysfunctions) are pointing to a relationship with the aetiology of schizophrenia. In spite of this knowledge, the diagnostic definitions of spectrum disorders (particularly schizotypal PD) are much more heterogeneous and probably involve multiple nosological entities.

Schizotypal PD subjects show neuropsychological and neurophysiological abnormalities similar to those in schizophrenia, and these impairments seem to be associated with negative schizotypal traits. Subjects from the population scoring high on questionnaires designed to assess schizotypal traits also show some of these impairments. The neuropsychological profile of schizoaffective patients is very close to that found in schizophrenic patients.

There is some evidence for hyperdopaminergia in schizophrenia spectrum disorders, especially schizotypal PD, which is correlated with positive symptoms and intermediate between schizophrenics and control subjects. Amphetamine challenge results in improved cognitive functioning without affecting other psychotic symptoms.

Structural brain imaging studies demonstrate sulcal and ventricular enlargement in schizophrenia spectrum disorders, which is intermediate between schizophrenia and control subjects. Preliminary evidence from functional imaging points to a pattern of changes which is similar to schizophrenia.

There is very little consolidated knowledge about the effective treatment of schizophrenia spectrum disorders. Using low-dose neuroleptics may be an effective way to improve or relieve psychotic-like symptoms in schizotypal PD. Lithium and/or antipsychotics are useful in schizomania, while the combination of antidepressants and antipsychotics is the first-line treatment in schizodepression. Lithium is proven to be effective in long-term treatment.

Phenomenology and Diagnosis

Consistent Evidence

Schizotypal features are clustering in subjects with elevated risk for schizophrenia and prodromal to the subsequent full manifestation of schizophrenia.

Incomplete Evidence

This evidence concerns:

- The taxonomy of schizotypal features. (Is schizophrenia-related disorder an appropriate diagnostic category or should it be broken down into three dimension traits which could also cover those features of paranoid PD and schizoid PD related to schizophrenia?);
- The boundary of the schizophrenic concept. (Do paranoid and schizoid PDs belong to the spectrum? Should subthreshold patterns, for example detectable by questionnaires, also be included in the spectrum? Are anhedonia or somatic complaints valid criteria for characterizing biological relatives of schizophrenics? Apparently, only a subgroup of schizoaffective/psychotic affective disorder as well as a subgroup of other non-schizophrenic psychoses belong to the spectrum; where may a valid delineation line be drawn?)

Areas Still Open to Research

- Is a one-dimensional or a multidimensional concept of the spectrum more appropriate than the combination of some diagnostic entities (as schizotypal PD, schizoaffective disorder)?
- What is an appropriate comprehensive genetic model of schizophrenia and its spectrum, given that schizophrenia is a multifactorial disease with a polygenic component? Schizotypal PD and schizoaffective disorder might: (a) be an attenuated variant of schizophrenia sharing only part of susceptibility genes with schizophrenia (severity model); (b) share all susceptibility genes with schizophrenia, with protective factors prohibiting the expression of the full syndrome; (c) be heterogeneous conditions, with some subgroups presenting with distinct aetiologies unrelated to schizophrenia.

Familial–Genetic Basis of Spectrum Concepts

Consistent Evidence

Schizotypal PD and a subgroup of schizoaffective disorders (preferentially mainly schizophrenic type) are strongly and consistently linked to schizophrenia by family studies; common genetic risk factors contribute considerably to this relationship; relationship to paranoid and schizoid PD is less strong.

Incomplete Evidence

Paranoid and schizoid PDs are linked to schizophrenia by common genetic factors; schizotypal PD and schizoaffective disorder among relatives are most common in families of probands with the same diagnosis but less common in families of schizophrenics. Which symptoms and signs are most sensitive and specific for distinguishing relatives of schizophrenics and of other disorders/controls?

Areas Still Open to Research

Are there subtypes of schizotypal PD or schizoaffective disorder with specific familial–genetic aetiology unrelated to schizophrenia? Are schizophrenia, schizoaffective disorder (DSM-III-R) and schizotypal PD and probably other psychotic disorders located on a single latent dimension of vulnerability with schizophrenia? If yes, what is the proper ordering?

Neuropsychology

Consistent Evidence

Most studies employing measures which are sensitive to cognitive abnormalities in schizophrenic patients and in their relatives have also shown cognitive impairments in schizotypal PD patients. Quite solid evidence exists for frontal lobe functions requiring flexibility and working memory (e.g. WCST, verbal fluency, spatial delayed response). Sustained attention (CPT) probably is also impaired in schizotypal PD. In general, where schizotypal PD and schizophrenic patients have been studied together, the neuropsychological impairments of schizotypal PD patients were found to be milder in degree but qualitatively similar to those found in schizophrenic patients. On most cognitive functions examined, schizoaffective patients cannot be discriminated from schizophrenic patients.

Incomplete Evidence

Some preliminary evidence suggests that spectrum disorders other than schizotypal PD may differ from schizotypal PD with regard to neuropsychological deficits, but this awaits further systematic study. More work is needed to corroborate the preliminary evidence of impaired declarative memory functioning in spectrum disorders. The relationship between schizotypal symptoms and neuropsychological measures may differ between spectrum disorders and psychometric high-risk subjects. In the latter group, most findings point towards more neuropsychological impairment when positive schizotypal symptoms are present (e.g. perceptual aberrations), while in the former group negative schizotypal symptoms (like anhedonia) are more often associated with neurocognitive deficits.

Areas Still Open to Research

Very few studies are available on the neuropsychological performance of paranoid and schizoid PDs, so that the overlap with schizotypal PD cannot be properly judged. It is important to use more comprehensive neuropsychological assessments in future studies in order to compare neuropsychological profiles between groups of patients within the spectrum and beyond. Furthermore, family studies should include self-report measures to complement the diagnostic interviews in order to assess schizotypal traits.

Neurophysiology

Consistent Evidence

An impaired smooth pursuit eye tracking in schizotypal PD and in relatives of schizophrenic patients has been found repeatedly. The changes in evoked potential amplitude or latencies do not seem to be pronounced in spectrum disorders.

Incomplete Evidence

Reflexive errors in the antisaccade task have not yet been studied in patients with spectrum disorders, but data from biological relatives of schizophrenics and from subjects who report unusual perceptual experiences suggest that this might be fruitful, especially because insufficient inhibition of saccades may be a core deficit leading to both reduced SPEM performance and involuntary reflexive saccades. Preliminary data also suggest that pre-pulse inhibition of the startle response is reduced in schizotypal PD subjects.

Areas Still Open to Research

Almost no data exist with regard to spectrum disorders other than schizotypal PD. At least for measures which have reliably revealed differences between schizotypal PD patients and controls, this seems to be an important issue for further research.

Neurochemistry/Neuroendocrinology

Consistent Evidence

Studies demonstrate increased dopamine metabolism in schizotypal PD, with values intermediate between schizophrenia and control subjects. The dexamethasone suppression test is undisturbed in schizophrenia-like schizoaffective disorder, where psychotic features are more prevalent than mood disturbances.

Areas Still Open to Research

The neurochemistry and neuroendocrinology of schizoid and paranoid PD is completely open to research.

Brain Imaging

Consistent Evidence

Enlarged ventricular and sulcal space are present in schizotypal PD, but sulcal enlargement prevails. The extent of enlargement is usually situated between schizophrenics and control subjects.

Incomplete Evidence

Regional specific enlargement of the ventricular system and genetic factors are more likely responsible for sulcal, while genetic and environmental (birth trauma) causes are responsible for ventricular pathology. Blood flow and biochemical profiles *in vivo* in schizotypal PD resemble the pattern in schizophrenia in an attenuated form.

Areas Still Open to Research

Brain imaging in paranoid and schizoid PDs is completely open to research.

Treatment Options

Consistent Evidence

Low-dose neuroleptics (1–2 mg haloperidol equivalent) are beneficial for the treatment of psychotic-like symptoms in schizotypal PD. In schizophrenia-like schizoaffective disorder, lithium and/or neuroleptics are the first-line drugs in acute (manic and psychotic symptoms) and long-term treatment.

Antidepressants and lithium are the first-choice drugs in depressive syndromes.

Incomplete Evidence

Should lithium or neuroleptics be given in acute schizomania? Are neuroleptics and/or antidepressants superior to a combination of both in acute schizodepression? What is the efficacy of mood stabilizers other than lithium on the long-term outcome of schizoaffective disorders?

Areas Still Open to Research

The psychotherapy of schizophrenia-spectrum PD and the pharmacotherapy of schizoid and paranoid PD are completely open to research.

REFERENCES

1. Kraepelin E. (1919) *Dementia Praecox and Paraphrenia.* Churchill Livingstone, Edinburgh.
2. Bleuler E. (1911) *Dementia Praecox or the Group of Schizophrenias.* International Universities Press, New York.
3. Hoch P., Polatin, P. (1949) Pseudoneurotic forms of schizophrenia. *Psychiatr. Quarterly*, **23**: 248–276.
4. Kretschmer E. (1925) *Physique and Character.* Kegan, Trench, and Trubner, London.
5. Kallmann F.J. (1946) The genetic theory of schizophrenia. An analysis of 691 schizophrenic twins index families. *Am. J. Psychiatry*, **103**: 309–322.
6. Rado S. (1953) Dynamics and classification of disordered behavior *Am J Psychiatry*, **110**: 406–416.
7. Meehl P.E. (1962) Schizotaxia, schizotypy, schizophrenia. *Am. Psychol.*, **17**: 827–838.
8. Meehl P.E. (1990) Toward an integrated theory of schizotaxia, schizotypy, and schizophrenia. *J. Pers. Disord.*, **4**: 1–99.
9. Kety S.S., Rosenthal D., Wender P.H. (1968) The types and prevalence of mental illness in the biological and adoptive families of schizophrenics. *J. Psychiatr. Res.*, **6**: 345–362.
10. Kety S.S. (1985) Schizotypal personality disorder: an operational definition of Bleuler's latent schizophrenia? *Schizophr. Bull.*, **11**: 590–594.
11. Spitzer R.L., Endicott J., Gibbon M. (1979) Crossing the border into borderline personality and borderline schizophrenia: the development of criteria. *Arch. Gen. Psychiatry*, **36**: 17–24.
12. Gunderson J.G., Siever L.J., Spaulding E. (1983) The search for a schizotype: crossing the border again. *Arch. Gen. Psychiatry*, **40**: 15–22.
13. Kavoussi R.J., Siever L.J. (1992) Overlap between borderline and schizotypal personality disorders. *Compr. Psychiatry*, **33**: 7–12.
14. Frances A. (1985) Validating schizotypal personality disorders: problems with the schizophrenia connection. *Schizophr. Bull.*, **11**: 595–597.

15. American Psychiatric Association (1987) *Diagnostic and Statistical Manual of Mental Disorder*, 3rd edn revised. American Psychiatric Association, Washington, DC.

16. American Psychiatric Association (1994) *Diagnostic and Statistical Manual of Mental Disorders*, 4th edn. American Psychiatric Association, Washington, DC.

17. World Health Organization (1992) *ICD: The ICD-10 Classification of Mental and Behavioural Disorders — Clinical Descriptions and Diagnostic Guidelines*. World Health Organization, Geneva.

18. Claridge G. (1987) The schizophrenias as nervous types revisited. *Br. J. Psychiatry*, **151**: 735–743.

19. Chapman L.J., Chapman J.P., Kwapil T.R., Eckblad M., Zinser M.C. (1994) Putatively psychosis-prone subjects 10 years later. *J. Abnorm. Psychol.*, **103**: 171–183.

20. Kwapil T.R., Miller M.B., Zinser M.C., Chapman J., Chapman L.J. (1997) Magical ideation and social anhedonia as predictors of psychosis proneness: a partial replication. *J. Abnorm. Psychol.*, **106**: 491–495.

21. Masons O., Claridge G., Williams L. (1997) Questionnaire measurement. In *Schizotypy* (Ed. G. Claridge), pp. 19–37. Oxford University Press, Oxford.

22. Kendler K.S., Gruenberg A.M., Kinney D.K. (1994) Independent diagnoses of adoptees and relatives as defined by DSM-III in the provincial and national samples of the Danish adoption study of schizophrenia. *Arch. Gen. Psychiatry*, **51**: 456–468.

23. Spitzer R.L., Endicott J., Robins E. (1978) *Research Diagnostic Criteria (RDC) for a Selected Group of Functional Disorders*, 3rd edn. New York State Psychiatric Institute, Biometrics Research, New York.

24. Coryell W., Tsuang M.T. (1986) Outcome after 40 years in DSM-III schizophreniform disorder. *Arch. Gen. Psychiatry*, **43**: 324–328.

25. Kasanin J. (1933) The acute schizoaffective psychoses. *Am. J. Psychiatry*, **13**: 97–126.

26. Kendler K.S., Lieberman J.A., Walsh D. (1989) The structured interview of schizotypy (SIS): a preliminary report. *Schizophr. Bull.*, **15**: 559–571.

27. Chapman L.J., Chapman J.P., Raulin M.L. (1976) Scales for physical and social anhedonia. *J. Abnorm. Psychol.*, **85**: 374–382.

28. Chapman L.J., Chapman J.P., Raulin M.L. (1978) Body image aberration in schizophrenia. *J. Abnorm. Psychol.*, **87**: 339–407.

29. Eckblad M., Chapman L.J. (1983) Magical ideation as an indicator of schizotypy. *J. Consult. Clin. Psychol.*, **51**: 215–225.

30. Raine A. (1991) The SPQ: a scale for the assessment of schizotypal personality based on DSM-III-R criteria. *Schizophr. Bull.*, **17**: 555–564.

31. Claridge G., Broks P. (1984) Schizotypy and hemisphere function. I. Theoretical considerations and the measurement of schizotypy. *Pers. Individ. Diffs.*, **5**: 633–648.

32. Kendler K.S., Thacker L., Walsh D. (1996) Self-report measures of schizotypy as indices of familial vulnerability to schizophrenia. *Schizophr. Bull.*, **22**: 511–520.

33. Raine A., Allbutt J. (1989) Factors of schizoid personality. *Schizophr. Bull.*, **20**: 191–201.

34. Rosenberger P.H., Miller G.A. (1989) Comparing borderline definition: DSM-III borderline and schizotypal personality disorders. *J. Abnorm. Psychol.*, **98**: 161–169.

35. Bergman A.J., Harvey P.D., Mitropoulou V., Aronson A., Marder D., Silverman J., Trestman R., Siever L.J. (1996) The factor structure of schizotypal symptoms in a clinical population. *Schizophr. Bull.*, **22**: 501–509.

36. Kendler K.S., Hewitt J. (1992) The structure of self-report schizotypy in twins. *J. Pers. Disord.*, **6**: 1–17.
37. Gruzelier J.H. (1996) The factorial structure of schizotypy: Part I. Affinities with syndromes of schizophrenia. *Schizophr. Bull.*, **22**: 611–620.
38. Kendler K.S., McGuire M., Gruenberg A.M., Walsh D. (1995) Schizotypal symptoms and signs in the Roscommon family study. Their factor structure and familial relationship with psychotic and affective disorders. *Arch. Gen. Psychiatry*, **52**: 296–303.
39. Torgersen S. (1985) Relationship of schizotypal personality disorder to schizophrenia: genetics. *Schizophr. Bull.*, **11**: 554–563.
40. McGlashan T.H. (1987) Testing DSM-III symptom criteria for schizotypal and borderline personality disorders. *Arch. Gen. Psychiatry*, **44**: 15–22.
41. Battaglia M., Cavallini M.C., Macciardi F., Bellodi L. (1997) The structure of DSM-III-R schizotypal personality disorder diagnosed by direct interview. *Schizophr. Bull.*, **23**: 83–92.
42. Raine A., Reynolds C., Lencz T., Scerbo A., Triphon N., Kim D. (1994) Cognitive-perceptual, interpersonal, and disorganized features of schizotypal personality. *Schizophr. Bull.*, **20**: 191–201.
43. Lenzenweger M.F., Dworkin R.H., Wethington E. (1991) Examining the underlying structure of schizophrenic phenomenology: evidence for a three-process model. *Schizophr. Bull.*, **17**: 515–524.
44. Kraepelin E. (1921) *Einführung in die psychiatrische Klinik*, 4. Aufl. Barth, Leipzig.
45. Freiman K., Widiger T. (1989) *Co-occurrence and diagnostic efficiency statistics.* Unpublished data, University of Kentucky, Lexington.
46. Kalus O., Bernstein D.P., Siever L.J. (1996) Schizoid personality disorder. In *DSM-IV Sourcebook*, vol. 2 (Eds T.A. Widiger, A.J. Frances, H.A. Pincus, R. Ross, M.B. First, W.W. Davis), pp. 675–684. American Psychiatric Association, Washington, DC.
47. Morey L.C. (1988) Personality disorders in DSM-III and DSM-III-R: convergence, coverage, and internal consistency. *Am. J. Psychiatry*, **145**: 573–577.
48. Pfohl B., Coryell W., Zimmerman M., Stangl D. (1986) DSM-III personality disorders: diagnostic overlap and internal consistency of individual DSM-III criteria. *Compr. Psychiatry*, **27**: 21–34.
49. Fulton M., Winokur G. (1993) A comparative study of paranoid and schizoid personality disorders. *Am. J. Psychiatry*, **150**: 1363–1367.
50. McGlashan T.H. (1986) Schizotypal personality disorder, Chestnut Lodge follow-up study, VI: long-term follow-up perspective. *Arch. Gen. Psychiatry*, **43**: 329–334.
51. Siever L.J., Bernstein D.P., Silverman J.M. (1996) Schizotypal personality disorder. In *DSM-IV Sourcebook*, vol. 2 (Eds T.A. Widiger, A.J. Frances, H.A. Pincus, R. Ross, M.B. First, W.W. Davis), pp. 685–702. American Psychiatric Association, Washington, DC.
52. Bernstein D.P., Useda D., Siever L.J. (1996) Paranoid personality disorder. In *DSM-IV Sourcebook*, vol. 2 (Eds T.A. Widiger, A.J. Frances, H.A. Pincus, R. Ross, M.B. First, W.W Davis), pp. 665–674. American Psychiatric Association, Washington, DC.
53. Levitt J.J., Tsuang M.T. (1990) Atypical psychoses. In *Manual of Clinical Problems in Psychiatry* (Eds S. Hyman, M. Jennike), pp. 45–52. Little Brown, Boston.
54. Marneros A., Rohde A., Deister A. (1989) Unipolar and bipolar schizoaffective disorders: a comparative study. II. Long-term course. *Eur. Arch. Psychiatry Neurol. Sci.*, **239**: 164–170.

55. Marneros A., Deister A., Rohde A. (1991) *Affektive, schizoaffektive und schizophrene Psychosen.* Springer, Berlin.
56. Baron M., Gruen R., Asnis L., Kane J. (1982) Schizoaffective illness, schizophrenia and affective disorders: morbidity risk and genetic transmission. *Acta Psychiatr. Scand.*, **65**: 253–262.
57. Maj M., Starace F., Pirozzi R. (1991) A family study of DSM-III-R schizoaffective disorder, depressive type, compared with schizophrenia and psychotic and nonpsychotic major depression. *Am. J. Psychiatry*, **148**: 612–616.
58. Coryell W., Keller M., Lavori P., Endicott J. (1990) Affective syndromes, psychotic features, and prognosis. I. Depression. *Arch. Gen. Psychiatry*, **47**: 651–657.
59. Coryell W., Keller M., Lavori P., Endicott J. (1990) Affective syndromes, psychotic features, and prognosis. II. Mania. *Arch. Gen. Psychiatry*, **47**: 658–662.
60. Maier W., Lichtermann D., Minges J., Heun R., Hallmayer J., Benkert O. (1992) Schizoaffective disorder and affective disorders with mood-incongruent psychotic features: keep separate or combine? Evidence from a family study. *Am. J. Psychiatry*, **149**: 1666–1673.
61. Baron M., Gruen R., Rainer J.D., Kane J., Asnis L., Lord S. (1985) A family study of schizophrenic and normal control probands: implications for the spectrum concept of schizophrenia. *Am. J. Psychiatry*, **142**: 447–455.
62. Zimmerman M., Coryell W.H. (1990) Diagnosing personality disorders in the community. A comparison of self-report and interview measures. *Arch. Gen. Psychiatry*, **47**: 527–531.
63. Maier W., Lichtermann D., Klingler T., Heun R., Hallmayer J. (1992) Prevalences of personality disorders (DSM-III-R) in the community. *J. Pers. Disord.*, **6**: 187–196.
64. Kendler K.S., McGuire M., Gruenberg A.M., O'Hare A., Spellman M., Walsh D. (1993) The Roscommon family study. III. Schizophrenia-related personality disorders in relatives. *Arch. Gen. Psychiatry*, **50**: 781–788.
65. Reich J.H., Yates W., Nduaguba M. (1989) Prevalence of DSM-III personality disorders in the community. *Soc. Psychiatry*, **24**: 12–16.
66. Häfner H., Maurer K., Löffler W., Nowotny B. (1996) Der Frühverlauf der Schizophrenie. *Z. Med. Psychol.*, **5**: 22–31.
67. Foerster A., Lewis S., Owen M., Murray R. (1991) Premorbid adjustment and personality in psychosis: effects of sex and diagnosis. *Br. J. Psychiatry*, **158**: 171–176.
68. Parnas J., Schulsinger F., Schulsinger H., Mednick S.A., Teasdale T.W. (1982) Behavioral precursors of schizophrenia spectrum. *Arch. Gen. Psychiatry*, **39**: 658–664.
69. Olin S.S., Mednick S.A. (1996) Risk factors of psychosis: identifying vulnerable populations premorbidly. *Schizophr. Bull.*, **22**: 223–240.
70. Freedman L.R., Rock D., Roberts S.A., Cornblatt B.A., Erlenmeyer-Kimling L. (1998) The New York High-Risk Project: attention, anhedonia and social outcome. *Schizophr. Res.*, **30**: 1–9.
71. Crow T.J., Done D.J., Sacker A. (1995) Birth cohort study of the antecedents of psychosis: ontogeny as witness to phylogenetic origins. In *Search for the Causes of Schizophrenia*, vol. 3 (Eds H. Häfner, W.F. Gattaz), pp. 3–20. Springer, Berlin.
72. Gross G., Huber G., Klosterkötter J., Linz M. (1987) *Bonner Skala für die Beurteilung von Basissymptomen (BSABS: Bonn Scale for the Assessment of Basic Symptoms).* Springer, Berlin.
73. Klosterkötter J., Ebel H., Schultze-Lutter F., Steinmeyer E.M. (1996) Diagnostic validity of basic symptoms. *Eur. Arch. Psychiatry Clin. Neurosci.*, **246**: 147–154.

74. Huber G. (1997) The heterogeneous course of schizophrenia. *Schizophr. Res.*, **28**: 177–185.
75. Peralta V., Cuesta M.J., de Leon J. (1991) Premorbid personality and positive and negative symptoms in schizophrenia. *Acta Psychiatr. Scand.*, **84**: 336–339.
76. Foerster A., Lewis S., Owen M., Murray R. (1991) Low birth weight and a family history of schizophrenia predict poor premorbid functioning in psychosis. *Schizophr. Res.*, **5**: 13–20.
77. Cornblatt B.A., Lenzenweger M.F., Dworkin R.H., Erlenmeyer-Kimling L. (1992) Childhood attentional dysfunctions predict social deficits in unaffected adults at risk for schizophrenia. *Br. J. Psychiatry*, **161** (Suppl. 18): 59–64.
78. Olin S.S., Raine A., Cannon T.D., Parnas J., Schulsinger F., Mednick S.A. (1997) Childhood behaviour precursors of schizotypal personality disorder. *Schizophr. Bull.*, **23**: 93–103.
79. Tsuang M.T., Levitt J.J., Simpson J.C. (1995) Schizoaffective disorder. In *Schizophrenia* (Eds S.R. Hirsch, D.R. Weinberger), pp. 46–57. Blackwell, Oxford.
80. Maj M., Staracc F., Kemali D. (1987) Prediction of outcome by historical, clinical and biological variables in schizoaffective disorder, depressed type. *J. Psychiatr. Res.*, **21**: 289–295.
81. Kendler K.S., McGuire M., Gruenberg A.M., O'Hare A., Spellman M., Walsh D. (1993) The Roscommon family study. I. Methods, diagnosis of probands, and risk of schizophrenia in relatives. *Arch. Gen. Psychiatry*, **50**: 527–540.
82. Kendler K.S., McGuire M., Gruenberg A.M., Spellman M., O'Hare A., Walsh D. (1993) The Roscommon family study. II. The risk of nonschizophrenic non-affective psychoses in relatives. *Arch. Gen. Psychiatry*, **50**: 645–652.
83. Siever L.J., Silverman J.M., Howarth T.B., Klas H., Coccaro E., Keefe R.S., Pinkham L., Rinaldi P., Mohs R.C., Davis K.L. (1990) Increased morbid risk for schizophrenia related disorders in relatives of schizotypal personality disordered patients. *Arch. Gen. Psychiatry*, **47**: 634–640.
84. Thaker G., Adami H., Moran M., Lahti A., Cassady S. (1993) Psychiatric illness in families of subjects with schizophrenia-spectrum personality disorders: high morbidity risks for unspecified functional psychoses and schizophrenia. *Am. J. Psychiatry*, **150**: 66–71.
85. Battaglia M., Bernardeschi L., Franchini L., Bellodi L., Smeraldi E. (1995) A family study of schizotypal disorder. *Schizophr. Bull.*, **21**: 33–45.
86. Kendler K.S., Gruenberg A.M., Tsuang M.T. (1986) A DSM-III family study of the nonschizophrenic psychotic disorders. *Am. J. Psychiatry*, **143**: 1098–1105.
87. Torgersen S. (1984) Genetic and nosological aspects of schizotypal and border-line personality disorders: a twin study. *Arch. Gen. Psychiatry*, **41**: 546–554.
88. McCabe M.S. (1975) Reactive psychoses. A family study. *Arch. Gen. Psychiatry*, **32**: 447–454.
89. Frangos E., Athanassenas G., Tsitourides S., Katsanou N., Alexandrakou P. (1985) Prevalence of DSM-III schizophrenia among the first-degree relatives of schizophrenic probands. *Acta Psychiatr. Scand.*, **72**: 382–386.
90. Coryell W., Zimmerman M. (1988) The heritability of schizophrenia and schizo-affective disorder: a family study. *Arch. Gen. Psychiatry*, **45**: 323–327.
91. Gershon E.S., DeLisi L.E., Hamovit J., Nurnberger J.I., Maxwell M.E., Schrei-ber J., Dauphinais D., Dingman C.W., Guroff J.J. (1988) A controlled family study of chronic psychoses. *Arch. Gen. Psychiatry*, **45**: 328–336.
92. Onstad S., Skre I., Edvardsen J., Torgersen S., Kringlen E. (1991) Mental disorders in first-degree relatives of schizophrenics. *Acta Psychiatr. Scand.*, **83**: 463–467.

93. Parnas J., Cannon T.D., Jacobsen B., Schulsinger H., Schulsinger F., Mednick S.A. (1993) Lifetime DSM-III-R diagnostic outcomes in the offspring of schizophrenic mothers: results from the Cobenhagen high risk study. *Arch. Gen. Psychiatry*, **50**: 707–714.

94. Torgersen S., Onstad S., Skre I., Edvardsen J., Kringlen E. (1993) "True" schizotypal personality disorder: a study of co-twins and relatives of schizophrenic probands. *Am. J. Psychiatry*, **150**: 1661–1667.

95. Maier W., Lichtermann D., Minges J., Heun R. (1994) Personality disorders among the relatives of schizophrenia patients. *Schizophr. Bull.*, **20**: 481–493.

96. Erlenmeyer-Kimling L., Squires-Wheeler E., Adamo U.H., Bassett A.S., Cornblatt B.A., Kestenbaum C.J., Rock D., Roberts S.A., Gottesman I.I. (1995) The New York High-Risk Project: Psychoses and cluster A personality disorders in offspring of schizophrenic patients at 23 years of follow-up. *Arch. Gen. Psychiatry*, **52**: 857–865.

97. Maier W., Lichtermann D., Minges J., Hallmayer J., Heun R., Benkert O., Levinson D. (1993) Continuity and discontinuity of affective disorders and schizophrenia. Results of a controlled family study. *Arch. Gen. Psychiatry*, **50**: 871–883.

98. Kety S.S., Wender P.H., Jacobsen B., Ingraham L.J., Jansson L., Faber B., Kinney D.K. (1994) Mental illness in the biological and adoptive relatives of schizophrenic adoptees. *Arch. Gen. Psychiatry*, **51**: 442–455.

99. Kendler K.S., Neale M.C., Walsh D. (1995) Evaluating the spectrum concept of schizophrenia in the Roscommon family study. *Am. J. Psychiatry*, **152**: 749–754.

100. Baron M., Gruen R.S. (1991) Schizophrenia and affective disorder: are they genetically linked? *Br. J. Psychiatry*, **159**: 267–270.

101. Kendler K.S., Gruenberg A.M., Tsuang M.T. (1985) Psychiatric illness in first-degree relatives of schizophrenic and surgical control patients: a family study using DSM-III criteria. *Arch. Gen. Psychiatry*, **42**: 770–779.

102. Kendler K.S., Gruenberg A.M. (1982) Genetic relationship between paranoid personality disorder and the "schizophrenic spectrum" disorders. *Am. J. Psychiatry*, **139**: 1185–1186.

103. Kendler K.S., Masterson C., Davis K.L. (1985) Psychiatric illness in first-degree relatives of patients with paranoid psychosis, schizophrenia, and medical illness. *Br. J. Psychiatry*, **147**: 524–531.

104. Winokur G. (1985) Familial psychopathology in delusional disorder. *Compr. Psychiatry*, **26**: 241–248.

105. Marino C., Nobile M., Bellodi L., Smeraldi E. (1993) Delusional disorder and mood disorder: can they coexist? *Psychopathology*, **26**: 53–61.

106. Kendler K.S., Karkowski-Shuman L., Walsh D. (1996) The risk for psychiatric illness in siblings of schizophrenics: the impact of psychotic and non-psychotic affective illness and alcoholism in parents. *Acta Psychiatr. Scand.*, **94**: 49–55.

107. Tsuang M.T. (1991) Morbidity risks of schizophrenia and affective disorders among first-degree relatives of patients with schizoaffective disorders. *Br. J. Psychiatry*, **158**: 165–170.

108. Squires-Wheeler E., Skodol A.E., Basett A., Erlenmeyer-Kimling L. (1989) DSM-III-R schizotypal personality traits in offspring of schizophrenic disorder, affective disorder, and normal control parents. *J. Psychiatr. Res.*, **23**: 229–239.

109. Silverman J.M., Pinkham L., Horvath T.B., Coccaro E.F., Klar H., Schear S., Apter S., Davidson M., Mohs R.C., Siever L.J. (1991) Affective and impulsive personality disorder traits in the relatives of patients with borderline personality disorder. *Am. J. Psychiatry*, **148**: 1378–1385.

110. Erlenmeyer-Kimling L., Adamo U.H., Rock D., Roberts S.A., Bassett A.S., Squires-Wheeler E., Cornblatt B.A., Endicott J., Pape S., Gottesman I.I. (1997) The New York High-Risk Project: prevalence and comorbidity of axis I disorders in offspring of schizophrenic patients at 25-year follow-up. *Arch. Gen. Psychiatry*, **54**: 1096–1102.

111. Lyons M.J., Toomey R., Faraone S.V., Tsuang M.T. (1994) Comparison of schizotypal relatives of schizophrenic versus affective probands. *Am. J. Med. Genet.*, **54**: 279–285.

112. Thaker G., Moran M., Adami H., Cassady S. (1993) Psychosis proneness scales in schizophrenia spectrum personality disorders: familial vs. nonfamilial samples. *Psychiatry Res.*, **46**: 47–57.

113. Clementz B.A., Grove W.M., Katsanis J., Iacono W.G. (1991) Psychometric detection of schizotypy: perceptual aberration and physical anhedonia in relatives of schizophrenics. *J. Abnorm. Psychol.*, **100**: 607–612.

114. Franke P., Maier W., Hardt J., Hain C. (1993) Cognitive functioning and anhedonia in subjects at risk for schizophrenia. *Schizophr. Res.*, **10**: 77–84.

115. Raine A., Lencz T., Mednick S.A. (1995) *Schizotypal Personality*. Cambridge University Press, Cambridge.

116. Trestman R.L., Keefe R.S., Mitropoulou V., Harvey P.D., deVegvar M.L., Lees-Roitman S., Davidson M., Aronson A., Silverman J., Siever L.J. (1995) Cognitive function and biological correlates of cognitive performance in schizotypal personality disorder. *Psychiatry Res.*, **59**: 127–136.

117. Tien A.Y., Costa P.T., Eaton W.W. (1992) Covariance of personality, neurocognition, and schizophrenia spectrum traits in the community. *Schizophr. Res.*, **7**: 149–158.

118. Battaglia M., Abbruzzese M., Ferri S., Scarone S., Bellodi L., Smeraldi E. (1994) An assessment of the Wisconsin Card Sorting Test as an indicator of liability to schizophrenia. *Schizophr. Res.*, **14**: 39–45.

119. Keefe R.S., Silverman J.M., Roitman S.E., Harvey P.D., Duncan M.A., Alroy D., Siever L.J., Davis K.L., Mohs R.C. (1994) Performance of nonpsychotic relatives of schizophrenic patients on cognitive tests. *Psychiatry Res.*, **53**: 1–12.

120. Lyons M., Merla M.E., Young L., Kremen W. (1991) Impaired neuropsychological functioning in symptomatic volunteers with schizotypy: preliminary findings. *Biol. Psychiatry*, **30**: 424–426.

121. Raine A., Sheard C., Reynolds G.P., Lencz T. (1992) Pre-frontal structural and functional deficits associated with individual differences in schizotypal personality. *Schizophr. Res.*, **7**: 237–247.

122. Miller L.S., Swanson-Green T., Moses J.A., Faustman W.O. (1996) Comparison of cognitive performance in RDC-diagnosed schizoaffective and schizophrenic patients with the Luria-Nebraska neuropsychological battery. *J. Psychiatr. Res.*, **30**: 277–282.

123. Park S., Holzman P.S. (1992) Schizophrenics show spatial working memory deficits. *Arch. Gen. Psychiatry*, **49**: 975–982.

124. Keefe R., Lees-Roitman S., Dupre R. (1997) Performance of patients with schizophrenia on a pen and paper visuospatial working memory task with short delay. *Schizophr. Res.*, **26**: 9–14.

125. Park S., Holzman P.S., Goldman-Rakic P.S. (1995) Spatial working memory deficits in the relatives of schizophrenic patients. *Arch. Gen. Psychiatry*, **52**: 821–828.

126. Park S., Holzman P.S., Lenzenweger M.F. (1995) Individual differences in spatial working memory in relation to schizotypy. *J. Abnorm. Psychol.*, **104**: 355–363.

127. Maier W., Franke P., Hain C., Kopp B., Rist F. (1992) Neuropsychological indicators of the vulnerability to schizophrenia. *Progr. Neuropsychopharmacol. Biol. Psychiatry*, **16**: 703–715.

128. Franke P., Maier W., Hardt J., Hain C., Cornblatt B.A. (1994) Attentional abilities and measures of schizotypy: their variation and covariation in schizophrenic patients, their siblings, and normal control subjects. *Psychiatry Res.*, **54**: 259–272.

129. Cornblatt B.A., Keilp J.G. (1994) Impaired attention, genetics, and the pathophysiology of schizophrenia. *Schizophr. Bull.*, **20**: 31–46.

130. Siever L.J., Bergman A.J., Keefe R.S.E. (1995) The schizophrenia spectrum personality disorders. In *Schizophrenia* (Eds S.R. Hirsch, D.R. Weinberger), pp. 87–185. Blackwell, Oxford.

131. Roitman S.E., Cornblatt B.A., Bergman A., Obuchowski M., Mitropoulou V., Keefe R.S., Silverman J.M., Siever L.J. (1997) Attentional functioning in schizotypal personality disorder. *Am. J. Psychiatry*, **154**: 655–660.

132. Chen W.J., Hsiao C.K., Hsiao L.L., Hwu H.G. (1998) Performance of the Continuous Performance Test among community samples. *Schizophr. Bull.*, **24**: 163–174.

133. Keefe R.S., Silverman J.M., Mohs R.C., Siever L.J., Harvey P.D., Friedman L., Roitman S.E., DuPre R.L., Smith C.J., Schmeidler J. *et al.* (1997) Eye tracking, attention, and schizotypal symptoms in nonpsychotic relatives of patients with schizophrenia. *Arch. Gen. Psychiatry*, **54**: 169–176.

134. Green M., Nuechterlein K., Breitmeyer B. (1997) Backward masking performance in unaffected siblings of schizophrenic patients. *Arch. Gen. Psychiatry*, **54**: 465–472.

135. Braff D.L. (1981) Impaired speed of information processing in nonmedicated schizotypal patients. *Schizophr. Bull.*, **7**: 499–508.

136. Cadenhead K.S., Perry W., Braff D.L. (1996) The relationship of information-processing deficits and clinical symptoms in schizotypal personality disorder. *Biol. Psychiatry*, **40**: 853–858.

137. Schubert D.L., Saccuzzo D.P., Braff D.L. (1985) Information processing in borderline patients. *J. Nerv. Ment. Dis.*, **173**: 26–31.

138. Saykin A.J., Shtasel D.L., Gur R.E., Kester D.B., Mozley L.H., Stafiniak P., Gur R.C. (1994) Neuropsychological deficits in neuroleptic naive patients with first-episode schizophrenia. *Arch. Gen. Psychiatry*, **51**: 124–131.

139. Voglmaier M.M., Seidman L.J., Salisbury D., McCarley R.W. (1997) Neuropsychological dysfunction in schizotypal personality disorder: a profile analysis. *Biol. Psychiatry*, **41**: 530–540.

140. Cannon T.D., Zorrilla L.E., Shtasel D., Gur R.E., Gur R.C., Marco E.J., Moberg P., Price R.A. (1994) Neuropsychological functioning in siblings discordant for schizophrenia and healthy volunteers. *Arch. Gen. Psychiatry*, **51**: 651–661.

141. LaPorte D.J., Kirkpatrick B., Thaker G.K. (1994) Psychosis-proneness and verbal memory in a college student population. *Schizophr. Res.*, **12**: 237–245.

142. Manschreck T.C., Maher B.A., Beaudette S.M., Redmond D.A. (1997) Context memory in schizoaffective and schizophrenic memory. *Schizophr. Res.*, **26**: 153–161.

143. Beatty W.W., Jocic Z., Monson N., Staton R.D. (1993) Memory and frontal lobe dysfunction in schizophrenia and schizoaffective disorder. *J. Nerv. Ment. Dis.*, **181**: 448–453.

144. Spitzer M., Weisker I., Winter M., Maier S., Hermle L., Maher B.A. (1994) Semantic and phonological priming in schizophrenia. *J. Abnorm. Psychol.*, **103**: 485–494.

145. Hurt S.W., Holzman P.S., Davis J.M. (1983) Thought disorder. The measurement of its changes. *Arch. Gen. Psychiatry*, **40**: 1281–1285.
146. Hain C., Maier W., Hoechst-Janneck S., Franke P. (1995) Subclinical thought disorder in first-degree relatives of schizophrenic patients. Results from a matched-pairs study with the Thought Disorder Index. *Acta Psychiatr. Scand.*, **92**: 305–309.
147. Coleman M.J., Levy D.L., Lenzenweger M.F., Holzman P.S. (1996) Thought disorder, perceptual aberrations, and schizotypy. *J. Abnorm. Psychol.*, **105**: 469–473.
148. Edell W.S. (1987) Role of structure in disordered thinking in borderline and schizophrenic disorders. *J. Pers. Assess.*, **51**: 23–41.
149. Duchene A., Graves R.E., Brugger P. (1998) Schizotypal thinking and associative processing: a response commonality analysis of verbal fluency. *J. Psychiatry Neurosci.*, **23**: 56–60.
150. Beech A., Baylis G.C., Smithson P., Claridge G. (1989) Individual differences in schizotypy as reflected in measures of cognitive inhibition. *Br. J. Clin. Psychol.*, **28**: 117–129.
151. Peters E.R., Pickering A.D., Hemsley D.R. (1994) "Cognitive inhibition" and positive symptomatology in schizotypy. *Br. J. Clin. Psychol.*, **33**: 33–48.
152. Moritz S., Mass R. (1997) Reduced cognitive inhibition in schizotypy. *Br. J. Clin. Psychol.*, **36**: 365–376.
153. Beech A., Powell T., McWilliam J., Claridge G. (1989) Evidence of reduced "cognitive inhibition" in schizophrenia. *Br. J. Clin. Psychol.*, **28**: 109–116.
154. Williams L. (1996) Cognitive inhibition and schizophrenic symptom subgroups. *Schizophr. Bull.*, **22**: 139–151.
155. Lipton R.B., Levy D., Holzman P.S., Levin S. (1983) Eye movement dysfunctions in psychiatric patients: a review. *Schizophr. Bull.*, **9**: 13–32.
156. Holzman P.S., Solomon C.M., Levin S., Waternauz C.S. (1984) Pursuit eye movement dysfunctions in schizophrenia: family evidence for specificity. *Arch. Gen. Psychiatry*, **41**: 136–139.
157. Ross R.G., Hommer D., Radant A., Roath M., Freedman R. (1996) Early expression of smooth-pursuit eye movement abnormalities in children of schizophrenic parents. *J. Am. Acad. Child Adolesc. Psychiatry*, **35**: 941–949.
158. Siever L.J., Coursey R.D., Alterman I.S., Buchsbaum M.S., Murphy D.L. (1984) Smooth pursuit eye movement impairment: a vulnerability marker for schizotypal personality disorder in a volunteer population. *Am. J. Psychiatry*, **141**: 1560–1566.
159. Siever L.J., Coursey R.D., Alterman I.S., Zahn T., Brody L., Bernad P., Buchsbaum M., Lake C.R., Murphy D.L. (1989) Clinical psychophysiological, and neurological characteristics of volunteers with impaired smooth pursuit eye movements. *Biol. Psychiatry*, **26**: 35–51.
160. Keefe R.S., Siever L.J., Mohs R.C., Peterson A.E., Mahon T.R., Bergman R.L., Davis K.L. (1989) Eye tracking, schizophrenic symptoms, and schizotypal personality disorder. *Eur. Arch. Psychiatry Neurol. Sci.*, **239**: 39–42.
161. Lencz T., Raine A., Scerbo A., Redmon M., Brodish S., Holt L., Bird L. (1993) Impaired eye tracking in undergraduates with schizotypal personality disorder. *Am. J. Psychiatry*, **150**: 152–154.
162. Siever L.J. (1991) The biology of the boundaries of schizophrenia. In *Advances in Neuropsychiatry and Psychopharmacology, vol. 1: Schizophrenia Research* (Eds C.A. Tamminga, S.C. Schulz), pp. 181–191. Raven, New York.
163. Thaker G.K., Ross D.E., Cassady S.L., Adami H.M., LaPorte D., Medoff D.R., Lahti A. (1998) Smooth pursuit eye movements to extraretinal motion signals:

deficits in relatives of patients with schizophrenia. *Arch. Gen. Psychiatry*, **55**: 830–836.

164. Simons R.F., Katkin W. (1985) Smooth pursuit eye movements in subjects reporting physical anhedonia and perceptual aberrations. *Psychiatry Res.*, **14**: 275–289.

165. Clementz B.A., McDowell J.E., Zisook S. (1994) Saccadic system functioning among schizophrenia patients and their first-degree biological relatives. *J. Abnorm. Psychol.*, **103**: 277–287.

166. Katsanis J., Kortenkamp S., Iacono W.G., Grove W.M. (1997) Antisaccade performance in patients with schizophrenia and affective disorder. *J. Abnorm. Psychol.*, **106**: 468–472.

167. McDowell J., Clementz B. (1997) The effect of fixation condition manipulations on antisaccade performance in schizophrenia: studies of diagnostic specificity. *Exp. Brain Res.*, **115**: 333–344.

168. O'Driscoll G.A., Lenzenweger M.F., Holzman P.S. (1998) Antisaccades and smooth pursuit eye tracking and schizotypy. *Arch. Gen. Psychiatry*, **55**: 837–843.

169. Ross R.G., Harris J.G., Olincy A., Radant A., Adler L.E., Freedman R. (1998) Familial transmission of two independent saccadic abnormalities in schizophrenia. *Schizophr. Res.*, **30**: 59–70.

170. Ross R.G., Olincy A., Harris J.G., Radant A., Adler L.E., Freedman R. (1998) Anticipatory saccades during smooth pursuit eye movements and familial transmission of schizophrenia. *Biol. Psychiatry*, **44**: 690–697.

171. Heinrichs D.W., Buchanan R.W. (1988) Significance and meaning of neurological signs in schizophrenia. *Am. J. Psychiatry*, **145**: 11–18.

172. Rossi A., De Cataldo S., Di Michele V., Manna V., Ceccoli S., Stratta P., Casacchia M. (1990) Neurological soft signs in schizophrenia. *Br. J. Psychiatry*, **157**: 735–739.

173. Fish B. (1987) Infant predictors of the longitudinal course of schizophrenic development. *Schizophr. Bull.*, **13**: 395–409.

174. Fish B., Marcus J., Hans S.L., Auerbach J.G., Perdue S. (1992) Infants at risk for schizophrenia: sequelae of a genetic neurointegrative defect. A review and replication analysis of pandysmaturation in the Jerusalem Infant Development Study. *Arch. Gen. Psychiatry*, **49**: 221–235.

175. Walker E.F., Savoie T., Davis D. (1994) Neuromotor precursors of schizophrenia. *Schizophr. Bull.*, **20**: 441–451.

176. Blackwood D.H., St Clair D.M., Muir W.J., Duffy J.C. (1991) Auditory P300 and eye tracking dysfunction in schizophrenic pedigrees. *Arch. Gen. Psychiatry*, **48**: 899–909.

177. Frangou S., Sharma T., Alarcon G., Sigmudsson T., Takei N., Binnie C., Murray R.M. (1997) The Maudsley Family Study, II: Endogenous event-related potentials in familial schizophrenia. *Schizophr. Res.*, **23**: 45–53.

178. Friedman D., Cornblatt B.A., Vaughan H., Erlenmeyer-Kimling L. (1988) Auditory event-related potentials in children at risk for schizophrenia: the complete initial sample. *Psychiatry Res.*, **26**: 203–221.

179. Schreiber H., Stolz-Born G., Kornhuber H.H., Born J. (1992) Event-related potential correlates of impaired selective attention in children at high risk for schizophrenia. *Biol. Psychiatry*, **32**: 634–651.

180. Simons R.F., MacMillan F.W., Ireland F.B. (1982) Reaction time crossover in preselected schizotypic subjects. *J. Abnorm. Psychol.*, **6**: 414–419.

181. Blackwood D.H.R., St Clair D.M., Kutcher S.P. (1986) P300 event-related potential abnormalities in borderline disorder. *Biol. Psychiatry*, **21**: 557–560.

182. Kutcher S.P., Blackwood D.H.R., Gaskell D.F., Muir W.J., St Clair D. (1989) Auditory P300 does not differentiate borderline personality disorder from schizotypal personality disorder. *Biol. Psychiatry*, **26**: 766–774.

183. Siever L.J., Kalus O.F., Keefe R.S.E. (1993) The boundaries of schizophrenia. *Psychiatr. Clin. North Am.*, **16**: 217–244.

184. Trestman R.L., Horvath T., Kalus O., Peterson A.E., Coccaro E., Mitropoulou V., Apter S., Davidson M., Siever L.J. (1996) Event-related potentials in schizotypal personality disorder. *J. Neuropsychiatry Clin. Neurosci.*, **8**: 33–40.

185. Swerdlow N.R., Geyer M.A. (1998) Using an animal model of deficient sensorimotor gating to study the pathophysiology and new treatments of schizophrenia. *Schizophr. Bull.*, **24**: 285–301.

186. Cadenhead K.S., Geyer M.A., Braff D.L. (1993) Impaired startle prepulse inhibition and habituation in patients with schizotypal personality disorder. *Am. J. Psychiatry*, **150**: 1862–1867.

187. Cadenhead K., Kumar C., Braff D. (1996) Clinical and experimental characteristics of "hypothetically psychosis prone" college students. *J. Psychiatr. Res.*, **30**: 331–340.

188. Siegel C., Waldo M., Mizner G., Adler L.E., Freedman R. (1984) Deficits in sensory gating in schizophrenic patients and their relatives. Evidence obtained with auditory evoked responses. *Arch. Gen. Psychiatry*, **41**: 607–612.

189. Clementz B.A., Geyer M.A., Braff D.L. (1998) Poor P50 suppression among schizophrenia patients and their first-degree biological relatives. *Am. J. Psychiatry*, **155**: 1691–1694.

190. Squires-Wheeler E., Friedman D., Amminger G.P., Skodol A., Looser-Ott S., Roberts S., Pape K., Erlenmeyer-Kimling L. (1997) Negative and positive dimensions of schizotypal personality disorder. *J. Pers. Disord.*, **11**: 285–300.

191. Erlenmeyer-Kimling L., Cornblatt B.A., Rock D., Roberts S., Bell M., West A. (1993) The New York High-Risk Project: Anhedonia, attentional deviance, and psychopathology. *Schizophr. Bull.*, **19**: 141–153.

192. Cassady S.L., Adami H., Moran M., Kunkel R., Thaker G.K. (1998) Spontaneous dyskinesia in subjects with schizophrenia spectrum personality. *Am. J. Psychiatry*, **155**: 70–75.

193. Pollak L., Klein C., Rabey J.M., Schiffer J. (1996) Posterior fossa lesions associated with neuropsychiatric symptomatology. *Int. J. Neurosci.*, **87**: 119–126.

194. Caplan R., Guthrie D. (1994) Blink rate in childhood schizophrenia spectrum disorder. *Biol. Psychiatry*, **35**: 228–234.

195. Blum K., Braverman E.R., Wu S., Cull J.G., Chen T.J., Gill J., Wood R., Eisenberg A., Sherman M., Davis K.R. *et al* (1997) Association of polymorphism of dopamine D2 receptor (DRD2), and dopamine transporter (DAT1) genes with schizoid/avoidant behaviors (SAB). *Mol. Psychiatry*, **2**: 239–246.

196. Owen F., Simpson M.D. (1995) The neurochemistry of schizophrenia. In *Schizophrenia* (Eds S.R. Hirsch, D.R. Weinberger), pp. 358–378. Blackwell, Oxford.

197. Siever L.J., Amin F., Coccaro E.F., Bernstein D., Kavoussi R.J., Kalus O., Horvath T.B., Warne P., Davidson M., Davis K.L. (1991) Plasma homovanillic acid in schizotypal personality disorder. *Am. J. Psychiatry*, **148**: 1246–1248.

198. Siever L.J., Trestman R.L., Coccaro E., Amin F., Lawrence T., Gabriel S., Mitropoulou V. (1992) Monoamines in personality disorder. *Clin. Neuropharmacol.*, **15** (Suppl. 1): 231A–232A.

199. Siever L.J., Amin F., Coccaro E.F., Trestman R., Silverman J., Horvath T.B., Mahon T.R., Knott P., Altstiel L., Davidson M. *et al.* (1993) CSF homovanillic acid in schizotypal personality disorder. *Am. J. Psychiatry*, **150**: 149–151.

200. Schulz S.C., Cornelius J., Schulz P.M., Soloff P.H. (1988) The amphetamine challenge test in patients with borderline disorder. *Am. J. Psychiatry*, **145**: 809–814.
201. Siegel B.V., Trestman R.L., O'Flaithbheartaigh S., Mitropoulou V., Amin F., Kirrane R., Silverman J., Schmeidler J., Keefe R.S., Siever L.J. (1996) D-amphetamine challenge effects on Wisconsin Card Sort Test. Performance in schizotypal personality disorder. *Schizophr. Res.*, **20**: 29–32.
202. Coccaro E.F., Prudic J., Rothpearl A., Nurnberg H.G. (1985) The dexamethasone suppression test in depressive, non-depressive and schizoaffective psychosis. *J. Affect. Disord.*, **9**: 107–113.
203. Raz S., Raz N. (1990) Structural brain abnormalities in the major psychoses: a quantitative review of the evidence from computerized imaging. *Psychol. Bull.*, **108**: 93–108.
204. Nelson M.D., Saykin A.J., Flashman L.A., Riordan H.J. (1998) Hippocampal volume reduction in schizophrenia as assessed by magnetic resonance imaging: a meta-analytic study. *Arch. Gen. Psychiatry*, **55**: 433–440.
205. Falkai P., Bogerts B. (1995) The neuropathology of schizophrenia. In *Schizophrenia* (Eds S.R. Hirsch, D.R. Weinberger), pp. 275–292. Blackwell, Oxford.
206. Siever L.J., Rotter M., Losonczy M., Guo S.L., Mitropoulou V., Trestman R., Apter S., Zemishlany Z., Silverman J., Horvath T.B. (1995) Lateral ventricular enlargement in schizotypal personality. *Psychiatry Res.*, **57**: 109–118.
207. Silverman J.M., Smith C.J., Guo S.L., Mohs R.C., Siever L.J., Davis K.L. (1998) Lateral ventricular enlargement in schizophrenic probands and their siblings with schizophrenia-related disorders. *Biol. Psychiatry*, **43**: 97–106.
208. Buchsbaum M.S., Yang S., Hazlett E., Siegel B.V. Jr, Germans M., Haznedar M., O'Flaithbheartaigh S., Wie T., Silverman J., Siever L.J. (1997) Ventricular volume and asymmetry in schizotypal personality disorder and schizophrenia assessed with magnetic resonance imaging. *Schizophr. Res.*, **27**: 45–53.
209. Schulsinger F., Parnas J., Peterson E.T., Schulsinger H., Teasdale T.W., Mednick S.A., Moller L., Silverton L. (1984) Cerebral ventricular size in the offspring of schizophrenic mothers. A preliminary study. *Arch. Gen. Psychiatry*, **41**: 602–606.
210. Cannon T.D., Mednick S.A., Parnas J. (1990) Antecedents of predominantly negative- and predominantly positive-symptom schizophrenia in a high risk population *Arch. Gen. Psychiatry*, **47**: 622–632.
211. Cannon T.D., Mednick S.A., Parnas J., Schulsinger F., Praestholm J., Vestergaard A. (1993) Developmental brain abnormalities in the offspring of schizophrenic mothers. I. Contributions of genetic and perinatal factors. *Arch. Gen. Psychiatry*, **50**: 551–564.
212. Cannon T.D., Mednick S.A., Parnas J., Schulsinger F., Praestholm J., Vestergaard A. (1994) Developmental brain abnormalities in the offspring of schizophrenic mothers. II. Structural brain characteristics of schizophrenia and schizotypal personality disorder. *Arch. Gen. Psychiatry*, **51**: 955–962.
213. Keshavan M.S., Montrose D.M., Pierri J.N., Dick E.L., Rosenberg D., Talagala L., Sweeney J.A. (1997) Magnetic resonance imaging and spectroscopy in offspring at risk for schizophrenia: preliminary studies. *Progr. Neuropsychopharmacol. Biol. Psychiatry*, **21**: 1285–1295.
214. Seidman L.J., Faraone S.V., Goldstein J.M., Goodman J.M., Kremen W.S., Matsuda G., Hoge E.A., Kennedy D., Makris N., Caviness V.S. *et al.* (1997) Reduced subcortical brain volumes in nonpsychotic siblings of schizophrenic patients: a pilot magnetic resonance imaging study. *Am. J. Med. Genet.*, **74**: 507–514.
215. Sharma T., DuBoulay G., Lewis S., Sigmundsson T., Gurling H., Murray R. (1997) The Maudsley family study I: Structural brain changes on magnetic

resonance imaging in familial schizophrenia. *Progr. Neuropsychopharmacol. Biol. Psychiatry*, **21**: 1297–1315.

216. Brooks W.M., Hodde-Vargas J., Vargas L.A., Yeo R.A., Ford C.C., Hendren R.L. (1998) Frontal lobe of children with schizophrenia spectrum disorders: a proton magnetic resonance spectroscopic study. *Biol. Psychiatry*, **43**: 263–269.

217. Hirsch S.R., Barnes T.R. (1995) The clinical treatment of schizophrenia with antipsychotic medication. In *Schizophrenia* (Eds S.R. Hirsch, D.R. Weinberger), pp. 443–468. Blackwell, Oxford.

218. Coccaro E.F. (1998) Clinical outcome of psychopharmacologic treatment of borderline and schizotypal personality disordered subjects. *J. Clin. Psychiatry*, **59** (Suppl. 1): 30–35.

219. Reyntjens A.M. (1972) A series of multicentric pilot trials with pimozide in psychiatric practice. I. Pimozide in the treatment of personality disorders. *Acta Psychiatr. Belg.*, **72**: 653–661.

220. Goldberg S.C., Schulz S.C., Schulz P.M., Resnick R.J., Hamer R.M., Friedel R.O. (1986) Borderline and schizotypal personality disorders treated with low-dose thiothixene versus placebo. *Arch. Gen. Psychiatry*, **43**: 680–686.

221. Soloff P.H., George A., Nathan R.S., Schulz P.M., Ulrich R.F., Perel J.M. (1986) Progress in the pharmacotherapy of borderline disorders: a double-blind study of amitriptyline, haloperidol and placebo. *Arch. Gen. Psychiatry*, **43**: 691–697.

222. Frankenburg F.R., Zanarini M.C. (1993) Clozapine treatment of borderline patients: a preliminary study. *Compr. Psychiatry*, **34**: 402–405.

223. Vilkin M.I. (1964) Comparative chemotherapeutic trial in treatment of chronic borderline patients. *Am. J. Psychiatry*, **120**: 1004.

224. Stone M. (1992) Treatment of severe personality disorder. In *Annual Review of Psychiatry* (Eds A. Tasman, M. Riba), pp. 98–115. American Psychiatric Association, Washington, DC.

225. MacFarlane W.F. (1990) Psychoeducational treatment of schizophrenia. In *Handbook of Schizophrenia*, vol. 4 (Eds M.L. Hertz, S.J. Keith, J.P. Docherty), pp. 167–189. Elsevier, New York.

226. Goodnick P.J., Meltzer H.Y. (1983) Lithium treatment of schizomania and mania. Presented at the APA Meeting, New York, 1–6 May.

227. Carman J.S., Bigelow L.B., Wyatt R.J. (1981) Lithium combined with neuroleptics in chronic schizophrenic and schizoaffective patients. *J. Clin. Psychiatry*, **42**: 124–128.

228. Möller H.J., Morin C. (1989) Behandlung schizodepressiver Syndrome mit Antidepressiva. In *Schizoaffektive Psychosen: Diagnose, Therapie und Prophylaxe* (Ed. A. Marneros), pp. 159–178. Springer, Berlin.

229. Müller-Oerlinghausen B., Thies K., Volk J. (1989) Lithium in der Prophylaxe schizoaffektiver Psychosen. Erste Ergebnisse der Berliner Lithium-Katamnese. In *Schizoaffektive Psychosen: Diagnose, Therapie und Prophylaxe* (Ed. A. Marneros), pp. 191–195. Springer, Berlin.

230. Lenz G., Wolf R., Simhandl C., Topitze A., Berner P. (1989) Langzeitprognose und Rückfallprophylaxe der schizoaffektiven Psychosen. In *Schizoaffektive Psychosen: Diagnose, Therapie und Prophylaxe* (Ed. A. Marneros), pp. 55–66. Springer, Berlin.

231. Mattes J.A., Nayak D. (1984) Lithium versus fluphenazine for prophylaxis in mainly schizophrenic schizoaffectives. *Biol. Psychiatry*, **19**: 445–448.

Commentaries

5.1
Extending the Schizophrenia Spectrum even Further

Gordon Claridge[1]

In their very detailed paper, Maier *et al* provide not only a comprehensive review of literature, but also a lucid framework for describing and investigating those disorders that present, not as schizophrenia, but as some apparent variation of it—or rather of "them", since it is clear that, as with the schizophrenias themselves, we are dealing here with a group of heterogeneous "borderline" conditions. The slant of the target paper is naturally clinical, the authors' priority being to use schizophrenia spectrum in its most obvious way: as a construct for linking together forms of *disorder* that may differ in severity but which might be linked aetiologically. The purpose of the present commentary is to suggest a broader view of the schizophrenia spectrum which, hopefully, will be seen, not as an alternative to, but as complementing, that offered by Maier *et al*, extending their model in theoretically and empirically useful ways.

The best starting point for my remarks is their model of multifactorial transmission. That summarizes a relatively uncontroversial set of conclusions from the reviewed evidence about the schizophrenia spectrum as a biological continuum of varying liability to the disorders listed. At least that is true at the *upper end* of the continuum, enclosing individuals whose risk for a schizophrenia-related illness varies from submaximal to severe. More ambiguous is the status of individuals falling somewhat outside that range, those about whose position on the continuum Maier *et al* comment: "Lower values are not associated with any impairment induced by etiological factors contributing to schizophrenia". The statement raises some interesting questions. Does it mean that people falling lower down in the continuum have too few of the multifactorial characteristics involved for them realistically ever to be expected to pass the threshold, even into subclinical schizophrenia? Or does it mean they will never do so, because they do not, for example, possess the single gene that writers like Meehl [1] believe is responsible for this spectrum

---

[1]*Department of Experimental Psychology, University of Oxford, OX1 3UD, U.K.*

of disorder? And if the latter, why is there not more discontinuity in the "continuum"?

The above ambiguity articulates a rarely aired subtext in the debate about the schizophrenia spectrum. It concerns the dual meaning of "dimensionality" as it relates to schizophrenia. The point, presented in more detail elsewhere [2, 3], is that it is possible to identify two (historically and theoretically distinct) ways in which dimensionality has been construed.

One, labelled "quasi-dimensional" (QD), refers to continuity that exists only within the illness domain; captured in the *forme fruste* notion of disease and permitting some variation in the severity of symptom expression. The other, termed "fully dimensional" (FD), is more personality centred and regards traits like schizotypy as merely features of normal individual difference, in the same sense as, say, anxiety: such traits are not in themselves pathological — indeed they may even be adaptive at optimum levels — but they can nevertheless predispose to illness under unfavourable circumstances.

Space does not permit a detailed comparison of these two views of dimensionality; suffice it to say that the evidence strongly supports the broader (FD) interpretation (see refs [2] and [3]). Here I will confine myself to a few observations about that, relevant to the target article.

One point concerns the many correlates of schizotypy. Some of these do not have any pathological content or consequence at all and can include: enhanced creativity (see ref. [4] for a recent review); positive spiritual experience [5]; and the ability to indulge without harm in such unusual psychological explorations as out-of-the-body-experiences [6]. Even where there is psychopathology, it can fall well outside the usually recognized boundaries of the schizophrenia spectrum and include obsessive–compulsive disorder [7], eating disorders [8], and dyslexia [9]. On the face of it, such evidence appears to make the task of understanding the so-called "schizophrenia spectrum" even greater than Maier *et al* already acknowledge. However, there is one consistent finding in all of the studies quoted that may be of some significance: signs of high schizotypy in these groups were always confined to the "positive symptom" (perceptual aberration, unusual experiences) component of the trait and never included raised levels on features like anhedonia. This agrees well with Maier *et al*'s conclusion that perhaps the uniquely *schizophrenic* indicators of risk are the "negative symptom" aspects of schizotypy.

Even so, as they imply, determining the likely outcome for schizotypal individuals will demand precise profiling with respect to several — perhaps many — biological and psychosocial influences on a person's life course. In this respect, the broadening of the schizophrenia spectrum suggested here has one advantage. It emphasizes the possibility of beneficial, instead of exclusively pathological, outcomes for schizotypy. This, in turn, has implications for prevention and the need to search as vigorously for factors that protect from illness as for those that encourage it.

REFERENCES

1. Meehl P. (1990) Toward an integrated theory of schizotaxia, schizotypy, and schizophrenia. *J. Pers. Dis.*, **4**: 1–99.
2. Claridge G. (Ed.) (1997) *Schizotypy: Implications for Illness and Health*. Oxford University Press, Oxford.
3. Claridge G. (1999) Schizotypy: theory and measurement. *Rev. Argentina. Clin. Psicol.* (in press).
4. Brod J. (1997) Creativity and schizotypy. In *Schizotypy: Implications for Illness and Health* (Ed. G. Claridge), pp. 274–298. Oxford University Press, Oxford.
5. Jackson M. (1997) Spiritual experience and schizotypy. In *Schizotypy: Implications for Illness and Health* (Ed. G. Claridge), pp. 227–250. Oxford University Press, Oxford.
6. McCreery C., Claridge G. (1993) Out-of-the-body experiences and personality. *J. Soc. Psychiat. Res.*, **60**: 129–148.
7. Enright S.J., Claridge G., Beech A.R., Kemp-Wheeler S.M. (1994) A questionnaire assessment of schizotypy in OCD. *Pers. Individ. Diffs.*, **16**: 191–194.
8. Murphy R. (1998) A relationship between eating disorders and psychosis-proneness. Unpublished research report, University of Oxford.
9. Richardson A.J., Stein J.F. (1993) Personality characteristics of adult dyslexics. In *Studies in Visual Information Processing* (Eds R. Groner, S. Wright), pp. 411–423. Elsevier, Amsterdam.

5.2
Schizotypy: Theoretical Considerations, Latent Structure, and the Expanded Phenotype

Mark F. Lenzenweger[1]

Contemporary models of the aetiology and pathogenesis of schizophrenia [1, 2] have been informed by the accumulating literature supporting an unambiguous linkage between schizotypic psychopathology and schizophrenia liability. Indeed, we [3, 4] have argued, based on a large series of empirical investigations, that schizotypic psychopathology is best viewed as an alternative expression of schizophrenia liability. The review by Maier *et al* provides a window on this exciting area of psychopathology research. Discussion of a variety of theoretical and definitional issues may facilitate assimilation of their review as well as point to other active areas of schizotypy research.

[1]*Department of Psychology, Harvard University, 33 Kirkland Street, Cambridge, Massachusetts 02138, USA*

To begin, the term "schizotype" was coined by Rado to represent a condensation of "schizophrenic *pheno*type" [5, 6]. It is interesting to note that Rado did *not* suggest schizotype as a condensation of the terms schizophrenic and genotype as has sometimes been thought to be the case. Meehl's model of schizotypy [7, 8] suggested that schizophrenia is the complex developmental result of a single major genetic factor relatively specific for schizophrenia operating against a background of other genetically determined potentiators (e.g. anxiety, hedonic potential, social introversion) and environmental stressors. One should note that this encompasses the notion of a "mixed model" of genetic influence, which is quite viable as a genetic model in schizophrenia, as Maier *et al* point out. Meehl hypothesized that the single major gene (schizogene) codes for a functional central nervous system synaptic control aberration termed *hypokrisia*, which results in *schizotaxia*, extensive synaptic slippage throughout the brain. Through social learning experiences, essentially all schizotaxia individuals develop *schizotypy*, a personality organization that harbours the latent liability for schizophrenia [8]. As a personality organization, *schizotypy cannot be observed directly per se*, however this latent personality organization gives rise to schizotypic psychological and behavioural manifestations and is also reflected in deviance on laboratory measures (e.g. eye tracking dysfunction, sustained attention deficits). Schizotypic individuals (*though not necessarily diagnosable as DSM-III-R schizotypic personality disorder*) exhibit cognitive slippage, interpersonal aversiveness, pan-anxiety, and mild depression. The majority remain only schizotypic throughout the lifespan, while a subset go on to develop diagnosable schizophrenia.

Assuming that schizotypy represents a *latent liability* construct and that current schizotypy indexes are valid, a basic question about the fundamental structure of schizotypy remains. Is it continuous (i.e. "dimensional") or is it truly discontinuous (or "qualitative") in nature? One surely cannot reason with confidence that schizotypy is dimensional in latent structure (i.e. a quantitative character) based on: (a) a *unimodal* distribution of phenotypic schizotypic traits; (b) the results of factor analytic studies of schizotypy; or (c) the fact that one measured it with a dimensional scale [9]. Regarding factor analytic results, one must always remember that factor analysis *always* provides evidence that data are dimensional in nature, it cannot do otherwise. There are no compelling data available to support the dimensionality of schizotypy as a latent liability construct. There are data, however, available from taxometric studies that speak to the latent structure question, and those data strongly support a qualitative latent structure for schizotypy. The prevalence of the latent class detected in these studies is approximately 10% [10, 11].

The schizotype can be defined and identified in one of three ways: (a) clinically (e.g. *DSM-IV*; see the review by Maier *et al*); (b) in terms of deviance on reliable laboratory measures or psychometric indexes of schizotypy; or (c) by virtue of having a first-degree biological relative affected with schizophrenia. We [3] have presented data based on the criterial facets of: (a) clinical phenomenology, (b) family history, (c) delimitation from other conditions, (d) follow-up study and (e) laboratory indexes, suggesting that the psychometrically identified schizotype can be viewed as a valid expression of schizotypy (i.e. the latent liability for schizophrenia). The laboratory findings associated with the psychometrically identified schizotype are particularly robust, including deviance on tasks of: sustained attention, smooth pursuit eye tracking, spatial working memory, thought disorder, antisaccade performance, executive functioning, negative priming and personality pathology [3]. Moreover, we have argued that the pattern of evidence supportive of the validity of psychometrically identified schizotypes provides a compelling case for expanding the schizophrenia phenotype in genetic analysis to include the schizotype.

REFERENCES

1. Lenzenweger M.F., Dworkin R.H. (Eds) (1998) *Origins and Development of Schizophrenia: Advances in Experimental Psychopathology*. American Psychological Association, Washington, DC.
2. Lenzenweger M.F. (1999) Schizophrenia: refining the phenotype, resolving endophenotypes. *Behav. Res. Ther.*, **37**: 281–295.
3. Lenzenweger M.F. (1998) Schizotypy and schizotypic psychopathology: mapping an alternative expression of schizophrenia liability. In *Origins and Development of Schizophrenia: Advances in Experimental Psychopathology* (Eds M.F. Lenzenweger, R.H. Dworkin), pp. 93–121. American Psychological Association, Washington, DC.
4. Lenzenweger M.F., Loranger A.W. (1989) Detection of familial schizophrenia using a psychometric measure of schizotypy. *Arch. Gen. Psychiatry*, **46**: 902–907.
5. Rado S. (1953) Dynamics and classification of disordered behavior. *Am. J. Psychiatry*, **110**: 406–416.
6. Rado S. (1960) Theory and therapy: the theory of schizotypal organisation and its application to the treatment of decompensated schizotypal behavior. In *The Outpatient Treatment of Schizophrenia* (Eds S.C. Scher, H.R. Davis), pp. 87–101. Grune and Stratton, New York.
7. Meehl P.E. (1962) Schizotaxia, Schizotypy, Schizophrenia. *Am. Psychologist*, **17**: 827–838.
8. Meehl P.E. (1990) Toward an integrated theory of schizotaxia, schizotypy, and schizophrenia. *J. Personality Dis.*, **4**: 1–99.
9. Lenzenweger M.F., Korfine L. (1995) Tracking the taxon: on the latent structure and base rate of schizotypy. In *Schizotypal Personality* (Eds A. Raine, T. Lencz, S.A. Mednick), pp. 135–167. Cambridge University Press, New York.
10. Lenzenweger M.F., Korfine L. (1992) Confirming the latent structure and base rate of schizotypy: a taxometric analysis. *J. Abnorm. Psychol.*, **101**: 567–571.
11. Lenzenweger M.F. (1999) Deeper into the schizotypy taxon: on the robust nature of maximum covariance analysis. *J. Abnorm. Psychol.*, **108**: 182–187.

5.3
Empirical Characterization of the Schizophrenia Spectrum

Loring J. Ingraham[1]

Diagnosis of psychopathology is based on clinical observation and choice of diagnostic criteria rather than on the empirical assessment of pathophysiology. In the absence of specific pathophysiology, competent clinicians may disagree over what constitutes a particular syndrome, which diagnostic criteria are relevant and whether a given case meets those criteria. The promise of evidence-based nosology is to help further the progress of diagnosis from the assessment of clinically observed syndromes to the identification of categories or dimensions that reflect the operation of specific physiological mechanisms.

Adoption studies of schizophrenia have established that the clinical observation of an increased risk for schizophrenia among the family members of affected individuals is due to the operation of shared genes [1]. The observation of a similar risk for schizophrenia among the biological relatives of adoptees with schizophrenia and among the biological relatives of non-adopted individuals with schizophrenia suggests the operation of similar mechanisms responsible for illness. The demonstration of the operation of genetic factors in no way rules out the operation of environmental contributions to the pathogenesis of schizophrenia, but indicates that such environmental contributions are present in the families of both adopted and non-adopted individuals with schizophrenia.

Adoption studies also offer an approach to the establishment of empirically based criteria for defining schizophrenia. Affected biological relatives of ill adoptees share genetic material but not specific family environments; thus the characteristics of illness observed among affected relatives reflect the operation of shared genes. Initial assessment of illness among the biological relatives of affected adoptees indicated that one form of clinically observed schizophrenia-like psychotic illness (acute schizophrenia) was not genetically related to chronic schizophrenia, but a less severe variant (latent schizophrenia) was related [2]. Confirmed by subsequent replication [1], these results helped to establish an objective somatic basis for schizophrenia and schizophrenia spectrum disorders.

Establishment of specific diagnostic criteria for schizophrenia spectrum disorders was built upon the results of adoption studies [3], but initial efforts did not rely exclusively on cases biologically related to individuals with schizophrenia. Gunderson et al [4] focused specifically on the characteristics of non-psychotic schizophrenia-like illness observed in the family members

[1]Center for Professional Psychology, George Washington University, 2300 M Street NW, Washington, DC 20037, USA

of affected individuals to develop more specific diagnostic criteria. Analyses of data from the provincial sample of the Danish adoption studies [1, 5], using different diagnostic criteria for schizophrenia spectrum disorders, demonstrate the sensitivity of analyses to alternative diagnostic criteria. It is important to note that the direct comparison of results of these analyses is hampered by the inclusion of hospital record data in one determination of diagnoses in relatives [1] and its exclusion in the other [5]. Work with adoption designs to determine relevant criteria for schizophrenia spectrum diagnoses is ongoing [6, 7].

Despite advances made in developing evidence-based criteria for defining schizophrenia spectrum disorders, several aspects require clarification.

As noted by Kendler [8], schizophrenia-like syndromes observed in patients treated by clinicians may be quite different from the schizophrenia-like syndromes seen among some of the family members of schizophrenia patients. In particular, it is important to determine the long-term course of non-treatment-seeking individuals and whether less severe schizophrenia-like syndromes should be considered as prodromal to schizophrenia.

From the earliest descriptions of a familial link between schizophrenia and less severe schizophrenia-like syndromes, the dimensional versus categorical nature of schizophrenia has been debated. While initial results from adoption studies did not find an excess of a diagnosis of schizoid personality among biological relatives of schizophrenia patients, more recent reports [7, 9] that some of the relatives of schizophrenia patients have distinctive personality characteristics encourages further exploration of the boundaries of the schizophrenia spectrum.

While genetic factors in psychopathology have traditionally been thought of as liability factors with environmental contributions modifying liability, the search for protective genetic factors in schizophrenia is supported by the existence of protective genes in other somatic illnesses and the report of a genetic protective factor in bipolar illness [10].

REFERENCES

1. Kety S.S., Wender P.H., Jacobsen B., Ingraham L.J., Jansson L., Faber B., Kinney D. (1994) Mental illness in the biological and adoptive relatives of schizophrenic adoptees: replication of the Copenhagen study in the rest of Denmark. *Arch. Gen. Psychiatry*, **51**: 442–455.
2. Kety S.S., Rosenthal D., Wender P.H., Schulsinger F., Jacobsen B. (1975) Mental illness in the biological and adoptive families of adopted individuals who have become schizophrenic: a preliminary report based upon psychiatric interviews. In *Genetic Research in Psychiatry* (Eds R. Fieve, D. Rosenthal, H. Brill), pp. 147–165. Johns Hopkins, Baltimore.
3. Spitzer R.L., Endicott J., Gibbon M. (1979) Crossing the border into borderline personality and borderline schizophrenia. *Arch. Gen. Psychiatry*, **36**: 17–24.

4. Gunderson J.G., Siever L.J., Spaulding E. (1983) The search for a schizotype. Crossing the border again. *Arch. Gen. Psychiatry*, **40**: 15–22.
5. Kendler K.S., Gruenberg A.M., Jacobsen B., Kinney D.K., Jansson L., Faber B. (1994) An independent analysis of the Provincial and National samples of the Danish adoption study of schizophrenia: the pattern of illness, as defined by DSM-III, in adoptees and relatives. *Arch. Gen. Psychiatry*, **51**: 456–468.
6. Ingraham L.J. (1995) Family–genetic research and schizotypal personality. In *Schizotypal Personality* (Eds A. Raine, T. Lencz, S. Mednick), pp. 19–42. Cambridge University Press, Cambridge.
7. Ingraham L.J. (1997) Characterizing heritable psychopathology among the biological relatives of individuals with schizophrenia. *Schizophr. Res.*, **24**: 43.
8. Kendler K.S. (1985) Diagnostic approaches to schizotypal personality disorder: a historical perspective. *Schizophr. Bull.*, **11**: 538–553.
9. Levy D.L., Bloom R., Matthysse S., Teraspulsky L., Mendell N.R., Holzman P.S. (1997) What clinical characteristics distinguish relatives of schizophrenics from normal controls? *Schizophr. Res.*, **24**: 45.
10. Ginns E.I., St Jean P., Philibert R., Galdzicka M., Damschroder-Williams P., Thiel B., Long R.T., Ingraham L.J., Dalwadi H., Murray M. *et al.* (1998) A genome-wide search for chromosomal loci linked to mental health wellness in relatives at high risk for bipolar affective disorder among the old order Amish. *Proc. Natl. Acad. Sci.*, **95**: 15531–15536.

5.4
Exploring Schizophrenia Across the Continuum

Elaine F. Walker[1]

The paper by Maier *et al* is a systematic and integrative overview of schizophrenia spectrum disorders. A discussion of the historical antecedents of the concept of spectrum disorders begins with the observations of Kraepelin and Bleuler. Writings by these historical figures illustrate how astute clinical observation has laid the groundwork for empirical inquiry into the boundaries of schizophrenia. Maier and his colleagues then go on to describe research findings that address phenomenological, genetic, neurobiological and cognitive aspects of spectrum disorders. At all of these levels of analysis, we see that individuals with spectrum disorders, especially schizotypal personality disorder (PD), manifest characteristics similar to those observed in diagnosed schizophrenia patients.

As described in the paper, the parallels between the brain abnormalities found in schizophrenia and schizotypal PD are especially important. They are consistent with a continuum of biological vulnerability. Future research in this area will undoubtedly elucidate in greater detail the specific structural anomalies associated with the schizotypal syndrome. There is now extensive evidence of hippocampal volumetric reductions in schizophrenia, and it will

[1]*Department of Psychology, Emory University, 532 North Kilgo Circle, Atlanta, GA 30322–2470, USA*

be of theoretical relevance to determine whether the same phenomenon is present in schizotypal PD.

It has become increasingly clear that the study of spectrum disorders has unique potential for elucidating the aetiology of schizophrenia. As pointed out by Maier and colleagues, one pragmatic advantage is that individuals with schizotypal and other spectrum personality disorders have typically not received psychopharmacologic treatment. Given the demonstrated effects of antipsychotic medication on cognitive and motor functions, as well as brain physiology, this obviates a significant methodologic problem. The study of spectrum disorders also lends itself to the exploration of the developmental origins of schizophrenia. The chapter reviews research which demonstrates that a significant proportion of schizophrenia patients show a behavioural syndrome similar to schizotypal PD prior to the onset of their symptoms. Thus, for many, the schizotypal syndrome is the prodromal phase of the clinical illness. Yet, it also appears that most individuals who meet diagnostic criteria for schizotypal PD never develop schizophrenia. This raises obvious questions about the factors that determine the progression of schizotypal PD. Is the developmental course predetermined, so that postnatal events have little impact on the trajectory? Alternatively, is there a critical developmental period during which experiential factors play a role in potentiating the expression of illness in vulnerable individuals?

The developmental precursors of spectrum disorders have only recently been the subject of systematic research. We initiated a study of adolescents with schizotypal personality disorder in 1995, and the findings to date support the assumption that research on spectrum disorders can shed light on the aetiology of schizophrenia. The chief objective was to determine whether these youths manifest some of the signs of risk that have been observed in schizophrenia patients. Of particular interest were the dysmorphic features, specifically minor physical and dermatoglyphic abnormalities, that occur at an elevated rate in schizophrenia. These dysmorphic signs are known to originate in the prenatal period, and their developmental course parallels that of the central nervous system (CNS). They are, therefore, viewed as indirect indicators of abnormalities in fetal brain development. We have found that schizotypal adolescents show significantly higher rates of minor physical anomalies than adolescents with no personality disorder [1]. They also manifest more dermatoglyphic asymmetry in finger ridge counts [1], and a higher rate of involuntary movements [2]. These findings are consistent with those from the neuroimaging studies, in that they suggest the presence of CNS dysfunction. Moreover, given the well-established prenatal origin of dysmorphic features, the results indicate that, like schizophrenia, the vulnerability to schizotypal PD has neurodevelopmental origins. This brings us back to the question why a presumably congenital vulnerability is not expressed as an illness until later in life.

Diathesis–stress models assume that environmental stressors trigger the expression of clinical symptoms in vulnerable individuals. Drawing on this framework, we have begun to focus on biological indicators of the stress response in schizotypal youngsters. Two noteworthy findings have emerged. First, schizotypal adolescents show a higher level of cortisol secretion than controls [1]. Second, consistent with some previous reports, we find that cortisol secretion shows a maturational increase during the pubertal period for both disturbed and normal children. Assuming adolescence is associated with a normative rise in activity of the hypothalamic–pituitary–adrenal axis, the pubertal period may be a critical one for stress-induced expression of latent vulnerabilities.

Maier and colleagues emphasize the importance of future research aimed at delineating the boundaries of spectrum disorders. The authors note that the paranoid and schizoid PDs are more homogeneous than schizotypal PD; the former are essentially defined on the basis of a single symptom dimension. Yet, paranoid and schizoid PDs have received little attention from investigators. Comparative studies of the developmental and biological correlates of these PDs hold great promise for enhancing our understanding of the boundaries of vulnerability for schizophrenia.

REFERENCES

1. Davis-Weinstein D., Diforio D., Schiffman J., Walker E., Bonsall R. (1999) Minor physical anomalies, dermatoglyphic asymmetries, and cortisol levels in adolescents with schizotypal personality disorder. *Am. J. Psychiatry*, **156**: 617–623.
2. Walker E., Lewis N., Loewy R., Paylo S. (1999) Motor dysfunction and risk for schizophrenia. *Dev. Psychopathol.*, **11**: 509–523.

5.5
Schizophrenia Spectrum Disorders and the Psychotic Continuum
Victor Peralta[1]

The review by Maier *et al* integrates and consolidates the existing evidence about the validity of the concept of schizophrenia spectrum disorders. This concept is mainly based on two factors: the phenomenological similarity between the disorders within the spectrum, and their common genetic risk factors. Thus, the schizophrenia spectrum concept seems to be a robust one in terms of phenomenology and aetiology.

[1] *Psychiatric Unit, Virgen del Camino Hospital, Irunlarrea 4, 31008 Pamplona, Spain*

Two recent studies from our group further support the validity of the schizophrenia spectrum concept in psychotic disorders at the phenomenological level. The first study refers to the diagnostic usefulness of first-rank symptoms (FRS) for diagnosing schizophrenia [1]. According to DSM-IV and ICD-10, these symptoms are among the most characteristic of schizophrenia. The high diagnostic value ascribed to FRS is probably due to the assumption that they are substantially more prevalent in schizophrenia than in other psychotic disorders. We examined this question in the full range of DSM-III-R functional psychotic disorders, using the Feighner criteria as the gold standard for diagnosing schizophrenia (as they do not cast particular diagnostic value to FRS). Results showed a similar prevalence of these symptoms in schizophrenia and in non-schizophrenic psychotic disorders. It was concluded that FRS are not useful in differentiating schizophrenia from other psychotic disorders.

The other study concerns the factor structure of symptoms of psychoses [2]. We reported that the well-known three-factor structure of schizophrenic symptoms (comprising the factors of psychosis, disorganization and negative) was also present in groups of patients with (a) schizophreniform, (b) schizoaffective and mood disorders, and (c) delusional, brief reactive, and atypical psychoses. These data clearly indicate a continuity in the internal structure of symptoms that cut across different types of psychoses, and they suggest some common pathological mechanism for individual dimensions which is unrelated to diagnostic categories. Furthermore, data from factor-analytic studies of scales measuring schizotypia indicate that schizotypal traits segregate in at least three factors roughly corresponding to the psychosis, disorganization and negative factors of the psychotic disorders. Based on this structural and phenomenological similarity, it has been suggested that schizotypal dimensions represent vulnerability states, which when exacerbated give rise to the clinical dimensions of psychotic disorders [3].

The review by Maier *et al* and our own data support Crow's [4] contention that there are not disease entities but continua of variation. This concept has been referred to as the psychotic continuum hypothesis. The schizophrenia spectrum concept and the continuity hypothesis seem to represent different perspectives of the same phenomenon. In turn, the two concepts seem to be also related to the old notion of "unitary psychosis". Although a single definition for these three concepts does not exist, they are compatible with either a quantitative variation along various dimensions of psychopathology or with clinical syndromes representing different stages in the longitudinal course of the illness.

No experienced clinician in the field of psychosis would deny that the boundaries among psychotic disorders set by the current nosological systems are artificial and arbitrary. Acknowledging that there are "pure cases" best represented by the extreme psychopathological states (i.e. core schizophrenia and non-psychotic affective disorders), it is also true that schizophrenia may present with manic and depressive syndromes and a relatively good outcome, and that affective syndromes may convey mood-incongruent psychotic features and poor outcome. However, with different degree of severity and/or prevalence, virtually every individual symptom or cluster of symptoms may be present in each type of psychosis. In addition, syndromal polymorphism appears to be the rule rather than the exception, particularly when the long-term course is considered, and syndromal stability seems to be limited only to cases lying at the end of the spectrum.

The current splitting of psychotic disorders into various subforms has been uncritically accepted and has become deeply influential in clinical practice, education and research. It has led us to believe that we are dealing with clear and discrete disorders, and as a consequence, the various types of psychoses are viewed as if they were separate nosological entities. This prevalent view is neither enough supported by empirical data nor by clinical practice, but how can we deal with the continuum of variation of psychoses? With regard to schizophrenia, and until more data on its differentiation from other psychoses are available, a wise research approach would be to use competing definitions of the disorder and to make them the focus of research (the polydiagnostic approach). On the other hand, evidence has accumulated supporting the notion that research strategy should be based on clinical dimensions rather than on diagnosis. Dimensions of psychopathology can be used as an alternative to the categorical diagnosis, since they seem to have clinical and neurobiological reality irrespective of diagnostic categories (the multidimensional approach). Dimensional and categorical approaches, however, are not antagonistic but complementary. Where more empirical work needs to be done is in the comparative testing of the dimensional versus categorical model of psychotic disorders, since the relationship between dimensions and diagnoses is at the heart of the matter. Both approaches have their advantages and drawbacks, therefore combining the two strategies into a polydiagnostic–multidimensional research paradigm [5] seems to be a promising method for systematizing clinical and aetiopathogenic information on psychotic disorders in general and schizophrenia in particular. It remains for future studies to search for the specific circumstances in which one approach is preferred over the other.

REFERENCES

1. Peralta V., Cuesta M.J. (1999) Diagnostic significance of Schneider's first-rank symptoms in schizophrenia. Comparative study between schizophrenic and non-schizophrenic psychotic disorders. Br. J. Psychiatry, 174: 243–248.
2. Peralta V., Cuesta M.J., Farre C. (1997) Factor structure of symptoms in psychotic disorders. Biol. Psychiatry, 42: 806–815.

3. Vollema M.G., van den Bosch R.J. (1995) The multidimensionality of schizotypy. *Schizophr. Bull.*, **21**: 19–31.
4. Crow T.J. (1995) A continuum of psychosis, one human gene and not much else: the case for homogeneity. *Schizophr. Res.*, **17**: 135–145.
5. Peralta V., Cuesta M.J. (2000) Clinical models of Schizophrenia: a critical approach to competing conceptions. *Psychopathology*, **33**: 252–258.

5.6
Dimensions of Schizotypy in Symptomatic, Neurocognitive and Psychophysiological Indicators

Keith H. Nuechterlein, Kenneth L. Subotnik and Robert F. Asarnow[1]

As Maier *et al* indicate in their review, increasing evidence suggests that proneness to schizophrenia at the clinical symptomatic level may involve several dimensions with limited or no intercorrelation, rather than a single coherent diagnostic entity as is implied in the concept of schizotypal personality disorder. Furthermore, several dimensions, rather than one dimension, of neurocognitive and psychophysiological dysfunction are likely to detect factors associated with genetic vulnerability to schizophrenia. We agree that the delineation of the dimensions of schizotypy will be greatly aided by additional research examining biological relatives of individuals with schizophrenia, and believe that it is particularly helpful at this point to combine symptomatic indicators with indicators at the neurocognitive and/or psychophysiological level, so that the phenotypes relevant to genetic susceptibility to schizophrenia can be better characterized.

At the symptomatic level, recent factor analytic evidence from biological relatives of schizophrenia patients in our Family Members Study at the University of California, Los Angeles (UCLA) indicates that symptoms of schizotypal personality disorder are distributed across four or five independent factors when considered in the context of symptoms from five DSM-III-R personality disorders [1]. This adds to prior evidence suggesting that the symptoms currently included in schizotypal personality disorder probably do not represent a single underlying dimension.

A related issue is whether the neurocognitive and psychophysiological anomalies found among biological relatives of schizophrenia patients are best viewed as underlying factors that characterize a diagnostic entity such as schizotypal personality disorder or whether at least some may be abnormalities that are broader than the symptom clusters that define schizophrenia

[1]*Department of Psychiatry and Biobehavioral Sciences, University of California, Los Angeles, USA*

spectrum disorders. Neurocognitive and psychophysiological abnormalities that can be detected among biological relatives of schizophrenia patients who do not manifest even schizotypal personality disorder or other symptomatically defined schizophrenia spectrum disorders may particularly extend the relevant phenotype for genetic transmission studies. Earlier evidence from studies of children born to schizophrenic parents suggested that attentional deficits and certain other cognitive performance deficits are detectable even before schizophrenia or schizophrenia spectrum disorders would typically have their onset. More recently, evidence from adult siblings of schizophrenia patients indicates that some neurocognitive abnormalities, such as excessive visual backward masking effects [2], are present even in those adult siblings who would not be characterized as having any schizophrenia spectrum disorder on symptomatic grounds. Combined with evidence of psychophysiological anomalies such as certain antisaccade task errors in likely genetic carriers for schizophrenia [3], the promise of neurocognitive and psychophysiological indicators for meaningful extension of the phenotype(s) relevant to genetic susceptibility to schizophrenia remains clear.

Another issue addressed by Maier *et al* is the association of neurocognitive and psychophysiological abnormalities with particular dimensions of schizotypal symptoms. To the extent that schizotypal personality disorder involves more than one symptom dimension, one might expect that each dimension would have characteristic neurocognitive and psychophysiological determinants. We agree that the evidence for such specific associations is mixed at this point. It remains possible that the associations within psychometric high-risk subjects can be differentiated into those involving the positive schizotypy and negative schizotypy components when specific neurocognitive and psychophysiological abnormalities are considered. In earlier work with individuals drawn from temporary employment agencies who had no history of treatment for psychiatric disorder, we found that impairments on a measure of vigilance level (a Degraded-Stimulus Continuous Performance Test) and on a measure of early perceptual encoding (the forced-choice Span of Apprehension Task) were both significantly associated with higher schizophrenia scale scores on the Minnesota Multiphasic Personality Inventory (MMPI) [4]. However, low vigilance level was significantly associated with higher scores on the Chapman's Physical Anhedonia scale, whereas low early perceptual encoding was significantly associated with higher Perceptual Aberration and Magical Ideation scale scores, suggesting that some differentiation of the schizotypal correlates is present. Similarly, using a startle eyeblink modulation paradigm, Schell *et al* [5] have shown that both high Physical Anhedonia and high Perceptual Aberration/Magical Ideation college students show deficient attentional modulation of startle eyeblink, similar to that observed in schizophrenia patients, but anhedonic individuals show delayed development of the attentional modulation rather than the full absence of modulation characteristic of schizophrenia patients and of the individuals high on perceptual aberration and/or magical ideation.

An alternative role for overall severity of neurocognitive deficits in schizotypy is that it may reflect genetic susceptibility factors but relate more strongly to severity of functional impairment than to either positive or negative schizotypal symptom dimensions. Within individuals with schizophrenia, increasing evidence suggests that severity of neurocognitive deficits is more closely tied to functional outcome than to either positive or negative symptoms [6, 7]. Thus, further research on the potential roles of neurocognitive and psychophysiological abnormalities in relationship to schizotypal symptom dimensions is clearly indicated.

REFERENCES

1. Fogelson D.L., Nuechterlein K.H., Asarnow R.F., Payne D.L., Subotnik K.L., Giannini C.A. (1999) The factor structure of schizophrenia spectrum personality disorders: signs and symptoms in relatives of psychotic patients from the UCLA Family Members Study. Submitted for publication.
2. Green M.F., Nuechterlein K.H., Breitmeyer B. (1997) Backward masking performance in unaffected siblings of schizophrenic patients: evidence for a vulnerability indicator. *Arch. Gen. Psychiatry*, **54**: 465–472.
3. Clementz B.A. (1998) Psychophysiological measures of (dis)inhibition as liability indicators for schizophrenia. *Psychophysiology*, **35**: 648–668.
4. Asarnow R.F., Nuechterlein K.H., Marder S.R. (1983) Span of apprehension performance, neuropsychological functioning and indices of psychosis-proneness. *J. Nerv. Ment. Dis.*, **171**: 662–669.
5. Schell A.M., Dawson M.E., Hazlett E.A., Filion D.L. (1995) Attentional modulation of startle in psychosis-prone college students. *Psychophysiology*, **32**: 266–273.
6. Green M.F. (1996) What are the functional consequences of neurocognitive deficits in schizophrenia? *Am. J. Psychiatry*, **153**: 321–330.
7. Green M.F., Nuechterlein K.H. (1999) Should schizophrenia be treated as a neurocognitive disorder? *Schizophr. Bull.*, **25**: 309–319.

5.7

The Role of Syndromes and Neurophysiology in Conceptualizing the Schizophrenia Spectrum and Predisposing Influences

John Gruzelier[1]

Maier *et al* provide a helpful overview of the poorly integrated field of research on the schizophrenia spectrum disorders. Grist to the mill is

[1]*Department of Behavioural and Cognitive Sciences, Division of Neuroscience and Psychological Medicine, Imperial College of Science, Technology and Medicine, St Dunstan's Road, London, W6 8RF, UK*

provided for the need to develop an integrative syndromal perspective of the spectrum by the sheer diversity of their conclusions. To wit, factor analytic studies do not correspond to the taxonomy which separates schizotypal, schizoid and paranoid personality disorders; these conditions cover overlapping personality traits. Follow-back studies report the full gamut of symptoms in the pre-schizophrenic, including negative symptoms, cognitive symptoms such as unusual speech, suspiciousness, perceptual aberrations, etc, as well as depression. There is a familial link between schizophrenia and delusional disorders, a clear nosological link between schizoaffective and schizophrenic disorders, and when a comprehensive range of symptoms is included the spectrum is found to encompass all psychotic disorders. Eccentricity, odd speech, cognitive slippage and negative features are not only the best discriminators of a familial relation with schizophrenia but also of a relation with affective disorders. There are within the spectrum differences in frontal executive impairments. Negative rather than positive symptoms more commonly characterize the relatives of chronic schizophrenic patients. Similarly, smooth pursuit eye movements are associated with more chronic enduring symptoms in schizophrenia and with deficit and not psychotic symptoms in schizotypy. Dopamine on the other hand is associated with florid symptoms of schizophrenia.

This brief commentary concerns a syndromal perspective of the spectrum together with the neurophysiological underpinnings, and due to brevity focuses mainly on only two syndromes characterized by activity and withdrawal [1, 2]. Converging evidence began by comparing in unmedicated schizophrenic patients whose clinical evaluation encompassed the full range of specific and non-specific symptoms, left > right versus right > left psychophysiological functional asymmetries. These delineated active and withdrawn syndromes, concepts central to schizophrenia in the 1960s. These were independent of nuclear symptoms forming an unreality syndrome. Subsequently similar syndromes were found in factor analyses of schizotypy personality dimensions along with neuropsychophysiological correlates. Active and withdrawn descriptors were consistent with social interaction (left) versus social withdrawal (right) theories of hemispheric specialization. An accumulation of evidence implicated as underlying mechanisms interhemispheric arousal systems, but especially lateral biases in the thalamocortical non-specific projection system [1].

Abnormalities at very early, subcortical stages of processing have been implicated in schizophrenia, schizotypal patients, their relatives, children at genetic risk for schizophrenia, and have been found in association with schizotypal personality traits. Two, often opposite, excitatory and inhibitory "profiles" have been found which can be loosely associated with positive/acute (active and unreality) versus negative/chronic (withdrawn) distinctions [2]. Some relations have been demonstrated with active and withdrawn syndromes. Evidence of opposite profiles has encompassed putative magnocellular versus parvocellular tasks, P50 suppression, slow/fast frequency resting EEG patterns, reduced N100, and delayed electrodermal habituation. In view of the dominance of cortical re-entrant pathways over thalamic cortical relay pathways, subcortical dysfunction in schizophrenia could theoretically be secondary to cortical impairment, particularly of the frontal lobe which is the more strongly innervated by the thalamic systems. But reviewed evidence [2] indicates that early processing deficits and thalamic involvement in schizophrenia may occur in the absence of deficits in higher processing, and secondly that the regional distribution of thalamic involvement occurs throughout the cortex involving the thalamic systems as a whole and not simply their anterior projections [1]. On the other hand, cortical dysfunction will to some extent mirror individual differences in biases within subcortical–cortical interactions. In this regard relations were reviewed between the low level deficits and between deficiencies in later/higher levels of processing, including the P200 and P300 evoked potential components, auditory signal detection, distractibility on the continuous performance test, lateralized inattention, figure-ground object recognition tests, a thought disorder index, and a range of frontal tests including the Wisconsin Card Sort [2].

The fact that functional asymmetries in schizophrenia reverse with successful antipsychotic treatment, and that these syndrome-related reversals could occur in either direction, has provided a clue to neurochemical mechanisms [1]. Neuroleptic-induced reversals in turning tendencies, which represent coordinated activity of attentional, motor and reinforcement systems, had in animals been utilized as a test of neuroleptic efficacy. Importantly, in both animals and schizophrenic patients, the effects of neuroleptics (assumed to be dopaminergic) can be seen to be bidirectional, reciprocal, and in animals were dependent on endogenous asymmetries while in patients they were dependent on syndrome. In the rat, drug-induced interhemispheric reciprocity relied on nigrostriatal dopaminergic input to the basal ganglia, which was mediated by the intralaminar nuclei of the non-specific thalamic system.

Developmental influences on subcortex are clear. Abnormal perceptions are characteristic of the preschizophrenic state, the prodrome and the early stages of schizophrenia, and visual symptoms are forerunners of first-rank symptoms. In schizophrenia there are reports of an absence of gliosis, cell loss and reduced volume of the mediodorsal nucleus of the thalamus, implying a failure of a normal developmental regressive event. Abnormalities in startle response pre-pulse inhibition found in schizophrenia and in association with the active schizotypy dimension follow the regressive event of puberty in animals in whom there were developmental lesions of the hippocampus. Extremes of pubertal timing have been shown to relate to active, withdrawn and unreality schizotypy syndromes along with EEG connectivity differences consistent with extremes of dendritic pruning in active and withdrawn schizotypy. In animals the direction of the endogenous turning preference was found dependent on genes, hormones, and early experience including stressors. Trevarthen [3] has shown in children that there are asymmetries in gesture and emotion which precede the development of language and visuoconstructive skills, and has posited that the approach/withdrawal balance in social encounters arises from early neurochemical asymmetries in the brainstem. Accordingly, in schizophrenia we propose that the active/withdrawn syndrome-related functional asymmetries represent modifiable lateral biases in non-specific thalamocortical activation which may be determined in part by developmental traits forming part of the vulnerability to psychosis [1–2].

REFERENCES

1. Gruzelier J.H. (1999) Functional neuropsychophysiological asymmetry in schizophrenia: a review and reorientation. *Schizophr. Bull.*, **25**: 91–120.
2. Gruzelier J.H. (1999) A review of the implications of early sensory processing and subcortical involvement for cognitive dysfunction in schizophrenia. In *Ann. Rev. of Psychiatry* 28 (Ed. J. Oldham). American Psychiatric Press, Washington, DC (in press).
3. Trevarthen C. (1996) Lateral asymmetries in infancy: implications for the development of the hemispheres. *Neurosci. Biobehav. Rev.*, **20**: 571–586.

5.8
Irremediable Flaws in the Schizophrenia Spectrum Concept
C. Robert Cloninger[1]

The spectrum concept of schizophrenia is historically a modification of the categorical concept of schizophrenia, adding cases that are considered to be milder forms or variable expressions of susceptibility to the core entity. It was developed in the Danish adoption studies of schizophrenia and gave rise to our current concept of schizotypal personality disorder. Consequently the crucial test is whether the putative spectrum disorder is found in excess in the relatives of schizophrenics compared to the relatives of non-schizophrenics. However, for a heritable disorder like schizophrenia, clinical conditions that are predictive of later onset of schizophrenia are also assumed to be spectrum conditions. These criteria are mutually consistent for a heritable

[1] *Department of Psychiatry, Washington University School of Medicine, 4940 Children's Place, St Louis, MO 63110, USA*

disorder like schizophrenia because the correlations between syndromes in different biological relatives are expected to be the same as those within an individual, allowing for attenuation by incomplete heritability. Thus much can be learned about a putative set of spectrum conditions by attention to the correlations that are known to exist between syndromes within individuals in any population [1].

Both the categorical and spectrum concepts of schizophrenia assume that there is a discontinuity defining the boundary between the schizophrenia-related disorders and other disorders. Remarkably, there is little evidence for such discontinuity. The only evidence for a boundary is partial, such that there remains substantial overlap with other non-schizophrenic syndromes within individuals and within families [2]. The boundaries even of the core entity of schizophrenia have been revised between DSM-IIIR and DSM-IV, with greater emphasis on negative symptoms more recently. Current DSM-IV criteria allow the diagnosis of definite schizophrenia in individuals who have neither hallucinations nor delusions.

Furthermore, the review of the schizophrenia spectrum by Maier *et al* provides thorough documentation for fundamental problems with the whole concept. In particular, cases of schizoaffective disorder have an excess of affective disorder not seen in the relatives of schizophrenics, and schizotypal personality disorder is more prevalent in the relatives of probands with the same diagnosis than in the relatives of schizophrenics. These are strong indications of heterogeneity and incomplete overlap in liability among putative spectrum conditions. The nosological problem is further underscored by the overlap among conditions that are supposed to be in the spectrum with disorders that are supposed not to be in the spectrum (mood disorders, non-odd personality disorders, and somatization).

I have examined methods for the diagnosis of personality disorders in detail in order to understand the strengths and weaknesses of our current categorical system of classification [3, 4]. My work using multiple quantitative dimensions of temperament and character to assess personality disorders has been widely translated and tested throughout the world [5]. Initially I took the view that schizotypy belonged with schizophrenia, as in ICD-10, and that criteria for other disorders would not be relevant or overlap with schizotypal personality disorder. However, empirically it turned out that schizotypal personality disorder can be reliably diagnosed as one configuration of the same seven dimensions that define all other personality disorders [6, 7]. The concept of personality disorders being organized as a hierarchical, branching set of clusters and categories is invalidated by the extensive overlap among clusters and among categories [6]. In other words, individuals with a diagnosis in one personality cluster often have another diagnosis in another cluster, or they may satisfy criteria for multiple categories within one cluster. What is now clear is that there is a set of quantitative dimensions that occur in all possible combinations, giving rise to a wide variety of syndromes, none of which is discrete. There is also predictable variation over time in the underlying configurations, which are predictable developmental events explained by non-linear dynamics [8, 9]. Thus, many intermediate and mixed forms are observed in longitudinal studies of the schizophrenia spectrum, as described in the review of Maier *et al*. Consequently categorical and spectrum concepts must be recognized as fuzzy approximations to the observed clinical variability, and have the disadvantage of misleading people into thinking categorically instead of quantitatively.

Recent work has suggested that these meta-stable configurations of multiple personality dimensions are systematically related to vulnerability to schizophrenic and affective psychoses [10]. This should not be surprising since Kraepelin originally identified personality variants as the basic rudiments that are stable and essential for the development of a psychotic disorder [11].

The use of biological markers to define a spectrum condition is the persistent hope of biological psychiatry, but it must be admitted that *no* biological marker for schizophrenia or any other categorical diagnosis in psychiatry has sufficient sensitivity and specificity to be of use as a diagnostic laboratory test. If something is not useful to diagnose the core, it is dubious that it can be used reliably to define a broader, more heterogeneous spectrum. This is not to say that there are not genetic factors or related neurobiological variables in schizophrenia. Rather it means that the categorical and spectrum concepts themselves may be inadequate to understand and characterize the phenotypic and aetiological covariation.

Overall our present categorical system of classification may be convenient for labelling in treatment and epidemiological work, but we should not make the error of thinking that the conceptual categories correspond to discrete entities that exist in nature. Both the core categories, and their extension into still more heterogeneous spectra, have severe limitations for rigorous descriptive and aetiological research. Modifications of the categorical system to a broader spectrum do not correct the fundamental flaws in the criterion core. Continued tinkering with the item-sets and efforts to define subtypes simply obscure or ignore the undeniable fact that the entire spectrum is made up of partly overlapping, heterogeneous syndromes. The observable phenotypic variation can be more aptly characterized in terms of quantitative variation in multiple dimensions that relate equally well to everyone in the general population, not only to relatives of schizophrenics. Tinkering with the item-sets, as in the shifts between various editions of DSM and ICD, is about as useful as moving around the chairs on the top deck of an ocean liner which is sinking because of a gaping hole in its bow. The addition of hundreds of new categories has not reduced the number of cases regarded as atypical or not otherwise specified, but has increased the redundancy or overlap among categorical labels. There is no evidence of any discrete boundary between individuals within the putative schizophrenia spectrum and those outside it. Consequently the spectrum concept itself is irremediably flawed.

REFERENCES

1. Maser J.D., Cloninger C.R. (Eds) (1990) *Comorbidity in Anxiety and Affective Disorders*. American Psychiatric Press, Washington, DC.
2. Cloninger C.R., Martin R.L., Guze S.B., Clayton P.J. (1985) Diagnosis and prognosis in schizophrenia. *Arch. Gen. Psychiatry*, **40**: 15–25.
3. Cloninger C.R. (1987) A systematic method for clinical description and classification of personality variants. *Arch. Gen. Psychiatry*, **44**: 573–588.
4. Cloninger C.R., Svrakic D.M., Przybeck T.R. (1993) A psychobiological model of temperament and character. *Arch. Gen. Psychiatry*, **50**: 975–990.
5. Cloninger C.R., Przybeck T.R., Svrakic D.M., Wetzel R.D. (1994) *The Temperament and Character Inventory (TCI): A Guide to its Development and Use*. Center for Psychobiology of Personality, Washington University, St Louis.
6. Svrakic D.M., Whitehead C., Przybeck T.R., Cloninger C.R. (1993) Differential diagnosis of personality disorders by the seven-factor model of temperament and character. *Arch. Gen. Psychiatry*, **50**: 991–999.
7. Bayon C., Hill K., Svrakic D.M., Przybeck T.R., Cloninger C.R. (1996) Dimensional assessment of personality in an outpatient sample: relations of the systems of Millon and Cloninger. *J. Psychiatr. Res.*, **30**: 341–352.
8. Svrakic N.M., Svrakic D.M., Cloninger C.R. (1996) A general quantitative theory of personality development: fundamentals of a self-organizing psychobiological complex. *Dev. Psychopathol.*, **8**: 247–272.
9. Cloninger C.R., Svrakic N.M., Svrakic D.M. (1997) Role of personality self-organization in development of mental order and disorder. *Dev. Psychopathol.*, **9**: 881–906.
10. Cloninger C.R., Bayon C., Svrakic D.M. (1998) Measurement of temperament and character in mood disorders: a model of fundamental states as personality types. *J. Affect. Disord.*, **51**: 21–32.
11. Kraepelin E. (1919) *Dementia Praecox and Paraphrenia*. Livingstone, Edinburgh.

5.9
Do Not Dismiss the Single Major Locus Hypothesis So Quickly

Philip S. Holzman, Deborah L. Levy and Steven Matthysse[1]

When Kraepelin included in a single diagnostic category Morel's Démence Précoce, Kahlbaum's Katatonie and Hecker's Hebephrenie [1], he began an almost unending process of redefining the disease we now call schizophrenia.

[1] *Harvard Medical School, Psychology Research Laboratory, McLean Hospital, 115 Mill Street, Belmont, MA 02178, USA*

As Maier *et al*'s review makes clear, the process of redrawing the boundaries of the category schizophrenia continued with Bleuler's [2] efforts to widen Kraepelin's unifying concept, and it continues with contemporary empirical efforts that include epidemiological surveys, family and genetic studies. Whatever else schizophrenia may be, it surely presents itself as more than the typical psychotic behaviours that careful naturalistic observers and compilers like Kraepelin described.

One great puzzle of schizophrenia is to describe its essential features and their interrelationships so that its aetiology and causal pattern become clear. Schizophrenia, however, like all natural categories, has fuzzy boundaries. Although the members of the category vary in their typicality, they are bound together by a family resemblance. There are no attributes that are true of all members of the category, yet there are attributes that are true of some. Some schizophrenic people, therefore, will escape detection, while others will leap to our awareness as prototypical. The task set by Maier *et al*'s paper is to discover the defining characteristics of schizophrenia. But schizophrenia is an arbitrary classification of behaviours that will turn out to be useful if it corresponds to a distinctive biological process. Only then, will we be certain of what it is that schizophrenia comprises.

As Maier *et al* indicate, there is overwhelming evidence that schizophrenia runs in families, although its phenotypic clinical manifestations vary even within families. And it shows no simple Mendelian pattern in its inter- and intra-generational appearance. But its protean presentations put a strain on the application of most models of genetic transmission, particularly if one confines the definition of schizophrenia to schizophrenic psychosis. That is one reason that the spectrum concept has heuristic value. Yet, a Mendelian mode of inheritance does not fit the distribution of affected cases well even when one also includes the various associated clinical pheno- types described in Maier *et al*'s review. The model these authors adopt is, therefore, not an unreasonable one. They accept the idea that there exists a predisposing "vulnerability" like Meehl's [3] schizotaxia—Meehl now dubs it hypokrisia [4]—that is present in all people with a schizophrenia spectrum disorder, or a "neurobiological indicator" that appears in these disorders. Inasmuch as there is a greater familial prevalence of schizotypal traits (as well as other spectrum traits like paranoid and schizoid charac- teristics) than of schizophrenia alone, the authors also assume that these traits are necessary antecedent conditions for all schizophrenias. Indeed, they propose that neuropsychological and neurophysiological abnormalities studied in schizophrenia, as well as the spectrum conditions, are all necessary preconditions for schizophrenia.

But the empirical data do not fit easily into this model. Here is the problem. There are some schizophrenic patients with no premorbid evidence of schizotypic traits who have non-psychotic relatives with such traits [5].

Indeed, M. Bleuler [5] found 30% of his schizophrenic probands to be without any premorbid pathological traits, and an additional 28% of his probands had schizoid characteristics within normal limits. A similar pattern is apparent in the distribution of co-familial psychophysiological and neuropsychological phenotypes. For example some schizophrenic patients with normal smooth pursuit eye movements (about 20% to 40% have normal pursuit movements) have relatives with abnormal smooth pursuit eye movements even when those relatives are neither schizophrenic nor schizotypic [6]. A similar pattern emerges in the "P50 inhibition failure" studied by Freedman's group [7]. If schizotypic personality disorders (or traits) or smooth pursuit eye movement abnormalities (or other non-clinical phenotypes) are necessary preconditions for schizophrenia, why do not all schizophrenic patients have them? And, if schizophrenia produces these traits, why do the clinically well relatives have them?

These data suggest a different model for both the relation of these phenotypes to each other and for their genetic transmission. The data suggest a genetic latent trait model. This model, which we proposed several years ago, still seems tenable. It is a taxometric one, much like that suggested by Meehl [3]. We [6] postulated that there is a latent trait that is not directly observable, but that can independently cause either schizophrenia, the neuropsychological and neurophysiological abnormalities, or the schizophrenia-related personality traits, or all of them. It is this latent trait that is to be regarded as genetically transmitted, rather than the phenotypes of schizophrenia or the laboratory measures of abnormal eye tracking, P50 inhibition, working memory or of vigilance (e.g. as measured by the Continuous Performance Test). Although the manifest traits may be said to be "genetic" along with the latent trait, we proposed that the transmission pattern of the latent trait might be close to that of a Mendelian gene with higher penetrance than any of the manifest traits alone.

There are similarities between our model and Meehl's. Both rely on the concept of pleiotropy, or variable expressivity with incomplete penetrance for any one manifestation. The model does not rule out that other genes may also be implicated in schizophrenia, although a purely polygenic model would fit the data poorly because it overestimates the MZ/DZ concordance ratio [8, 9], and the affected offspring of dual matings [9].

The implications of this model for research strategy are important. The model highlights the value of studying the clinically asymptomatic members of the families of schizophrenic patients. This strategy will take the investigator beyond the usual nosological categories subsumed under the spectrum diagnoses, which is a desideratum, since there is no reason to believe that the categories of ICD-10 or DSM-IV correspond to distinct aetiological processes. It will further direct the investigator to a study of the underlying physiology of the laboratory indicators of abnormality, and thus closer to the pathophysiology of schizophrenia.

REFERENCES

1. Kraepelin E. (1896) *Psychiatrie. Ein lehrbuch für Studierende und Ärzte. 5 Auflage.* Abel, Leipzig.
2. Bleuler E. (1911) Dementia praecox oder die Gruppe der Schizophrenien. In *Handbuch der Geisteskrankheiten* (Ed. G. Aschaffenburg). Deuticke, Leipzig.
3. Meehl P.E. (1962) Schizotaxia, schizotypy, schizophrenia. *Am. Psychol.*, **17**:827–838.
4. Meehl P.E. (1990) Toward an integrated theory of schizotaxia, schizotypy, and schizophrenia. *J. Personality Dis.*, **4**: 1–99.
5. Bleuler M. (1978) *The Schizophrenic Disorders. Long Term Patient and Family Studies.* Yale University Press, New Haven.
6. Matthysse S., Holzman P.S., Lange K. (1986) The genetic transmission of schizophrenia: application of Mendelian latent structure analysis to eye tracking dysfunctions in schizophrenia and affective disorder. *J. Psychiatr. Res.*, **20**: 57–65.
7. Freedman R., Adler L.E., Waldo M.C., Pachtman E., Frands R.D. (1983) Neurophysiological evidence for a defect in inhibitory pathways in schizophrenia. *Biol. Psychiatry*, **18**: 537–551.
8. Risch N. (1990) Linkage strategies for genetically complex traits. I. Multilocus models. *Am. J. Hum. Genet.*, **46**: 222–228.
9. Matthysse S., Kidd K.K. (1976) Estimating the genetic contribution to schizophrenia. *Am. J. Psychiatry*, **133**: 185–191.

5.10
Schizophrenia Spectrum: Where to Draw the Boundary?

Gisela Gross and Gerd Huber[1]

Besides schizophrenia, schizophreniform, schizoaffective and schizotypal disorders, including their prodromal and residual symptoms (PRS), some abortive variants belong in our view to the schizophrenia spectrum [1]. The definition of the PRS in DSM-IV, limited to negative symptoms (NS) and positive symptoms (PS) "in attenuated form", is not satisfactory. The PRS of DSM-III-R and DSM-IV are behavioural symptoms, observed by others, unlike the PRS described by us as basic symptoms (BS), experiential in kind and only ascertainable by the self-reports of patients [1–4]. BS and NS reveal essential differences, important for theory, diagnostics, therapy and

[1]*Department of Psychiatry, University of Bonn, D-53105 Bonn (Venusberg), Germany*

early intervention in schizophrenia [5]. Schizophrenia spectrum disorders represent a susceptibility to a dysfunction of information processing, manifesting itself also in PRS, as in abortive courses, described, for example, as latent, pseudoneurotic, larvate or coenaesthetic schizophrenia, as endogenous juvenile–aesthenic failure syndromes and endogenous obsessive–compulsive disorders [1, 5, 6]. A categorical distinction into negative and positive or type II and type I schizophrenia is not possible, but a typological differentiation can be proposed with a dimensional continuum between the two symptom groups as stages of the same disorder imperceptibly merging into one another and a spectrum from schizophrenia through schizophreniform, schizoaffective and schizotypal disorders to a large variety of formes frustes [1, 5, 7–9]. BS, PS and NS develop mainly in this chronological sequence, except for a small subgroup (11%) of primary negative schizophrenics with anosognosia, lacking the common criteria of BS, that is self-perception of deficiencies, preserved insight and ability to develop coping strategies against the BS [3–5].

Behavioural symptoms preceding schizophrenia found in follow-back and high-risk studies, are only rarely premorbid personality traits, but mainly BS, recognizable with the Bonn Scale for the Assessment of BS (BSABS) [2]; only 11% of schizophrenics reveal unambiguously personality disorders [10]. The Bonn Study [10], the prospective early recognition study of schizophrenia [3, 4, 11] and the transition rows study [12] have shown that prodromes and outpost syndromes precede the first psychotic episode by 3.3 and 10 years respectively on average and that cognitive level-2-BS, out of which distinct FRS arise, are predictive for the schizophrenic psychosis. The results of the BS research enabled the development of new BS-orientated pharmacopsychiatric and psychological treatment concepts [1, 3, 5, 13]. The sensitivity and specificity of some predictive BS is sufficient enough [4, 11] to justify an early intervention in the initial prodromes, making it possible to inhibit an increase of the process activity of the cognitive BS, before the threshold for the shift into psychosis is reached. The model of "psychoeducation", presented by McFarlane et al [14], corresponds to the BS-orientated prevention concept of our group [1, 3, 5, 13].

The detailed knowledge of the phenomenology of the pre- and postpsychotic basic stages made it possible to overcome the doctrine of a radical heterogeneity and "numinous singularity" of schizophrenia [5, 7, 15, 16]. Because in the abortive courses typical schizophrenic symptoms appear only after many years and then in short episodes, while uncharacteristic level-1-BS determine the psychopathological picture in long lasting periods, here the relationship of the BS with schizophrenia can only be recognized by course observation for years [1, 5, 6, 8, 15]. A pilot study on this issue has been the first description of coenaesthetic schizophrenia, because here prodromes persisting on the average 7 years, determined only by BS, preceded the first psychotic episode [6]. In coenaesthetic as in other schizophrenics neuroimaging findings show correlation not with disease duration, but with irreversible basic stages (pure residues) and a progression of ventricular enlargement parallel to the psychopathological changes [6, 16–19].

REFERENCES

1. Süllwold L., Huber G. (1986) *Schizophrene Basisstörungen*. Springer, Berlin.
2. Gross G., Huber G., Klosterkötter J., Linz M. (1987) *BSABS. Bonn Scale for the Assessment of Basic Symptoms*. Springer, Berlin.
3. Gross G., Huber G. (1996) The true onset of schizophrenia and its meaning for the view of the disorder. *Neurol. Psychiatry Brain Res.*, 4: 93–102.
4. Gross G., Huber G., Klosterkötter J. (1992) Early diagnosis of schizophrenia. *Neurol. Psychiatry Brain Res.*, 1: 17–22.
5. Huber G. (1999) *Psychiatrie*, 6th edn. Schattauer, Stuttgart.
6. Huber G. (1957) Die coenästhetische Schizophrenie. *Forschr. Neurol. Psychiatrie*, 25: 491–520.
7. Huber G. (1992) Die Konzeption der Einheitspsychose aus der Sicht der Basisstörungslehre. In *Für und Wider die Einheitspsychose* (Eds C. Mundt, H. Sass), pp. 61–72. Thieme, Stuttgart.
8. Huber G. (Ed.) (1985) Basisstadien Endogener Psychosen und das Borderline-Problem. 6th Weißenauer Schizophrenia Symposion. Schattauer, Stuttgart.
9. Gross G., Huber G., Sass H. (Eds) (1998) Moderne Psychiatrische Klassifikationssysteme. 11th Weißenauer Schizophrenia Symposion. Schattauer, Stuttgart.
10. Huber G., Gross G., Schüttler R. (1979) *Schizophrenie. Eine verlaufs- und sozialpsychiatrische Langzeitstudie*. Springer, Berlin.
11. Klosterkötter J., Gross G., Huber G., Wieneke A., Steinmeyer E.M., Schulze-Lutter F. (1997) Evaluation of the Bonn Scale for the Assessment of Basic Symptoms (BSABS) as an instrument for the assessment of schizophrenia proneness: a review of recent findings. *Neurol. Psychiatry Brain Res.*, 5: 137–150.
12. Klosterkötter J. (1988) *Basissymptome und Endphänomene der Schizophrenie*. Springer, Berlin.
13. Gross G. (1987) Basic symptoms and coping behavior in schizophrenia. In *Psychosocial Treatment of Schizophrenia* (Eds J.S. Strauss, W. Böker, H.D. Brenner), pp. 126–135. Huber, Bern.
14. McFarlane W.R., Lukens E., Link B., Dushay R., Deakins S.A., Newmark M., Dunne E.J., Horen B., Toran J. (1995) Multi-family groups and psychoeducation in the treatment of schizophrenia *Arch. Gen. Psychiatry*, 52: 679–687.
15. Huber G. (1966) Reine Defektsyndrome und Basisstadien endogener Psychosen. *Fortschr. Neurol. Psychiatrie*, 34: 409–426.
16. Gross G, Huber G, Armbruster B. (1986) Schizoaffective psychoses — long-term prognosis and symptomatology. In *The Schizoaffective Psychoses* (Eds A. Marneros, M.T. Tsuang), pp. 188–203. Springer, Berlin.
17. Gross G., Huber G., Schüttler R. (1982) Computerized tomography studies on schizophrenic diseases. *Arch. Psychiat. Nervenkr.*, 231: 519–526.
18. Huber G. (1957) *Pneumencephalographische und Psychopathologische Bilder bei Endogenen Psychosen*. Springer, Berlin.
19. Gross G., Huber G. (1997) Is schizophrenia a neurodevelopmental disorder? *Neurol. Psychiatry Brain Res.*, 5: 57–70.

5.11
Is There a Place for the Nature–Nurture Hypothesis in the Aetiology of Schizophrenia Spectrum Disorders?

Allan F. Mirsky[1] and Connie C. Duncan[2]

The review by Maier *et al* emphasizes that the cutting edge of research in schizophrenia has shifted from imaging the brains of patients and their more-or-less vulnerable relatives to investigations of genetic factors in the disorder. This latest development continues the tradition of applying the newest techniques from biotechnology to the study of the most enigmatic of all disorders. Thus, in the past 100 years, we have seen emphasis on the following factors (among others) in the aetiology of schizophrenia: infection, hormones, neurotransmitters, autoimmune function, viruses, brain disease, and now, genes [1, 2]. And each of these approaches to the disorder has generated unique treatment strategies. We are aware that none of these factors necessarily excludes the others, that some of the older hypotheses are still viable and, moreover, that some investigators have been studying genetic factors for years. Nevertheless, the idea that the actual schizophrenic gene (or more likely, genes) may be identified in the foreseeable future has caused many to put aside their 2- and 3-Tesla magnetic coils and take up with electrophoresis plates.

In our view, a factor that is relatively unrepresented in current theorizing (and research) is the role that environment may play in interaction with a schizophrenic diathesis in producing the variety of phenotypes that are recognized as schizophrenia spectrum disorders.

Some years ago, we suggested that environmental factors, and specifically, harsh and punitive treatment could interact with a schizophrenic diathesis to increase the severity of the phenotypic expression of a disorder [3]. We later expanded on this theme, citing other data that support the view of an interaction between experience and diathesis in terms of outcome severity. The data came from a number of sources, including studies of communication deviance, affective style and expressed emotion in the nuclear families of patients [4]; these indicate that more chaotic, punitive family environments were associated with higher incidences of schizophrenia spectrum disorders. In addition, in a study of 184 adopted-away offspring of schizophrenic mothers, it was found that in families with relatively good mental health there was a low incidence (7%) of psychiatric disorder in the adoptees, whereas in families with poor mental health, the incidence rose to 52% [5]. In a reanalysis of the Danish adoption study data, Lowing and Mirsky [6]

[1] *Section on Clinical and Experimental Neuropsychology, Laboratory of Brain and Cognition, National Institute of Mental Health, 15 North Drive, Bethesda, MD 20982–2668, USA*
[2] *Clinical Psychophysiology and Pharmacology Laboratory, Department of Psychiatry, Uniformed Services University of the Health Sciences, 4301 Jones Bridge Road, Bethesda, MD 20814, USA*

found that among 20 subjects with DSM-III diagnoses of schizophrenia spectrum, the 10 with diagnoses of schizophrenia or schizotypal personality disorder had significantly more stress reported in childhood that the 10 with diagnoses of schizoid, borderline, or mixed personality disorders. The stresses that were reported included harsh treatment, intrusiveness and restriction of autonomous functioning by parents, as well as feelings of alienation and chronic arguments. Finally, in the Israeli high-risk study, it was found that there was a significantly greater incidence of psychopathological outcomes (from two- to ten-fold, depending on the disorder) in the offspring of schizophrenic parents raised in kibbutzim than in the offspring raised by their own parents in cities and towns throughout Israel. This result was attributed to the hypercritical, intrusive and deviance-intolerant nature of kibbutz life [7]. These studies are summarized in Mirsky and Duncan [2], where a model was presented hypothesizing that the interaction between the degree of stress and the severity of the schizophrenogenic brain abnormalities determined the severity of the schizophrenic spectrum disorder. A similar model was proposed earlier by Zubin and Steinhauer [8]. Our point is evident, we think; although it is easier and more "scientific" to think of the schizophrenic spectrum disorders simply in terms of varying degrees of penetrance of one or more schizophrenogenic genes, if we ignore the effects of stress during development, we do so at our peril. This accounts for an unknown portion of the variance of the inheritance of schizophrenia, and should become a part of the routine investigation of spectrum disorders.

REFERENCES

1. Mirsky A.F. (1969) Neuropsychological bases of schizophrenia. *Ann. Rev. Psychol.*, **20**: 321–348.
2. Mirsky A.F., Duncan C.C. (1986) Etiology and expression of schizophrenia: neurobiological and psychosocial factors. *Ann. Rev. Psychol.*, **37**: 291–319.
3. Mirsky A.F., Duncan-Johnson C.C. (1984) Nature vs. nurture in schizophrenia: the struggle continues. *Integr. Psychiatry*, **2**: 137–141.
4. Goldstein M.J. (1985) Family factors that antedate the onset of schizophrenia and related disorders: the results of a fifteen year prospective longitudinal study. *Acta Psychiatr. Scand.*, **72** (Suppl. 319): 7–18.
5. Tienari P., Sorri A., Lahti I., Naarala M., Wahlberg K.E., Pohjala J., Moring J. (1985) Interaction of genetic and social factors in schizophrenia. *Acta Psychiatr. Scand.*, **72** (Suppl. 319): 19–30.
6. Lowing P.A., Mirsky A.F., Pereira R. (1983) The inheritance of schizophrenia spectrum disorders: a reanalysis of the Danish Adoptee Study data. *Am. J. Psychiatry*, **140**: 1167–1171.
7. Mirsky A.F., Silberman E.K., Latz A., Nagler S. (1985) Adult outcomes of high-risk children: differential effects of town and kibbutz rearing. *Schizophr. Bull.*, **11**: 150–154.
8. Zubin J., Steinhauer S. (1986) How to break the logjam in schizophrenia. A look beyond genetics. *J. Nerv. Ment. Dis.*, **159**: 477–492.

5.12
Schizophrenia Spectrum — a "Terra Flexibilis"

Andreas Marneros[1]

If we accept that a schizophrenic spectrum, as described by Maier *et al*, really exists, is it difficult to define it exactly? Or is it impossible to do so? Or impossible now, but perhaps possible in decades to come? The crucial question is: what is the most reliable way of defining schizophrenia spectrum?

The most usual means of defining schizophrenia-like or schizophrenia spectrum disorders is through the phenomenology, the aetiology, the long-term prognosis, or a combination of two or all of the above. Grouping disorders according only or mainly to their phenomenology is the path delineated by Jaspers (hierarchical principle), Schneider (first-rank symptoms) and, to some extent, Eugen Bleuler (fundamental symptoms). But the phenomenological approach is not sufficiently reliable. Symptoms and signs of mental disorders are usually non-specific. The prognostic aspect of mental disorders, especially their long-term outcome, as a defining issue — suggested by Kraepelin but also by his opponents, such as the Wernicke–Kleist–Leonhard school — proved only weakly reliable. The opinion of Maier *et al*, that the spectrum disorders share symptoms, causes and risk factors with schizophrenia, is correct. However, the cause of schizophrenia is still shadowy, so it remains risky to put the whole weight of the specificity of a criterion on the assumed common or related aetiology.

Both of the widely accepted international diagnostic systems, ICD-10 and DSM-IV, distinguish from schizophrenia, but at the same time associate with it, a group of "schizophreniform" or "brief" or "acute and transient" psychotic disorders. Some authors assume that the only relevant difference between these disorders and schizophrenia concerns chronicity: schizophrenic disorders are chronic; "schizophreniform" or "acute" disorders are not. Recent research, however, shows some relevant differences between schizophrenia and "acute/transient" or "schizophreniform" disorders which theoretically can be extended to the "specific criterion" of the schizophrenic spectrum, namely the cause. Our research [1] shows that acute transient psychotic disorders differ significantly from schizophrenia not only regarding gender (significantly more females) and age at onset (significantly higher) — both of these factors can be assumed to be indirectly "biological" — but also in some other important parameters, such as the

[1]*Department of Psychiatry and Psychotherapy, Martin-Luther-University Halle-Wittenberg, 06097 Halle, Germany*

prevalence of anxiety and bipolarity of symptoms (significantly higher) and of social withdrawal (significantly lower). The question which arises considering such findings is: how strong is the relation of "acute/transient", "brief" or "schizophreniform" disorders, to mood disorder? Or: how weak is the relation of the above disorders to schizophrenia? Our still ongoing family study of "acute/transient psychosis", and other studies, may provide more evidence.

Schizoaffective disorders are undoubtedly a heterogeneous group. Yet it is certainly possible to distinguish between unipolar and bipolar types according to the affective symptomatology which is always present [2, 3]. Perhaps it might be possible also to distinguish between "schizodominant" and "affectively dominant" types. But according to what criteria? According to phenomenology, prognosis, treatment response, or family risk, or according to occurrence of pure schizophrenic episodes in the course? None of them furnishes a sufficiently reliable distinction [4]. Even in the families of schizoaffective patients with schizophrenia-like prognosis or with a dominance of schizophrenic symptoms, we find cases with affective disorders, and vice versa [1]. Family studies as well as other genetic investigations require homogeneity of samples. Homogeneity requires reliable and consistent definitions. But this is not the case in schizoaffective disorders. Nevertheless, it seems that in addition to the (strongly reliable) dichotomy "unipolar–bipolar", the (weakly reliable) dichotomy "schizodominant–affectively dominant" can contribute to the homogeneity of the group of schizoaffective disorders, separating them into a schizophrenia spectrum and an affective spectrum disorder [5].

We believe that there are many more uncertainties than certainties surrounding schizophrenia spectrum disorders.

REFERENCES

1. Marneros A., Pillmann F., Haring A., Zänker S. Acute and transient psychosis. A comparison with schizophrenic, bipolar schizoaffective and mentally healthy people (unpublished manuscript).
2. Marneros A., Deister A., Rohde A. (1989) Unipolar and bipolar schizoaffective disorders: a comparative study. I. Premorbid and sociodemographic features. *Eur. Arch. Psychiatry Neurol. Sci.*, **239**: 158–163.
3. Marneros A., Deister A., Rohde A. (1990) The concept of distinct but voluminous groups of bipolar and unipolar diseases. Part I: Bipolar diseases. *Eur. Arch. Psychiatry Clin. Neurosci.*, **240**: 77–84.
4. Marneros A., Deister A., Rohde A. (1991) *Affektive, Schizoaffektive und Schizophrene Psychosen: Eine Vergleichende Langzeitstudie.* Springer, Berlin.
5. Marneros A. (1999) *Handbuch der Unipolaren und Bipolaren Erkrankungen.* Thieme, Stuttgart.

5.13
Some Open Research Issues Concerning Schizophrenia
Spectrum Disorders

J.D. Guelfi[1]

Schizotypal, paranoid and schizoid personality disorders are the three "odd cluster" personality disorders described in the DSM-IV. Empirical data on these disorders remain scarce.

Schizoid personality disorder is distinguished from the other personality disorders by the prominence of social withdrawal with interpersonal deficits. It seems to be a very heterogeneous disorder. Schizotypal personality disorder (SPD) is distinguished from the other personality disorders by eccentricity, odd thinking, suspiciousness and paranoid ideation. This particular disorder with chronic psychotic-like characteristics is described and defined partly by its presumably genetic relationship to schizophrenia. Nevertheless, the genetic specificity of SPD is not clearly established yet. The comorbidity of this disorder has recently been explored in several studies, whose results remain inconsistent. For example, the percentage of patients with SPD receiving a concomitant diagnosis of borderline personality disorder ranges from 33% to 91%, and the comorbidity of SPD in borderlines ranges from 0% to 53%. The overlap between SPD, affective disorders and borderline personality disorders may be an artefact of diagnostic criteria.

More empirical data are needed in this field. As stated by Siever *et al* [1], external validating studies are required "to determine whether schizotypal patients with a concomitant borderline personality disorder differ from pure schizotypal patients in genetic, biological, outcome and treatment–response parameters".

Numerous questions about schizoaffective disorder also remain open. This disorder overlaps with both affective and schizophrenic disorder. The heterogeneity of this group of patients may be limited by treatment response, family history, long-term course and biological studies. The results of the most recent family studies can be summarized as follows. According to Aubert and Rush [2], schizoaffective disorder "did not seem to be directly transmitted as a separate entity. Schizoaffective, mainly affective disorder (and more so for the manic than the depressed type) had high family loading for affective disorder (bipolar more than unipolar). Schizoaffective disorder (mainly schizophrenic or depressed type) was associated with higher familial loadings for schizophrenia."

Finally, there is no real consensus in France about the nature of schizophrenia spectrum disorders. The validity of DSM criteria for schizoid and

[1]University Paris XI, Hôpital Paul Brousse, 12 Avenue P. Vaillant-Couturier, 94804 Villejuif, France

schizotypal disorders and for schizoaffective disorders is not well established. The boundaries between these disorders and borderline disorder, affective disorders or some mild forms of schizophrenia are not really known.

REFERENCES

1. Siever L.J., Bernstein D.P., Silverman J.M. (1996) In *DSM-IV Sourcebook*, vol. 2 (Eds T.A. Widiger, A.J. Frances, M.A. Pincus, R. Ross, M.B. First, N.W. Davis), pp. 685–702. American Psychiatric Association, Washington, D.C.
2. Aubert J.L., Rush A.J. (1996) Schizoaffective disorder. In *DSM-IV Sourcebook*, vol. 2 (Eds T.A. Widiger, A.J. Frances, H.A. Pincus, R. Ross, M.B. First, N.W. Davis), pp. 65–96. American Psychiatric Association, Washington, DC.

5.14
Schizophrenia Spectrum Disorders Revisited

Muhammed Afzal Javed[1]

Schizophrenia, possibly the most common serious mental illness, is recognized all over the world and has been described in almost all cultures. Since its description by Emil Kraepelin, this disorder has been the subject of extensive investigations [1]. The issues relating to phenomenology and the dimensionality of schizophrenia have always remained of remarkable interest to the mental health professionals and, despite the advent of DSM and ICD classifications, considerable controversy still prevails regarding the most appropriate way to classify and categorize this disorder.

It is true that the adoption of descriptive approaches has helped to conceptualize many psychiatric syndromes to a large extent, but it is fair to say that diagnosis in psychiatry is still more of an art than a science. Current efforts, both in theory and research, to understand the development and pathogenesis of schizophrenia also fall in the same domain. Following Kraepelin's attempt to bring together different clinical types, present-day psychiatry is still faced with the dilemma of subdividing this illness into distinctive forms which represent a diverse and broad range of cognitive, emotional and behavioural disturbances [2].

Generally, use of a single word or phrase in medicine for a specific illness refers to a condition that is aetiologically and pathophysiologically homogeneous. Unfortunately the situation for schizophrenia presents with several paradoxes. Researchers and investigators have thus always been aware of

[1] *University of Warwick Medical Centre, 2 Manor Court Avenue, Nuneaton CV11 5HX, UK*

the diagnostic confusions and nosological chaos and have been continuously attempting to resolve such issues. The present era has witnessed a number of efforts in refining the phenomenological aspects of schizophrenia, mainly searching for the pathognomonic symptoms, discovering or rediscovering the concepts of positive and negative symptoms, defining various subtypes and even moving from categories to dimensions and individual symptoms [3].

The concept of schizophrenia spectrum disorder also reflects such an attempt and emphasizes the diversities in the recognition of different boundaries of this mental illness. This term, however, provides some advantages over many other terms which have been used to describe different aspects of schizophrenia in the past. Originally, this term included conditions which were related to schizophrenia, but were different in terms of presentation. Historically, the spectrum disorders encompassed some specific personality traits (or states) and certain conditions sharing clinical features with schizophrenia, but often with an episodic course and variable outcome. The last few decades have witnessed an increasing interest in this area. As mentioned in Maier et al's paper, further support has been given to this approach by many recent studies. Given the evidence for genetic determination of schizophrenia, an excess of schizophrenia-like personality features (e.g. schizoid, paranoid and schizotypal traits) has been found among the probands and siblings of schizophrenic patients. Similarly, schizophrenia-like symptomatology has been described in first-degree relatives of patients suffering from these personality disorders. Identical neurobiological and neuropsychological changes in schizophrenia and similar disorders also strengthen the case of a spectrum of disorders.

Phenomenological work is again consistent with the above-mentioned model, suggesting similarities among different clinical presentations of the spectrum. This issue gets further support from work in developing countries, as clinical presentations like acute brief psychosis, excess of affective symptoms in female schizophrenics and association of different personality traits with schizophrenia have all been well documented. It is interesting to know that all these conditions can be conveniently classified under the heading of schizophrenia spectrum disorders [4, 5]. When it comes to treatment, the rational use of neuroleptics is upheld for schizophrenia as well as schizophrenia-related disorders. Keeping in view the mode of action of antipsychotics (typical as well as atypical), it can be postulated that the effectiveness of these drugs can be explained on the basis of the underlying aetiological similarities of these clinical conditions.

It is thus fair to conclude that schizophrenia constitutes a group of multiple and diverse presentations which overlap in different ways. As the predispositions and clinical presentations are shared, refinements in the nosology of this illness are required. For practical and therapeutic purposes, and despite some conceptual and empirical caveats, it may be justified to use the term schizophrenia spectrum disorders which may include conditions like schizophrenia, brief psychotic states, schizophreniform disorders, schizoaffective disorders (mainly schizophrenic) and personality states (traits) of schizotypal, schizoid and paranoid types. It may be the case that some of these spectrum disorders be conceptualized as less severe variants of schizophrenia, but this model does combine contributing aetiological factors into a hypothetical dimension.

This proposed model, therefore, needs thoughtful discussions. As evidence suggests strong similarities of aetiology, genetic predisposition, biological correlates and treatment options for schizophrenia spectrum disorders, it will be fair to include these conditions under one major nosological heading. This will help not only in consolidating different clinical conditions, but also in setting priorities for future work in this area.

REFERENCES

1. Javed M.A. (1998) Schizophrenia: moving to the 21st century. *Pakistan J. Med. Sci.,* **14**: 277–279.
2. Lenzenweger M.F., Dworkin R.H. (1996) The dimensions of schizophrenia symptomatology: not one or two, at least three, perhaps four. *Br. J. Psychiatry,* **168**: 432–440.
3. Copolov D. (1996) Diagnosis and phenomenology of schizophrenia and related disorders. *Curr. Opin. Psychiatry,* **9**: 63–67.
4. Susser E., Varma V.K., Mattoo S.K., Finnerty M., Mojtabai R., Tripathi B.M., Misra A.K., Wig N.N. (1998) Long term course of acute brief psychosis in a developing country. *Br. J. Psychiatry,* **173**: 226–230.
5. Javed M.A. Phenomenology of schizophrenias across two cultures (in preparation).

6

Economics of Schizophrenia: A Review

Martin Knapp, Judit Simon, Mauro Percudani and Stephen Almond

London School of Economics, and Institute of Psychiatry, University of London, London, UK

INTRODUCTION

Burdens and Costs

Schizophrenia often has a considerable impact not only on patients, but also on their families, the health care system and the wider society. The health outcomes of the illness are variable and for some people can be relatively mild, with the patient suffering one (16%) or several (32%) episodes and little or no lasting impairment [1]. But a majority experience repeated episodes with worse outcomes, 9% suffering lasting impairment and 43% enduring increasingly severe symptoms and no periods of complete remission [2].

The debilitating symptoms of schizophrenia clearly require specialist health care interventions and targeted treatments. Poor personal and social functioning often associated with the illness generates a need for support in the activites of daily living. People with schizophrenia may find it difficult to secure paid employment, or to hold on to jobs when they get them, with implications for their own income and for the economy's productivity. Consequently, many people with schizophrenia face impoverished lives and lifestyles, and their families and other caregivers may carry a large responsibility, providing or paying for some services themselves. Caregivers' own employment chances and quality of life may be compromised. On a wider scale, society at large may carry intangible "costs" associated with the perceived suffering of those with the illness and the fear that mentally disturbed people may be a danger to themselves or others.

These are all costs of schizophrenia. Some are direct and immediately recognized by health care and other service decision-makers, others are more indirect and nebulous. Some of the broad societal fears about "dangerous people" may only be "costs" in a colloquial sense, although of course their relevance for policy should not be underestimated. When summed, these

Schizophrenia, Second Edition. Edited by Mario Maj and Norman Sartorius.
© 2002 John Wiley & Sons Ltd.

various costs quickly mount up and they can endure for long periods [3]. The large aggregate financial impact of the illness is one reason for growing concern about the costs of schizophrenia and the cost effectiveness of treating it.

Demands for Economic Analyses

How do demands for economic insights manifest themselves in mental health care systems, either at the macro level of the whole system or at the micro level of individual treatment settings? At the macro level we can see the nature and origins of some of these demands simply by comparing two contrasting types of health care system: a predominantly private insurance system as in the USA and a national or public health care system as in the UK.

The US health care system is heavily reliant on private health insurance, but has recently been dominated by the growth of "managed care" in both the private and public systems. Managed care seeks to control or manage service access, quality and costs. The USA has had an historically high proportion of national income devoted to health care. As provider costs and insurance premiums escalated during the 1970s and 1980s [4, 5], so the search for cost containment drove many funders to introduce a variety of managed care initiatives. Controversy swiftly followed [6]. Utilization reviews, case management, capitated payments and a host of other measures have been employed to try to arrest increases in expenditure and costs [7]. At the same time, patients and their families — and, of course, the professionals who treat them — continue to want to secure the best health outcomes they can. One consequence is rationing of a more overt (and controversial) kind than hitherto experienced.

A contrasting system of health care is provided by Britain's tax-funded, public sector National Health Service (NHS). Although, compared to the situation in the USA, different incentives may appear to be at work, and different operational objectives to prevail, in fact there are many similar underlying aims and shared consequences. Cost containment has been explicitly a core objective for longer in the UK than in the USA, and has also been easier to achieve. Rationing has always been quite overt. The Blair Government is committed to formally-constituted health improvement programmes and evidence-based medicine, shifting the emphasis away from costs and more on to quality and outcomes. However, such a shift only serves to make plain the difficult choices that always have to be made about resource deployment.

At the macro level, therefore, the scarcity of available resources relative to the many demands and needs for them necessitates careful consideration of the alternative uses to which society's resources may be put and the resultant consequences for outcomes. This is the prompt for economic evaluation. Economic arguments and analyses at this macro level examine how mental health care systems operate, the effects of different incentive structures and funding arrangements and so on.

At a narrower, micro level there are different questions to be addressed: how do treatments and policies impact upon the lives of individual people and the activities and resource flows of different organizations? At the micro level, therefore, economic analysis should aim to assist the individual clinician or care professional who has to decide how to spread limited treatment resources across a large number of competing uses. How is consultation time to be rationed between the many people wanting to see a primary care doctor? How are inpatient beds to be allocated when need exceeds capacity? If pharmacy budgets only allow a limited number of schizophrenia patients to be prescribed the more expensive atypical antipsychotics, which patients must go without? These are examples of micro-level resource allocation questions, and individual care professionals cannot and should not be expected to find answers without information on the consequences of their choices. Economic evaluations help to provide some of this information.

Criteria for Choices

Decision-makers in every mental health care system in the world and at almost every level in the organizational and care hierarchies need evaluative evidence to help them predict the consequences of their actions. Those consequences should be judged in terms of both outcomes and resources. Indeed, a number of criteria are used by decision-makers to underpin or to justify their decisions. Commonly used criteria include effectiveness, resource targeting on priority needs, patient and public safety, protection of civil liberties, patient autonomy, continuity of care and economy. Economics has concerned itself primarily, although not exclusively, with two particular criteria: efficiency and equity.

Efficiency is a measure of the extent to which a particular resource configuration achieves patient and other outcomes; it is most certainly not synonymous with "cheap". An efficient configuration would be one that leads to the best level of effectiveness (highest level of outcomes) achieved from a given set of resources (level of costs), or one that minimizes the cost of producing a given set of outcomes. Equity refers to the fairness or justice of an allocation of either outcomes (benefits) or costs (burdens). Both efficiency and equity therefore refer to optimal balances between outcomes and costs. These two criteria may sometimes be in conflict. However, they underpin and indeed *justify* economic studies of mental health care systems and treatment arrangements.

Structure of the Chapter

The next section of this chapter looks at the overall costs of schizophrenia, particularly those revealed in cost-of-illness evaluations. We then turn our attention to some of the principal cost drivers within these overall estimates: relapse, inpatient services, specialist residential care, mortality, lost employment, family impact, and public safety and concern. Each of these might be seen as generating potentially high costs in relation to schizophrenia sufferers, and each has attracted attention from various quarters, including from those stakeholders seeking to improve the efficiency and equity with which mental health care services and systems support vulnerable people.

In the fourth section we briefly describe the main evaluative modes of economic evaluation (cost-offset, cost-minimization, cost-effectiveness, cost-consequences, cost-benefit and cost-utility analyses). We then use these evaluative techniques in the search for cost-effectiveness, or — to use a more generic terminology — for an improved balance between outcomes and costs. One section looks at pharmacotherapies, one at psychosocial therapies and one at care arrangements. Can available financial, human and other resources be deployed more efficiently or more equitably in schizophrenia care? For example, can we improve the return (in terms of changes in patient symptoms and quality of life) from a given set of resources? Can the distribution of outcomes and burdens be made fairer?

In this chapter we cannot attempt a formal systematic review of the international evidence, although such reviews can be enormously helpful, nor can we even begin to analyse the implications of the available evidence for every health care system in the world. Our aims are more modest but indicative: to identify the main economic issues relating to schizophrenia and its treatment and to summarize the main economic evidence. The material we bring together in pursuit of these aims will inevitably be a personal selection, although hopefully a useful one.

THE OVERALL COSTS OF SCHIZOPHRENIA

Translating the overall burden of schizophrenia into economic terms can be helpful in a number of ways. It allows us to gain a better understanding of schizophrenia's relative magnitude in comparison to the burdens imposed by other chronic illnesses. It also has the signal virtue of drawing attention to what could be a very wide-ranging impact of an illness or disorder. *Cost-of-illness* or *burden-of-disease* studies, as these global measurement exercises are called, may or may not offer useful guides to policy makers about the best use of resources, for they do not tell us very much about efficiency or equity attainment. Cost-of-illness (COI) estimates can in fact be misleading. The extent of service use will be a function not only of the severity and duration of an illness but also the availability of services. The heterogeneous nature of supply side factors can make it difficult to derive a standard global account. Comorbidities make cost attribution quite challenging. Nevertheless, there are quite well-developed methods for this kind of exercise [8].

COI estimates are either constructed "top-down", by disaggregating national or regional budgets by diagnostic group, or they are constructed "bottom-up", by building on prevalence or incidence figures. Prevalence-based COIs calculate the direct and indirect economic burden of illness according to the current time period in which the illness takes place — usually a year. Incidence-based COIs represent the full lifetime costs of an illness from its onset. The majority of COI studies are prevalence based. The "bottom-up" approach would follow a standard series of questions: What is the prevalence or incidence of schizophrenia? What services are used by people with schizophrenia in the cross-section (prevalence estimate) or at different stages of their illness (incidence estimate)? What is the unit cost of each of these services? What other costs (not related directly to services) need to be included in the calculations such as family burden or lost employment? Finally, how representative are these total costs?

Most COI studies calculate both direct and indirect costs, and do so from a broad societal perspective (i.e. not restricting the analysis to, say, health care expenditures) in order to reflect the full social costs of schizophrenia. Ideally all resource impacts would be *opportunity costs*, that is, the values forgone by not using these resources in their next best employment. Direct costs cover services such as hospital inpatient days, outpatient visits, specialist supported accommodation, etc. Indirect costs, broadly defined, usually focus on lost employment, but can and should also include costs such as the victim costs of crime and the support from caregivers. There are some disputes about what it is legitimate to include and how it is to be valued [9] but we do not dwell on those methodological issues here, except to note that apparently modest methodological differences can produce quite wide discrepancies in overall cost estimates [10]. The distinction between direct and indirect costs is not unambiguous nor is it consistently made, and some health economists no longer use it.

Recent Cost-of-illness Estimates

Fein [11] conducted the first cost-of-illness study in the mental health field, since which time there have been many such estimates. The most comprehensive indications of the overall economic impact of schizophrenia have been constructed in the USA, based on the informative Epidemiologic Catchment Area (ECA) survey conducted by the National Institute of Mental Health. Using a prevalence approach, total direct and indirect costs for schizophrenia were estimated by Rice and Miller [12] to be $32.5 billion in 1990 (22% of total mental illness costs). Direct costs were obtained using national household surveys and accounted for $17.3 billion, reflecting the high costs of institutionalization as well as a large number of ambulatory visits per person. About 2.5% of national health care expenditure went on schizophrenia patients.

Indirect costs in this widely-cited US study were based on the human capital approach—the value of labour at market prices forgone as a direct result of illness, using average incomes—and accounted for $12.0 billion. Regression analysis predictions reduced income effects by adjusting for socio-economic variables. This partly explains the relatively low level of morbidity costs compared with findings from other studies (other estimates suggest "indirect" costs are three to four times higher than direct costs) [13–15]. On the other hand, it has been argued that the indirect costs are over-estimated because of errors in the calculated prevalence rate [16]. As found for other countries (see below), mental health organizations and nursing homes made up the bulk of direct costs (approximately 68%). Costs for the homeless and military population were excluded.

The first robust COI in the UK came from Davies and Drummond [14]. Total direct costs of treating schizophrenia in 1990/91 were estimated to be £397 million, or 1.6% of the total health care budget. Hospital-based and community-based residential care accounted for almost 75% of these costs. Almost all of the direct costs (97%) were incurred by less than 50% of the patients. A conservative estimate of annual indirect costs—based on lost productivity using unemployment and average wage statistics—was approximately £1.7 billion. Subsequent UK studies suggest that these direct cost estimates are somewhat low, partly due to the limited range of services included in the cost calculations and partly because lower bound estimates were taken for frequency of service use. For example, Knapp [17] suggested figures of £810 million for direct costs—approximately 2.8% of all NHS expenditure—and £2.6 billion for both direct and indirect costs. Even this total is an underestimate, because it excludes caregiver time.

The unevenness of the cost impact has been noted by others [18]. Mean annual costs for a cohort of newly diagnosed patients over the first five years in the UK were £172.5 million, representing approximately only 1.5% of the whole schizophrenia population.

A retrospective cross-sectional survey of patients treated by public and private hospital and community psychiatrists was the basis for a French study [19]. Costs in 1992 amounted to fr12.4 billion, or 2% of total annual health care expenditure. Again the largest contributor to costs was hospitalization (55%) and then intermediate care facilities, such as day hospitals and occupational therapy centres (30%). Indirect costs for lost employment were measured by social assistance allowances and accounted for fr5.2 billion, although this could be seen as an underestimate of lost productivity unless allowances are close to the average wage.

Using comprehensive data from most health care sectors in the Netherlands — and boosted by the fact that more than 99% of the population have full health insurance cover — Meerding *et al* [20] computed all health care costs for all individual illnesses. Costs were based on prevalence but included only direct costs. Schizophrenia was the twenty-third most expensive illness to treat over all age groups, but was much more important for the 15–44 age group. Overall, schizophrenia costs represented 1.4% of total health care spending, but 3.5% for the population aged 15–44.

Several other studies from European countries have calculated the COI for schizophrenia, as recently reviewed [21]. Although estimates vary between and even within countries, all of the studies point to the large social and economic impacts of schizophrenia, especially the important indirect costs related to lost employment and premature mortality. The use of mental health services in three areas of Spain — Burlada, Cantabria and Barcelona — illustrates how patterns and apparent impacts can vary regionally *within* countries [22]. Costs were higher in the two centres with greater community mental health service development. A good illustration of how the applied methodology influences the calculation comes from Puerto Rico. Rubio-Stipec *et al* [23] found huge differences between the results of prevalence-based ($60 million) and incidence-based methods ($266.1 million).

Most COI studies include an estimate of the cost of lost employment based on the human capital approach, which uses average wage levels to value production losses. But an individual's inability to work may not reduce national productivity by an amount equal to the average national wage (which is the usual assumption). It may be more sensible to use "friction cost" estimates [24] rather than human capital-based estimates on the assumption that productivity losses arise only until such time as a sick employee is fully replaced. Health economists continue to debate this issue, not least because the two methods can produce markedly different results [25].

It is clear that COI estimates can be informative. At the national level, COI estimates can provide policy-makers with valuable information to aid decision making on macro-level resource allocation. But the total costs of schizophrenia can really only be interpreted relative to other demands on health care services, and are consequently context bound [26]. We must also reiterate that COI studies are not evaluations as such.

PRINCIPAL COST DRIVERS

The global costs of schizophrenia have generated a number of concerns. What, then, are the principal cost drivers? We now briefly consider eight topics which have attracted particular attention when the costs of schizophrenia are discussed, and which feature regularly in the empirical evaluations described later in the chapter: relapse; inpatient services; specialist community accommodation; medication; mortality; lost employment; family impact; and public safety and concern.

Relapse

A prominent feature of schizophrenia is its long-term debilitating effects, associated with a high rate of relapse. Historically, relapse was closely associated with inpatient readmission, but the advent of more intensive, better targeted *community* services in some health care systems has broken that association: relapse today might result in the mobilization of a crisis intervention team rather than admission to an acute ward. Nevertheless, relapse usually means an exacerbation of symptoms and deterioration in social functioning, followed by full or partial remission, and consequently the long-term pattern of repeated, intensive service usage is likely to be similar whether the mental health care system is predominantly hospital or community based. Relapse will be costly whatever the system.

A helpful perspective on the resource consequences of relapse comes from a meta-analysis of a number of studies [27], linking the relapse probability to poor medication efficacy, and non-concordance with medication programmes (identifying the respective contributions to each). For example, relapse rates for patients who do not take their medications were found to be three times higher than for those who do. Second, the analysis separated the cost of inpatient care for first-episode patients and relapsing patients. First-episode inpatient care was estimated to have cost $2.3 billion in the USA, while the direct costs of readmission in the 2 years following first episode were only slightly less at around $2 billion. This latter "cost of relapse" was attributed mainly (63%) to loss of medication response, and partly (37%) to medication non-concordance. Another study suggested that people with repeated episodes of schizophrenia requiring hospitalization or intensive community care could incur direct costs more than 100 times greater than the cost of treating a single episode [14].

Inpatient Services

Hospitals have been the mainstay of schizophrenia care for a long time, and they are expensive. Whether they are *too* expensive is a moot point. Is it the case, for example, that hospital inpatient services are relied upon for too many people with schizophrenia and are periods of admission too long? Concern about hospitalization costs has energized searches for community care arrangements which can either reduce cost or improve patient health and quality of life. Nevertheless, the historically dominant contribution of inpatient services to total cost (see above) has been so marked that many research studies have even taken avoidance or reduction of hospital admissions as a criterion of success in its own right.

Different countries rely to different degrees on inpatient services as a component of the portfolio of provision for serious mental illness. Countries like the USA and Italy — and, increasingly, many other Western European countries — have reduced their numbers of inpatient beds quite markedly, but hospitalization is still a major cost factor (as high as 75% of direct health care costs in a Danish study, and also quite high in some other countries [28]). In Central and Eastern Europe countries, which still rely heavily on this form of care, and in countries like Japan and China, which have seen increases in per capita bed numbers, the contribution to proportional total cost could well be much larger [29, 30]. *Within* countries, of course, reliance on inpatient services varies markedly; for instance, a recent Spanish study found that 76% of direct health care costs in Cantabria were accounted for by inpatient care, compared to only 31% in Barcelona [22].

What is common across all countries and regions, however, is a funding "imbalance". This can be illustrated by data from England. In a study of treated prevalence, based on a patchwork of cross-sectional surveys, Kavanagh *et al* [30] found that 14% of people with schizophrenia were resident as short- or long-stay inpatients in 1992, but they accounted for 51% of total public sector expenditure on schizophrenia care. Another English study estimated that 97% of the total lifetime direct treatment costs of the illness are incurred by the 41% of patients experiencing episodes requiring hospitalization for more than 2.5 years [14]. Equivalent expenditure distributions have been noted elsewhere [31]. Consequently, treatments or care arrangements which can reduce the need for inpatient stays while maintaining outcomes will look attractive to strategic decision-makers, although they may not *necessarily* be more cost-effective.

Specialist Community Accommodation

Many people with schizophrenia do not need to be in hospital but nevertheless have a short-term or continuing need for a structured living environment, often in specialist staffed accommodation, ranging from facilities with nurse-qualified staff on duty 24 hours a day to unstaffed group homes with occasional peripatetic supervision. Developing an appropriate array of community accommodation and managing the interface with inpatient services have become essential ingredients of an efficient mental health care system [32], yet many systems fall some way short [33]. One of the readily observable consequences is the large number of homeless mentally ill people in many cities across the world [34], although cause and effect can be hard to disentangle [35].

From the ECA, Cohen and Thompson [35] estimated that nursing home expenditure accounted for 31% of direct health care costs of schizophrenia, and 16% of the total cost. An English and Welsh survey of almost 400 community accommodation facilities found them to be significantly less costly than ongoing inpatient care (on long-stay or acute wards) even after adjusting for the fact that hospitals tend to accommodate people with more severe symptomatology and greater needs [36, 37]. There were 1050 people in the sample with schizophrenia, living either in hospital or in community residential accommodation. The total costs of their care varied markedly by type of accommodation: from an annual average of £51 000 for an acute inpatient bed in London in 1994 to an average of £10 000 for a group home outside London.

Medication

The proportion of the total direct costs of schizophrenia attributable to drugs has been estimated to be quite modest in many countries, at 2.3% in the USA [8], 4.0% in the UK [38], 5.6% in France [19] and 1.1% in the Netherlands [39], although as high as 9% in Hungary [29] and up to 13% in Spain [22]. The proportion is generally greater in countries where the service range is more limited and the cost of in-patient treatment lower. For example, a Nigerian study found the cost of drugs to be 61.8% of the direct costs of schizophrenia, partly because the typical treatment is inpatient care [40]. The proportion of the total cost of schizophrenia attributable to medications is expected to increase in the short term with the development and more widespread use of atypical antipsychotics, partly because these drugs have higher acquisition costs than those they replace, and partly because they are likely to lead to reductions in hospitalization, thereby reducing the overall cost (the denominator in the proportional calculation).

Mortality

Mortality among people with schizophrenia is 1.6 times that expected in a general population of similar age and gender (standardized mortality rate of 156 for males and 141 for females, both statistically significant differences from the general population rates) [42]. These figures come from a substantial pooled analysis of 20 studies, covering 36 000 people from nine countries. While there are some differences between countries, the mortality risk from schizophrenia is universal. The mortality risk from suicide is particularly high (nine times higher than expected) and other violent incidents 2.3 times higher than expected. Suicide was most likely "close to the time of treatment inception ... during inpatient care ... and among current outpatients" [42].

In Denmark mortality among schizophrenia patients was found to have grown over time, with suicides being a particular cause [43]. Many people who commit suicide have no contact with mental health services.

With above-average mortality rates, especially among younger people, there are inevitably cost consequences associated with lost productivity. Many cost-of-illness studies make allowance for this loss, although — as we show below — there is some dispute about the appropriate value to attach. The highest estimates suggest that mortality accounts for around 10% of all the value of lost productivity due to schizophrenia [8, 29].

Lost Employment

A large part of the global economic impact of the illness is due to the difficulties that sufferers encounter in finding and keeping paid employment. We previously noted the methodological debate currently underway among health economists about how to value this lost employment. If the arguments of the "friction cost" school are valid [24], the associated productivity loss to the economy is much smaller than most COI studies have maintained, with their estimates based on "human capital" assumptions. A Canadian study concluded that the human capital method to cost forgone productivity or employment — which was the method used to derive some of the better known estimates (such as $10.7 billion in the USA [8] and £1.7 billion in the UK [14]) — produces a figure vastly greater than the friction cost method [25].

People with schizophrenia who are unable to earn a decent wage are quite likely to be both economically and socially marginalized. Even with welfare or income support payments from the state or elsewhere their disposable incomes will be low, and the social and personal consequences could be numerous.

Family Impact

The policy of deinstitutionalizing psychiatric patients has highlighted the role of the family as one of the main providers of care. Although the situation differs from country to country, it is estimated that between one third and one half of patients live with their families in developed countries [30, 43, 44]. The caring role in schizophrenia could affect most aspects of family functioning. Families live with behaviour that often involves profound mood swings and unpredictability, bizarre ideation, attentional deficit, non-communicativeness, withdrawal and apathy [45, 46]. They may have to contend with disruptions to established patterns of household living, social embarrassment, destruction of property, immature or demanding behaviour, verbal and physical abuse and self-destructive acts [47]. While it is true that not all of the effects will be negative [48, 49], the family impact of schizophrenia is usually seen in this light [50]. Many caregivers have ambivalent relationships with mental health professionals, feeling unsupported, uninformed, misinformed and blamed, in turn reinforcing feelings of guilt.

Results from a five-country study describe the burden, coping strategies and social networks of 236 relatives of patients with schizophrenia in Italy, England, Germany, Greece and Portugal [51]. Relatives reported restrictions to their social activities, negative effects on family life and feelings of loss. Family burden and coping strategies were somewhat different across sites, and clearly could be influenced by cultural factors. To anticipate a later discussion, family interventions should also have a social focus, aiming to increase family social networks and reduce stigma. In Nigeria, a study of 44 rural and urban families found the greatest burden fell on family routine, followed by the effect on family interaction [52].

Material costs include household and travel expenditure and lost earnings. There is also the value of lost leisure time. Although these costs may constitute only a small proportion of the total costs of schizophrenia, their impact on some families could obviously be large, although difficult to measure accurately [53]. Caregiving may force relatives to work less or to give up their jobs altogether, often precisely at a time when they face expenses for psychiatric or other health care and medication. A study of 408 families in the USA with a mentally ill family member (80% with schizophrenia) showed that caregiving absorbed most of their spare time (67 hours per month) [9], with knock-on employment and financial difficulties. The ECA estimate of the total value of time committed by family caregivers for the care of schizophrenia sufferers was $2.5 billion (17% of all indirect costs) in 1990 [12]. In Italy, the family impact was found to be rather higher, at 41% of all indirect costs [54], similar to the 48% computed in Nigeria [40].

Public Safety and Concern

As we noted earlier, in some countries there is growing public concern, perhaps fanned by the media, about violent incidents involving psychiatric patients who are insufficiently supported or supervised. Although many suicides and incidents of self-harm occur in hospital settings, community-based care is seen by many members of the public as an inappropriately dangerous location for the treatment of acutely mentally ill people. Taylor and Gunn [55] reviewed the myths and evidence on the links between homicide and mental health problems. They suggested that "about 10% of those convicted of homicide in England and Wales suffer from schizophrenia". Figures for other parts of the world are comparable: for example, 15% of homicide convictions in Iceland 1900–79 were people with schizophrenia [56] and 8% of those convicted in North Sweden and Stockholm had schizophrenia and 4% schizophreniform psychosis [57]. The societal concern about violent incidents and the growth of community-based care — whether well founded or not — is itself an (intangible) cost, an "externality" in economic parlance.

A follow-on consequence of violent or other crime is the involvement of criminal justice agencies in dealing with people with schizophrenia. Costs to the criminal justice system amounted to $464 million in Rice and Miller's estimates for the USA [12] (2.7% of all direct costs, or 1.4% of total costs). A national survey in Great Britain found high rates of functional psychosis among prisoners: 7% of sentenced men; 10% of remanded men (unconvicted); and 14% of both sentenced and remanded women [58].

ECONOMIC EVALUATIONS

Evaluation Aims

The most frequently posed micro-level questions asked of economic evaluations relate to the cost effectiveness of interventions. And as we noted in the introduction, one macro-level aim of health care decision-makers is to contain the various expenditures associated with schizophrenia or to improve the patient outcomes achieved from them. Economists employ a range of evaluative tools to address these micro and macro questions, the best known being cost-effectiveness, cost-benefit and cost-utility analyses. Each of these is concerned with the relationship between costs and outcomes. In contrast, the cost-of-illness studies described above focus exclusively on costs.

As we describe below, the methods used to measure the impact or effectiveness of a policy approach, care arrangement or treatment mode vary from one type of economic evaluation to another (see Table 6.1). However, the approach to costing is more or less the same. While there may occasionally be justification in looking only at the cost to individual patients, or to a particular health care funder, comprehensiveness of cost measurement is an important aim for most economic evaluations. If nothing else, the broad social impact of mental illness, and also the broad societal responsibility often assumed for tackling it, demand that a comprehensive costing be included in an economic evaluation.

Modes of Evaluation

The simplest of economic evaluations are concerned only with costs, not (usually) because they see outcomes as irrelevant but because health and quality of life outcomes have been well established from other research, or are (currently) not measurable because of conceptual difficulties or research funding limitations. *Cost-minimization analysis* concentrates exclusively on costs. It seeks to find precisely what its name suggests: which of a

TABLE 6.1 Economic evaluations — measurement of costs and outcomes

Mode of evaluation	Cost measurement	Outcome measurement	Feasibility/usefulness?
Cost-minimization analysis	Comprehensive	No outcomes measured	Limited use unless it follows an outcome evaluation
Cost-effectiveness analysis	Comprehensive	Only one outcome measured	Powerful if there is one dominant outcome dimension
Cost-consequences analysis	Comprehensive	Multiple outcomes measured	Needs multiple clinical and other measures. Difficult but realistic decision algorithm
Cost-benefit analysis	Comprehensive	Monetary valuation of outcomes	Powerful but rarely feasible today — few monetary benefit measures in mental health
Cost-utility analysis	Comprehensive	Summary utility score of outcomes	Feasible once a satisfactory health-related utility measure is developed for mental health contexts

number of treatment options has the lowest cost? It often proceeds in the knowledge that previous research has shown outcomes to be identical in the treatment or policy alternatives being evaluated. One illustration would be the randomized controlled trial of case management for homeless mentally ill people by Gray *et al* [59], which found lower costs for the case-managed group (although the difference was not statistically significant, raising some important methodological issues). This cost analysis followed some months after the clinical evaluation [60].

The other modes of economic evaluation seek to include not only cost but also outcome evidence. This makes them more interesting and informative, but correspondingly more complex to conduct. Nowadays, they are commonly but not exclusively carried out alongside clinical trials (which has numerous advantages, but some disadvantages too — see Design Issues below).

Probably the most intuitive and straightforward modes of economic evaluation from the perspective of clinical research are *cost-effectiveness* and *cost-consequences analyses*. Both measure outcomes using instruments and scales familiar from clinical trials. Both are employed to help decision-makers choose between alternative interventions available to or aimed at specific patient groups: If two care options are of equal cost, which provides the greater effectiveness? Or if two options have been found to be equally effective in terms of reduced symptoms, improved functioning or enhanced quality of life, which costs the smaller amount? In the strict sense in which the term is used, a cost-effectiveness analysis (CEA) looks at a *single* effectiveness dimension—such as the number of life years saved, the number of symptom-free days or the duration of time to relapse—and then computes and compares the ratios of cost to effectiveness for each of the treatments being evaluated. The option with the lowest cost-effectiveness ratio is the most efficient. For example, Essock *et al* [61] computed costs and scores on the Brief Psychiatric Rating Scale (BPRS) for patients given clozapine and those given usual medication in three US state hospitals.

An obvious weakness with the strict cost-effectiveness methodology is the enforced focus on a single outcome dimension (in order to compute ratios) when most people with schizophrenia have multiple needs for support and when most clinicians would expect to achieve improvements in more than one area (Essock and her colleagues themselves went on to look at a wider set of outcomes). Carrying multiple outcomes forward in an analysis is less tractable analytically, but three options are available, associated with the other three modes of economic evaluation identified earlier. One option—cost-consequences analysis—is to retain all outcome dimensions (using standard clinical scales). The other two options, discussed below, weight the outcomes, either in terms of money (cost-benefit) or in terms of utility (cost-utility).

A *cost-consequences analysis* has the ability to evaluate policies and practices in a way which arguably comes close to everyday reality. For each treatment alternative the evaluation would compute total (and component) costs and measures of change along each of the relevant outcome dimensions. The cost and outcome results would need to be reviewed by decision-makers, the different outcomes weighed up (informally and subjectively), and compared with costs. The decision calculus may therefore be less tidy and more complicated than when using cost-effectiveness ratios or monetary or utility measures of impact (see below), but decision-makers in health care systems—from strategic policy-makers at macro level to individual professionals at micro level—face these kinds of decisions daily.

On the other hand, the weighting of the various outcomes is implicit and subjective, whereas the choice of the single outcome dimension in a CEA and the weighting algorithms in other evaluative modes are explicit and potentially less susceptible to influence from the value positions of one or two individuals (of course the evaluators must not simply impose their own values in the analysis). The term "cost-consequences analysis" is relatively new, although the technique is long established. One example is a study [62] of motivational interviewing to improve compliance with medication which looked at costs, insight, attitudes to medication, global functioning, symptoms and of course compliance. Other examples of cost-consequences analyses are given below.

Cost-benefit analysis (CBA) addresses the extent to which a treatment or policy is socially worth while in the broadest sense: Do the benefits exceed the costs? All costs and benefits are valued in the same (monetary) units. If benefits exceed costs, the evaluation would recommend providing the treatment, and vice versa. With two or more alternatives, the treatment with the greatest net benefit would be deemed the most efficient. CBAs are thus intrinsically attractive, but conducting them is problematic in mental health care because of the difficulties associated with valuing all outcomes in monetary terms. Some CBAs have chosen to focus on a subset of the outcomes.

A good example of a CBA is the classic evaluation of assertive community treatment (ACT) by Weisbrod *et al* [63], which compared a quite wide measure of costs with patient earnings from employment (see the section on community-based care below). A CBA of this kind can describe only a part of the overall impact of an intervention, in this case the employment effect of ACT, but fortunately Weisbrod and colleagues also used what we would now call a cost-consequences approach, covering a larger set of outcome domains. Methodological advances offer a way to obtain *direct* valuations of health outcomes by patients, relatives or the general public. These "willingness-to-pay" techniques ask an individual to state the amount they would be prepared to pay (hypothetically) to achieve a given health state or health gain, or observe actual behaviour and impute the implicit values [64].

Another evaluative mode which seeks to reduce outcomes to a single dimension is *cost-utility analysis* (CUA), which measures and then values the impact of an intervention in terms of improvements in preference-weighted, health-related quality of life. The value of the quality of life improvement is measured in units of "utility", usually expressed by a combined index of the mortality and quality of life effects of an intervention. The best known index is the Quality Adjusted Life Year (QALY). CUAs have a number of distinct advantages, including using a unidimensional measure of impact, a generic measure which allows comparisons to be made across diagnostic or clinical groups, and a fully explicit methodology for weighting preferences and valuing health states. But these same features are sometimes seen as disadvantages: the utility measure may be too reductionist, the generic quality of life indicator may not be sufficiently sensitive to the kinds of change expected in schizophrenia treatment, and a transparent approach to scale construction paradoxically opens the approach to criticism from those who question the values thereby obtained [65]. But CUAs avoid the potential ambiguities with multidimensional outcomes in cost-consequences studies and are obviously more general than the single-outcome CEA. The result is a series of cost-utility ratios (such as the cost per QALY gained) which can then inform health care resource allocation decisions or priority setting.

Design Issues

Several types of research design have been employed in economic analyses. In common with their clinical evaluator colleagues, many economists see the prospective randomized controlled trial as the gold standard. Randomized designs can straightforwardly collect cost-effectiveness information, but they assess the impact of a new drug or psychological therapy in an experimental rather than a naturalistic setting, which can be a particular limitation for economic evaluations. In addition, some non-drug trials include an economics component at the risk of "breaking the blind" (for example collecting data about service contacts in a study of a psychological therapy might reveal to the evaluator whether a particular patient was in the experimental group). Another practical problem is that some of the main cost consequences of a policy or practice may not occur for some time, so that a prospective randomized trial may be a slow way to obtain economic insights.

A different approach is to use existing data or past experiences, as in retrospective or mirror designs. These are generally easier to carry out, faster to produce results, but more difficult to interpret. Mirror designs are vulnerable to influence from confounding variables that cannot be controlled. On the other hand, they are inexpensive to conduct and can be tailored so as to generate findings applicable to a local area. They certainly have the advantage of being naturalistic, but they are likely to be of value only if conducted alongside prospective trials. The analysis of large databases (such as those held by service-providing or funding agencies) offers another non-experimental route to evaluation.

Perhaps the most ambiguous evidence about cost effectiveness comes from those non-experimental studies using clinical decision analysis and modelling [66]. Hypothetical routes through successive phases of an illness and its treatment are mapped out, based on expected or estimated probabilities of clinical and/or administrative outcomes and the costs associated with each. The empirical basis is usually a review of completed studies plus expert clinical opinion about practice patterns [67]. Modelling is helpful in the absence of prospective trial data on the economic consequences of an intervention or for making longer-term projections, but it has its limitations. Models are usually restricted to specific types of schizophrenia patient and treatment (for example dual diagnosis patients and depot treatments are usually excluded). The parameters of the model are not always readily estimated from the published literature, and the choice of parameter values may be seen by some people as open to bias. Moreover, the models only produce or project *theoretical* and not actual cost savings.

There are in fact many design issues to be faced when conducting any evaluation, but an *economic* evaluation can raise particular difficulties. These include the need for a naturalistic setting, the time elapse before the full economic consequences can be observed, the selection of comparator treatments, the measurement of health-related quality of life, achievement of sufficient sample size for statistical power with skewed cost data, and data analysis and interpretation [68, 69].

COST–OUTCOME EVIDENCE: PHARMACOTHERAPIES

Given the overall high costs of schizophrenia, and the concern about some of the principal cost drivers within this total, can we improve cost effectiveness? That is, can we improve the cost–outcome balance? The evaluative methods just outlined have been used in a number of empirical studies of different treatments and care arrangements. In this and the next two sections we summarize the evidence from these studies, looking first at pharmacotherapies, then psychological therapies, and thirdly care arrangements.

Side Effects and Non-concordance

Pharmacotherapy is the first-line treatment for patients presenting with acute psychotic symptoms. It reduces both the incidence of positive symptoms and the risk of subsequent relapse. However, a problem with conventional neuroleptics is that many patients do not want to take them, and non-cordance (or non-compliance) can push up costs: "Noncompliant patients consume more resources; they are more severely ill at the point of admission than those who are readmitted despite compliance, they are more likely to be admitted compulsorily, they have longer in-patient stays, and they have a higher long-term readmission rate" [70].

Many factors are associated with non-concordance with drug therapy, including symptomatology, culture and ethnic group, low response to treatment, a poor patient–doctor relationship and limited insight [71–73]. Depot neuroleptics have been used in the past to improve concordance but are associated with extrapyramidal symptoms (EPS) and other side effects [72, 74, 75].

The new (atypical or novel) antipsychotics are different from traditional therapies in their effects on positive symptoms and they appear to be associated with lower levels of EPS. Unlike the conventional antipsychotics, some of the newer drugs may also reduce negative symptoms, such as emotional withdrawal and blunted affect, albeit probably only modestly. The objectives in developing new medications for schizophrenia are generally seen as threefold:

1. Improved control of positive symptoms (particularly in refractory patients), thereby decreasing the duration of in-hospital care and the rates of relapse and rehospitalization, and improving the effectiveness of community care programmes.
2. Improved control of negative symptoms, which should decrease overall morbidity and increase patient involvement in rehabilitative and community programmes.
3. Reduced EPS, which may improve compliance, thereby reducing the rates of relapse and rehospitalization, as well as improving the quality of life and productivity of patients [76].

These newer drugs have been called "atypical" because of their impacts on the brain chemistry, but—colloquially—they might also be seen as "atypical" because of their high acquisition costs (high prices). These higher prices are a major bone of contention in some health care systems. Pharmacy managers and some other budget holders have been reluctant to sanction the prescribing of the atypicals, and some national governments have declined to include them on the lists of drugs eligible for partial or full patient reimbursement. The consequences might be quite the opposite of that intended. In an earlier period, cost-saving measures by Medicaid in one US state that limited schizophrenia patients to three prescriptions per month (saving $5 per patient) led to patients using more mental health services at an increased cost of roughly 17 times the amount saved on drugs [77].

Improved tolerability of the new drugs is expected to lead to improved concordance and reduced relapse rates. In turn, this should reduce costs. One of the most pressing questions, therefore, is whether the atypical antipsychotics are cost-effective.

Hypotheses

Figure 6.1 summarizes a number of hypothesized links between treatments (on the left-hand side), their intermediate effects (for example on side effect profiles and compliance), their impacts on patient and other outcomes (from symptoms and social functioning through to societal outcomes) and, finally, their longer-run cost consequences. One hypothesis is that higher costs on the left-hand side of the diagram (as a result of greater usage of atypical antipsychotics or equivalently the wider availability of psychological therapies) will be outweighed by downstream resource savings (on the right-hand side of the diagram). A cost-offset analysis would test this hypothesis. Another possibility is that higher treatment costs might improve patient and other outcomes sufficiently to make the newer treatment modalities more cost-effective.

| Treatments | Intermediate effects | Outcomes | Longer-term costs |

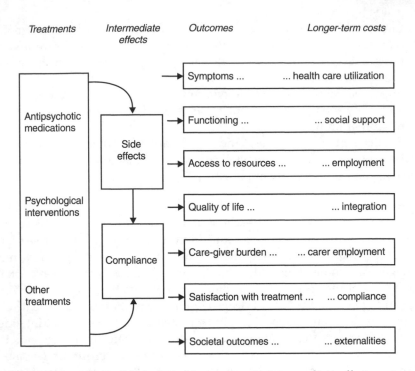

FIGURE 6.1 Hypothesized links between treatments, intermediate effects, outcomes and longer-term costs

Depot treatments

Despite the continued widespread use of depot antipsychotics in the treatment of schizophrenia in some countries, the quantity and the quality of the available cost-effectiveness evidence are limited. Systematic reviews of clinical evidence suggest that, although depot administration has advantages over oral administration for patients who are not well engaged with services or do not regularly take their oral medication, the international evidence on effectiveness is mixed [78, 79]. Although it has been argued that depot medication is cost saving compared to oral conventional antipsychotics under certain assumptions [80, 81], the cost-effectiveness evidence is too poor to draw firm conclusions [82, 83]. However, the non-concordance problem, which has often in the past led to the prescription of a depot medication, generates challenges for evaluative research in this area: patients who do not take their oral medication may also be hard to recruit into, or keep in trials.

Clozapine

The first of the atypical antipsychotics was clozapine, which has now been the subject of many clinical evaluations. The early evaluations of clozapine did not include an economic dimension. One of the earliest demonstrated the superior efficacy of clozapine over chlorpromazine in treatment-resistant schizophrenia in a 6-week, double-blind, randomized controlled trial involving a total of 319 severely ill schizophrenic patients who had failed to respond to at least three standard medications [84]. At the end of the study, 30% of clozapine patients versus 4% of chlorpromazine patients had clinically significant improvements. A Cochrane Collaboration systematic review of clinical effectiveness has concluded that "clozapine reduces relapse and symptoms and produces clinically meaningful improvement in patients with schizophrenia" [85].

Most published studies of clozapine cost and cost-effectiveness are naturalistic, retrospective, non-experimental analyses or decision models [86], although long-term prospective randomized trial evidence has now emerged. Here we focus on the most important studies, since recently published reviews address this topic in some detail [87, 88].

The first economic evaluation was an open, non-randomized study conducted by Revicki et al [89]. In the clozapine group, 65% of patients responded to the therapy and 35% discontinued therapy after a mean period of 80 days (14% for non-compliance, 15% for lack of response, and 6% for adverse events). After one year of treatment the clozapine group had improved (significant reduction in BPRS) and the inter-group difference had narrowed. Total mean medical costs in the pretreatment year were about $10 000 higher per patient in the clozapine group than in the comparator group, although pretreatment hospital costs for the two groups were similar. Clozapine patients had lower hospital costs during the two post-treatment years. However, the costs for non-hospital services for this group, excluding drug therapy, increased during the first post-treatment year. The clozapine group averaged $10 040 more in total costs than the comparator group in the first year after start of treatment, but costs were lower during the second year. Various criticisms have been levelled at this study, relating to the failure to follow up drop-outs (35% of the original clozapine group), the narrow measurement of costs, the inability to match patients at baseline (the clozapine group was more severely ill) and the different measurement approaches employed for the two groups [90, 91]. Nevertheless, after some re-analysis of the data, Revicki [92] concluded that clozapine produced net cost savings.

There have been numerous similar studies in the USA and in other countries over the past 8 years, some focused exclusively on treatment-resistant patients. Most used modelling, mirror design or other retrospective evaluations to conclude that clozapine improves symptoms (usually BPRS and/or Clinical Global Impression, CGI) and quality of life, and reduces either hospitalization or total costs compared to the pretreatment period [93–98]. All reach similar conclusions: clozapine improves symptoms and reduces costs.

Two prospective randomized trials in the USA have examined the comparative effectiveness of clozapine and conventional neuroleptics. Economic evaluations were conducted alongside these trials. Essock *et al* [99] conducted a randomized open-label study of clozapine therapy versus usual care among patients in three large Connecticut state hospitals ($n = 227$ patients). The study continued for 2 years on an intention-to-treat basis (there were a number of cross-overs) and found no differences between the groups in relation to symptoms or functioning. However, clozapine had a comparative advantage with respect to avoidance of hospital readmissions, total time in community settings, EPS side effects and disruptiveness. Compared to the usual care group, the clozapine sample had $1112 higher costs in the first year after randomization but $7149 lower costs in the second year. These differences (or their sum) did not reach statistical significance. Consequently, clozapine was found to produce better outcomes at a cost that was no different, and was therefore more cost-effective than a range of conventional antipsychotic medication for long-stay patients in state hospitals [100].

The other North American randomized controlled trial compared clozapine and haloperidol treatments for refractory patients who had been hospitalized for 30–364 days in the previous year. The study was based in 15 Veteran Administration (VA) medical centres across the USA. The results have been reported in a series of papers by Rosenheck *et al* [101–103]. The clozapine group had better concordance lower symptom levels (as measured by the Positive and Negative Syndrome Scale, PANSS) and improved quality of life (among those who did not cross over to the other treatment, but not in the intention-to-treat analysis). The clozapine group had fewer days of hospitalization for psychiatric reasons, but used more outpatient services, and had fewer problems with tardive dyskinesia and akathisia. Health care costs were included (inpatient, outpatient and drug therapy) and unusually the study also included many non-health care costs (accommodation, lost productivity, criminal justice, family burden and administration of transfer payments). Costs were higher in the clozapine group for antipsychotic drugs and outpatient care, but these higher costs were more than offset by reductions in hospitalization costs. Overall, the costs for the clozapine group were $2734 per patient year lower than for the haloperidol group over a 1-year study period [101].

In a second paper a cost-utility analysis was carried out based on the Composite Health Index for Schizophrenia (CHIS) and confirmed the results obtained in the cost-effectiveness study [102]. A further analysis split the sample into "high hospital users" and "low hospital users" [103]. Clozapine use for the low hospital users did not produce cost savings (mean annual saving of $759 by intent-to-treat analysis and $4140 after excluding crossovers), although there was a significant difference in QALYs gained (2–3%). For the high hospital users there was a large cost saving ($7134 and $4806, respectively), and QALY improvements were greater than for the low hospital users (3.7–4.7%). The authors concluded that clozapine is more cost-effective than treatment with haloperidol for patients suffering from refractory schizophrenia, and especially for patients with high prior levels of hospital use.

Risperidone

A systematic review of the effectiveness of risperidone concluded that this atypical antipsychotic "produces greater clinical improvement than conventional neuroleptic agents in patients with schizophrenia and is associated with fewer extrapyramidal side effects" [104, 105]. There are no prospective randomized trials which examine the cost effectiveness of this atypical antipsychotic, but mirror-design and observational studies which point to cost-offset advantages.

Retrospective analysis of an open-label clinical trial of risperidone in Canada found that the number of days spent in hospital was reduced by 20% following treatment for those who responded to risperidone, although 64% of patients were non-responders. The resultant sample size was small ($n = 27$), the economic analysis confined to inpatient days, and the conclusions only preliminary [106]. An unusual retrospective cost-utility evaluation of a sub-population of patients from this trial revealed that risperidone provided more than double of QALYs compared with haloperidol. However, the analysis was so complex that it is impossible to evaluate the robustness of the findings [107]. Most economic studies of risperidone have employed similar mirror-designs and reached the same conclusion that inpatient days fall, even after making allowance for the general downward trend in psychiatric hospitalizations [108–111].

All of these studies suggest that risperidone may be a cost-effective alternative to conventional neuroleptics, but they are open to the same reservations as other uncontrolled mirror-design studies, including being susceptible to sample selection artefacts and historical bias [87]. Costs in some studies were quite narrowly measured and outcomes were sometimes not included in the analyses, although of course there are powerful effectiveness results from a recently published randomized trial [112].

Risperidone is almost certainly more cost-effective than conventional neuroleptic treatment, but the economic evidence is not as strong as for some other atypicals. Recent reviews summarize this evidence (83, 87, 88).

Olanzapine

Olanzapine first became available on prescription for treating schizophrenia in 1996. In the absence of long-term economic data alongside clinical trials,

Lilly Industries commissioned the development of a decision model to compare the cost effectiveness of alternative therapies. Published results from this model compare olanzapine with haloperidol in the UK [113], Germany [114] and Spain [115] with the addition of risperidone in the USA [116]. The 5-year model evaluates the expected direct costs of treatment for patients with schizophrenia. Looking across these models, the higher acquisition costs of olanzapine (and risperidone in the US model) compared to haloperidol, are largely offset by a reduction in (assumed) service utilization associated with better health outcomes — mainly because olanzapine reduces negative and positive symptoms, and also lowers relapse rates. Over 1 year, the comparison of costs looks to be at least cost neutral.

An independent study in the UK has modelled the cost consequences of prescribing olanzapine as first and second line treatment [117]. A simple model estimated the costs of schizophrenia according to disease severity by estimating resource use by the different groups of people distinguished previously by Davies and Drummond [14]: those with a single episode (average duration 22 weeks); episodes of major disorder lasting up to 1 year; episodes for 1 to 2.5 years; and episodes lasting for more than 2.5 years, stratified by whether receiving community care or hospital care. Resource use was restricted to inpatient and outpatient services, day care and community support. The results projected cost savings associated with olanzapine use compared with haloperidol.

Economic evidence is now available from a 17-country RCT comparing olanzapine ($n = 1336$) and haloperidol ($n = 660$) over a 6-week treatment period. Half the sample continued into a responder extension for another 46 weeks. The clinical evaluation found superior outcomes for olanzapine over haloperidol in relation to negative symptoms, EPS profile, prolactin levels and response rate [118]. The economic evaluation, which is reported by Hamilton *et al* [119] and focused on the US subsample, found monthly medication costs to be $209 higher for olanzapine than for haloperidol in both the acute and maintenance phases, but outpatient and inpatient costs were lower in both phases. Total monthly medical costs in the acute phase were $431 lower with olanzapine ($p = 0.026$) and $345 lower in the maintenance phase ($p = 0.160$). No other costs were included in the evaluation. Analysis of the French subsample reached a similar conclusion of cost-effectiveness [120].

Other Atypicals

A number of other atypical antipsychotics have been licensed for the treatment of schizophrenia. Few economic evaluations have been published [121, 122], but no review is possible at this stage.

Comparisons of different atypical antipsychotics

There are few direct comparisons between the different atypical medications, and most are methodologically a little weak, often based on naturalistic designs, collecting data retrospectively, and sometimes employing rather narrow measures of cost. Their findings do not point consistently in any one direction. Most of these studies have compared olanzapine and risperidone, some pointing to relative hospitalization and cost advantages for risperidone [123–125], and others pointing to relative advantages for olanzapine [126, 127]. In another naturalistic study, Lewis et al [128] found no significant cost differences between risperidone, olanzapine and clozapine patients.

Only one cost-effectiveness study based on a randomized controlled trial design has yet been published. Based on analysis of data for 150 US patients included in a multi-country randomized controlled trial, Edgell et al [129] concluded that medication and inpatient costs were lower for olanzapine compared to risperidone patients, but total costs were not significantly different. Superior outcomes led them to conclude that olanzapine was the more cost-effective treatment for this patient group. A recently completed European study, again based on the prospective collection of data over six months within a randomized controlled trial design, found amilsulpride and risperidone to be equally cost-effective. Interestingly, there were differences between Eastern and Western European sites in service use pattern, relative costs and the balance between costs and outcomes [130].

The methodological limitations of some of these studies and the draft status of some papers make it difficult to reach overall conclusions as to comparative cost-effectiveness of the various atypical antipsychotics.

COST–OUTCOME EVIDENCE: PSYCHOLOGICAL THERAPIES

An increasingly studied area of schizophrenia therapy covers the often complementary psychological treatments. There are many psychological and psychosocial approaches to the management of schizophrenia [131, 132], but few have been studied by economists. However, because most psychological treatments, even group sessions, are labour-intensive and sometimes continue for long periods, they may look expensive. An important question to be addressed is whether they have counter-balancing outcomes or whether they reduce longer-term costs. A recent global systematic review found evidence of no effectiveness in the case of several widely applied psychological interventions [83]. Two areas that *have* been studied also from an economic viewpoint are concentrated on improving patient concordance with medication treatment and improving family support in community settings.

Improving Concordance

We noted earlier that relapse is one of the principal cost "drivers" or concerns in schizophrenia, and can have high cost implications, especially if a patient needs readmission to hospital. More than one third of the costs of schizophrenia relapse are attributable to non-concordance with treatment [27]. Not surprisingly, therefore, care professionals are keen to improve concordance with recommended drug treatment regimes, both to improve the health and quality of life of schizophrenia sufferers in the short term and to reduce the probability of relapse in the longer term. Psychological therapies have an important role to play.

Many approaches have been tried to improve concordance or adherence [133]. Education about the nature of the disease and its management has been found to achieve, among other things, significant improvements in taking medications compared with control groups. However, there appears to be no published economic evaluation of a formal psychoeducation programme [83]. Boczkowski *et al* [134] found that concordance with antipsychotic medication could be improved by measures that built the treatment into patients' everyday activities, and other studies have found similar effects [135].

A recently published study shows that a short counselling intervention based on cognitive behaviour therapy, called *compliance therapy* by the clinicians who devised it, can achieve better outcomes at the same cost as standard counselling. Patients were invited to discuss first their attitude towards their illness, and subsequently the drawbacks and advantages of drug treatment. A randomized controlled trial of 74 people with psychosis about to move from inpatient residence found that patients counselled in this way were five times more likely than a control group to take their medication without prompting, and over an 18-month follow-up period had better global functioning, insight, compliance and attitudes to their medication [136].

The economic analysis covered all health and social care services, education, social security and housing supports, and criminal justice contacts, but excluded caregiver and lost employment costs. The cost-consequences analysis found costs to be the same for compliance therapy as for standard counselling during each of the three 6-month follow-up phases and over the full 18 months. Costs were higher for patients with greater symptomatology. Significant correlations were found between greater compliance and higher costs over the first 6 months. That is, improving compliance will initially *increase* costs, although over time there is an offsetting reduction [62].

Another UK study reported the cost-effectiveness of cognitive behaviour therapy (more broadly focused) when compared to standard care [137, 138]. The cost-consequence analysis was based on a randomized controlled trial of 54 patients with schizophrenia spectrum disorders, and covered all health care, community care and accommodation costs. Cognitive behaviour therapy was found to be more effective (in relation to BPRS, delusional distress) and perhaps less costly than standard care, although the small sample made it difficult to reach firm conclusions on the cost difference.

Both of these studies, evaluating treatments based on cognitive behavioural approaches, thus concluded that this therapeutic mode is not costly in relative terms and that it appears to be efficient when looking at its outcome and resource implications.

Family Intervention

A wide range of responses can be expected from families in the caregiving role. Brown et al [139] described how patients discharged from hospital to their families were more likely to be readmitted than those discharged to live alone or with private landlords. This stimulated interest in the role of the family in the course of schizophrenia and led to the work on expressed emotion (EE) [140]. Stress, hostility and emotional over-involvement may result in a family with a high level of EE, which may cause further deteriora-tion in the situation, as patients living in high-EE households have a worse prognosis than those in low-EE households.

Family interventions aim to reduce the impact of family stress and conflict often seen in high-EE households [141]. A recent systematic review of randomized trial findings whittled down the international literature to 18 studies, employing quite tight selection criteria, particularly in relation to methodology and design, to make the selection. The reviewers concluded that family interventions reduce relapse and readmission rates, improve concordance with medication and decrease carer burden [142].

Family interventions may also reduce costs. The most recent economic review identified nine economic studies from the USA, the UK, Germany and China [83]. Generally, they were not as comprehensive in their coverage of direct and indirect costs as would now be expected, but they complemented the clinical evidence well. Falloon et al [143] conducted their randomized trial in Los Angeles, comparing a psychoeducational family programme combined with maintenance drug treatment against drug treatment alone. The relapse rate was substantially lower in the family therapy group — a result which has been replicated in other studies — and there were greater improvements in household tasks, work or study activities and social relations. Caregiver burden was also reduced over both the initial 9 months and the full 2 years of the follow-up period. Three economic studies based their analyses on these trial data [144–146]. A (limited) cost-benefit analysis compared costs with earnings from employment [146], but the more interesting results came from the cost-effectiveness analysis (outcomes measured in terms of symptoms, social functioning and family functioning were crudely weighted into a single effectiveness index) [144]. A basic cost-offset analysis found also possible cost savings by family therapy [145]. This led the authors to conclude that family therapy was more cost effective than "traditional individual-based management".

Tarrier *et al*'s economic study in Salford [147] built on the previously reported benefits of a behavioural intervention with families of schizophrenic patients in terms of lower relapse rates [148]. The evaluation found that any increased cost associated with the family intervention was outweighed by reduced utilization of other mental health services. Other costs were not examined. The other, most recent UK study by Leff *et al* [149] confirmed this finding in circumstances where also costs of training of staff were included in the analysis. In Norway, Rund *et al* [150] reached a similar conclusion from a small sample of adolescent schizophrenia patients ($n = 24$), non-randomized trial. Costs were again measured quite narrowly.

Evidence from China [151] comes from a randomized trial ($n = 63$) comparing standard post-hospitalization care (which is effectively just a prescribed medication with possibly some outpatient contact) and family intervention. The latter was tailored to the complex family relationships and unique social environment in China, and involved monthly counselling on a range of topics, particularly management of social and work problems, medication, family education and crisis intervention. The 18-month RCT found that family intervention was associated with reductions in hospital readmissions, duration of inpatient stay, duration of unemployment and family burden. There were also some advantages as measured using standard clinical scales. Both treatment costs and lost income from employment were measured, and the trial found lower costs for the family intervention group.

McFarlane *et al* [152] compared two different ways of delivering family therapies, and demonstrated that a multi-family group intervention is more cost-effective than a single-family intervention. Compared to the weight of evidence on the atypical antipsychotics, there is only a modest amount of economic data on family interventions. Most of the completed studies have some methodological weakness, but—notwithstanding the different approaches to family intervention studied—there appear to be grounds for believing that this kind of psychological therapy can be not only effective but also less costly than standard care. However, a word of caution is needed. Schooler *et al* [153] compared two types of family intervention—the form examined in some previous studies and a simpler version—and found no effectiveness differences between them, but similar to those found in earlier research. The research sites also practised "an intensive and assertive clinic model ... [and] an intensive family intervention may have been unnecessary" [154].

COST-OUTCOME EVIDENCE: CARE ARRANGEMENTS

Changing the Hospital/Community Balance

The development of improved pharmacotherapies and psychosocial thera-pies has been one of the contributory factors in the shifting balance between inpatient and community-based care. It is by no means the only reason [155]. Communities have become more tolerant, and there is generally a better understanding of the needs and preferences of mentally ill people. Old psychiatric hospitals have become increasingly unacceptable, associated as they are with "institutionalism" and restrictions on civil liberties. Even today, in a mature and fairly well-funded system such as Britain's there are unacceptable standards in some inpatient settings [156].

Many countries have seen quite marked reductions in the per capita numbers of inpatient psychiatric beds, although there are countries (such as China, Japan and Korea) where the trend has been in the opposite direction or where there has been little change for many years. The financing structure of some health care systems can generate resistance to changes in the hospital–community balance (such as in Germany, France, Belgium and The Netherlands). As we noted above, the high *per diem* costs of inpatient care provide another explanation for moves to reduce the number of hospital beds in favour of what are sometimes thought to be cheaper alternatives in the community. On the other hand, good quality community mental health care often requires support services from a range of agencies. What, then, is the economic evidence on community-based care?

There have been few studies of community care compared to hospital care which concentrate *exclusively* on people with schizophrenia or psychosis. Most studies have looked at a range of diagnostic groups, and although schizophrenia is often the most common condition, the findings from these studies should be seen as providing fairly broad indications of the consequences of changing the locus of care specifically for people with schizophrenia.

Many countries share a common pattern not just of dehospitalization (policy and/or practice) but also of associated professional and public concerns. In the initial years of hospital rundown and closure, the focus has tended to be on whether and how *long-stay*, chronically ill residents of the facilities could move to community settings. Financial transfers have often been contentious issues, and new modes of inter-service and inter-agency coordination have had to be established. In some countries case management has been encouraged, although not often delivered to these kinds of patients. Misgivings have been expressed in some professional and public quarters about hospital closures and the policy of community rehabilitation, but criticism of community-based care for the long-term mentally ill has generally dissipated as it has become apparent that most long-stay hospital residents are able to move successfully to the community (see below).

It is the acutely ill rather than the chronically ill who generate most concern. Patients with recurring florid symptoms of schizophrenia, it is often argued, are a danger to themselves and to others. They face ridicule and stigma. They may lose contact with their families, become destitute and homeless. They may fail to take their medications or to turn up for outpatient appointments. As psychiatric bed numbers are reduced, they may find it harder to gain admission, or to remain in hospital for as long as they really need. New care arrangements for acutely ill patients such as crisis interventions and acute day hospitals have been introduced.

One of the pressing questions of today in many mental health systems, therefore, is how to build up effective community-based services which can provide continuous, high-quality support. In many countries attention has turned to care arrangements such as the assertive community treatment model, and various forms of case management and community mental health teams. The economic evidence on these is discussed below.

Figure 6.2 gives a highly simplified representation of a mental health care system, showing stylized routes through community and hospital-based services. Imposed upon the diagram are six broad types of research study. It is immediately clear that even a highly simplified model of a care system and a short selection of potential research studies suggests a large research

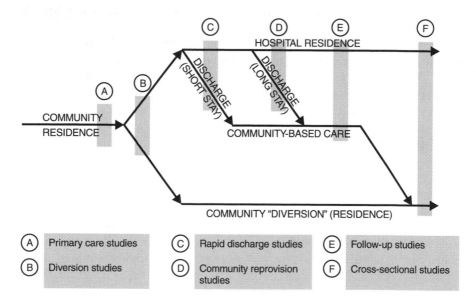

FIGURE 6.2 Simplified representation of a mental health care system and of potential research studies

agenda. Not surprisingly, the ratio of completed to potential economics research is rather low: relatively little formal evidence has yet accumulated. What evidence there is tends to be scattered across the diagram. The evidence is often robust, but it is clearly context specific [36, 157–161]. However, there are two specific areas where evidence has come together in sufficient quantity to allow conclusions to be drawn: (a) community provision for former long-stay hospital residents; and (b) intensive community support for people with acute illnesses who would otherwise face hospitalization.

We focus the remainder of this section on these two fields. We should emphasize again that most studies cover people with a range of mental health problems, generally not being restricted to schizophrenia.

Community Provision for Long-stay Inpatients

The changing hospital–community balance has obviously been one of the major themes of recent times and in large part has been achieved by relocating long-stay inpatients to suitably staffed community facilities. The controversy surrounding this often enforced rehabilitation and the practical difficulties of building or converting care facilities in the community have made it very difficult for researchers to set up randomized trials in this area. Consequently most economic, clinical and social evaluations have had to exercise imagination and caution in designing and interpreting empirical studies. One challenge, for example, is the tendency for hospital closure programmes to move the most independent, least symptomatic people first [162, 163], requiring adjustments to be made to outcome and cost findings before generalizations are possible [164].

Many studies of the rehabilitation of long-stay inpatients have found community-based care to be more cost effective than hospital care for most people, such as in the USA [165–167], Canada [168], the UK [169–171] and Germany [172]. This result applies particularly to those with less severe mental illness or fewer dependencies [173]. However, many long-stay inpatients with very challenging needs are more costly to accommodate in the current range of community settings than in hospital, even though their clinical and social outcomes do show improvements. Success depends on having sufficient staffing intensity [174], that is, it depends on expending sufficient resources.

The most comprehensive and long-running (10-year) evaluation of community-based care for former long-stay inpatients has looked at the closure of two North London hospitals [175]. The outcome findings suggest that former inpatients were enjoying a quality of life at least as good as in hospital 1 and 5 years after discharge (initially this was by comparison with matched controls in hospital, but later became a mirror-image design). There were no problems with higher-than-normal mortality, or with homelessness and crime. Accommodation stability in the community was impressive, and care environments were rated by researchers and residents as much better than hospital. Social networks were stable; a minority gained in this respect, but most were not socially integrated into local communities. Hospital readmissions were common (38% had at least one readmission over a 5-year period). Careful examination of clinical outcomes revealed striking stability over time in both psychiatric symptoms and social behaviour. Patients strongly preferred community living to hospital.

The associated economic evaluation found that many services were used in the community, with patterns of service use changing over time. The full costs were no different between community and long-stay hospital care [171]. Pooling the cost and outcome findings suggested that community care was more cost effective. Higher cost community care packages appear to be associated with better individual outcomes. Care appeared to be more cost effective in the public than in the private sector [176].

Intensive community support

A vast number of models of intensive, community-based care have been developed and implemented across the world, all with the intention of supporting people with acute mental health problems outside inpatient settings if possible, but facilitating hospital admissions when appropriate. This wide range of models has been given a bewildering array of names, with a great deal of terminological inexactitude. Recent reviews of evidence on effectiveness and cost-effectiveness have rightly bemoaned the looseness with which labels have been attached to models, with the potential to confuse and unwittingly mislead decision-makers [83, 177, 178]. These reviews have also worked carefully through the evidence and sought to employ a more robust framework to organize the evidence. One review grouped all services aiming to treat patients outside the hospital under the single heading of "home treatment", arguing that "the lack of a clear definition of different community-based models undermines any attempt to evaluate specific services through meta-analysis" [178].

Notwithstanding that argument, with which we have great sympathy, we will here nevertheless describe the economic evidence under three heads: assertive community treatment, case management and community mental health teams. It should be borne in mind, however, that the models discussed under each of these headings will vary. It should also be emphasized that, in this area as much as in any other, evidence collected in one health system may not generalize well to another [179].

Assertive community treatment

The assertive community treatment (ACT) or assertive outreach model associated with developments in Madison, Wisconsin has been one of the most important approaches in community psychiatry [180].

ACT provides a comprehensive range of treatment, rehabilitation, and support services through a multidisciplinary team based in the community. Basic characteristics of ACT programs include assertive engagement, in vivo delivery of services, a multi-disciplinary team approach, continuous responsibility and staff continuity over time, caseloads with high staff-to-client ratios, and brief but frequent contacts (high service intensity) [181].

The ACT approach has been quite widely copied across the world, although outside the USA usually only in demonstration sites [182, 183]. Where evaluations have been conducted they have usually concluded that the approach can significantly improve outcomes [181, 184], although this is not always the case [185, 186]. What are the economic consequences?

The original Training in Community Living model can be seen as a variant of ACT. It was evaluated in a cost-benefit framework [63]. Patients ($n = 130$) were randomly assigned either to the experimental community programme or to inpatient hospital treatment and community aftercare. Over 14 months, a range of input costs (spanning hospital, social services, criminal justice, social security services, plus informal carers' forgone earnings) were compared to the monetized benefits of care (patient earnings). The additional benefits of the experimental programme ($1200 per patient year) were greater than the additional costs incurred ($800 per patient year), providing a clear cost-benefit advantage. Non-monetized indicators of patients' mental health (symptoms and satisfaction) were also significantly better in the community group.

A London modification of the ACT model — the Maudsley's Daily Living Programme (DLP) — looked at seriously mentally ill people facing crisis admission to the Maudsley Hospital. A randomized controlled trial recruited 189 people, many of them with schizophrenia. The DLP produced better outcomes, higher patient and family satisfaction and lower costs than standard care in the short term [187, 188], but after 4 years all of the earlier clinical gains and the cost advantage to the community programme were lost [189, 190]. Nevertheless, over the full 4-year period the DLP was more cost effective than the standard hospital-based care with which it was compared.

Other studies confirm the cost-effectiveness of community-based crisis interventions, which may be seen to have ACT-like characteristics [191, 192]. Although a multi-centred study in the US found discrepancies between the cost-saving characteristics of the different sites [193], the overall weight of evidence is that forms of ACT that adhere more closely to the original Wisconsin model are more cost effective than conventional hospital-based services or other community arrangements [83, 178, 194–198]. Research has also begun to examine the patient characteristics associated with greater cost effectiveness [184].

Case Management

Moving away from the assertive outreach model, the organization of community care generally could have a bearing on cost effectiveness. Of special interest has been the general theme of case management — which generally does not involve multi-disciplinary teams. In the case of the intensive form of case management, caseloads are small, as in the assertive community treatment approach. The efficiency evidence is equivocal. There are etymological and organizational difficulties that partly explain why it is difficult to reach firm conclusions [199], and there are rather different research designs. Some studies find variants of case management to be effective and cost effective [200, 201], while others do not [202]. When comparing the cost-effectiveness of the standard and intensive forms of case management, two studies found standard form to be more cost-effective [203, 204]. However, a large randomized controlled trial in the UK showed the two approaches to be equally cost-effective, and confirmed that reduced caseloads have no clear beneficial effect on the efficiency of case management [205].

Community mental health teams

Service provision by community mental health teams is well represented by the care programme approach (CPA) in the UK, which promises close supervision by nominated keyworkers from a multi-disciplinary team. Compared to standard care, contact is more likely to be maintained with vulnerable patients under the CPA, but psychiatric inpatient admissions have been found to be higher [206]. Another study compared CPAs administered by community-based and hospital-based teams following discharge from inpatient care, finding higher costs for the latter without any difference in outcomes [207]. However, the high use of placements in private hospitals in one locality confounded the findings. Other studies of community mental health teams give equivocal results [208–210], and the overall evidence suggests no real cost savings by this form of care arrangement [83].

Numerous studies have compared the cost-effectiveness of the different community care arrangements, but no firm conclusions can be drawn about the superiority of one setting over the others, since the evidence is neither unambiguous nor robust [83].

Looking across the range of experiences, Tyrer [208] has concluded that:

> the exact model of community care being offered, whether assertive, intensive or standard, is really unimportant. The key to the success lies in having a

coordinated team approach to the care of the severely mentally ill in which each member has the requisite skills to intervene appropriately and at an opportune time to produce the maximum benefit. Supporting the team's skills is therefore more important than reducing the case loads of individual workers. Our preoccupation with the bureaucracy of care—case load size, care programme levels, independent needs assessment—has prevented us from examining the more difficult task of what makes a team function badly or well, or in another sense, what allows it to be effective and assertive even if relatively deprived of resources.

SUMMARY

Schizophrenia is a costly illness. There are potentially high costs for patients, their families, service systems and the broader society. These high costs partly explain the interest in the economic consequences of different treatments for the illness. Another reason has been the development of more effective pharmacological and psychological treatments which generally have higher acquisition costs (higher prices) than the treatments they are targeted to replace. A commonly voiced question is whether the newer, more expensive treatments are nevertheless cost effective.

Economic evaluations of the costs of schizophrenia and the cost effectiveness of its treatment are inherently context bound. These evaluations describe the consequences of both the illness and its treatment for service systems and social relations, and these latter will vary from country to country, and often from region to region. Making generalizations across countries is therefore more hazardous than with, say, clinical evaluations.

Nevertheless, there are some cost-raising events or features associated with schizophrenia which surface in almost all systems and societies. Relapse in schizophrenia is a particularly costly event, and mortality has major economic consequences given that it tends to occur in younger adults. Loss of employment is strongly associated with acute phases of the illness. All of these have economic consequences. Additionally, there are some service components which frequently dominate estimates of total expenditure. Inpatient services, specialist community accommodation and family caregiver support feature large in the overall impact of the disease. Another important "cost" associated with schizophrenia is public concern about safety.

Consistent Evidence

The accumulated economic research provides consistent evidence on some fronts. For the full range of serious mental illnesses, and particularly for schizophrenia, arrangements have been developed for community-based care which have proved cost effective. Particular examples would be the assertive community treatment model and the well-planned community rehabilitation of people who would otherwise remain for years in psychiatric hospitals.

Economic evidence on two psychological approaches to treatment is also consistent in pointing to the potential for cost effectiveness advantages. Family interventions appear capable not only of improving clinical profiles and reducing family burden, but also reducing the overall costs of care, and a short counselling intervention has been found to improve concordance with medication plans and clinical outcomes while not costing any more than standard care.

It has been the licensing of atypical antipsychotic drugs which has prompted so much of the recent economics research. For clozapine the accumulated weight of evidence points to a cost effectiveness advantage over conventional neuroleptics. The published evidence is remarkably consistent in finding that clozapine produces better outcomes and lower costs compared to older drugs.

Incomplete Evidence

The strictest interpretation of the available economic evidence would suggest that the cost effectiveness of later atypicals remains to be established without ambiguity. None has yet been the subject of as much economic research as clozapine. Nevertheless, once again the balance of data points to a cost effectiveness advantage over conventional drug treatments. Evidence here is uncertain not because the results of the completed evaluations are equivocal within their own designs, but because the short time elapse since licensing has not allowed sufficient evidence to accumulate.

Another uncertainty is the true size of the indirect costs of schizophrenia. In many societies, the family is almost the first line of treatment for schizophrenia. Certainly the family is relied upon heavily for ongoing support across the world. The absolute or relative weight of this burden is by no means clear. Yet without an appreciation of its importance relative to the direct service costs of treatment and support, future policies in this area may make over-optimistic assumptions about the future availability of caregiver support.

Most people with schizophrenia live in community settings, not in hospitals. We still know very little about the cost-effectiveness of the different organizational arrangements for community care. It is not clear whether the body of international evidence provides the right pointers to practitioners to guide them towards the *best* model for their local circumstances.

Areas Still Open to Research

What, then, remains to be researched? Obviously many of the uncertainties need further attention, and hopefully greater attention will encourage convergence on robust methodologies and produce consistent findings. Many of the currently practised psychological approaches have not been evaluated by economists, nor have the newest of the atypical antipsychotics. There have been very few head-to-head comparisons between two or more atypical antipsychotics. There is little evidence on the economic consequences of first-line treatment with atypicals or the relative cost-effectiveness of oral atypical antipsychotics compared to depots. Another almost empty box is evaluation of specific combinations of pharmacological and psychological therapies. We have little evidence on the economic consequences of side effects or non-compliance, yet one would suspect these to be important drivers of longer-term costs. Another underdeveloped research area relates to the distributional consequences of different treatments and care arrangements. Although there is scarcity of evidence on cost-effectiveness (efficiency), much less is known about equity.

Finally, the body of completed research signals areas where cost savings may be achieved, but these are cost savings *in principle*, and they may not lead to cost savings *in practice*. In particular, with the growth of community-based care involving multiple agencies with their own budgets and their own ways of working, the available evidence still tells us little about the incentives and constraints that might help or hinder *integrated* responses to schizophrenia. It thus cannot tell us whether the cost-effectiveness gains uncovered in empirical research can be turned into real cost-effectiveness gains on the ground. This last issue is clearly central to the operationalization of research findings.

REFERENCES

1. Shepherd M., Watt D., Falloon I., Smeeton N. (1989) The natural history of schizophrenia: a five year follow-up study of outcome and prediction in a representative sample of schizophrenics. *Psychol. Med. Monograph*, **15**: 1–44.
2. Watt D.C., Katz K., Shepherd M. (1983) The natural history of schizophrenia: a five-year prospective follow-up of a representative sample of schizophrenics by means of a standardised clinical and social assessment. *Psychol. Med.*, **13**: 663–670.
3. Fenton W.S. (1996) Longitudinal course and outcome of schizophrenia. In *Handbook of Mental Health Economics and Policy: Schizophrenia* (Eds M. Moscarelli, A. Rupp, N. Sartorius), pp. 79–91. Wiley, London.
4. Dorwart R.A. (1990) Managed mental health care: myths and realities in the 1990s. *Hosp. Commun. Psychiatry*, **41**: 1087–1091.
5. Frank R.G., Salkever D., Sharfstein S. (1991) A new look at rising mental health insurance costs. *Hlth Affairs*, **10**: 116–123.
6. Geraty R.D., Hendren R.L., Flaa C.J. (1992) Ethical perspectives on managed care as it relates to child and adolescent psychiatry. *J. Am. Acad. Child Adolesc. Psychiatry*, **31**: 398–402.
7. Ünutzer J., Tischler G.L. (1996) The many faces of managed care. In *Handbook of Mental Health Economics and Policy: Schizophrenia* (Eds M. Moscarelli, A. Rupp, N. Sartorius), pp. 493–502. Wiley, London.

8. Rice D.P., Miller L.S. (1996) The economic burden of schizophrenia: conceptual and methodological issues, and cost estimates. In *Handbook of Mental Health Economics and Policy: Schizophrenia* (Eds M. Moscarelli, A. Rupp, N. Sartorius), pp. 321–334. Wiley, London.

9. McGuire T. (1991) Measuring the economic costs of schizophrenia. *Schizophr. Bull.*, **17**: 375–378.

10. Wyatt R.J., Henter I., Leary M.C., Taylor E. (1995) An economic evaluation of schizophrenia — 1991. *Soc. Psychiatry Psychiatr. Epidemiol.*, **30**: 196–205.

11. Fein R. (1958) *Economics of Mental Illness*. Basic Books, New York.

12. Rice D.P., Miller L.S. (1998) Health economics and cost implications of anxiety and other mental disorders in the United States. *Br. J. Psychiatry*, **173** (Suppl. 34): 4–9.

13. Gunderson J.G., Mosher L.R. (1975) The cost of schizophrenia. *Am. J. Psychiatry*, **132**: 901–906.

14. Davies L.M., Drummond M.F. (1994) Economics and schizophrenia: the real cost. *Br. J. Psychiatry*, **165** (Suppl. 25): 18–21.

15. Andrews G., Hall W., Goldstein G., Lapsey H., Bartels R., Silove D. (1985) The economic costs of schizophrenia. *Arch. Gen. Psychiatry*, **42**: 537–543.

16. Warner R., de Girolamo G. (1995) *Epidemiology of Mental Disorders and Psychosocial Problems*. World Health Organisation, Geneva.

17. Knapp M.R.J. (1997) Cost of schizophrenia. *Br. J. Psychiatry*, **171**: 509–518.

18. Guest J.F., Cookson R.F. (1999) Cost of schizophrenia to UK society. *PharmacoEconomics*, **15**: 597–610.

19. Rouillon F., Toumi M., Dansette G.Y., Benyaya J., Auquier P. (1997) Some aspects of the costs of schizophrenia. *PharmacoEconomics*, **11**: 578–594.

20. Meerding W.J., Bonneux L., Polder J.J., Koopmanschap M.A., van der Mnass P.J. (1998) Demographic and epidemiological determinants of healthcare costs in Netherlands: cost of illness study. *Br. Med. J.*, **317**: 111–115.

21. Knapp M., Mangalore R., Simon J. (2002) The global costs of schizophrenia. Submitted for publication.

22. Haro J.M., Salvador-Carrulla L., Cabases J., Madoz V., Vazquez-Barquero J.L. (1998) Utilisation of mental health services and costs of patients with schizophrenia in three areas of Spain. *Br. J. Psychiatry*, **173**: 334–340.

23. Rubio-Stipec M., Stipec B., Canino G. (1994) The costs of schizophrenia in Puerto Rico. *J. Ment. Hlth Administration*, **21**: 136–144.

24. Koopmanschap M.A., Rutten F.F.H., van Ineveld B.M., van Roijen L. (1995) The friction cost method for measuring indirect costs of disease. *J. Hlth Economics*, **14**: 171–189.

25. Goeree R., O'Brien B.J., Goering P., Blackhouse G., Agro K., Rhodes A., Watson J. (1999) The economic burden of schizophrenia in Canada. *Can. J. Psychiatry*, **44**: 464–472.

26. Rupp A., Gause E.M., Regier D.A. (1998) Research policy implications of cost-of-illness studies for mental disorders. *Br. J. Psychiatry*, **173** (Suppl. 36): 19–25.

27. Weiden P.J., Olfson M. (1995) Cost of relapse in schizophrenia. *Schizophr. Bull.*, **21**: 419–429.

28. Knapp M., Chisholm D., Leese M., Amaddeo F., Tansella M., Schene A., Thornicroft G., Vasquez-Barquero J., Knudson H.C., Becker T. (2002) Comparing patterns and costs of schizophrenia care in five European countries: the EPSILON study. *Acta Psychiatr. Scand.*, **105**: 42–54.

29. Shinfuku N. (1998) Mental health services in Asia: international perspective and challenge for the coming years. *Psychiatry Clin. Neurosci.*, **52**: 269–274.

30. Kavanagh S.M., Opit L., Knapp M.R.J., Beecham J.K. (1995) Schizophrenia: shifting the balance of care. *Soc. Psychiatry Psychiatr. Epidemiol.*, **30**: 206–212.
31. Andrews G., Teesson M. (1996) Some get more than they pay for: mental health services in Australia. In *Handbook of Mental Health Economics and Policy: Schizophrenia* (Eds M. Moscarelli, A. Rupp, N. Sartorius), pp. 447–451. Wiley, London.
32. Carling P.J. (1996) Emerging approaches to housing and support for people with psychiatric disabilities. In *Handbook of Mental Health Economics and Policy: Schizophrenia* (Eds M. Moscarelli, A. Rupp, N. Sartorius), pp. 239–259, Wiley, London.
33. Shepherd G., Beardsmoore A., Moorse C., Hardy P., Muijen M. (1997) Relation between bed use, social deprivation and overall bed availability in acute adult psychiatric units, and alternative residential options. *Br. Med. J.*, **314**: 262–266.
34. Lamb R.H., Lamb D.M. (1990) Factors contributing to homelessness among the chronically and severely mentally ill. *Hosp. Comm. Psychiatry*, **41**: 301–305.
35. Cohen C.I., Thompson K.S. (1992) Homeless mentally ill or mentally ill homeless? *Am. J. Psychiatry*, **6**: 816–822.
36. Knapp M.R.J., Chisholm D., Astin J., Lelliott P., Audini B. (1997) The cost consequences of changing the hospital-community balance: the mental health residential care study. *Psychol. Med.*, **27**: 681–692.
37. Lelliott P., Audini B., Knapp M.R.J., Chisholm D. (1996) The mental health residential care study: classification of facilities and description of services. *Br. J. Psychiatry*, **169**: 139–147.
38. National Health Service Executive (1996) *Burden of Disease*. NHSE, Leeds.
39. Evers S.M.A.A., Ament A.J.H.A. (1995) Costs of schizophrenia in the Netherlands. *Schizophr. Bull.*, **21**: 141–153.
40. Suleiman T.G., Ohaeri J.U., Lawal R.A., Haruna A.Y., Orija O.B. (1997) Financial cost of treating out-patients with schizophrenia in Nigeria. *Br. J. Psychiatry*, **171**: 344–368.
41. Harris E.C., Barraclough B. (1998) Excess mortality of mental disorder. *Br. J. Psychiatry*, **173**: 11–53.
42. Munk-Jørgensen P., Mortensen P.B. (1992) Incidence and other aspects of the epidemiology of schizophrenia in Denmark, 1971–1987. *Br. J. Psychiatry*, **161**: 489–495.
43. Lamb R., Oliphant E. (1978) Schizophrenia through the eyes of families. *Hosp. Commun. Psychiatry*, **29**: 803–806.
44. Fisher G.A., Benson P.R., Tessler R.C. (1990) Family response to mental illness. developments since deinstitutionalisation. *Res. Commun. Ment. Hlth*, **6**: 203–236.
45. Gibbons J.S., Horn S.H., Powell J.M., Gibbons J.L. (1984) Schizophrenic patients and their families. A survey in a psychiatric service based on a DGH unit. *Br. J. Psychiatry*, **144**: 70–77.
46. MacCarthy B., Lesage A., Brewin C.R., Brugha T.S., Mangen S., Wing J.K. (1989) Needs for care among the relatives of long-term users of day care. A report from the Camberwell High Contact Survey. *Psychol. Med.*, **19**: 725–736.
47. Leftley H.P. (1997) The consumer recovery vision: will it alleviate family burden? *Am. J. Orthopsychiatry*, **67**: 210–219.
48. Perring C., Twigg J., Atkin K. (1990) *Families Caring for People Diagnosed as Mentally Ill. The Literature Examined*. HMSO, London.
49. Szmukler G. (1996) From family "burden" to caregiver. *Psychiatr. Bull.*, **20**: 449–451.
50. Kuipers E. (1993) Family burden in schizophrenia: implication for services. *Soc. Psychiatry Psychiatr. Epidemiol.*, **28**: 207–210.

51. Magliano L., Fadden G., Madianos M., Caldas de Almeida J.M., Held T., Guarneri M., Marasco C., Tosini P., Maj M. (1998) Burden on the families of patients with schizophrenia: results of the BIOMED I study. *Soc. Psychiatry Psychiatr. Epidemiol.*, **33**: 405–412.
52. Martyns-Yellowe I.S. (1992) The burden of schizophrenia on the family: A study from Nigeria. *Br. J. Psychiatry*, **161**: 779–782.
53. Franks D.D. (1990) Economic contribution of families caring for persons with severe and persistent mental illness. *Admin. Policy Ment. Hlth*, **18**: 9–18.
54. Tarricone R., Gerzeli S., Montanelli R., Frattura L., Percudani M., Racagni G. (2000) Direct and indirect costs of schizophrenia in community psychiatric services in Italy. The GISIES study. *Health Policy*, **51**: 1–18.
55. Taylor P.J., Gunn J. (1999) Homicides by people with mental illness: myth and reality. *Br. J. Psychiatry*, **174**: 9–14.
56. Petursson H., Gudjonsson G.H. (1981) Psychiatric aspects of homicide. *Acta Psychiatr. Scand.*, **64**: 363–372.
57. Lindqvist P. (1989) *Violence Against a Person. The role of Mental Disorder and Abuse*. Medical Dissertation, University of Umeå, Sweden.
58. Singleton N., Meltzer H., Gatward R., Coid J., Deasy D. (1998) *Psychiatric Morbidity Among Prisoners*. HMSO, London.
59. Gray A.M., Marshall M., Lockwood A., Morris J. (1997) Problems in conducting economic evaluations alongside clinical trials: lessons from a study of case management for people with mental disorders. *Br. J. Psychiatry*, **170**: 47–52.
60. Marshall M., Lockwood A., Gath D. (1995) How effective is social services case management for people with long-term mental disorders? *Lancet*, **345**: 409–412.
61. Essock S., Hargreaves W.A., Covell N.H., Goethe J. (1996) Clozapine effectiveness for patients in state hospitals: results from a randomized trial. *Psychopharmacol. Bull.*, **323**: 683–697.
62. Healey A., Knapp M.R.J., Astin J., Beecham J.K., Kemp R., Kirov G., David A. (1998) Cost-effectiveness evaluation of compliance therapy for people with psychosis. *Br. J. Psychiatry*, **172**: 420–424.
63. Weisbrod B.A., Test M.A., Stein L.I. (1980) An alternative to mental hospital treatment. 2: Economic cost–benefit analysis. *Arch. Gen. Psychiatry*, **37**: 400–405.
64. Olsen J.A., Smith R.D. (2001) Theory versus practice: a review of 'willingness to pay' in health and health care. *Health Economics*, **10**: 39–52.
65. Chisholm D., Healey A., Knapp M.R.J. (1997) QALYs and mental health care. *Soc. Psychiatry Psychiatr. Epidemiol.*, **32**: 68–75.
66. Sheldon T. (1996) Problems of using modelling in the economic evaluation of health care. *Hlth. Econ.*, **5**: 1–12.
67. Hargreaves W.A., Shumway M. (1996) Pharmacoeconomics of antipsychotic drug therapy. *J. Clin. Psychiatry*, **57** (Suppl. 9): 66–76.
68. Drummond M.F., Knapp M.R.J., Burns T.P., Miller K.D., Shadwell P. (1998) Issues in the design of studies in the economic evaluation of new atypical antipsychotics: the ESTO study. *J. Ment. Hlth. Policy Econ.*, **1**: 15–22.
69. Hargreaves W.A., Shumway M., Hu T-W., Cuffel B. (1998) *Cost–Outcome Methods for Mental Health*. Academic Press, London.
70. Hale A. (1993) Will the new antipsychotics improve the treatment of schizophrenia? *Br. Med. J.*, **307**: 749–750.
71. Buchanan A. (1992) A two-year prospective study of treatment compliance in patients with schizophrenia. *Psychol. Med.*, **22**: 787–797.

72. Kemp R., David A. (1996) Psychological predictors of insight and compliance in psychotic patients. *Br. J. Psychiatry*, **169**: 444–450.
73. McPhillips M.A., Sensky T. (1998) Coercion, adherence or collaboration? Influences on compliance with medication. In *Outcome and Innovation in Psychological Treatment of Schizophrenia* (Ed. T. Wykes). Wiley, Chichester.
74. Van Putten T. (1974) Why do schizophrenic patients refuse to take their drugs? *Arch. Gen. Psychiatry*, **31**: 67–72.
75. Frances A., Weiden P. (1987) Promoting compliance with outpatient drug treatment. *Hosp. Commun. Psychiatry*, **38**: 1158–1160.
76. Wasylenki D.A. (1994) The costs of schizophrenia. *Can. J. Psychiatry*, **39** (Suppl. 2): 65–69.
77. Soumerai S.B., McLaughlin T.J., Ross-Degnan D. (1994) Effects of limiting Medicaid drug-reimbursement benefits on the use of psychotropic agents and acute mental health services by patients with schizophrenia. *N. Engl. J. Med.*, **331**: 650–655.
78. Adams C.E., Fenton M.K.P., Quraishi S., David A.S. (2001) Systematic meta-review of depot antipsychotic drugs for people with schizophrenia. *Br. J. Psychiatry*, **179**: 290–299.
79. David A.S., Adams C.E. (2001) Depot antipsychotic medication in the treatment of patients with schizophrenia: meta-review. *Hlth Technol. Assess.*, **5**.
80. Glazer W.M., Ereshefsky L. (1996) A pharmacoeconomic model of outpatient antipsychotic therapy in "revolving door" schizophrenic patients. *J. Clin. Psychiatry*, **57**: 337–345.
81. Hale A.S., Wood C. (1996) Comparison of direct treatment costs for schizophrenia using oral or depot neuroleptics: a pharmacoeconomic analysis. *Br. J. Med. Economics*, **10**: 37–45.
82. Knapp M., Ilson S., David A. (2002) Depot antipsychotic preparations in schizophrenia: the state of the economic evidence. *Int. Clin. Psychopharmacol.*, **17**: 135–140.
83. National Collaborating Centre for Mental Health (2002) *Schizophrenia: The Treatment and Management of Schizophrenia in Primary and Secondary Care*. National Clinical Practice Guideline-No.1, National Institute for Clinical Excellence, London.
84. Kane J.M., Honigfeld G., Singer J., Meltzer H., and the Clozaril Collaborative Group (1988) Clozapine for the treatment-resistant schizophrenic. *Arch. Gen. Psychiatry*, **45**: 789–796.
85. Wahlbeck K., Cheine M., Essali M.A. (1998) Clozapine vs. typical, neuroleptic medication for schizophrenia (Cochrane review). In *The Cochrane Library*, Issue 4. Update Software, Oxford.
86. Morris S., Hogan T., McGuire A. (1998) The cost-effectiveness of clozapine: a survey of literature. *Clin. Drug Invest.*, **15**: 137–152.
87. Taylor D. (2002) Schizophrenia. In *Pharmacoeconomics in Psychiatry* (Eds D. Taylor, M. Knapp, R. Kerwin). Dunitz, London, (in press).
88. NICE (2002) Guidance on the Use of Newer (Atypical) *Antipsychotic Drugs for the Treatment of Schizophrenia*. Technology Appraisal Guidance 43, NICE, London.
89. Revicki D.A., Luce B.R., Weschler J.M. (1990) Cost-effectiveness of clozapine for treatment-resistant schizophrenics. *Hosp. Commun. Psychiatry*, **41**: 850–854.
90. Frank R.G. (1991) Clozapine's cost benefits (Letter). *Hosp. Commun. Psychiatry*, **42**: 92.

91. Goldman H.H. (1991) Clozapine's cost benefits (Letter). *Hosp. Commun. Psychiatry*, **42**: 92–93.
92. Revicki D.A., Luce B.R., Weschler J.M., Brown R.E., Adler M.A. (1990) Cost-effectiveness of clozapine in treatment-resistant schizophrenic patients. *Hosp. Commun. Psychiatry*, **41**: 850–854.
93. Honigfeld G., Patin J. (1990) A two-year clinical and economic follow-up of patients on clozapine. *Hosp. Commun. Psychiatry*, **41**: 882–885.
94. Meltzer J.Y., Cola P., Way L., Thompson P.A., Bastani B., Davies M.A., Snitz B. (1993) Cost-effectiveness of clozapine in neuroleptic-resistant schizophrenia. *Am. J. Psychiatry*, **150**: 1630–1638.
95. Davies L.M., Drummond M.F. (1993) Assessment of costs and benefits of drug therapy for treatment-resistant schizophrenia in the United Kingdom. *Br. J. Psychiatry*, **162**: 38–42.
96. Jönsson D., Wälinder J. (1995) Cost-effectiveness of clozapine treatment in therapy-refractory schizophrenia. *Acta Psychiatr. Scand.*, **92**: 199–201.
97. Geronimi-Ferret D., Lesay M., Barges-Bertocchio M.H., Cornet Bonnefont M., Robert H. (1997) Evaluation medico-economique du traitement par la clozapine versus les traitements neuroleptiques anterieurs. *Encephale*, **23** (Suppl. 4): 24–31.
98. Percudani M., Fattore G., Galletta J., Mita P.L., Contini A., Altamura A.C. (1999) Health care costs of therapy-refractory schizophrenic patients treated with clozapine: a study in a community psychiatric service in Italy. *Acta Psychiatr. Scand.*, **99**: 974–980.
99. Essock S., Hargreaves W.A., Covell N.H., Goethe J. (1996) Clozapine effectiveness for patients in state hospitals: results from a randomized trial. *Psychopharmacol. Bull.*, **323**: 683–697.
100. Essock S.M., Frisman L.K., Covell N.H., Hargreaves W.A. (2000) Cost-effectiveness of clozapine compared with conventional antipsychotic medication for patients in state hospitals. *Arch. Gen. Psychiatry*, **57**: 987–994.
101. Rosenheck R., Cramer J., Xu W., Thomas J., Henderson W., Frisman L., Fye C., Charney D. (1997) A comparison of clozapine and haloperidol in hospitalized patients with refractory schizophrenia. *N. Engl. J. Med.*, **337**: 809–852.
102. Rosenheck R., Cramer J., Xu W., Grabowski J., Douyon R., Thomas J., Henderson W., Charney D. (1998) Multiple outcome assessment in a study of the cost-effectiveness of clozapine in the treatment of refractory schizophrenia. *Hlth Serv. Res.*, **33**: 1237–1261.
103. Rosenheck R., Cramer J., Allan E., Erdos J., Frisman L.K., Xu W., Thomas J., Henderson W., Charney D. (1999) Cost-effectiveness of clozapine in patients with high and low levels of hospital use. *Arch. Gen. Psychiatry*, **56**: 565–572.
104. Kennedy E., Song F., Hunter R. (1998) Review: risperidone produces more clinical improvement and causes fewer extrapyramidal side effects. *Evidence-Based Ment. Hlth*, **1**: 15.
105. Kennedy E., Song F., Hunter R. (1997) Risperidone versus conventional antipsychotic medication for schizophrenia. In *Cochrane Database of Systematic Reviews* (updated 29 August 1997). *The Cochrane Collaboration.* Issue 4. Update Software, Oxford.
106. Addington D.E., Jones B., Bloom D., Chouinard G., Remington G., Albright P. (1993) Reduction of hospital days in chronic schizophrenic patients treated with risperidone: a retrospective study. *Clin. Ther.*, **15**: 917–926.
107. Chouinard G., Albright P.S. (1997) Economic and health state utility determinations for schizophrenic patients treated with risperidone or haloperidol. *J. Clin. Psychopharmacol.*, **17**: 298–307.

108. Lindström E., Eriksson B., Hellgren A. (1995) Efficacy and safety of risperidone in the long-term treatment of patients with schizophrenia. *Clin. Ther.*, **17**: 402–412.
109. Guest J.F., Hart W.M., Cookson R.F. (1996) Pharmacoeconomic evaluation of long-term treatment with risperidone for patients with chronic schizophrenia. *Br. J. Med. Economics*, **10**: 59–67.
110. Albright P.S., Livingstone S., Keegan D.L. (1996) Reduction of health care resource utilisation and costs following the use of risperidone for patients with schizophrenia previously treated with standard antipsychotic therapy. *Clin. Pharmacoeconomics*, **11**: 289–299.
111. Finley P.R., Sommer B.R., Corbitt J.L., Brunson G.H., Lum B.L. (1998) Risperidone: clinical outcome predictors and cost-effectiveness in a naturalistic setting. *Psychopharmacol. Bull.*, **34**: 75–81.
112. Csernansky J.G., Mahmoud R., Brenner R. (2002) A comparison of risperidone and haloperidol for the prevention of relapse in patients with schizophrenia. *N. Engl. J. Med.*, **346**: 16–22.
113. Almond S., O'Donnell O. (1998) Cost analysis of the treatment of schizophrenia in the UK: a comparison of olanzapine and haloperidol. *PharmacoEconomics*, **13**: 575–588.
114. Spannheimer A., Clouth J. (1999) Pharmacoeconomic evaluation of the treatment of schizophrenia in Germany: a comparison of olanzapine and haloperidol. Presented at the CINP Congress, London, September 21-25.
115. Sacristan J.A., Gomez J.C., Salvador-Carulla L. (1997) Analisis coste-efectividad de olanzapina frente a haloperidol en el tratamiento de la esquizofrenia en España. *Actas Luso-Esp. Neurol. Psiquiatr.*, **24**: 225–234.
116. Palmer C.S., Revicki D.A., Genduso L.A., Hamilton S.H., Brown R.E. (1998) A cost-effectiveness clinical decision analysis model for schizophrenia. *Am. J. Managed Care*, **4**: 345–355.
117. *Development and Evaluation Committee Report No. 84*, March 1998, Department of Public Health and Epidemiology, Birmingham University.
118. Tollefson G.D., Beasley C.M., Tran P.V., Street J.S., Krueger M.B.A., Tamura R.N., Graffeo K.A., Thieme M.E. (1997) Olanzapine versus haloperidol in the treatment of schizophrenia and schizoaffective and schizophreniform disorders: results of an international collaborative trial. *Am. J. Psychiatry*, **154**: 457–465.
119. Hamilton S.H., Revicki D.A., Edgell E.T., Genduso L.A., Tollefson G. (1999) Clinical and economic outcomes of olanzapine compared with haloperidol for schizophrenia. Results from a randomised clinical trial. *PharmacoEconomics*, **15**: 469–480.
120. Le Pen C., Lilliu H., Allicar M.P., Olivier V., Gregor K.J. (1999) Comparaison economique de l'olanzapine versus haloperidol dans le traitement de la schizophrenie en France. *Encephale*, **25**: 281–286.
121. Ereshefsky L., Nabulsi A., Silber C. (1997) Reduction of hospital days in sertindole treated patients: one year findings. *Schizophr. Res.*, **24**: 201–202.
122. Souêtre E., Martin P., Lelanu J.P. (1992) Évaluation médico-économique des neuroleptiques dans la schizophrénie: amisulpride versus halopéridol. *Encéphale*, **18**: 263–269.
123. Kelly D.L., Nelson M.W., Love R.C., Yu Y., Conley R.R. (2001) Comparison of discharge rates and drug costs for patients with schizophrenia treated with risperidone or olanzapine. *Psychiatr. Serv.*, **52**: 676–678.
124. Rabinowitz J., Lichtenberg P., Kaplan Z. (2000) Comparison of cost, dosage and clinical preference for risperidone and olanzapine. *Schizophr. Res.*, **46**: 91–96.

125. Kasper S., Jones M., Duchesne I. (2001) Risperidone Olanzapine Drug Outcomes studies in Schizophrenia (RODOS): health economic results of an international naturalistic study. *Int. Clin. Psychopharmacol.*, **16**: 189–196.

126. Zhao Z. (2002) A retrospective economic evaluation of olanzapine versus risperidone in the treatment of schizophrenia. *Managed Care Interface*, **15**: 75–81.

127. Russo P.A., Smith M.W., Namjoshi M. (2002) Expenditures in schizophrenia: a comparison of olanzapine and risperidone. Presented at the CINP Congress, Montreal, June 23–27.

128. Lewis M., McCrone P., Frangou S. (2001) Service use and costs of treating schizophrenia with atypical antipsychotics. *J. Clin. Psychiatry*, **62**: 749–756.

129. Edgell E.T., Andersen S.W., Johnstone B.M., Dulisse B., Revicki D., Breier A. (2000) Olanzapine versus risperidone. A prospective comparison of clinical and economic outcomes in schizophrenia. *PharmacoEconomics*, **18**: 567–579.

130. Knapp M., Spiesser J., Carita P. (2002) The comparative cost-effectiveness of amilsulpride and risperidone in schizophrenia care in Western and Eastern Europe. Presented at the CINP Congress, Montreal, June 23–27.

131. Tarrier N. (1996) A psychological approach to the management of schizophrenia. In *Handbook of Mental Health Economics and Policy: Schizophrenia* (Eds M. Moscarelli, A. Rupp, N. Sartorius), pp. 271–285. Wiley, London.

132. Wykes T., Tarrier N., Lewis S. (Eds) (1998) *Outcome and Innovation in Psychological Treatment of Schizophrenia.* Wiley, London.

133. McPhillips M., Sensky T. (1998) Coercion, adherence or collaboration? Influences on compliance with medication. In *Outcome and Innovation in the Psychological Treatment of Schizophrenia* (Eds T. Wykes, N. Tarrier, S. Lewis), pp. 161–177. Wiley, London.

134. Boczkowski J.A., Zeicher A., DeSanto N. (1985) Neuroleptic compliance among chronic schizophrenic outpatients: an intervention outcome report. *J. Consult. Clin. Psychol.*, **53**: 666–671.

135. Kuipers E. (1996) The management of difficult to treat patients with schizophrenia, using non-drug therapies. *Br. J. Psychiatry*, **169** (Suppl. 31): 41–51.

136. Kemp R., Kirov G., Everitt B., Hayward P., David A. (1998) A randomised controlled trial of compliance therapy: 18 month follow-up. *Br. J. Psychiatry*, **172**: 413–419.

137. Kuipers E., Garety P., Fowler D., Dunn G., Freeman D., Bebbington P., Hadley C. (1997) London East-Anglia randomised controlled trial of cognitive behavioural therapy for psychosis: I. Effects of treatment Phase. *Br. J. Psychiatry*, **171**: 319–327.

138. Kuipers E., Fowler D., Garety P., Chisholm D., Freeman D., Dunn G., Bebbington P., Hadley C. (1998) London-East Anglia randomised controlled trial of cognitive-behavioural therapy for psychosis. III: Follow-up and economic evaluation at 18 months. *Br. J. Psychiatry*, **173**: 61–68.

139. Brown G.W., Monck E.M., Carstairs G.M., Wing J.K. (1962) Influence of family life on the course of schizophrenic illness. *Br. J. Prevent. Soc. Med.*, **16**: 55–68.

140. Vaughn C.E., Leff J.P. (1976) The measurement of expressed emotion in the families of psychiatric patients. *Br. J. Clin. Soc. Psychiatry*, **15**: 157–165.

141. Leff J.P. (1996) Working with families of schizophrenic patients: effects on clinical and social outcomes. In *Handbook of Mental Health Economics and Policy: Schizophrenia* (Eds M. Moscarelli, A. Rupp, N. Sartorius), pp. 261–270. Wiley, London.

142. Pilling S., Bebbington P., Kuipers E., Garety P., Geddes J., Martindale B., Orbach G., Morgan C. (2002) Psychological treatments in schizophrenia: I. Meta-analysis of family intervention and cognitive behaviour therapy. *Psychol. Med.*, (in press).
143. Falloon I.R.H., Boyd J.L., McGill C.W. (1982) Family management in the prevention of exacerbations of schizophrenia. *N. Engl. J. Med.*, **306**: 1437–1440.
144. Cardin V.A., McGill C.W., Falloon I.R.H. (1986) An economic analysis: costs, benefits and effectiveness. In *Family Management of Schizophrenia* (Ed. I.R.H. Falloon). Johns Hopkins University Press, Baltimore.
145. Goldstein M.J. (1996) Psychoeducational family programs in the United States. In: *Handbook of Mental Health Economics and Health Policy* (Eds M. Moscarelli, A. Rupp, N. Sartorius), Vol. 1, pp. 287–297. Wiley, New York.
146. Liberman R.P., Cardin V., McGill C.W., Falloon I.R. (1987) Behavioral family management of schizophrenia: clinical outcome and costs. *Psychiatr. Ann.*, **17**: 610–619.
147. Tarrier N., Lowson K., Barrowclough C. (1991) Some aspects of family interventions in schizophrenia. II: Financial considerations. *Br. J. Psychiatry*, **159**: 481–484.
148. Tarrier N., Barrowclough C., Vaughn C. (1988) The community management of schizophrenia: a controlled trial of behavioural intervention with families to reduce relapse. *Br. J. Psychiatry*, **153**: 532–542.
149. Leff J., Sharpley M., Chisholm D., Bell R., Gamble C. (2001) Training community psychiatric nurses in schizophrenia family work: a study of clinical and economic outcomes for patients and relatives. *J. Ment. Hlth*, **10**: 189–197.
150. Rund B.R., Moe L.C., Sollien T., Fjell A., Borchgrevink T., Hallert M., Naess P.O. (1994) The psychosis project: an efficiency study of a psychoeducational treatment for schizophrenic adolescents. *Acta Psychiatr. Scand.*, **89**: 211–218.
151. Xiong W., Phillips M.R., Hu X., Wang R., Dai Q., Kleinman J., Kleinman A. (1994) Family-based intervention for schizophrenic patients in China: a randomized controlled trial. *Br. J. Psychiatry*, **165**: 239–247.
152. McFarlane W.R., Lukens E., Link B., Dushay R., Deakins S.A., Newmark M., Dunne E.J., Horen B., Toran J. (1995) Multiple-family groups and psychoeducation in the treatment of schizophrenia. *Arch. Gen. Psychiatry*, **52**: 679–87.
153. Schooler N.R., Keith S.J., Severe J.B. (1997) Relapse and rehospitalisation during maintenance treatment of schizophrenia: the effects of dose reduction and family treatment. *Arch. Gen. Psychiatry*, **54**: 453–463.
154. Hargreaves W.A. (1998) Commentary: Patterns of usual care for schizophrenia. *Schizophr. Bull.*, **24**: 23–24.
155. Goodwin S. (1997) *Comparative Mental Health Policy: From Institutional to Community Care.* Sage, London.
156. Ford R., Durcan G., Warner L., Hardy P., Muijen M. (1998) One day survey by the Mental Health Act Commission of acute adult psychiatric inpatient wards in England and Wales. *Br. Med. J.*, **317**: 1279–1283.
157. Creed F., Mbaya P., Lancashire S., Tomenson B., Williams B., Holme S. (1997) Cost effectiveness of day and inpatient psychiatric treatment. Results of a randomised controlled trial. *Br. Med. J.*, **314**: 1381–1385.
158. Fenton J.R., Tessier L., Contandriopoulous A.P. (1982) A comparative trial of home and hospital psychiatric treatment: financial costs. *Can. J. Psychiatry*, **27**: 177–187.

159. Dickey B., Cannon N.L., McGuire T.G., Gudeman J.E. (1986) The quarter-way house: a two-year cost study of an experimental residential programme. *Hosp. Commun. Psychiatry*, **37**: 1136–1143.

160. Endicott J., Hertz M., Gibbon M. (1978) Brief versus standard hospitalization: the differential costs. *Am. J. Psychiatry*, **135**: 707–712.

161. Linn M.W., Caffey E.M., Klett C.J., Hogarty G.E., Lamb H.R. (1979) Day treatment and psychotropic drugs in the aftercare of schizophrenic patient. *Arch. Gen. Psychiatry*, **36**: 1055–1066.

162. Dorwart R.A. (1988) A ten-year follow-up study of the effects of deinstitutionalisation. *Hosp. Commun. Psychiatry*, **39**: 287–290.

163. Jones D. (1993) The selection of patients for reprovision. *Br. J. Psychiatry*, **162** (Suppl. 19): 36–39.

164. Knapp M.R.J. (1996) From psychiatric hospital to community care; reflections on the English experience. In *Handbook of Mental Health Economics and Policy: Schizophrenia* (Eds M. Moscarelli, A. Rupp, N. Sartorius), pp. 473–484. Wiley, Chichester.

165. Rothbard A.B., Kuno E., Schinnar A.P., Hadley T.P., Turk R. (1999) Service utilization and cost of community care for discharged state hospital patients: a three year follow up study. *Am. J. Psychiatry*, **156**: 920–927.

166. Wright E.R., Holmes A., Deb P., Blunt B., Duzan J. (1997) *Treatment Costs of the Former Central State Hospital Patients: A Comparison of Institutionalized and Community-based Care*. Indiana Consortium for Mental Health Services Research.

167. Murphy J.P., Datel W.E. (1976) A cost–benefit analysis of community versus institutional living. *Hosp. Commun. Psychiatry*, **27**: 165–169.

168. Cassel W.A., Smith C.M., Grunberg F., Boan J.A., Thomas R.F. (1972) Comparing costs of hospital and community care. *Hosp. Commun. Psychiatry*, **23**: 197–200.

169. Knapp M.R.J., Cambridge P., Thomason C., Beecham J., Allen C., Darton R. (1992) *Care in the Community: Challenge and Demonstration*. Ashgate, Aldershot.

170. Donnelly M., McGilloway S., Mays N., Perry S., Knapp M.R.J., Kavanagh S., Beecham J., Fenyo A., Astin J. (1994) *Opening New Doors: An Evaluation of Community Care for People Discharged from Psychiatric and Mental Handicap Hospitals*. HMSO, London.

171. Beecham J.K., Hallam A., Knapp M.R.J., Baines B., Fenyo A., Asbury M. (1997) Costing care in the hospital and in the community. In *Care in the Community: Illusion or Reality?* (Ed. J. Leff), pp. 93–108. Wiley, Chichester.

172. Salize H.J., Rössler W. (1996) The cost of comprehensive care of people with schizophrenia living in the community: a cost evaluation from a German catchment area. *Br. J. Psychiatry*, **169**: 42–48.

173. Knapp M.R.J., Beecham J.K., Fenyo A., Hallam A. (1995) Community mental health care for former hospital in-patients; predicting costs from needs and diagnoses. *Br. J. Psychiatry*, **166** (Suppl. 27): 10–18.

174. Trieman N., Leff J. (1996) The most difficult to place long-stay psychiatric in-patients: outcome one year after relocation. *Br. J. Psychiatry*, **169**: 289–292.

175. Leff J. (Ed.) (1997) *Care in the Community: Illusion or Reality?* Wiley, Chichester.

176. Knapp M.R.J., Hallam A., Beecham J.K., Baines B. (1999) Private, voluntary or public? Comparative cost-effectiveness in community mental health care. *Policy and Politics*, **27**: 25–41.

177. Burns T., Knapp M., Catty J., Healey A., Henderson J., Watt H., Wright C. (2001) Home treatment for mental health problems: a systematic review. *Hlth Technol. Assess.*, **5**: 1–129.

178. Catty J., Burns T., Knapp M., Watt H., Wright C., Henderson J., Healey A. (2002) Home treatment for mental health problems: a systematic review. *Psychol. Med.*, **32**: 383–401.

179. Burns T., Catty J., Watt H., Wright C., Knapp M., Henderson J. (2002) International differences in home treatment for mental health problems: the results of a systematic review. *Br. J. Psychiatry*, (in press).

180. Marx A.J., Test M.A., Stein L.I. (1973) Extra-hospital management of severe mental illness: feasibility and effects of social functioning. *Arch. Gen. Psychiatry*, **29**: 505–511.

181. Scott J.E., Dixon L.B. (1995) Psychological interventions for schizophrenia. *Schizophr. Bull.*, **21**: 621–630.

182. De Cangas J.P.C. (1994) Le "case management" affirmatif: une evaluation complete d'un programme du genre en milieu hospitalier. *Sante Mentale au Quebec*, **19**: 75–92.

183. Preston N.J., Fazio S. (2000) Establishing the efficacy and cost effectiveness of community intensive case management of long-term mentally ill: a matched control group study. *Aust. N. Z. J. Psychiatry*, **34**: 114–121.

184. Mueser K.T., Bond G.R., Drake R.E., Resnick S.G. (1998) Models of community care for severe mental illness: a review of research on case management. *Schizophr. Bull.*, **24**: 37–74.

185. Chamberlain R., Rapp C.A. (1991) A decade of case management: a methodological review of outcome research. *Commun. Ment. Hlth J.*, **27**: 171–188.

186. Holloway F., Carson J. (1998) Intensive case management for the severely mentally ill: controlled trial. *Br. J. Psychiatry*, **172**: 19–22.

187. Marks I.M., Connolly J., Muijen M. (1994) Home-versus hospital-based care for people with serious mental illness. *Br. J. Psychiatry*, **165**: 179–194.

188. Knapp M.R.J., Beecham J.K., Koutsogeorgopoulou V., Hallam A., Fenyo A.J., Marks I.M., Connolly J., Audini B., Muijen M. (1994) Service use and costs of home-based versus hospital-based care for people with serious mental illness. *Br. J. Psychiatry*, **165**: 195–203.

189. Audini B., Marks I.M., Laurence R.E. (1994) Home-based versus out-patient/in-patient care for people with serious mental illness: phase II of a controlled trial. *Br. J. Psychiatry*, **165**: 204–210.

190. Knapp M.R.J., Marks I.M., Wolstenholme J., Beecham J.K., Astin J., Audini B., Connolly J., Watts V. (1998) Home-based versus hospital-based care for serious mental illness: controlled cost-effectiveness study over four years. *Br. J. Psychiatry*, **172**: 506–512.

191. Ford R., Minghella E., Chalmers C., Hoult J., Raftery J., Muijen M. (2001) Cost consequences of home-based and in-patient-based acute psychiatric treatment: Results of an implementation study. *J. Ment. Hlth*, **10**: 467–476.

192. Fenton F.R., Tessier L., Struening E.L., Smith F.A., Benoit C., Contandriopoulos A.P., Nguyen H. (1984) A two-year follow-up of a comparative trial of the cost-effectiveness of home and hospital psychiatric treatment. *Can. J. Psychiatry*, **29**: 205–211.

193. Bond G.R., Miller L.D., Krumwied R.D., Ward R.S. (1988) Assertive case management in three CMHCs: a controlled study. *Hosp. Commun. Psychiatry*, **39**: 411–418.

194. Hoult J., Reynolds I. (1985) Schizophrenia: a comparative trial of community-oriented and hospital-oriented psychiatric care. *Acta Psychiatr. Scand.*, **69**: 359–372.

195. Santos A.B., Thrasher J.W.J., Ballenger J.C. (1988) Decentralised services for public hospital patients: a cost analysis. *Hosp. Commun. Psychiatry*, **39**: 827–829.

196. Essock S.M., Frisman L.K., Kontos N.J. (1998) Cost-effectiveness of assertive treatment models. *Am. J. Orthopsychiatry*, **68**: 179–190.
197. Test M.A., Knoedler W.H., Allness D.J. (1985) The long-term treatment of young schizophrenics in a community support program. In *The Training in Community Living Model: A Decade of Experience* (Eds L.I. Stein, M.A. Test). Jossey-Bass, San Francisco.
198. Marshall M., Lockwood A. (1998) *Assertive Community Treatment for People with Severe Mental Disorders* (Cochrane Review). The Cochrane Library.
199. Burns T. (1997) Case management, care management and care programming. *Br. J. Psychiatry*, **170**: 393–395.
200. McCrone P., Beecham J.K., Knapp M.R.J. (1994) Community psychiatric nurse teams: cost-effectiveness of intensive support versus generic care. *Br. J. Psychiatry*, **165**: 218–221.
201. Quinlivan R., Hough R., Cromwell A., Beach C., Hofstetter R., Kenworthy K. (1995) Service utilization and costs of care for severely mentally ill clients in an intensive case management program. *Psychiatr. Serv.*, **46**: 365–371.
202. Ford R., Raftery J., Ryan P., Bearsmoore A., Craid T., Muijen M. (1997) Intensive case management for people with serious mental illness-site 2: cost-effectiveness. *J. Ment. Hlth*, **6**: 191–199.
203. Galster G.C., Champney T.F., Williams Y. (1995) Costs of caring for persons with long-term mental illness in alternative residential settings. *Evaluation & Program Planning*, **17**.
204. Johnston S., Salkeld G., Sanderson K., Issakidis C., Teesson M., Buhrich N. (1998) Intensive case management: a cost effectiveness analysis. *Aust. N. Z. J. Psychiatry*, **32**: 551–559.
205. UK700 Group (2000) Cost-effectiveness of intensive vs. standard case management for severe psychotic illness. UK700 case management trial. *Br. J. Psychiatry*, **176**: 537–543.
206. Tyrer P., Morgan J., Van Horn E., Jayokody M., Evans K., Brummell R., White T., Baldwin D., Harrison-Read P., Johnson T. (1995) A randomised controlled study of close monitoring of vulnerable psychiatry patients. *Lancet*, **345**: 756–759.
207. Tyrer P., Evans K., Gandhi N., Lamont A., Harrison-Read P., Johnson T. (1998) Randomised controlled trial of two models of care for discharged psychiatric patients. *Br. Med. J.*, **316**: 106–107.
208. Gates R., Goldsberg D., Jackson G., Jennett N., Lawson K., Ratcliffe J., Saraf T., Warner R. (1997) The care of patients with chronic schizophrenia: a comparison between two services. *Psychol. Med.*, **27**: 1325–1336.
209. Merson S., Tyrer P., Carlen D., Johnson T. (1996) The cost of treatment of psychiatric emergencies: a comparison of hospital and community services. *Psychol. Med.*, **26**: 727–734.
210. Burns T., Raftery J. (1993) A controlled trial of home-based acute psychiatric services II: Treatment patterns and costs. *Br. J. Psychiatry*, **163**: 55–61.
211. Tyrer P. (1998) Whither community care? *Br. J. Psychiatry*, **173**: 359–360.

Commentaries

6.1
Is Schizophrenia Worth the Cost?

Gavin Andrews[1]

To quote Knapp *et al*, "difficult choices always have to be made about resource deployment... ideally all resource impacts would be opportunity costs, that is, the values forgone by not using these resources in their next best employment".

Schizophrenia is a relatively rare disease with a 12-month prevalence of 0.5%. As the 12-month prevalence for any mental disorder is of the order of 25% [1–3], only one in 50 people with a mental disorder have schizophrenia. According to Knapp *et al*, schizophrenia consumes a median of 2% of the health budgets of economically developed countries. Mental health budgets are typically 5–10% of the total health budget, so schizophrenia accounts for 10 times the amount that would be appropriate if prevalence was the only issue. In Australia [4], 2% of the health budget for schizophrenia would mean that schizophrenia consumed 40% of the mental health budget, a figure that is not improbable, despite the fact that Australia has divested itself of most high cost options, has only 40 inpatient psychiatric beds per 100 000 population, and has a well-developed system of community mental health clinics and private psychiatrists.

Is schizophrenia expensive because it is so severe? Mental disorders account for 22% of the burden of disease in economically developed countries, and schizophrenia is estimated to account for about one tenth of this [5], with anxiety, depressive and substance use disorders each accounting for more. In the recent Australian national mental health survey [3], a similar picture emerged. Anxiety and depressive disorders were common and accounted for 55% of the total disability days reported that month, whereas schizophrenia accounted for only 2%. People in the community identified as psychotic on a screening interview may be atypical, but even if all had reported being disabled every day, the disability due to schizophrenia would still have been

[1] School of Psychiatry, University of New South Wales at St Vincent's Hospital, 299 Forbes Street, Darlinghurst, NSW 2010, Australia

only one tenth of the total, which suggests that the Murray and Lopez figure [5] is an upper bound.

Bobadilla *et al* [6] argued that, as no country could afford to treat all who demanded it, resources would have to be rationed in terms of the burden of the disease and the cost effectiveness of dealing with the disease. Is the budget for schizophrenia large because treatment is such a good buy? Probably not. The treatment of schizophrenia is, in comparison with the treatment of other mental disorders, expensive. Knapp *et al* agree that schizophrenia is a chronic relapsing disorder, have said that hospitalization is not necessarily cost effective [7] and do not use the word cure. In contrast, the psychological treatments of chronic anxiety disorders are very cost effective [8], and the economical termination of an episode of depression by medication is expected rather than remarked upon. Given the disability associated with both these conditions, they may well represent better buys for the health dollar than treating people with schizophrenia.

Why then, does a relatively rare disease like schizophrenia continue to consume 20–40% of the mental health budget? It is easy to attribute this to historical reasons as many were once the people who inhabited mental hospitals, and care in the community has continued to mean help with accommodation, finances, recreation and employment—care that is not provided for people with other disorders. But this is probably not the whole story. In economically developed countries, the important costs are strongly related to the decision to admit to hospital. In Australia some admissions assuage the very real affront and pain of families with a disturbed member, others respond to the concern of the wider society that persons with schizophrenia may be a danger to themselves or others. Surprisingly few admissions are due to a need for a treatment that cannot be offered in a community setting. For instance, family intervention studies have been shown to reduce the need for admission by half, and when used proactively these techniques are cost effective [9]. Second, the judgement of risk of dangerousness is an enormously complex matter, and admission is by no means the only option [10]. Third, as admission to hospital can engender a career of hospital admissions [11], it can be an expensive, and not necessarily cost-effective decision. The admission decision is usually made by junior doctors, and it has been demonstrated that they err on the side of caution and admit patients, whereas senior consultants are more conservative. Perhaps we should have senior consultants on duty at all times. I note that the prognosis in schizophrenia, and hence the relative cost, is better in the undeveloped world where patients live with families and seldom go to hospital [12].

Calman [13] argued that a health service could not afford to provide everything. While people might have a right to shelter, primary care and emergency care when sick, specialist medicine would not be available to all, but be prioritized in terms of cost effectiveness of the intervention (see ref. [14] for a worked example for mental disorders). The Netherlands is also approaching this problem by the establishment of separate budgets for prevention, cure and care [15]. Perhaps it is time for a sectoral costing of the treatment of all mental disorders to discover the best deployment of resources, for only then will we be able to assess the meaning of cost estimates for the treatment of schizophrenia. Estimates provided in isolation [7, 9] simply say that schizophrenia is costly, treated or not. We need comparative data to allow proper decision making.

REFERENCES

1. Kessler R.C. (1994) The National Comorbidity Study of the United States. *Int. Rev. Psychiatry*, **6**: 365–376.
2. Meltzer H., Jenkins R. (1994) The National Survey of Psychiatric Morbidity in Great Britain. *Int. Rev. Psychiatry*, **6**: 349–356.
3. Andrews G. (2000) Meeting the unmet need through disease management. In *Unmet Need in Psychiatry* (Eds G. Andrews, A.S. Henderson), pp. 11–38. Cambridge University Press, Cambridge.
4. Andrews G., Issakidis C. (1998) Mental health services in the city of Sydney. In *Mental Health in Our Future Cities* (Eds D. Goldberg, G. Thornicroft), pp. 195–216. Psychological Press, London.
5. Murray C.J.L., Lopez A.D. (Eds) (1996) *The Global Burden of Disease*. Harvard University Press, Cambridge.
6. Bobadilla J.L., Cowley P., Musgrove P., Saxenian H. (1994) Design, content and financing of an essential national package of health services. In *Global Comparative Assessments in the Health Sector* (Eds C.J. Murray, A.D. Lopez), pp. 171–180. World Health Organization, Geneva.
7. Knapp M. (1977) Costs of schizophrenia. *Br. J. Psychiatry*, **171**: 509–516.
8. Ginsberg G., Marks I. (1977) Costs and benefits of behaviour therapy. *Psychol. Med.*, **7**: 685–700.
9. Andrews G., Hall W., Goldstein G., Lapsley H., Bartels R., Silove D. (1985) The economic costs of schizophrenia. *Arch. Gen. Psychiatry*, **42**: 537–544.
10. Buchanan A. (1997) The investigation of acting on delusions as a toll for risk assessment in the mentally disordered. *Br. J. Psychiatry*, **170** (Suppl. 32): 12–16.
11. Kiesler C.A. (1982) Mental hospitals and alternative care. *Am. Psychol.*, **37**: 349–360.
12. Jablensky A., Sartorius N., Ernberg G., Anker M., Korten A., Cooper J.E., Day R., Bertelsen A. (1992) Schizophrenia: manifestations, incidence and course in different cultures. *Psychol. Med. Monogr. Suppl.*, **20**: 1–97.
13. Calman K.C. (1994) The ethics of allocation of scarce health resources: a view from the centre. *J. Med. Ethics*, **20**: 71–74.
14. Andrews G. (1997) Managing scarcity: a worked example using burden and efficacy. *Australasian Psychiatry*, **5**: 225–228.
15. Netherlands Scientific Council for Government Policy (1997) *Priorities and a Sound Financial Basis for Health Care in the 21st Century*. Netherlands Scientific Council for Government Policy, The Hague.

6.2
Morality and Cost in the Management of Schizophrenia
Paul Bebbington[1]

The style and content of health organizations is always informed by ethical principles, although these may not always be clear. Thus in pay-per-service or insurance-based services, the moral imperative is the right of choice: the right of citizens to spend their money in their own way, choosing perhaps to spend it on health care or insurance. This right cuts across other imperatives, and is rarely implemented fully because good health is seen as a right in most countries.

Health organizations paid for by the taxpayer are mainly guided by other principles: in the UK, the National Health Service (NHS) is strongly influenced by the related ideas of *equity* and *proportionality*. Briefly, these assert that people should receive health care according to their level of need, and that each person with a given level of need should be equally entitled to treatment.

In the UK, my own area of knowledge, these principles are often breached. Thus, middle class people are typically more practised in accessing health care than their less fortunate fellow citizens. Likewise, major regional variations in health needs and in the availability of treatment have always militated against the ideals of the NHS.

To these twin pillars of the NHS, we must add a third, of cost effectiveness, or even better, cost utility. Decisions about health service allocation should of course be both principled and rational. Given the principles of equity, of proportionality and of appropriateness, rational decisions must be based on judgements of need, effectiveness and cost effectiveness. Providing an effective treatment where it is not needed will not be cost effective, nor will failing to provide it where it is needed.

Rationing within the UK NHS has been the phenomenon that dared not speak its name. The new Labour Government's attempts to shift emphasis from costs to quality and outcome are laudable. However, it has been forced recently to admit that rationing does and must exist, even though it may be more covert and informal in a nationally funded health service.

Questions of cost are almost always seen as a hindrance and an embarrassment to those working in publicly funded services. However, the imperative behind health economics has always been a moral one: it is only ethical to spend scarce funds in the best way possible. This shifts the problem of cost control from cost minimization to the possibility of measuring relative health benefits. This is difficult, but cannot be avoided.

---

[1] *Department of Psychiatry and Behavioural Sciences, Whittington Hospital, Highgate Hill, London N19 5NF, UK*

The study of variations in uptake of services and treatment may indicate potential breaches of all three principles. There are a number of obvious indications of this type. Thus, Haro *et al* [1] showed a range of regional variations in health service utilization by people with schizophrenia. While there are clear differences in the prevalence of schizophrenia between urban and rural locations, with schizophrenia being between two and three times commoner in inner city than in rural areas [2], this cannot possibly be used to discount the Spanish regional variations, which are so large that they probably indicate an inequitable distribution.

There are also notable variations — about which we know very little — in response uptake between different people with schizophrenia. Certainly in the British National Survey of Psychiatric Morbidity [3] over 20% of people with psychosis were *not* receiving psychotropic medication, over 40% were not in contact with secondary services and a similar proportion had not seen their family doctor for a year. The hope is that these variations are explicable in terms of varying need, but this is unlikely.

Thus, a simple examination of the distribution of resources in schizophrenia raises questions about both equity and cost effectiveness. The data to resolve them are probably relatively easy to acquire. However, this relates to the deployment of resources within one illness group. Ideally, we would wish to make rational decisions between illness groups. For instance, in the UK, there is a deliberate policy to target severe mental illness (effectively psychosis) at the expense of less severe disorders like depression. This decision is based on the principle of proportionality rather than cost effectiveness, but there is no real empirical basis to it.

The allocation of resources between different sorts of illness is usually done on the basis of the champion with the loudest voice. Ideally, the judgement should be based on cost–utility comparisons, as those based on cost–benefit may be somewhat harsh. However, this is very difficult within one group of illnesses, and virtually infeasible between illness groups. Imagine the problem of choosing between allocating treatment for diabetic leg ulcers and for schizophrenia. The overall consequences are that we just muddle along in our allocation of health services resources between different disorders. The sad result in Britain is that mental illness has had a declining share of the cake.

REFERENCES

1. Haro J.M., Salvador-Carulla L., Cabases J., Madoz V., Vazquez-Barquero J.L. and the PSICOST Group (1998) Utilisation of mental health services and costs of patients with schizophrenia in three areas of Spain. *Br. J. Psychiatry*, **173**: 334–340.
2. Meltzer H., Gill B., Petticrew M., Hinds K. (1995) The prevalence of psychiatric morbidity among adults living in private households. OPCS Survey of Psychiatric Morbidity in Great Britain, Report 1. HMSO, London.

3. Foster K., Meltzer H., Gill B., Hinds K. (1996) Adults with a psychotic disorder living in the community. OPCS Survey of Psychiatric Morbidity in Great Britain, Report 8. HMSO, London.

6.3
Caveat Emptor: Pitfalls in Measuring the Costs of Schizophrenia
Richard Warner[1]

In health cost studies, the devil is in the details, but the reader who is alert to the inherent actuarial and statistical problems may still draw valuable conclusions.

It is unfortunate, for example, that research on the costs of schizophrenia in the USA relies extensively for prevalence data on the Epidemiologic Catchment Area (ECA) study. Adequate though these data may be for other diagnoses, they have been shown to be quite inaccurate for schizophrenia. The ECA study used a diagnostic instrument (the DIS) which, in the hands of lay interviewers, produced a high false-positive rate for schizophrenia. In some areas, the identified occurrence rates were several times the US mean, and, overall, ECA data overestimate the prevalence of schizophrenia by a factor of two or more [1].

This problem becomes important in Rice and Miller's [2] calculation of the economic burden of schizophrenia in the USA. Their figure of $17.9 billion in direct costs of schizophrenia in 1990 may well be reliable since it is based on actual costs; their estimate of $14.6 billion in indirect costs, however, could be greatly inflated, as it is based on ECA prevalence data. This bias more than offsets the authors' methodological rigour in incorporating in their model socioeconomic variables which tend to reduce income effects.

Indirect cost analyses are difficult to interpret when we note the differences in categorization and calculation of costs. For example, whereas Rice and Miller [2] place incarceration and family caregiving under indirect costs, Hu and colleagues [3], in another American study, assign these resources to direct costs. Again, lost productivity from patient disability amounts to 37% of the total economic impact in Rice and Miller's study, but only 0.5% in Hu *et al*'s study (because they reason that most patients are not in the labour force). Consequently, where Rice and Miller attribute 45% of costs to indirect resources, Hu *et al* assign less than 1% to this area. To make sense of these figures one must be aware of how categories are derived and on what data they are based.

---

[1]*Mental Health Center, Boulder County, 1333 Iris Avenue, Boulder, Colorado 80304–2296, USA*

If we accept the higher, and more usual, estimates of indirect costs from lost patient productivity, it becomes clear that certain policy interventions could reduce costs and improve outcomes. Employment of the mentally ill, for example, is substantially greater in northern Italy than in the USA or Britain. In recent studies, 50–60% of people with schizophrenia in Bologna and Verona were in stable employment, around a quarter full-time. By contrast, in Boulder, Colorado, where employment of the mentally ill is twice the expected US rate, the figures for people with schizophrenia were substantially lower — less than 30% employed and only 8% full-time [4].

Why is there such a wide variation between industrialized countries? In part, the answer lies in obstacles to employment inherent in the different national disability pension schemes. In Italy, work disincentives are much less severe than in the USA or Britain, because Italian patients may usually retain their disability benefits while working. In Colorado, on the other hand, the income of mentally ill people who work part-time is little more than that of unemployed subjects, due to deductions from their disability pension and rent subsidy. For the average part-time worker the loss amounts to, what economists term, an "implicit tax" of 64% on earned income [5]. In Britain, disincentives to work are worse, as disabled people run the risk of losing all benefits if they earn as little as £15 ($25) a week. Since a full benefits package, including pension, housing subsidy and prescriptions, is worth about £13 000 a year, and a full-time minimum-wage job yields only £9000 a year of taxable income, there is little incentive to work.

When we see, then, that the cost of government entitlements amounts to only 15% of the total treatment and support costs of people with schizophrenia in the USA [3], whereas the amount ascribed to lost patient productivity accounts for 36% of total costs [2], it becomes clear that a relaxation of disability pension regulations to eliminate disincentives to work could be covered by the economic benefits of increased employment.

It is evident that health economics is not a dark science useful only to cost-cutting bureaucrats. As Knapp *et al* point out, the goal of health economics is not to pare costs, but to improve the efficiency and equity with which we target scarce resources and provide the greatest benefit to the most needy clients. If we use these data to establish rational social policies, schizophrenia may become a less disabling illness.

REFERENCES

1. Warner R., de Girolamo G. (1995) *Epidemiology of Mental Disorders and Psychosocial Problems: Schizophrenia*. World Health Organization, Geneva.
2. Rice D.P., Miller L.S. (1996) The economic burden of schizophrenia: conceptual and methodological issues and cost estimates. In *Handbook of Mental Health Economics and Health Policy, vol. 1: Schizophrenia* (Eds M. Moscarelli, A. Rupp, N. Sartorius), pp. 321–334. John Wiley, New York.

3. Hu T.-W., Hargreaves W.A., Shumway M. (1996) Estimating costs of schizo-phrenia and its treatment. In *Handbook of Mental Health Economics and Health Policy, vol. 1: Schizophrenia* (Eds M. Moscarelli, A. Rupp, N. Sartorius), pp. 359–371. John Wiley, New York.
4. Warner R., de Girolamo G., Belelli G., Bologna C., Fioritti A., Rossini G. (1998) The quality of life of people with schizophrenia in Boulder, Colorado, and Bologna, Italy. *Schizophr. Bull.*, **24**: 559–568.
5. Polak P., Warner R. (1996) The economic life of seriously mentally ill people in the community. *Psychiatr. Serv.*, **47**: 270–274.

6.4

The Economic Consequences of Schizophrenia

Steven S. Sharfstein[1]

The review by Knapp *et al* is an excellent contribution to the health care field on the economic impact of schizophrenia, a serious, long-term, debili-tating brain disorder that affects millions of individuals, and the economic consequences of differing medical and non-medical interventions that might change the course and duration of this disorder. At the end of the twentieth century, breakthroughs in our understanding of brain function and dysfunc-tion are being matched by an increasingly economically-driven, sophisticated approach in understanding the choices that we must make as a compassionate society in the provision of scarce resources to alleviate suffering and return people to productive lives.

There is hardly another clinical and public health problem that matches the devastating economic consequences of schizophrenia — a condition that most often strikes individuals in late adolescence or early adulthood and affects the organ which allows all of us to cope with the realities of daily living: that is, the brain. Significant brain impairment leads immediately to the consequence of high direct treatment costs, especially 24-hour inpatient hospital-level care and expensive diagnostic tests. The psychotic symptoms of schizophrenia require urgent crisis intervention, safe and secure surroundings, and highly trained medical and nursing professionals. The psychopharmacologic treat-ment options now available to us and an increasing array of available psychosocial interventions in the hospital and in the community, including various levels of therapeutic housing and rehabilitation, add other direct costs for caring for individuals with this condition. These direct costs, however, pale in comparison to the lifetime of indirect costs of lost vocational and social functioning, and the costs related to social control problems including homelessness and crime.

[1]*Sheppard Pratt Health System, 6501 N. Charles St, Baltimore, MD 21204, USA*

The economic consequences of schizophrenia are felt most directly by the individual and the family. The burden of treatment and home care can be so great on families as to have devastating consequences for the overall economic health of the household. Studies on these consequences need to be pursued more vigorously, as society must support the family first and foremost, given the long-term nature of the disorder and the impoverishment that occurs as a result. Sometimes we see these consequences in rather abstract terms, such as numbers of lost productivity days, welfare costs, criminal justice costs. The cost to the family who must get a second mortgage on a home or give up their primary place of residence to support an ill family member, or the sacrifice of other members of the family should be studied further.

The main drivers of high, preventable costs relate to relapse and non-compliance. Knapp *et al*'s review shows that, to the extent that we can prevent relapse and ensure compliance with effective treatment regimens combining psychopharmacology and psychosocial treatment, we can have a major impact on these direct costs. Continuity of care and the continuum of care are critical, as well as the psychosocial education for families and individuals on the importance of staying in treatment. As we learn more and more about how to get patients and families to follow through with clinicians and treatment systems as a result of understanding the illness well, we will see a major impact on the reduction of relapse rates and on the high direct and indirect costs of schizophrenia due to hospitalization, homelessness, incarceration in jail and suicide.

Cost-effectiveness research is also an important guide to policy makers and clinicians on the appropriate use of scarce resources. Today, unfortunately, the major policy concern is not cost effectiveness, but cost shifting. In today's managed care marketplace, the spreading of risks through traditional insurance has given way to the shifting of risks through managed care and not on cost effective approaches established by scientific studies. For example, if one can get the highest cost patients out of one's health maintenance organization in the USA, one can show a profit. And much, if not most, managed care is a for-profit enterprise with stockholder's financial interests as a first priority. Certainly individuals with psychotic disorders, such as schizophrenia, are among the highest cost users that any health system can be expected to manage. The consequences of this cost shifting of schizophrenia from the private to the public sector is another area that requires urgent study. As a compassionate society, we must rely more on cost effectiveness and less on cost shifting to avoid the tragedies that occur every day in our communities.

Perhaps the best way to get resources devoted to cost-effective interventions is to show the economic benefits (or reduced economic costs) of such interventions in the long run. The ability to find long-term care for individuals with schizophrenia in the community depends on the studies cited in this review and done by the authors. Multi-year studies encompassing long-term outcomes with associated total costs in the context of understanding the risks of non-intervention must continue.

The best cost–benefit occurs with rehabilitation and recovery, and a long-term perspective is essential to achieve fully what we can do today for individuals with schizophrenia and their families. Let us focus on these economic consequences as we struggle with the costs of schizophrenia over a lifetime.

6.5
The Many and the Few: Evidence-based Mental Health in a Primary-care-led Health Service
Linda Gask[1]

Professor Knapp *et al*'s review elegantly highlights many of the conflicts and dilemmas faced by those who attempt to plan or to provide services for people with schizophrenia and other severe mental illnesses. Economic evaluations seek to provide answers, and indeed in some cases have contributed valuable evidence to support or refute claims for particular approaches to care provision. However, much work remains to be done.

In the UK, the division of care provision between primary and secondary care and the gate-keeping function of the general practitioner (GP) have ensured that the cost of health care remains relatively low in comparison with other developed countries. The GP remains the doctor of first contact for patients with all health problems, including mental disorders, making the decision about who should be referred to the specialist. However, evaluation has yet to be carried out in order to assist in decision making about who is best treated at which "level" of the National Health Service (NHS).

Although there is increasing evidence that it is probably more cost effective to treat the majority of people with neurotic illness and adjustment disorders in primary care, ring-fencing the specialist services for people with major disorders, there is still a dearth of good economic research [1]. Secondary care policy makers seek both to promote spending on proven approaches to care for the seriously mentally ill, such as assertive community treatment teams, and to involve the GP in the care of the significant number of people with psychotic illness who are out of contact with the specialist mental health services [2]. Meanwhile, primary care policy moves inexorably towards the concept of a "primary-care led NHS", in which those working in primary care are increasingly involved at a local level in planning how services will

[1] *Royal Preston Hospital, Sharoe Green Lane, Preston PR2 8HT, UK*

develop and therefore how money will be spent. Their priority has not been the smaller number of people with major disorders such as schizophrenia, but the much larger number of people with neurotic, substance misuse and personality disorders in the community at large, who are considerably more of a burden to primary care.

The last years of the Conservative Government saw successive experiments in "fundholding". British GPs were provided with increasing control over their local health budgets, resulting in the "total purchasing" experiments of the mid-1990s, in which groups of GPs obtained effective control of all or much of their health budget, including the cost of inpatient care. The theory behind such development was that it sought to ensure that decision making was "nearer the patient", as GPs were perceived to be closer to the community, and more informed about its needs.

In research carried out at the National Primary Care Research and Development Centre in Manchester [3], we have evaluated the impact of such changes on mental health services, and sought to explore, using qualitative methods, the incentives and barriers to such "total purchasing" groups achieving the change that they set out to do. What has been most striking has been the lack of understanding, at a local level, of the evidence base for mental health service development, some of which Martin Knapp and his colleagues have delineated. This, combined with a dearth of needs assessment and any real attempt at involvement of service users themselves in planning services, does not bode well for future developments, unless there is a real attempt made to educate those in a position to make such decisions about service development and evaluation.

However, to assert this view too stridently is to be unfair to the clinician, particularly the primary care doctor, who is viewed by all specialities as being "ideally placed" to carry more of the burden of routine care. The front-line practitioner has to balance the need for evidence-based practice with the, sometimes incompatible, practice of "patient-centred medicine"[4]. Health care systems vary considerably in what they expect the generalist to be able to deal with. For example, the degree to which a GP in Australia might be expected to manage alone a first episode of schizophrenia would be viewed with some surprise by a British GP who would view this as the remit of the specialist. Who is to say, without appropriate evaluation being carried out, which is the more efficient model of service delivery? Health economics will assist us enormously if it is able to provide us with essential information about the most efficient configurations of service. However, as working clinicians, we are often faced with a range of conflicting demands, not least our duty to provide the best possible care for the patient sitting in front of us. It is here, in our daily work, that "academic" conflicts between the criteria of efficiency and equity come to life.

REFERENCES

1. Gask L., Sibbald B., Creed F. (1997) Evaluating models of working at the interface between mental health services and primary care. *Br. J. Psychiatry*, **170**: 6–11.
2. Jenkins R., Bebbington P., Brugha T.S., Farrell M., Lewis G., Meltzer H. (1998) British psychiatric morbidity survey. *Br. J. Psychiatry*, **173**: 4–7.
3. Gask L., Lee J., Donnan S., Roland M. (1998) *Total Purchasing and Extended Fund-holding of Mental Health Services*. King's Fund, London.
4. Stewart M., Belle Brown J., Weston W.A., McWhinney I., McWilliam C.L., Freeman T.R. (1995) *Patient-Centered Medicine: Transforming the Clinical Method*. Sage, Thousand Oaks.

6.6
The Long-term Course of Schizophrenia and its Economic Consequences

Durk Wiersma[1]

The International Study of Schizophrenia (ISoS) [1, 2] aims at describing the long-term clinical and social course and outcome of schizophrenia and related psychotic disorders in different sociocultural settings and countries. This study combines study populations from the World Health Organization (WHO), International Pilot Study on Schizophrenia (IPSS), Determinance of Outcome of Severe Mental Disorders (DOSMeD), and Disability. The follow-up period varies on average from 15 years for incidence cohorts to 26 years for prevalence cohorts and comprises more than 1000 patients or 62% of the original study population, who from the very beginning were assessed with standardized instruments for psychopathology, negative symptomatology, disability, and work and living situation.

Long-term outcome seems rather favourable: according to Bleuler's scale or a global assessment of symptomatological functioning over the last month, about 60% of the patients fared relatively well with no or minimal symptomatology. However, the main course of the illness over the last 2 years for incidence as well as prevalence cohorts showed that half of them were all the time or episodically psychotic and that many other patients had suffered from non-psychotic episodes. This is at least an indication that the disease process had not yet stopped. Social functioning as measured by the Global Evaluation in the WHO-Disability Assessment Schedule looks somewhat less favourable: only 40% was reported as excellent to good socially adjusted. But, the great majority was living in the community with family or alone, while only a small proportion (12% in the

[1]*Department of Social Psychiatry, University Hospital of Groningen, P.O. Box 30.001, 9700 RB Groningen, The Netherlands*

incidence and 6% in the prevalence cohorts) needed shelter in hospital or other residential settings. Half of the patients of both types of cohorts were more or less employed or worked in the household during last assessment, indicating that employment among these patients is not lost for ever.

Concerning the development of social disabilities in incidence cohorts in six European countries [3], it can be concluded that social disability among patients with schizophrenia or related psychotic disorders follows a rather fluctuating course but appears to be a very persistent phenomenon. Disability in some specific role areas such as self-care, household participation, and social friction were even on the increase; nearly 60% of the patients were more or less disabled in the occupational role. From the longitudinal perspective, however, the conclusion must be that the severity of the disability is significantly decreasing among the majority of patients, although its course is fluctuating. For some, one out of seven, the schizophrenic "process" did not get better in the longer term. Community mental health care should take into account this long-term perspective and should be sensitive to the many needs these patients still have.

The economic burden of schizophrenia is considerable, as shown in recent cost-of-illness estimates in various countries (USA, UK, France, The Netherlands): about 2% of the total health care is spent on these disorders, of which at least two-thirds goes to hospital and residential care. The ISoS demonstrates in all cohorts that this kind of care is spent on a minor part of the total population in need. It is therefore well justified to ask for criteria of efficiency and equity as Knapp *et al* have argued. They review excellently the modes of economic evaluations and economic evidence regarding cost–outcome balance of pharmacotherapy, psychological therapy and care arrangement in the community. The most appropriate way of evaluating treatment and care in schizophrenia is probably the cost–consequences analysis, in which multiple clinical and social outcomes, like symptoms, functioning, quality of life, and family burden are measured together with a comprehensive direct and indirect medical and social cost measurement. There are still many areas open to investigate for further evidence of cost effectiveness: for example, a comparison between the new atypical antipsychotics, cognitive therapy for persistent delusions and hallucinations, various kinds of case management, duration of short-term versus long-term pharmacological prophylaxis, a combination of pharmacological and psychological therapies. An appealing approach for economic research could also be the development of an evidence-based disease management programme for schizophrenia in which patient care with all medical resources across the entire health care delivery system are combined and integrated with best evidence, clinical expertise and guidelines, pathophysiological knowledge and patient preferences [4]. The use of such a management programme has been tested among patients with minor and major depressions in primary care with demonstrated satisfaction, compliance and symptomatological improvement. Improving the process of care in schizophrenia in this way, while optimizing health outcomes and controlling costs, is a worth-while undertaking, because:

> the key task in community care for the seriously mentally ill is to organize functions comparable with those available in the hospital in a context where there is less control over patients and their whereabouts, and more difficulty in bringing together in a coordinated way the range of services these patients may need at various points in their lives; patients with serious mental illness have many needs requiring different services at varying times, and a long-term approach is required for effective care [5].

REFERENCES

1. Sartorius N., Gulbinat W., Harrison G., Laska G., Siegel C. (1996) Long-term follow-up of schizophrenia in 10 countries. *Soc. Psychiatry Psychiatr. Epidemiol.*, **31**: 249–258.
2. Hopper K., Harrison G., Janca A., Sartorius N. (1999) *The International Study of Schizophrenia (ISoS)*. Psychosocial Press, New York.
3. Wiersma D., Wanderling J., Dragomirecka E., Ganev K., Harrison G., an der Heiden W., Nienhuis F.J., Walsh D. (2000) Social disability in schizophrenia: its development and prediction over 15 years in incidence cohorts in six European centers. *Psychol. Med.*, **30**: 1155–1167.
4. Ellrodt G., Cook D.J., Lee J., Cho M., Hunt D., Weingarten S. (1997) Evidence-based disease management. *JAMA.*, **278**: 1687–1692.
5. Mechanic D. (1995) Challenges in the provision of mental health services: some cautionary lessons from US experience. *J. Public Health*, **17**: 132–139.

6.7
Health Economics in Schizophrenia: Clouding or Clarifying?

Tom Burns[1]

Knapp *et al* have provided a broad review of the costs of schizophrenia which does justice to the complexities of the disorder and gives an overview of current techniques in economic analysis. Such a detailed exposition of mental health economics could be heavy going for clinicians. However, the authors have identified the areas of research most relevant to care (the new antipsychotics, psychological treatments and care arrangements) and reviewed the

[1]*Department of Psychiatry, St. George's Hospital Medical School, Cranmer Terrace, London SW17 0RE, UK*

published studies. Their reference list is vast and comprehensive, permitting the interested reader to pursue individual issues at greater depth.

The costs of schizophrenia go far beyond the costs of specific treatments. The extent of societal costs of schizophrenia, both across agencies and over time, is thoroughly explored. The importance of "burden of disease" or "cost of illness" estimates for "macro" decision making is emphasized. Though of little direct obvious interest to the clinician, such studies establish the context of "macro" decision making and policy setting. Knapp *et al* stress that health economics research will not make policy or clinical decisions, but can ensure that those decisions can be better informed. In particular, they can contribute to greater equity in care by guiding the rational distribution of limited resources.

National evaluations of costs of schizophrenia confirm a generally similar pattern, but with tantalizing hints at cultural differences. What leads a handful of countries to research extensively and some to publish almost nothing in this area? The main "drivers" of cost in schizophrenia are identified — relapse, inpatient services, specialist community accommodation, mortality, lost employment, family impact, and (last but not least) public safety and concern. Their relative impact is clearly context dependent, so much so that the same change in the balance of services used can yield reversed cost outcomes when local costs for different countries are employed. What is cost effective in one country, at one time, may not be cost effective in another — a point often overlooked in hasty attempts to transport "successful" care packages between quite disparate health care systems.

Knapp *et al*'s review provides an invaluable and concise summary of the six major methodologies of economic evaluation. For the clinician, cost-effectiveness analyses are currently of most interest. This summary helps place them in perspective, both strengths and weaknesses.

In pharmacotherapy, cost–outcome for the economic impact of clozapine is examined in most detail, that of the newer atypicals less so, as the evidence is still thin. The potential strengths of decision modelling and more naturalistic quasi-experimental approaches are advanced, for example, US treatment histories reformulated using expert groups to identify probable UK treatments at critical clinical transition points. However, the use of varied sensitivity analyses in such studies can be as confusing as it is illuminating and the authors are refreshingly candid about the continuing need for careful judgement in interpreting them.

Psychological therapies have received much less attention from economic analyses because of the absence of commercial interest. From a UK perspective they are in more urgent need, not only because they are expensive, but because they draw on our supply of skilled staff which is severely restricted. Their efficient use ought to be of the utmost importance to health care planners. Compliance therapy and behavioural family management are subjected here to close scrutiny. Both are clearly generally cost effective but accumulating evidence on family interventions across cultures and care systems provides a natural sensitivity analysis. Where general services are very well developed, psychoeducation was found to add little. The issue of the quality of controls in studies is only touched on here tangentially. It is clearly of greater importance in the last section of the review dealing with care arrangements.

Forms of intensive case management and reprovision for discharged long-stay patients are the subjects of care arrangement comparisons. The methodological problems of reprovision studies — the unacceptability of randomized controlled trials (RCTs) for political reasons and the gradual discharge of increasingly disabled patients — are reviewed critically and usefully. Assertive community treatment (ACT), as it is called in the USA, and intensive case management in Europe have been the most extensively studied of all such programmes of care. Knapp *et al* address the mixed results in this field by focusing on issues of model fidelity and context but perhaps skate rather lightly over the relevance of the control service. A large UK RCT of 700 psychotic patients currently in press [1] lends support to coordination of care rather than model fidelity to the original Wisconsin approach (in particular caseload size) as the main driver of differential resource use, and hence treatment costs.

Currently in the UK it is almost impossible to get a mental health services research proposal funded without a health economics component. Policy makers and grant-awarding bodies should read this review. While Knapp and his colleagues have demonstrated eloquently why their profession has such influence, they emphasize that they can only address the question of efficiency (and indirectly equity). It is no use looking to health economics to tell us which treatment to use. For that we have to establish efficacy and effectiveness. Only when we have a range of effective treatments can health economics help us decide in which to invest our limited resources.

Mental health economics is a complex new discipline and schizophrenia is a complex disorder. The authors do not shrink from presenting the potential of their field while emphasizing the difficulties of interpretation and integration that their data bring. Including economic analyses of schizophrenia care in our thinking will lead to better-informed decisions, though not necessarily easier ones.

REFERENCES

1. Burns T., Creed F., Fahy T., Thompson S., Tyrer P., White I. and the UK 700 Group (1999) Intensive versus standard case management for severe psychotic illness: a randomised trial. *Lancet*, **353**: 2185–2189.

6.8
The Economic Burden of Schizophrenia
Marc De Hert[1] and Joseph Peuskens[1]

With its early age of onset and its chronic course, schizophrenia generates a large amount of burden and costs for patients, families and society. Schizophrenia is probably the most costly illness treated by psychiatrists.

In this era of economic uncertainty and budget cuts, treatment cost has become a major issue. Governments try to contain costs, while researchers and clinicians aim at the most cost-effective treatments.

Studies evaluating costs use the distinction between direct and indirect costs. Direct costs are those associated with medical care expenditure for diagnosis and treatment. The indirect costs are usually confined to the earnings that are forgone on account of the illness, loss of productivity and increased mortality. The intangible costs of pain and suffering for both patients and families are often forgotten in research [1].

Comparing costs between countries with different organization and funding of health care is difficult. All studies agree that the economic burden of schizophrenia is important; direct treatment costs are 2% of the total health care budget.

The losses due to indirect costs are dramatic and often higher than direct costs. A majority of patients suffering from schizophrenia are unemployed and are dependent on disability or social security incomes. Schizophrenic patients have a high risk of premature death, mainly due to suicide.

Schizophrenia also inflicts an important burden and financial strain on families. Most financial support is used to pay for lodging, treatment, food, clothing and transportation.

Hospitalization or community residential services are responsible for the majority of direct treatment costs. Treatment of the most severely ill and impaired patients will have the strongest impact on total direct treatment costs. In various countries, much of the burden of care has been transferred from services provided collectively back to the patients and their families. Deinstitutionalization may appear as direct cost savings for governments; it results in higher direct and indirect costs for patients and families. This shift in burden does not necessarily result in a net reduction of costs and might partly explain the rise in the number of people suffering from schizophrenia in the homeless population. Adequate delivery of community care is probably as expensive as residential care.

Only about 5% of direct expenditure is spent on medication [2]. Antipsychotics are the cornerstone in the treatment of psychotic symptoms, acute episodes and the prevention of relapse. New antipsychotics produce fewer

[1] University Centre St Jozef, Leuvensesteenweg 517, B-3070 Korteberg, Belgium

side effects and are possibly more effective on both cognitive and negative symptoms. They improve compliance and thus prevent relapse and rehospitalization. Psychoeducation of both patients and families is also important to improve compliance with medication and treatment as a whole.

Antipsychotic treatment needs to be integrated in a comprehensive psychosocial package of care, with continuity of care, individual support, family intervention and rehabilitation strategies [3]. Adequate relapse prevention will also decrease indirect costs through better functional outcomes, higher quality of life and reduction of suicide. Strategies of early detection and early intervention could lead to more positive long-term outcomes.

The enormous costs related to schizophrenic psychosis are in contrast with the limited expenditure on schizophrenia research. The current growing interest in cost of illness studies could increase awareness of clinicians, society and policy makers.

The Government's interest is containment or reduction of health care costs when resources are scarce. However, providing adequate accessible care for every patient is clearly expensive. The goal for further research on the treatment of schizophrenia should aim for cost-effective treatments (both pharmacological and psychosocial), improving global outcome, psychosocial functioning and quality of life, thereby reducing indirect costs and suffering.

REFERENCES

1. De Hert M., Thys E., Peuskens J. (1998) The costs of schizophrenia. *Acta Psychiatr. Belg.*, **98** (Suppl. 1): 9–16.
2. De Hert M., Thys E., Boydens J., Gilis P., Kesteloot K., Verhaegen L., Peuskens J. (1998) Health care expenditure on schizophrenia patients in Belgium. *Schizophr. Bull.*, **24**: 519–527.
3. Peuskens J. (1996) Proper psychosocial rehabilitation for stabilised patients with schizophrenia. *Eur. Neuropsychopharmacol.*, **6**: 7–12.

6.9
Lack of Comprehensive Care for Schizophrenic Patients: Is it Due to Prohibitive Costs or Insufficient Advocacy?

Thomas Detre[1]

The exceptionally well-written essay by Knapp *et al* begins with the statement that schizophrenia "often imposes a considerable burden not only on the

[1]*University of Pittsburgh, 3811 O'Hara Street, Pittsburgh, PA 15213, USA*

patients, but also on their families, the health care system and the wider society". After reviewing the principal cost drivers, the authors conclude that schizophrenia is indeed a costly illness, and the advances made in the pharmacotherapeutic and psychosocial management of this illness do not yet provide us with clear evidence for where cost savings may be achieved.

The difficulties in sorting out what is cost effective have to do with the fact that schizophrenia is in many ways similar to other chronic central nervous system (CNS) disorders of unknown aetiology. Like multiple sclerosis and epilepsy, schizophrenia is a syndrome rather than a discrete disease entity. As a result, it is not possible to predict with any degree of certainty the course of, or the response to, treatment. Some patients, after an acute episode, recover quickly and remain well for extended periods; others relapse repeatedly but remit quickly; still others require repeated and extensive hospitalization.

Where patients suffering from schizophrenic disorders differ from those with other CNS disorders is the degree to which the disease, in addition to producing cognitive dysfunction, interferes with the development or maintenance of social and vocational skills. For this reason, even patients who manage to join the workforce have trouble keeping their jobs, especially when relapses are preceded by prolonged periods of social withdrawal or odd or bizarre behaviour, making employers reluctant to rehire them.

The difficulties encountered in schizophrenia are further compounded by the fact that patients taking conventional neuroleptic drugs act better but feel worse. Preliminary evidence based on relatively short-term studies suggests that clozapine (and perhaps some of the recently marketed "atypical" drugs) is better tolerated by patients, leading to a higher level of compliance. It should be noted, however, that while relapse is most often caused by non-compliance (or attributed to the loss of therapeutic effects), one of the little studied reasons for relapse is the reluctance displayed by physicians to keep patients on a therapeutic dose of a drug when they complain of side effects, as has been shown in patients receiving cancer chemotherapy.

In any case, reducing relapse rates, or at least mitigating their severity, is of considerable importance, since frequent hospitalization and the use of intermediate facilities (such as day and night hospitals, specialist community-based accommodation) are the most expensive components in the overall care of schizophrenic patients. Relapse is also the time when patients are at the highest risk for suicide and other impulsive acts.

Obviously, treating patients with drugs that are better tolerated is desirable but probably insufficient by itself, and pharmacotherapy should be combined with psychosocial and other rehabilitative interventions. There is growing evidence that deficits in social cognition and the attendant ability to act wisely and display good judgement, whether they precede or follow the clinical manifestations of the illness, are factors that limit recovery, adjustment to community living and employability. The psychoeducational approach proposed by Anderson *et al* [1], which focuses on educating both the patient and his or her caregivers (be they family members or friends) about the nature of the patient's illness; the manner in which they can assist the patient in assuming increasing responsibility when he or she recovers from the psychotic decompensation; and other interventions aimed at improving compliance and increasing the adaptive social repertoire of patients, described in some detail by Knapp and his colleagues, together with increased use of atypical neuroleptics, have shown sufficient promise to be tried in a large-scale community-based controlled clinical trial. A coordinated approach, however, must also take into account the substantial burden schizophrenic illness places on the family. The deinstitutionalization that got underway in the 1970s in the United States and Western Europe further increased family burden. While patients clearly prefer living in the community, even under substandard conditions, families had to take over as crisis managers when other community facilities were lacking. This responsibility caused caregivers to earn less or give up their jobs altogether, and if the patient displayed bizarre behaviour, it also led to social isolation of carers and patients and a substantial decrease in their quality of life.

Major pharmaceutical companies are, for obvious reasons, ready to support controlled clinical trials on novel drugs, as well as economic research on their cost effectiveness, but have little interest in psychosocial approaches. Failure to finance major multicentre studies on these approaches is usually explained by talking about limited resources. Yet, we provide funds for liver transplants and show little reluctance to expend the funds necessary to keep alive infants with multiple handicaps or people with cancer; thus, these decisions are not based solely on the scarcity of resources but also on the priority assigned by policy makers to chronic mental illnesses. Advocacy groups (particularly in the United States) like the National Alliance for the Mentally Ill (NAMI), are making concerted efforts to change the situation and have done a great deal to eliminate inequities. While they enthusiastically support biologic therapies, perhaps because the psychological management of schizophrenic patients during the heydays of psychoanalysis deposited the responsibility for the illness on the family's doorstep, they are wary of psychosocial approaches involving family members. Clearly, governments will have to become the economic engine to ensure that further progress is made in treating this debilitating disease.

REFERENCE

1. Anderson C., Hogarty G., Reiss D. (1980) Family treatment of adult schizophrenic patients: a research based psycho-educational approach. *Schizophr. Bull.*, **6**: 490–505.

6.10

The Role of Cost-effectiveness Analysis in Improving the Treatment of Schizophrenia

Herbert Y. Meltzer[1]

Knapp *et al*'s excellent synthesis of the literature on the economic costs of schizophrenia and the cost effectiveness of various treatment approaches and policy matters shows that most Western societies are spending between 1.5% and 2.5% of their entire health budget on the direct costs of schizophrenia and an equivalent amount on indirect costs. The new atypical antipsychotic drugs (AAPD) should, in my view, be the major focus of the treatment of schizophrenia at the current time. About 55% of patients in the USA are receiving these medications and about 10% in Europe—percentages which are far too low given the number of neuroleptic-resistant patients and the undisputed advantages of the AAPD for a wide range of outcome measures beyond positive symptoms, as well as their reduced side effects. An accurate assessment of the economic costs of schizophrenia and the impact of treatment on these costs can, if used properly, be an invaluable tool in increasing utilization of the newer medications and necessary psychosocial supports. Knapp *et al* provide a useful critique of the evidence for greater cost effectiveness of the AAPD compared to the conventional neuroleptic drugs (CND). However, studies which compare the AAPD with each other, with and without psychosocial support and rehabilitation programmes, to determine their incremental benefits, are needed to facilitate choice of medication and are underway in the USA and elsewhere.

Why are there such discrepancies between the USA and Europe in the utilization of these medications, if, in fact, total expenditures are fairly similar? There is no uniform policy in the USA about access to the AAPD, with wide differences in availability based upon varying views with regard to drug expenditures by managed care or governmental agencies. Many systems which restrict access seek only cost minimization and neglect the differences in benefits of these agents. Ease of access was facilitated as long as the cost of medication could be retrieved by decreased hospitalization. As the average number of hospital days for those treated with CND decreased due to changes in the criteria for admission, shortened length of stay, regardless of symptoms, and more effective outpatient programmes, the cost of the AAPD could not be completely offset.

Knapp *et al* describe the various types of cost-effectiveness analysis which should be considered in medical decision making. While, ideally, cost minimization should not be the determining issue with regard to medication

[1]*Department of Psychiatry, Vanderbilt University School of Medicine, 1601 23rd Avenue South, Nashville, TN 37212, USA*

choice, one must recognize that many who should be able to consider other factors will not. Thus, it is important to establish, if possible, that these newer agents can still achieve cost minimization when used properly. I suggest that the major area to concentrate on is savings in indirect costs, that is, lost income, disability transfer payments, costs associated with courts and incarceration, and family burden, which may be anticipated based upon the superior efficacy and tolerability of the atypical antipsychotic drugs. Specifically, there is evidence that the newer agents improve cognitive function, the major cause of inability to work for many patients with schizophrenia [1, 2]. For example, clozapine enables up to 40% of patients with schizophrenia to work [3, 4], which is twice the rate for patients treated with typical neuroleptic drugs. Comparable results are possible with risperidone and olanzapine based upon their ability to improve verbal learning and memory and executive function. Increased funding of rehabilitation programmes and utilization of the most effective pharmacologic and cognitive rehabilitation methods to preserve and restore cognitive function in patients with schizophrenia are needed to achieve these savings. Secondly, these agents reduce aggression and violence, which should impact on the frequency with which the criminal justice system is confronted with patients with schizophrenia who have committed acts of aggression or property destruction [5]. There have been four highly publicized murders by patients with schizophrenia in the last 12 months, including the Unabomber murders and attacks, which have alerted the US public to the dangers of poorly treated schizophrenia.

A true appreciation of the costs of schizophrenia also requires attention to the lifetime costs of this illness, including non-medical as well as medical costs [6]. A societal perspective on this matter can provide additional stimulus to the full utilization of the best available treatments.

Finally, I would like to emphasize my belief that utilization of cost utility analysis should be greatly increased in schizophrenia research. Research in this area has been restricted by limited success in developing a quality adjusted life year (QALY) merit that reliably reflects the preferences of patients with schizophrenia. Comparisons with other treatments in medicine would, in my view, suggest that the AAPD have merit comparable to many other commonly used treatments in medicine for chronic illnesses.

REFERENCES

1. Green M.F. (1996) What are the functional consequences of neurocognitive deficits in schizophrenia? *Am. J. Psychiatry*, **153**: 321–330.
2. Davidson M., Keefe R.S.E. (1995) Cognitive impairment as a target for pharmacological treatment in schizophrenia. *Schizophr. Res.*, **17**: 123–129.

3. Lindstrom L.H. (1988) The effect of long-term treatment with clozapine in schizophrenia: a retrospective study in 96 patients treated with clozapine for up to 3 years. *Acta Psychiatr. Scand.*, **77**: 524–529.
4. Meltzer H. (1992) Dimensions of outcome with clozapine. *Br. J. Psychiatry*, **160** (Suppl. 17): 46–53.
5. Collaborative Working Group in Clinical Trial Evaluation (1998) Treatment of special populations with the atypical antipsychotics. *J. Clin. Psychiatry*, **59** (Suppl. 12): 46–52.
6. Meltzer D.O. (1997) Accounting for future costs in medical cost-effectiveness analysis. *J. Health Econ.*, **16**: 33–64.

6.11
Medical Cost Outcomes of the Atypical Antipsychotics
Dennis A. Revicki[1]

Schizophrenia is a chronic and often disabling psychiatric disorder associated with significant costs to society [1]. Clozapine's introduction into the United States for the treatment of refractory schizophrenia increased attention to both the costs and therapeutic effects of antipsychotic medications. Clinicians and health care decision-makers need evidence of safety and efficacy and cost effectiveness to determine the place for new, expensive antipsychotic treatments within the health care system [2, 3]. This commentary provides more recent information on the cost effectiveness of the new atypical antipsychotics, efficacy versus effectiveness clinical trials for answering health economic questions, and case management and psychosocial rehabilitation services.

Other than for clozapine [3, 4], there have been few prospective studies evaluating the cost effectiveness of the new atypical antipsychotics (i.e. olanzapine, quetiapine, risperidone) [2]. Most economic evaluations of atypical antipsychotics are based on non-controlled, mirror-image studies, often with very small sample sizes [2]. Several prospective studies have been recently reported evaluating the impact of clozapine [4, 5], olanzapine [6], and risperidone [7] on medical costs and outcomes. Rosenheck *et al* [4] completed a randomized clinical trial comparing clozapine and haloperidol in hospitalized, treatment refractory schizophrenia patients. They found few differences in clinical and quality of life outcomes between the treatments, except when treatment crossovers were excluded. The clozapine group had slightly lower total medical costs compared with the haloperidol group ($57 785 versus $60 225). Essock *et al* [5], in a clinical trial comparing clozapine with standard neuroleptics in treatment-resistant schizophrenia, found

[1]*Center for Health Outcomes Research, 7101 Wisconsin Avenue, Suite 600, Bethesda, MD 20814, USA*

reduced rehospitalization rates in those clozapine patients discharged from the hospital. However, the complete economic evaluation results have not yet been reported.

Hamilton *et al* [6] compared the medical cost and patient outcomes in US schizophrenia patients enrolled in a randomized clinical trial comparing olanzapine and haloperidol. Olanzapine-treated patients showed improved clinical and quality of life outcomes compared with haloperidol [6, 8]. Cost comparisons favoured olanzapine during short-term treatment ($6114 versus $6502) and, for treatment responders, olanzapine resulted in $636 fewer medical costs over maintenance treatment [6]. These long-term cost outcomes were based only on treatment responders and, since this was an efficacy clinical trial, there was incomplete follow-up of patients discontinuing treatment.

Mahmoud *et al* [7] conducted a naturalistic (effectiveness) clinical trial comparing risperidone with usual neuroleptic treatment in patients with schizophrenia with 1-year follow-up. Although the patient and mental health cost outcomes have only been incompletely reported, the results suggest greater improvement in clinical and quality of life outcomes, with slightly higher mental-health-related costs in the risperidone group. This study also observed significant variations in treatment for patients with schizophrenia, with many patients receiving incomplete antipsychotic treatment over the course of the 1-year follow-up.

Randomized clinical (efficacy) trials and naturalistic (effectiveness) trials have been used to evaluate the economic costs and outcomes of the atypical antipsychotics versus standard neuroleptics. There are recognized limitations to cost-effectiveness analyses based on randomized clinical trials [9, 10]. Clinical trials are conducted in carefully controlled research centres with rigorous treatment regimens and systematic assessment of highly selected, homogeneous patient populations. This artificial clinical practice setting, restricted patient population, and often incomplete follow-up of non-responders and drop-outs results in limitations to generalizability. The effectiveness studies also have recognized limitations, but often produce findings that are more generalizable (by design) to community practice settings [10]. There are trade-offs between internal validity and external validity in the design of prospective health economic evaluations. These limitations must be taken into consideration when interpreting the findings of cost-effectiveness studies. There is no simple solution to evaluating the economic impact of a novel antipsychotic, and we need to examine the mosaic of results from various different study designs to build greater or reduced confidence about cost effectiveness.

As pointed out by Knapp *et al*, the existing evidence on the cost effectiveness of case management and psychosocial interventions for patients with schizophrenia is inconsistent and mixed. Part of the reason for the poor performance of patients in rehabilitation therapy interventions may be the inefficacy of standard neuroleptics on negative symptoms and cognitive impairments associated with schizophrenia. There is some research suggesting that the atypical antipsychotics may improve neurocognitive function [11]. If this cognitive improvement, especially in memory and information processing, is demonstrated, schizophrenia patients may be more able to benefit from psychosocial and rehabilitative interventions. Currently, there is very limited information on the cost effectiveness of interventions involving case management, atypical antipsychotics and comprehensive rehabilitative programmes. It is expected that efficacy of these novel antipsychotics on negative symptoms and cognitive function may result in improved rehabilitation outcomes and patient quality of life, and fewer costs associated with hospitalizations and intensive outpatient services. Future research is needed to evaluate the benefits of combined atypical antipsychotic and psychosocial interventions on patient outcomes and costs.

The clinical and economic research evidence on the atypical antipsychotics is encouraging, especially in comparison to the older neuroleptic medications. Compared with standard neuroleptics, the newer antipsychotics have slightly better clinical efficacy, fewer extrapyramidal symptoms and other serious side effects, and less treatment discontinuation. The economic studies completed to date suggest that the total medical costs for the atypical antipsychotics are at best slightly lower (or at worst, no different) than the total costs for the standard neuroleptics. No studies have been completed comparing the cost effectiveness of the different atypical antipsychotics to each other. This research is needed to inform clinicians and health care decision-makers about the relative advantages and disadvantages of the novel antipsychotics. It remains to be demonstrated whether the introduction of the newer atypical antipsychotics will result in beneficial economic outcomes for the health care system in the United States and the rest of the world. The expectation is that the newer treatments will have benefits in terms of patient quality of life and functioning, but the question that remains to be answered is: what are the costs to the health care system?

REFERENCES

1. Wyatt R.J., Henter I., Leary M.C., Taylor E. (1995) An economic evaluation of schizophrenia. *Soc. Psychiatry Psychiatr. Epidemiol.*, **30**: 196–205.
2. Revicki D.A. (1999) Pharmacoeconomic studies of atypical antipsychotic drugs for the treatment of schizophrenia. *Schizophr. Res.*, **35** (Suppl.): S101–S109.
3. Revicki D.A. (1998) Pharmacoeconomic evaluation of treatments for refractory schizophrenia: clozapine-related studies. *J. Clin. Psychiatry*, **60** (Suppl. 1): 7–11.
4. Rosenheck R., Cramer J., Xu W., Thomas J., Henderson W., Frisman L., Fye C., Charney D. (1997) A comparison of clozapine and haloperidol in hospitalized patients with refractory schizophrenia. *N. Engl. J. Med.*, **337**: 809–815.

5. Essock S.M., Hargreaves W.A., Dohm F.A., Goethe J., Carver L., Hipshman L. (1996) Clozapine's effectiveness for patients in state hospitals: results from a randomized trial. *Psychopharmacol. Bull.*, **32**: 683–697.
6. Hamilton S.H., Revicki D.A., Edgell E., Genduso L., Tollefson G. (1999) Clinical and economic outcomes of olanzapine compared with haloperidol for schizophrenia: results from a randomized clinical trial. *PharmacoEconomics*, **15**: 469–480.
7. Mahmoud R.A., Englehart L.M., Oster G., Stevens M.C., Meredith C., Lee D.M. (1997) Risperidone vs. conventional antipsychotics: a prospective randomized naturalistic effectiveness trial of outcomes in chronic schizophrenia. Presented at the 36th Annual Meeting of the American College of Neuropsychopharmacology, Kanuela, Hawaii, 8–12 December.
8. Revicki D.A., Genduso L., Hamilton S.H., Ganozcy D., Beasely C.M., Beasely C.M. Jr (1999) Olanzapine versus haloperidol in the treatment of schizophrenia and other psychotic disorders: quality of life and clinical outcomes of a randomized clinical trial. *Qual. Life Res.*, **8**: 417–426.
9. Wells K.B. (1999) Treatment research at the crossroads: the scientific interface of clinical trials and effectiveness research. *Am. J. Psychiatry*, **156**: 5–10.
10. Revicki D.A., Frank L. (1999) Pharmacoeconomic evaluation in the real world: Effectiveness versus efficacy studies. *PharmacoEconomics*, **15**: 423–434.
11. Purdon S. (1997) Neuropsychological change in early phase schizophrenia over twelve months of treatment with olanzapine, risperidone or haloperidol. *Schizophr. Res.*, **29**: 152–153.

6.12

The Costs of Schizophrenia — New Treatments and New Economics

Melvin Sabshin[1]

As the twentieth century draws to a close, empiricism has achieved great success in facilitating psychiatry's therapeutic advances. Despite large gaps in our understanding of the pathogenesis of many psychiatric illnesses, much can be done to alleviate psychiatric symptomatology and to provide a better quality of life for patients with severe psychiatric illnesses. The best illustration of this situation can be found in the treatment of patients with schizophrenia. While the aetiology of schizophrenia is not yet clearly elucidated, a tremendous amount has been learned about biopsychosocial treatment of people with this severe disorder. There are thousands of reports about such treatments, and assisting in the understanding of such reports across the world is an important function of the World Psychiatric Association.

The paper by Knapp *et al* is an excellent example of an outcome analysis related to the treatment of schizophrenic patients. Remarkably, however, this

[1] 2801 New Mexico Avenue, NW 301, Washington, DC 20007, USA

paper ventures far beyond the ordinary outcome analysis and confronts the full panoply of economic issues related to the care of schizophrenic patients, their families, and the institutions necessary for such care. The authors entitle their paper "Costs of Schizophrenia". This title would have had particular meaning during each decade of the century, but it has very special meaning as the century comes to the end. Indeed, the basic thrust of the paper deals with economic data related to the treatment of schizophrenic patients. For the past quarter-century, economic analyses related to the treatment outcomes in psychiatry have become increasingly sophisticated. The empiricism at the centre of late-twentieth-century psychiatry has extended to economic empiricism, so that more valid costs can be estimated for treatment and their outcomes. Such analyses are useful in all parts of medicine, but in psychiatry they have special importance. Indeed, an expertise has now emerged to estimate costs of all of the socioeconomic variables, implicit and explicit, in the treatment of schizophrenic patients. Furthermore, this expertise has transcended national borders and included considerable comparative analyses of the "costs of schizophrenia" in different national and economic contexts. Indeed, the paper by Knapp *et al* contributes greatly to transnational psychiatry per se. The authors are fully aware of the impact of varying economic contexts in assessing the costs of schizophrenia. Loss of productivity by patients may have different costs in China from the United Kingdom. And family interaction may also be quite different. Social and economic variables are central to a full understanding of psychiatric treatment outcomes and multiple variables are involved. In the last half of the twentieth century the shift from hospital-based to community-based care requires special economic attention including the start-up costs for community care. Short-range versus long-range costs require careful attention.

In many ways, the psychopharmacological revolution of the late twentieth century has stimulated and facilitated economic analysis in psychiatry. Obviously, pharmaceutical industries have paid a great deal of attention to the costs and opportunities of developing new medications. Psychiatry and its related governmental agencies must also pay great attention to these variables. The authors illustrate this question very well by the discussion of economic factors related to the use of clozapine, risperidone, olanzapine, and psychosocial treatments of schizophrenic patients. Clozapine and other new atypical neuroleptics have had a strikingly positive impact in the treatment of schizophrenic patients, which has been superior to standard older products. The analysis of these effects, as in the complex use of clozapine, needed to be factored in so that the medication costs and required expensive laboratory tests may be understood. Patients on this medication must be watched very closely in order to protect them from the medication's toxicity. Despite all of these additional costs, the use of clozapine still reduces overall costs and is an economically sound treatment. When the ministers of health of developing nations ask about the cost benefits of including clozapine in their formularies, this paper would be useful as a basis for understanding why and how the decision should be made.

Psychiatry has matured to the point that each new treatment should be studied from an economic perspective as well as a clinical standpoint. The accumulation of economic data will be very important in decision making. At times, of course, psychiatry must argue for approaches that require greater initial expenditures. In many cases these costs will lead to ultimate savings over time. A psychiatry that advocates with good economic data as well as good clinical data is likely to be more effective in obtaining support. Empiricism helps to convince decision-makers and society as a whole that treatment is rational, useful and accountable. We understand much more about the costs of schizophrenia as we enter a new millennium.

Acknowledgements for the First Edition

The Editors would like to thank Drs Paola Bucci, Umberto Volpe, Pasquale Saviano, Andrea Dell'Acqua, Massimo Lanzaro, Vincenzo Scarallo, Enrico Tresca, Mariangela Masella and Giuseppe Piegari, of the Department of Psychiatry of the University of Naples, for their help in the processing of manuscripts.

The publication has been supported by an unrestricted educational grant from Janssen–Cilag Italy, which is hereby gratefully acknowledged.

Index

Note: Page numbers in **bold** refer to Tables

Index compiled by Annette Musker